Veterinary Anesthetic and Monitoring Equipment

Veterinary Anesthetic and Monitoring Equipment

Edited by

Kristen G. Cooley, BA, CVT, VTS (Anesthesia & Analgesia)
Instructional Specialist
School of Veterinary Medicine
University of Wisconsin
Madison, WI, USA

Rebecca A. Johnson, DVM, PhD, DACVAA
Clinical Associate Professor
Anesthesia and Pain Management
Department of Surgical Sciences
School of Veterinary Medicine
University of Wisconsin
Madison, WI, USA

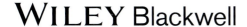

Registered Office
John Wiley & Sons, Inc., 111 River Street, Hoboken, NJ 07030, USA

Editorial Office
111 River Street, Hoboken, NJ 07030, USA

For details of our global editorial offices, customer services, and more information about Wiley products visit us at www.wiley.com.

Wiley also publishes its books in a variety of electronic formats and by print-on-demand. Some content that appears in standard print versions of this book may not be available in other formats.

Library of Congress Cataloging-in-Publication Data

Names: Cooley, Kristen G., editor. | Johnson, Rebecca A. (Rebecca Ann),
  editor.
Title: Veterinary anesthetic and monitoring equipment / edited by Kristen G.
  Cooley, Rebecca A. Johnson.
Description: Hoboken, NJ : John Wiley & Sons, Inc., 2018. | Includes
  bibliographical references and index. |
Identifiers: LCCN 2018013994 (print) | LCCN 2018014611 (ebook) | ISBN
  9781119277170 (pdf) | ISBN 9781119277163 (epub) | ISBN 9781119277156
  (cloth)
Subjects: | MESH: Anesthesia–veterinary | Monitoring,
  Intraoperative–veterinary | Anesthesiology–instrumentation | Monitoring,
  Intraoperative–instrumentation
Classification: LCC SF914 (ebook) | LCC SF914 (print) | NLM SF 914 | DDC
  636.089/796–dc23
LC record available at https://lccn.loc.gov/2018013994

Cover Design: Wiley
Cover Images: (left, right, and bottom images) © Rebecca A. Johnson; (middle image) © Kristen G. Cooley

Set in 10/12pt WarnockPro by SPi Global, Chennai, India

Printed and bound in Singapore by Markono Print Media Pte Ltd

10 9 8 7 6 5 4 3 2 1

This book is dedicated to our animal friends and their families – many of which require the use of anesthetic and monitoring equipment from time to time!

James Harrington (obscure English 25th century philosopher):

"Measurement is the first step that leads to control and eventually to improvement. If you can't measure something, you can't understand it. If you can't understand it, you can't control it. If you can't control it, you can't improve it."

Contents

List of Contributors

Turi Aarnes, *DVM, MS, DACVAA*
Associate Professor, Anesthesiology and
Pain Management
Department of Veterinary Clinical Sciences
College of Veterinary Medicine
The Ohio State University
Columbus, OH, USA

Molly Allen, *DVM*
Anesthesiologist
Lakeshore Veterinary Specialists
Glendale, WI, USA

Jonathan Bach, *DVM, DACVIM (SAIM), DACVECC*
Clinical Associate Professor, Emergency and
Critical Care
Department of Medical Sciences
School of Veterinary Medicine
University of Wisconsin
Madison, WI, USA

Caroline Baldo, *DVM, DACVAA*
Assistant Professor, Anesthesiology and Pain Medicine
Department of Veterinary Clinical Sciences
College of Veterinary Medicine
University of Minnesota
St Paul, MN, USA

Mario Arenillas Baquero, *DVM*
Resident, Anesthesia and Pain Management
Veterinary Clinical Teaching Hospital
Veterinary Faculty
Complutense University of Madrid
Madrid, Spain

Carl Bradbrook, *BVSc, CertVA, DipECVAA, MRCVS, RCVS*
European Specialist in Veterinary Anaesthesia &
Analgesia
Consultant Veterinary Anaesthetist
ACE Vets Ltd
Rossett, UK

David Brunson, *DVM, MS, DACVAA*
Veterinary Anesthesia Consultants, LLC
Adjunct Associate Professor, Anesthesia and
Pain Management
Department of Surgical Sciences
School of Veterinary Medicine
University of Wisconsin
Madison, WI, USA

Stephen Cital, *RVT, SRA, RLAT, VTS (Laboratory Animal Medicine)*
Private Consultant, Training Manager
Silicon Valley Veterinary Specialists
San Jose, CA, USA

Stuart Clark-Price, *DVM, MS, DACVIM-LA, DACVAA*
Associate Professor, Anesthesia
Department of Clinical Sciences
College of Veterinary Medicine
Auburn University
Auburn, AL, USA

Andrew Claude, *DVM, DACVAA*
Associate Professor and Section Chief, Anesthesiology
Department of Small Animal Clinical Sciences
College of Veterinary Medicine
Michigan State University
East Lansing, MI, USA

Kristen G. Cooley, *BA, CVT, VTS (Anesthesia & Analgesia)*
Instructional Specialist
School of Veterinary Medicine
University of Wisconsin
Madison, WI, USA

Anderson Favaro da Cunha, *DVM, MS, DACVAA*
Professor and Service Chief, Veterinary Anesthesia and
Analgesia
School of Veterinary Medicine
Louisiana State University
Baton Rouge, LA, USA

Cristina de Miguel Garcia, *DVM, MVetMed, MRCVS, DECVAA*
Clinical Instructor, Anesthesia and Pain Management
Department of Surgical Sciences
School of Veterinary Medicine
University of Wisconsin
Madison, WI, USA

Trish Anne Farry, *CVN, AVN, VTS (Anesthesia & Analgesia, ECC), TAA, GCHEd*
School of Veterinary Science
The University of Queensland
Gatton, Queensland, Australia

Tatiana H. Ferreira, *DVM, MSc, PhD, DACVAA*
Clinical Assistant Professor, Anesthesia and Pain Management
Department of Surgical Sciences
School of Veterinary Medicine
University of Wisconsin
Madison, WI, USA

Sharon Fornes, *MBA, RVT, VTS (Anesthesia & Analgesia)*
Regional Technician Training Coordinator
Veterinary Centers of America (VCA)
Bay Area Veterinary Specialists
San Leandro, California, USA

Alanna Johnson, *DVM, DACVAA*
Clinical Assistant Professor, Anesthesiology & and Pain Management
Department of Comparative, Diagnostic & Population Medicine
College of Veterinary Medicine
University of Florida
Gainesville, FL, USA

Rebecca A. Johnson, *DVM, PhD, DACVAA*
Clinical Associate Professor and Section Head, Anesthesia and Pain Management
Department of Surgical Sciences
School of Veterinary Medicine
University of Wisconsin
Madison, WI, USA

Stephanie Keating, *DVM, DVSc, DACVAA*
Clinical Assistant Professor
College of Veterinary Medicine
University of Illinois at Urbana Champaign
Urbana, IL, USA

Carolyn Kerr, *DVM, DVSc, PhD, DACVAA*
Professor and Chair, Clinical Studies
Ontario Veterinary College
University of Guelph
Guelph, ON, Canada

Kris Kruse-Elliott, *DVM, PhD, DACVAA*
Medical Director – AnimalScan SF
Redwood City, CA, USA

Katrina Lafferty, *BFA, CVT, VTS (Anesthesia & Analgesia)*
Office of the Vice Chancellor for Research and Graduate Education
Anesthesia and Surgery Department
Wisconsin National Primate Research Center
University of Wisconsin
Madison, WI, USA

Tracey Lawrence, *RVT, VTS (Anesthesia & Analgesia, ECC)*
Anesthesia and Cardiology Departments
Toronto Veterinary Emergency and Referral Hospital
Toronto, ON, Canada

Christoph Mans, *Dr Med. Vet., DACZM*
Assistant Clinical Professor, Zoological Medicine
Department of Surgical Sciences
School of Veterinary Medicine
University of Wisconsin
Madison, WI, USA

Craig Mosley, *DVM, MSc, DACVAA*
National Medical Director, Specialty Medicine
VCA Canada
Calgary, AB, Canada

Odette O, *DVM, DACVAA*
Anesthesiology
Canada West Veterinary Specialists
Vancouver, BC, Canada

Louise O'Dwyer, *MBA, BSc(Hons), VTS (Anesthesia & Analgesia and ECC), DipAVN (Medical & Surgical), RVN*
Clinical Support Manager VetsNow
Dunfermline, UK

Darci Palmer, *BS, LVT, VTS (Anesthesia & Analgesia)*
Anesthesia Technician
Southeastern Veterinary Surgery Center
Columbus, GA, USA

Denise Radkey, *DVM*
Anesthesiologist
MedVet Medical and Cancer Center for Pets
Worthington, OH, USA

Heidi Reuss-Lamky, *LVT, VTS (Anesthesia & Analgesia, Surgery), FFCP*
Surgery Technician
Oakland Veterinary Referral Services
Bloomfield Hills, MI, USA

Thomas Riebold, *DVM, DACVAA*
Professor, Anesthesiology
College of Veterinary Medicine
Oregon State University
Corvallis, OR, USA

Jennifer Sager, *BS, CVT, VTS (Anesthesia & Analgesia, ECC)*
Veterinary Hospital Anesthesiology Supervisor,
Anesthesia and Pain Management
College of Veterinary Medicine
University of Florida
Gainesville, FL, USA
and
Independent Contractor, Trainer
Midmark Anesthesia/Monitoring Training and
Education Network
Dayton, OH, USA

Carrie Schroeder, *DVM, DACVAA*
Clinical Instructor, Anesthesia and Pain Management
Department of Surgical Sciences
School of Veterinary Medicine
University of Wisconsin
Madison, WI, USA

Amanda Shelby, *BS, CVT, RVT, VTS (Anesthesia & Analgesia)*
Anesthesia Solution Coordinator
Jurox Animal Health
Kansas City, MO, USA
and
Anesthesia Nurse
IndyVet Emergency & Referral Hospital
Indianapolis, IN, USA

Kurt Sladky, *MS, DVM, DACZM, DECZM (Herpetology)*
Clinical Professor, Zoological Medicine
Department of Surgical Sciences
School of Veterinary Medicine
University of Wisconsin
Madison, WI, USA

Lesley Smith, *DVM, DACVAA*
Clinical Professor, Anesthesia and Pain Management
Department of Surgical Sciences
School of Veterinary Medicine
University of Wisconsin
Madison, WI, USA

Lindsey Snyder, *DVM, MS, DACVAA, CVA*
Clinical Instructor, Anesthesia and Pain Management
Department of Surgical Sciences
School of Veterinary Medicine
University of Wisconsin
Madison, WI, USA

Geoffrey Truchetti, *DMV, MSc, DES, DACVAA*
Centre Vétérinaire Rive Sud
Brossard, QC, Canada
and
Centre Vétérinaire Laval
Laval, QC, Canada

Julie Walker, *DVM, DACVECC*
Clinical Assistant Professor, Emergency and
Critical Care
Department of Medical Sciences
School of Veterinary Medicine
University of Wisconsin
Madison, WI, USA

Erin Wendt-Hornickle, *DVM, DACVAA*
Assistant Professor, Anesthesiology and Pain Medicine
Department of Veterinary Clinical Sciences
College of Veterinary Medicine
University of Minnesota
St Paul, MN, USA

Allan Williamson, *DVM, MS, DACVAA*
Clinical Instructor, Anesthesia and Pain Management
Department of Surgical Sciences
School of Veterinary Medicine
University of Wisconsin
Madison, WI, USA

Preface

In human anesthesiology, classic textbooks concerning anesthetic and monitoring equipment have been published since 1975 (*Understanding Anesthesia Equipment*, 1st ed. Dorsch, J.A. and Dorsch, S.E. (eds), currently on its 5th edition). *Veterinary Anesthetic and Monitoring Equipment* is the first attempt to compile similar information into one source. It was developed to present the most current equipment and techniques available to the field of veterinary anesthesia, specifically directed at our unique veterinary species.

No longer is veterinary anesthesia just a "spin off" of human anesthesia. Our field has developed quickly and specialized equipment and techniques have become imperative to current practice. To this end, knowledge concerning veterinary anesthesia and anesthetic monitoring is greatly expanding and continually developing as the breadth and depth of anesthetic procedures increase as well. It is not enough in modern-day practice to know that a specific piece of equipment is used in a specific situation; professionals must also know why it is used and how the equipment functions. This book was established to provide foundational information for all veterinary professionals to build upon, including laboratory animal anesthetists, private practice veterinary assistants and technicians, veterinarians, specialized anesthesia technicians, anesthesia residents, and ACVAA/ECVAA-boarded diplomates. Thus, the overall purpose of this book is to concisely assemble all necessary resources on equipment, in order to manage each individual veterinary case appropriately, safely and successfully.

Disclaimer

Although this compilation is quite comprehensive concerning available products and equipment, inclusion of every monitor and piece of equipment in existence is an impossible task; purposeful exclusion of certain equipment was not intended. We anticipate that this book will evolve with each new edition as our dynamic field continues to unfold.

1

Medical Gas Cylinders and Pipeline Systems

Carl Bradbrook

European Specialist in Veterinary Anaesthesia & Analgesia, Consultant Veterinary Anaesthetist, ACE Vets Ltd, Rossett, UK

1.1 Medical Gas Cylinders

Gas cylinders are used to store and supply medical gases to clinical areas of the veterinary hospital, including anesthetic machines, mechanical ventilators and surgical instruments. Cylinders are attached, either directly or using a pipeline and distribution system to the anesthetic machine or outlet. Cylinders are available in a number of sizes, described by the letters A–J. Their designated letter is dependent on their size; A is the smallest and J the largest (British Oxygen Company 2016). The size used is dependent on the intended use and region of the world. For example, in the United Kingdom (UK) and European Union (EU), the most commonly used sizes are E, F and J, whereas in North America, E and H are more usual. Table 1.1 details the sizes and volumes of the these cylinders.

Cylinders are available containing a number of different medical gases. The medical gases most used in veterinary practice include oxygen, nitrous oxide and medical air, although carbon dioxide may also be found in certain situations. For example, carbon dioxide is used for body cavity insufflation during minimally invasive procedures.

1.1.1 Gas Pressures

A pressure gauge, most commonly of the Bourdon type (Figure 1.1), should be associated with the cylinder connection to the system. A Bourdon gauge consists of a coiled tube that changes shape, dependent on gas pressure. As the coil changes shape, an attached pointer moves over the scale to display the pressure (Davis and Kenny 2007). The gauge reads the pressure generated within the cylinder or pipeline distribution system, dependent on the amount of gas or vapor supplied. The term "gas" is used to describe the contents of a cylinder

containing a non-liquefied compressed gas. Examples include oxygen and medical air (Davis and Kenny 2007). The cylinder contents are present in this state when the gas does not change into a liquid at room temperature regardless of pressure applied, since room temperature is above the critical temperature of gas. The critical temperature is the temperature above which a substance cannot be liquefied, regardless of the pressure applied. The term "vapor" is the gaseous state of a substance when, at ambient temperature, it is present below its critical temperature (Davis and Kenny 2007). The liquid phase is present in the cylinder with the vapor phase remaining on top; nitrous oxide is an example of a medical gas stored in this state.

The International System of Units (SI) used for pressure is the pascal (Pa) which, for convenience, is commonly expressed as kilopascal (kPa). However, conversion to other commonly used pressure units is frequently performed and is as follows:

$$100 \text{ kPa} = 1000 \text{ mbar} = 1 \text{ bar} = 750 \text{ mmHg}$$
$$= 1000 \text{ cmH}_2\text{O} = 14.5 \text{ psi} = 1 \text{ atm} \quad (1.1)$$

1.1.2 Medical Gases

Oxygen and medical air are stored as compressed gases (Highley 2009; Westwood and Rieley 2012), whereas nitrous oxide and carbon dioxide are stored as a liquid with a vapor phase above. The gauge pressure will depend on the particular gas. For example, those stored as compressed gases will have a gauge pressure that is directly related to cylinder contents at all times, whereas those stored in their liquid phase will only have a gauge pressure directly related to cylinder contents once all of the liquid has vaporized as the cylinder empties. This concept is discussed further below.

Veterinary Anesthetic and Monitoring Equipment, First Edition. Edited by Kristen G. Cooley and Rebecca A. Johnson.
© 2018 John Wiley & Sons, Inc. Published 2018 by John Wiley & Sons, Inc.

Table 1.1 Gas cylinder dimensions and capacity.

	UK				US			
	E	F	G	J	E	F	G	H
Dimensions (inches)	34 × 4	36 × 5½	54 × 7	56½ × 9	26 × 4½	51 × 5½	51 × 8½	51 × 9¼
Oxygen (L)	680	1360	3400	6800	650	2062	5300	6900
Nitrous oxide (L)	1800	3600	9000	18 000	1590	5260	13 800	15490

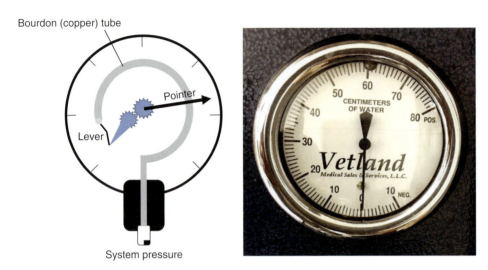

Figure 1.1 Left: Interior schematic of a Bourdon type pressure gauge including the expandable copper tubing and pointer. Right: Example of a common Bourdon gauge routinely located on an anesthetic machine.

1.1.3 Cylinder Components

Cylinders are traditionally composed of molybdenum steel, although lighter weight cylinders made from aluminum with non-magnetic valves are becoming more common and are magnetic resonance imaging (MRI) compatible (Dorsch and Dorsch 2008a; Highley 2009). Smaller aluminum cylinders with an epoxy resin coating may be used for patient transport (Figure 1.2). Cylinders are tested by the manufacturer every 5 years to ensure they are safe for continued use and a colored disc (Figure 1.3) may be placed around the neck (UK) of the valve to indicate when testing is next due. Information detailing the results of the safety tests is printed onto a sticker placed on the plastic collar surrounding the neck of the cylinder. Tests may be performed to check the strength of the cylinder, including subjecting them to greater than normal working pressures and endoscopically detecting any imperfections that may affect performance. Approximately 1 in every 100 cylinders is randomly subjected to impact testing and has its structural integrity checked by strip testing. Strip testing involves a piece of the tested cylinder being examined in depth for any damage and imperfections. Information

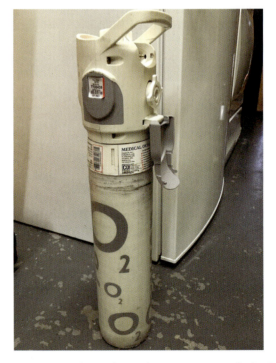

Figure 1.2 Lightweight CD aluminum oxygen cylinder for use during patient transport.

an appropriate outlet and facilitates cylinder opening and closing. The valve type depends on the cylinder size (Dorsch and Dorsch 2008a; Highley 2009; Alibhai 2016). Size E oxygen cylinders have a pin index valve (Figure 1.5), whereas the larger J oxygen and medical air cylinders have a side spindle pin index valve (Figure 1.6). Cylinders

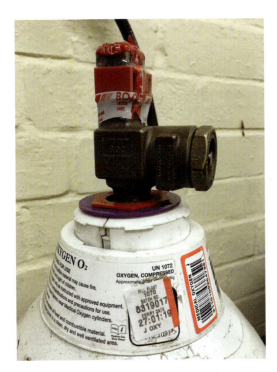

Figure 1.3 Cylinder safety information on the colored disc and printed sticker on the cylinder neck.

regarding the cylinder working pressure, serial number and testing may also be permanently etched onto the cylinder shoulder.

A valve block (Figure 1.4) is present at the top of the cylinder. The valve allows the cylinder to be connected to

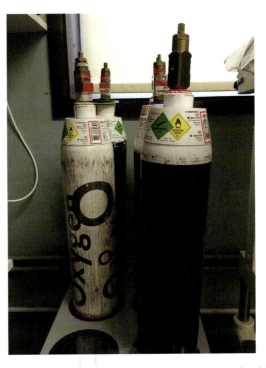

Figure 1.5 Size E (UK) oxygen cylinders in a vertical racking system with pin index valve.

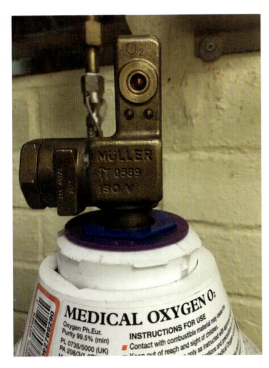

Figure 1.4 Side spindle pin index valve on a size J cylinder (UK).

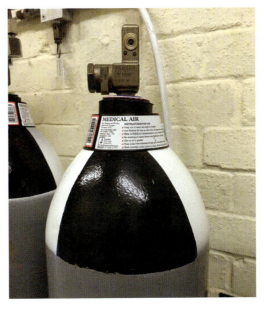

Figure 1.6 Medical grade air cylinder with a side spindle pin index valve.

fitted with the pin index system require a specific key or handle to open the valve. Size F oxygen cylinders have a bullnose valve (Figure 1.7), size G nitrous cylinders have a hand wheel side outlet (Figure 1.8) and size H cylinders have a bullnose valve, similar to F tanks. The valve allows either direct connection to an anesthetic machine or distribution pipeline supply. Unused, full cylinders frequently have a wrapping to ensure dust does not block the valve outlet port. This should always be checked for integrity and removed prior to use. The valve should always be opened slowly prior to use, as this prevents an adiabatic change from occurring (Davis and Kenny 2007). An adiabatic process is defined as one that occurs without an exchange of heat energy with the surroundings. For example, the pressure in the pipeline and gauge may rise rapidly, subsequently compressing the gas contained within the system, which may result in an increase in temperature and pose a potential fire risk. The valve should also not be over tightened when closed to prevent damage to the valve itself. A safety pressure release device is integrated within the valve housing and prevents cylinder over-pressurization and the subsequent risk of an explosion.

1.1.4 Safety

All cylinders are color coded (Dorsch and Dorsch 2011; Alibhai 2016) according to their constituent medical gas

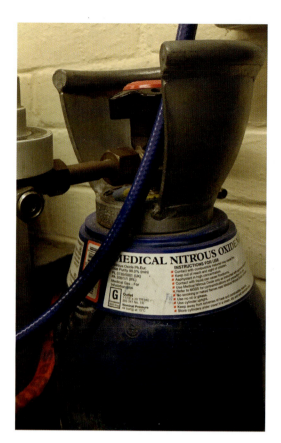

Figure 1.8 Nitrous oxide size G cylinder with a wheel valve.

to minimize accidental misconnections. An international code exists between some countries, but it is not universally adopted. The cylinder color depends on the country where it is used and therefore should always be checked if working outside of the practitioner's normal environment. The color coding used in the UK, EU and North America is detailed in Table 1.2. The new EU standard cylinders (British Oxygen Company) all have a white body, with different colored shoulders and the constituent medical gas clearly written on the cylinder body to further improve safety. All cylinders are identified either by the color of their body and/or shoulders (Figure 1.9A–C).

Pin indexing (International Standards Organization 2004; Dorsch and Dorsch 2011, Westwood and Rieley 2012; Moseley 2015) is incorporated within the valve block, or stem, of size E and J cylinders, to prevent connection to the incorrect gas yoke on an anesthetic machine or yoke on a distribution system. The pin index system is specific to the medical gas contained within the cylinder (Figure 1.10A, B, C), and corresponding holes on the yoke (Figure 1.11) only allow the specific gas cylinder to be attached. A compressible washer, "O" ring or Bodok seal (Figure 1.12), is placed between the valve outlet and yoke to ensure a gas-tight fitting. The pin index

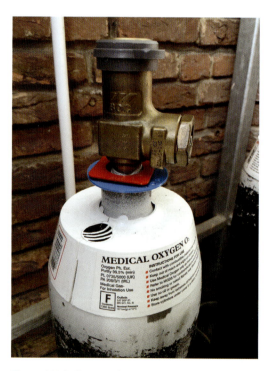

Figure 1.7 Bull nose valve on a size F (UK) oxygen cylinder. This type is similarly seen on size H (US) cylinders.

Table 1.2 Gas cylinder identification.

Gas	Gas Symbol	Color Code (US)	Color Code (UK)	New color code (EU standard)	Pin Index System	Physical state
Oxygen	O_2	Green/ Green and white	Black with white shoulders	White	2, 5	Gas
Nitrous oxide	N_2O	Blue	Blue	White with blue shoulders	3, 4	Liquid/vapor
Medical air	None	Yellow	Grey with black/white quarter shoulders	White with black/white quarter shoulders	1, 5	Gas
Carbon dioxide	CO_2	Grey	Grey	White with grey shoulders	1, 6	Gas
Entonox (50% O_2:50% N_2O)	O_2, N_2O	Blue	Blue with blue/white quarter shoulders	White with blue/white quarter shoulders	7	Gas/liquid/ vapor

and washer, ring or Bodok seal should be checked prior to cylinder connection and never have grease or oil applied to them.

As previously mentioned, cylinders should always be inspected prior to use, looking for any obvious external damage. The plastic valve wrapping or cap should be checked to ensure that it is intact and removed prior to attachment to the yoke, bull nose valve or distribution system. The yoke or similar attachment and any seal used should be checked for its integrity. Connections should not be over tightened, and once attached, the cylinder valve should be opened slowly to allow gas to be released. Any leaks should be identified and corrected at this time. The valve should be opened a minimum of two full turns to ensure complete gas flow and the pressure gauge read to check the cylinder capacity (appropriate for all cylinders to ensure they are not empty, but only reads quantity left for oxygen and medical air cylinders, see above). Cylinders attached to an anesthetic machine should be labeled as "in-use" or "full" as appropriate, to ensure that a cylinder containing a gas in its liquid state (e.g. nitrous oxide) is known to be either full or empty (Dorsch and Dorsch 2011).

Cylinder storage is dependent on size. Size E cylinders may be stored horizontally or vertically in appropriate restraints, so they cannot move or be tipped over (Figure 1.13).

Larger cylinders (size F and greater) should be stored vertically and chained to a wall or attached to the

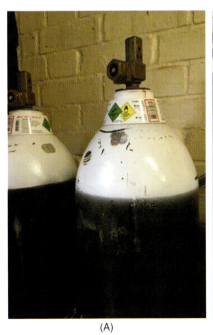
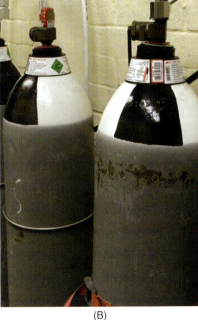
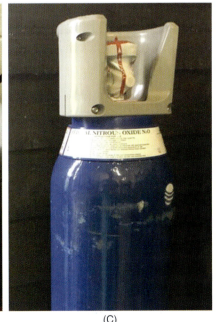

(A)   (B)   (C)

Figure 1.9 Examples of larger cylinder color identification. (A) Oxygen cylinders are white (UK) or have white shoulders and a black body (US). (B) Medical air cylinders can be gray with white or black shoulders (UK and EU) or yellow (US). (C) Nitrous oxide cylinders are commonly associated with a blue body or shoulders, in many geographical locations.

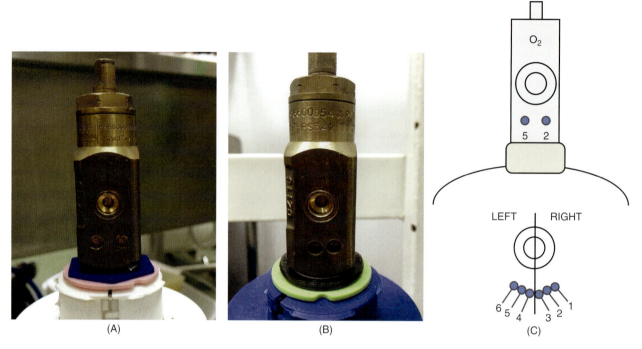

(A) (B) (C)

Figure 1.10 Pin index system on cylinder valves. The pins are placed at positions 2 and 5 on an E cylinder of oxygen (A) and at positions 3 and 5 on an E cylinder of nitrous oxide (B). The pin index system for an oxygen tank (positions 2, 5) and a complete schematic diagram showing all positions referred to in Table 1.2 are shown (C).

anesthetic machine using a permanent mount. Although not recommended, cylinders may be kept outside if extreme temperatures are not encountered, but should be protected from direct sunlight and rain. When stored outside, they should be kept in a locked area that is tamper proof. Careful storage is required to prevent cylinder damage and also to prevent injury to personnel. Large cylinders should be moved with the aid of a trolley or dolly, and gloves should be worn when handling them (Highley 2009).

Personal safety should be considered when working with gas cylinders. For example, smoking and flames are prohibited in proximity to any cylinders containing flammable

gases or liquid oxygen tanks due to risk of explosion. Cylinders should not be exposed to extreme temperatures, particularly high temperatures, should be handled with care, and should not be dropped due to risk of explosion from high pressures. All areas used for storage of cylinders

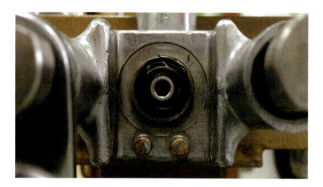

Figure 1.11 Close-up photo demonstrating the pin index system on the corresponding machine yoke for attachment of an E cylinder of oxygen.

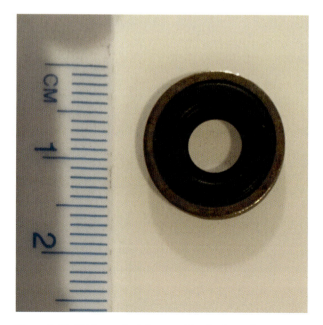

Figure 1.12 "O" ring or Bodok seal, with ruler for scale.

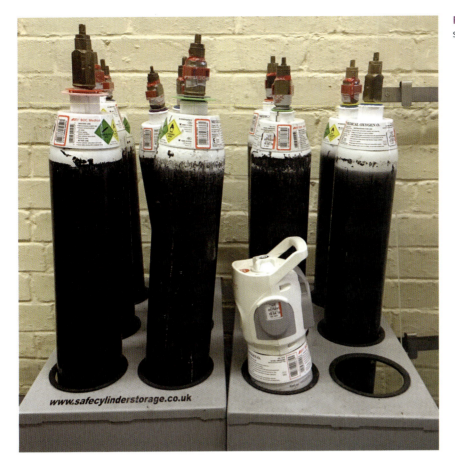

Figure 1.13 Cylinder storage rack for small size cylinders (e.g. E and CD).

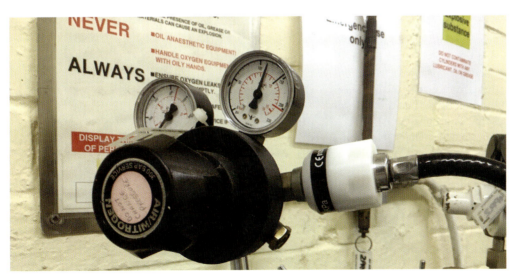

Figure 1.14 Safety warning signs clearly posted on the wall in a gas cylinder storage area.

and liquid oxygen tanks should be clearly signposted with safety warnings (Figure 1.14). Appropriate staff training should be undertaken by all personnel involved in using medical gases and attention paid to any local or regional regulations regarding their use (Moseley 2015).

1.1.5 Connections

Cylinders are either connected directly to an anesthetic machine using a yoke, by hosing to an anesthetic machine, or to a pipeline distribution system (Dorsch and Dorsch 2008a,b; Highley 2009; Westwood and Rieley 2012).

As mentioned above, Size E cylinders are attached directly to an anesthetic machine using a yoke with the integrated pin index safety system (Figure 1.5). Size F cylinders are attached from their bull nose valve (Figure 1.7) to the first stage regulator that has flexible tubing to connect to the anesthetic machine by a non-interchangeable screw thread (NIST; Highley 2009). Size G cylinders have a hand wheel valve (Figure 1.8) and size J cylinders a side spindle pin index system (Figure 1.6) for connection to a distribution system

1.1.6 Gas Cylinder Volume, Contents and Filling Ratio

The volume of gas (Dorsch and Dorsch 2008a; Moseley 2015) contained within a cylinder is dependent on the cylinder size and the physical state of the constituent gas (Table 1.1). For example, oxygen is present as a compressed gas (Table 1.2) and therefore its remaining volume within a cylinder is directly proportional to the pressure displayed on the gauge. For example, an E oxygen cylinder (UK) contains approximately 680 L oxygen when full at a pressure of 13 700 kPa. As the cylinder empties, the pressure displayed will be directly proportional to the cylinder contents; that is, at a pressure of 6850 kPa (50% full) there will be 340 L oxygen remaining.

Nitrous oxide and carbon dioxide (Table 1.2) are supplied as liquids with vapor above, therefore the pressure gauge does not denote volume remaining until all of the liquid has vaporized. Nitrous oxide cylinders contain a volume calculated according to the filling ratio (Highley 2009; Westwood and Rieley 2012), defined as the mass of liquid (i.e. nitrous oxide) in the cylinder divided by the mass of water required to fill the cylinder. In the EU and North America, this ratio is 0.75; in tropical climates, this is reduced to 0.67 to ensure the pressure generated by the vaporizing liquid does not exceed the cylinder specification. Thus, in contrast to oxygen or medical gas, an E nitrous oxide cylinder (UK) contains approximately 1800 L when full, but maintains a constant pressure of 4400 kPa until all of the liquid contents vaporize. At this point, the pressure gauge will fall as the remaining gas is delivered to the system. Therefore, there is no correlation between cylinder contents and gauge pressure and the cylinders must be weighed to determine the quantity of nitrous oxide remaining in the tank.

Readers are referred to the documents available from the British Oxygen Company (BOC) on cylinder types, valves, pin index, medical gases and capacities in the UK (http://www.bocmedical.co.uk).

1.2 Liquid Oxygen Tanks

In a large hospital with high oxygen demands, liquid oxygen stored in tanks may be used to supply the distribution system. Liquid oxygen is stored at −150 to −170 °C, below its critical temperature (−119 °C) and at a pressure of 5–10 atm within a double insulated tank (Howell 1980; Dorsch and Dorsch 2008b; Alibhai 2016). Storage of oxygen in its liquid state allows a larger quantity to be contained within the same volume compared to when in its gaseous state, making it more economical for the practitioner, especially if a nearly constant supply is required. One liter of liquid oxygen produces 842 L of gaseous oxygen at room temperature (Howell 1980). If demand is not constant, then wastage will occur due to atmospheric venting, which prevents excessive pressure from building within the tank.

The storage container is a vacuum insulated evaporator (VIE: Howell 1980; Dorsch and Dorsch 2008b; Al-Shaikh and Stacey 2013; Alibhai 2016) (Figure 1.15). Insulation is present between the two container walls and a vacuum is present to maintain its low temperature. The liquid oxygen continually draws heat from its surroundings, resulting in its vaporization (this is the latent heat of vaporization). Vaporized oxygen is removed from the VIE along the pipeline at the top of the container, where it passes through a heated coil, expanding as it does so. When demand is high and in excess of the normal vaporization processes, a control valve directs liquid from the bottom of the tank through a vaporizer and then to a super-heated coil. This gas then combines with the vaporized oxygen to supply the distribution system (Howell 1980). A pressure regulator is used to ensure

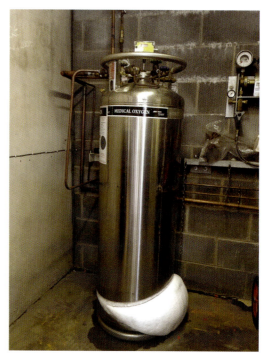

Figure 1.15 Vacuum insulated evaporator for liquid oxygen storage.

that a constant pressure (400 kPa; 3000 cmH$_2$O) is supplied to the pipeline and delivered to the hospital distribution system (Howell 1980).

Safety surrounding the storage and use of liquid oxygen is extremely important. Contact of liquid oxygen with skin may cause thermal burns, and pressure build-up within the system without appropriate venting may lead to explosion. A pressure relief valve is present to allow for excess pressure to be released to the environment due to continuous liquid oxygen vaporization when demand is low. The tank may be covered in ice and therefore presents a hazard if made contact with, due to condensing and subsequent freezing of water vapor on its cold surface. However, a liquid oxygen supply allows for remote filling away from the main hospital site and therefore is less disruptive. The VIE sits on a weigh scale to allow calculation of volume, which is displayed on an electronic screen. This may also be remotely connected to the gas supply company to alert them to fill the tank when it drops below a certain volume.

1.3 Oxygen Concentrators

Oxygen concentrators (Figure 1.16) filter and extract room air to produce oxygen for medical use. This may prove to be a cost-effective method for supplying oxygen, although it requires an electricity supply. Concentrators

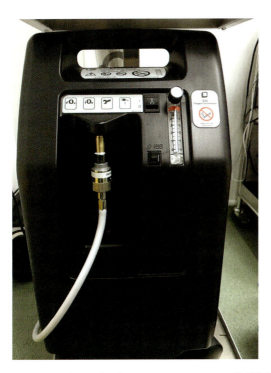

Figure 1.16 Example of an oxygen concentrator (DeVilbiss Healthcare, Tipton, UK).

consist of two zeolite molecular sieves in parallel. Zeolite retains nitrogen, some of the argon, and other unwanted components of air (Westwood and Rieley 2012; Al-Shaikh and Stacey 2013). Oxygen is released and pressurized by a compressor to approximately 137 kPa (1028 cmH$_2$O) for delivery to an anesthetic machine or other patient delivery system. An electronic valve switches between the two columns to ensure a constant oxygen supply. A maximum of approximately 10 L/min may be delivered at up to 92–95% oxygen. If used with a circle breathing system, higher gas flows must be delivered to ensure excessive argon (a small component of room air) concentrations do not accumulate within a low flow system. Argon accumulates due to its similar molecular size to oxygen and therefore it is able to pass through the molecular sieve (Al-Shaikh and Stacey 2013, Dorsch and Dorsch 2008c). Different types of zeolite have been utilized to reduce the amount of argon that passes through the sieve and increase the amount adsorbed. Appropriate gas monitoring in the anesthetic system should be available to ensure minimum oxygen delivery within the inspired gas mixture.

1.4 Medical Gas Pipeline Systems

Gas pipelines (Howell 1980) allow the supply of gases and vacuum from a central point to sites throughout the veterinary clinic, without the need for large pieces of apparatus at each outlet. Gas is supplied at 400 kPa (4 bar; 3000 cmH$_2$O), although medical air for surgical instruments may be delivered at 700 kPa (7 bar; 5250 cmH$_2$O). Special outlets are installed in clinical areas, allowing connections for anesthetic machines or other equipment. Oxygen, nitrous oxide, medical air and medical vacuum/ suction may all be supplied through a pipeline system. Active gas scavenging systems (AGSS) may also be provided in combination with gas pipeline systems.

1.4.1 Components

Gas pipeline systems (Howell 1980, Westwood and Rieley 2012) begin with a supply source, consisting of a bank of gas cylinders or liquid oxygen tanks. As previously mentioned, pipeline systems may be used for multiple gases as well as medical vacuum and suction, if available. A primary pressure regulator that ensures a constant supply to the distribution system controls the gas source. At this central supply point, there is a control panel displaying the status of the pipeline and each medical gas in use (Figure 1.17A,B). If a bank of cylinders is used as the supply source, then a secondary bank should also be available to switch to when the pressure from the primary bank falls below usable quantities. This apparatus is known as a cylinder manifold,

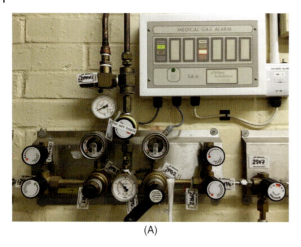 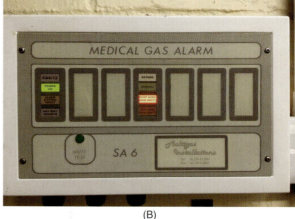

(A)   (B)

Figure 1.17 Pipeline system central control panel. (A) Control panel at the cylinder manifold with associated gauges and valves. (B) Medical gas alarm control panel.

and often comprises an automatic changeover between cylinder banks with subsequent activation of an electronic alarm, alerting staff that one bank is depleted and requires changing. Similarly, if liquid oxygen is used, then a reserve bank of cylinders should be available if the primary supply becomes depleted or fails. From the pressure regulator and corresponding pressure gauge, the distribution pipeline supplies the medical gas to the terminal outlet, consisting of a socket which accepts a matching quick connect and disconnect or Schrader probe (Figure 1.18). These components are detailed below.

1.4.2 Cylinder Manifold

A cylinder manifold (Howell 1980, Westwood and Rieley 2012) consists of two groups of large cylinders (Figure 1.19),

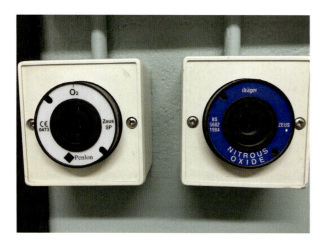

Figure 1.18 Terminal outlet with gas specific indexing collar; Schrader style, quick connect-disconnect type. The outlet is color coded to match the specific gas being supplied. The oxygen outlet is to the left and nitrous oxide outlet to the right, depicting the UK standard.

which alternate to supply medical gases to the distribution system. In the UK, size J cylinders are most commonly used for oxygen and medical air and size G for nitrous oxide. In the US, size H cylinders or liquid oxygen tanks are most commonly used. The manifold should be protected from the weather, being kept in a building or other suitable environment. One-way or non-return valves (Figure 1.20) using copper alloy pipework, connected to a common pressure regulator and gauge, connect each bank of cylinders. This ensures that the supply to the distribution system is kept constant. When the detected pressure is low from the "in use" cylinder bank, it automatically switches to the second full bank of cylinders. This switching triggers an electronic audible and visual alarm on the display to inform the user. Generally, the user is then required to move the in-use lever to the full bank (Figure 1.21) and arrange to replace the exhausted cylinders. Some manifolds may have a third, reserve bank of one or two cylinders to ensure the supply is not lost if both banks fail. If the gas source supply is a liquid oxygen tank, then a reserve cylinder bank should similarly be available.

1.4.3 Distribution System Connections

Gas cylinders connect to the pipeline at a central point, as part of a manifold or directly with connectors (i.e. side spindle pin index valve, wheel valve, etc.), depending on cylinder size and constituent gas. From the cylinder, manifold gases are distributed via the pipeline system to the terminal outlets in the treatment areas of the clinic.

1.4.3.1 Cylinder and Manifold Attachments

As described above, if demand is relatively high, an automatic supply system, such as a cylinder manifold, provides a constant supply to the clinic. Gas cylinders are connected to the manifold in two banks by flexible

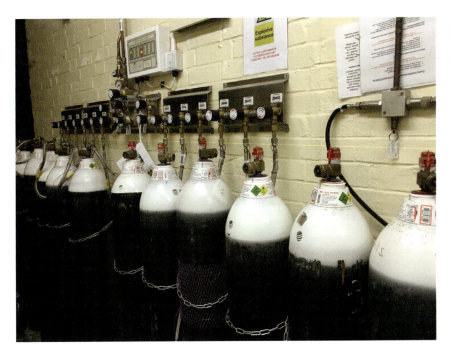

Figure 1.19 Cylinder manifold for supply to a pipeline distribution system. This is comprised of a left and right bank, 6-cylinder oxygen manifold.

pipework (Figure 1.22) to a common distribution system. Each cylinder supplying the manifold has a separate one-way or non-return valve feeding its supply to the central system (Howell 1980). All valves on the in-use cylinder bank should be fully open to ensure uniform emptying across the bank. These valves are easy to turn and may display a colored red or green line to denote their status. On the secondary bank, at least one cylinder should be fully open to ensure consistency of supply at switchover. At the start of the common distribution system, a pressure gauge is fitted (Howell 1980) after the regulator to display and monitor gas supply to the distribution system (Figure 1.23). The user may manually adjust the

pipeline pressure if required. There is also a pressure relief valve associated with the common part of the system (Figure 1.24). Each bank of cylinders has a vent valve to allow depressurizing when switching over to the secondary bank.

Copper alloy pipework is used to supply the individual medical gases to the required locations within the hospital, ending at self-sealing terminal outlets. Copper alloy is used as it does not interact with the medical gases and is also bacteriostatic (Howell 1980). Pipework diameter may vary, depending on position within the distribution system; for example, between the central supply point and dividing areas, piping will be of a larger diameter than after branching to supply individual rooms.

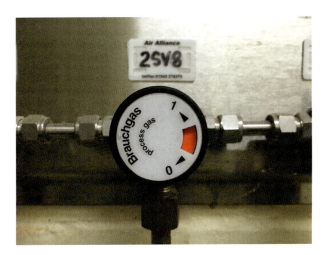

Figure 1.20 Non-return or one-way valve associated with cylinder connections to a manifold. The red/orange indicates that the valve is closed.

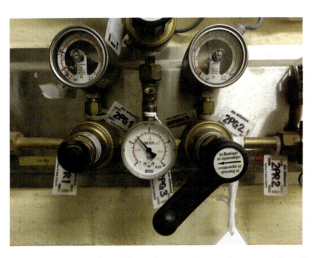

Figure 1.21 Manual switchover lever to discern between left and right cylinder banks in use following automatic changeover.

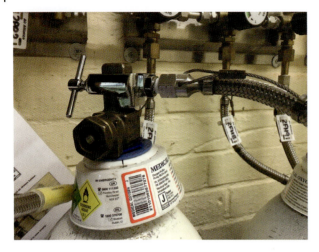

Figure 1.22 Cylinder connections to a manifold using the flexible tubing.

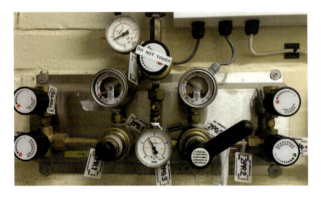

Figure 1.23 Pipeline pressure gauge and valve for manual adjustment of pipeline pressure. The manual pressure adjustment valve is labeled as "do not touch" to avoid inadvertent alterations to pipeline pressure.

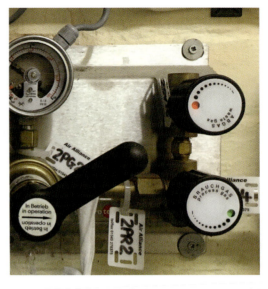

Figure 1.24 Pressure relief valves to vent one side of the manifold.

An alternative to a manifold is to use a pressure regulator and gauge fitted directly to the cylinder (Figure 1.25A,B). Flexible hosing with a Schrader probe or appropriate screw connection (Highley 2009) is directly attached to the regulator and then supplies the distribution system. This is less expensive than a cylinder manifold, but requires manual changeover between cylinders; supply may therefore be interrupted. This may be more useful for the supply of gases other than oxygen, in facilities with a lower gas demand or those places not requiring constant delivery.

1.4.3.2 Terminal Outlets and Machine Connections

Connections between the gas cylinders/manifolds and the terminal outlet or the anesthetic machine have a number

Figure 1.25 (A) Medical air size J cylinder connected to a pipeline directly from a side spindle pin index pressure regulator and gauge. (B) Size G nitrous oxide cylinder connected to a pipeline directly from a side port hand wheel valve.

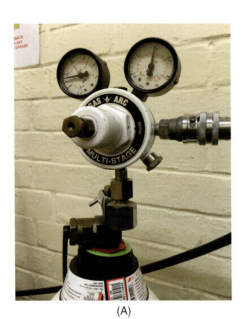

(A)

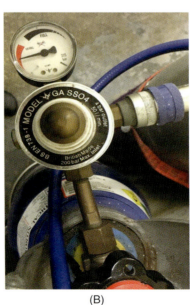

(B)

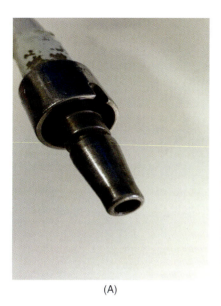
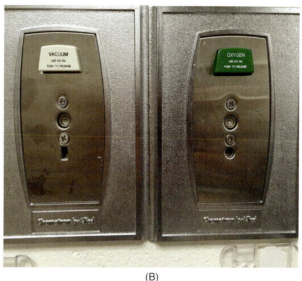

(A)   (B)

Figure 1.26 Examples of terminal gas outlets. (A) Schrader probe with gas specific (oxygen) index collar for insertion into the terminal outlet (UK). (B) Standard terminal vacuum (left, white) and oxygen (right, green) wall outlets (US).

of safety features to ensure correct gas supply. The safety system is based on threaded and non-threaded connections that are gas specific, to minimize risk of incorrect gas supply (Highley 2009; Moseley 2015; Alibhai 2016).

Terminal outlets (Howell 1980; Highley 2009) vary in type but always consist of a socket with an indexing collar that is specific to the gas supplied and therefore only a probe with the appropriate collar (Figure 1.26A) or pin system (Figure 1.26B) can be connected. The terminal units are also color coded and matched to the specific gas supplied. This avoids inadvertent connection of the wrong gas supply to the anesthetic machine or other piece of equipment. The terminal outlets are self-sealing and allow for easy and rapid connection and disconnection of hoses (Highley 2009). Once connected, a "tug test" should be performed to ensure the connection is secure and will not inadvertently detach. Different types of outlet are available, depending on where they are positioned. They may be wall mounted, on a hose dropped from the ceiling (Figure 1.27), or on a ceiling mounted unit. Terminal outlets for AGSS (Figure 1.28) usually have diameter index safety system (DISS) connections, again as a further safety feature to minimize risk of incorrect connection.

The anesthetic machine is connected to the terminal outlet using static-free, color-coded flexible tubing (Figure 1.29). This may have a Schrader probe and collar for attachment to the outlet at one end and a DISS with NIST (Highley 2009, Westwood and Rieley 2012; Moseley 2015) to attach to the anesthetic machine itself (Figure 1.30) at the other end, especially in the UK. The color coding is the same as the color of the appropriate

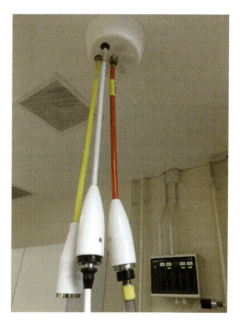

Figure 1.27 Available mounting types for terminal outlets. This is a ceiling mounted system with flexible tubing suspended from the ceiling mount.

medical gas cylinder. Each medical gas is assigned a DISS number, which is unique to the gas being supplied, and along with the NIST avoids inadvertent connection to the incorrect outlet. Only single, continuous hoses should be used for connections, as this avoids the risk of misconnection if a junction were present. If any tubing is found to be damaged, it should be replaced with a new unit and in no circumstances should it be attached with any connections to a second hose.

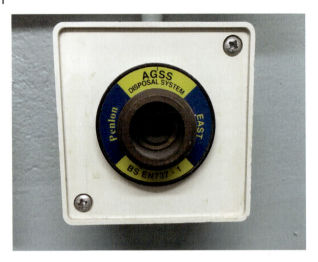

Figure 1.28 Active gas scavenging system (AGSS) terminal outlet.

1.4.4 Safety Features and Alarms

Pipeline distribution systems have a number of safety alarms (Howell 1980, Dorsch and Dorsch 2008b) to ensure they function correctly and to alert the user to any faults. The gas pressure being supplied to the distribution system is regulated from the cylinder or liquid

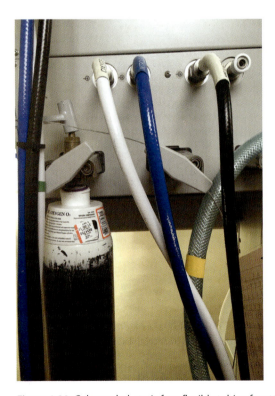

Figure 1.29 Color-coded, static free, flexible tubing for attachment of an anesthetic machine to the terminal outlet. In the UK, white connects oxygen, blue connects nitrous oxide, black connects medical air, and pale blue connects the AGSS. These colors may differ in other geographical locations (i.e. North America).

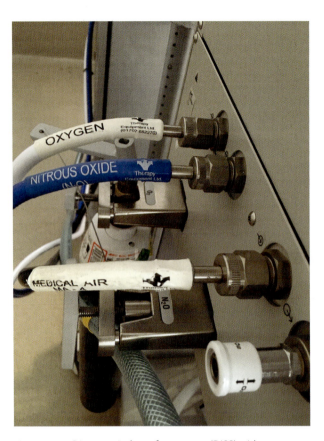

Figure 1.30 Diameter index safety system (DISS) with non-interchangeable screw threads (NIST) for attachment of gas specific tubing to the anesthetic machine.

oxygen tank as it enters the central control point. A pressure relief valve is present to prevent excess pipeline pressure, usually set at 50% above the normal working pressure. An electronic central display unit and control panel (Figures 1.17A, B) senses low gas pipeline pressures and sounds an audible and visual alarm. It informs the user which medical gas supply is low, which cylinder bank is empty, and if any faults within the system require troubleshooting. This unit should be located in a prominent position within the clinic to ensure that appropriate personnel are aware of any changes to the system status. Although the secondary cylinder bank and reserve cylinders are responsible for providing adequate oxygen supply back up, each anesthetic machine supplied by a gas pipeline should also be fitted with an oxygen cylinder, usually size E (Figure 1.31), in case of pipeline failure or another emergency situation.

Isolating or shut-off valves (Figure 1.32) should be strategically placed in the facility to enable the user to cut the supply to a specific area of the hospital, either in an emergency or for planned maintenance (Highley 2009). Emergency shut-off valves should also be fitted at the manifold to ensure the entire supply can be stopped if required.

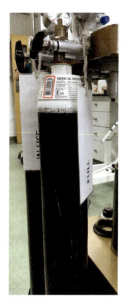

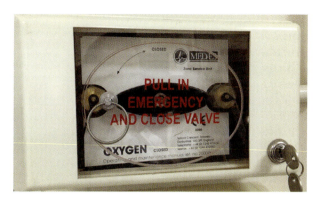

Figure 1.32 Isolating valves to shut off supply to a specific area of the distribution system.

A qualified engineer should only carry out testing and maintenance on the gas distribution system to ensure patient and personnel safety. A servicing contract will usually be in place to ensure the safe working of any medical gas pipeline.

Figure 1.31 Size E oxygen cylinder attached to an anesthetic machine as an emergency backup should the pipeline supply fail.

References

Alibhai, H.I.K. (2016) The anesthetic machine and vaporizers. In: Duke-Novakowski. T., de Vries. M., Seymour. C. (eds). *BSAVA Manual of Canine and Feline Anaesthesia and Analgesia*, 3rd ed. Gloucester, UK: BSAVA, pp. 24–44.

Al-Shaikh, B. and Stacey, S.G. (2013) Medical gas supply. In: *Essentials of Anaesthetic Equipment*, 4th ed. Edinburgh, UK: Churchill Livingston Elsevier, pp. 1–18.

British Oxygen Company Group PLC. *Cylinder Data Chart*. Available from: http://www.bocmedical.co.uk [accessed October 2016].

Davis, P.D. and Kenny, G.N.C. (2007) Pressure. In: *Basic Physics and Measurement in Anaesthesia*, 5th ed. Edinburgh, UK: Elsevier, pp. 1–11.

Dorsch, J.A. and Dorsch, S.E. (2008a) Medical gas cylinders and containers. In: *Understanding Anaesthesia Equipment*, 5th ed. Philadelphia, PA: Lippincott Williams & Wilkins, pp. 1–24.

Dorsch, J.A. and Dorsch, S.E. (2008b) Medical gas pipeline systems. In: *Understanding Anaesthesia Equipment*, 5th ed. Philadelphia, PA: Lippincott Williams & Wilkins, pp. 25–50.

Dorsch, J.A. and Dorsch, S.E. (2008c) Gas oxygen concentrators. In: *Understanding Anaesthesia Equipment*, 5th ed. Philadelphia, PA: Lippincott Williams & Wilkins, pp. 76–80.

Dorsch, J.A. and Dorsch, S.E. (2011) Medical gas sources. In: *A Practical Approach to Anesthesia Equipment*, 1st ed. Philadelphia, PA: Lippincott, Williams & Wilkins, pp. 3–28.

Highley, D. (2009) Medical gases, their storage and delivery. *Anaesth Intensive Care Med*, 10, 523–527.

Howell, R.S. (1980) Piped medical gas and vacuum systems. *Anaesthesia*, 35, 676–698.

International Standards Organization (2004) *Small Medical Gas Cylinders – Pin Index Yoke-type Valve Connections (ISO 407:2004)*. Available from: https://www.iso.org [accessed October 2016].

Mosley, C.A. (2015) Anaesthesia Equipment. In: Grimm. K.A., Lamont, L.A., Tranquilli, W.J., Greene, S.A. and Robertson, S.A. (eds) *Veterinary Anaesthesia and Analgesia, The Fifth Edition of Lumb and Jones*. Ames, IA: John Wiley & Sons Inc., pp. 23–85.

Westwood, M-M. and Rieley, W. (2012) Medical gases, their storage and delivery. *Anaesth Intensive Care Med*, 13, 533–538.

2

Oxygen Concentrators

Allan Williamson

School of Veterinary Medicine, University of Wisconsin, Madison, Wisconsin, USA

2.1 Introduction

Oxygen concentrators are a commonly-used piece of equipment, where cylinders or liquid oxygen storage would be impractical or prohibitively expensive, especially in remote areas or in small practices. They function by extraction of oxygen from the surrounding environment and as such only require ambient air and a source of electricity. They have been successfully used for the provision of anesthesia to dogs (Burn *et al.* 2016), as well as for oxygen delivery during field anesthesia of larger animals, including equids and wildlife (Fahlman *et al.* 2012; Coutu *et al.* 2015).

Low maintenance requirements, a small footprint and reliable function have made these a popular choice for small animal practitioners with limited surgical caseload (Shrestha *et al.* 2002; Burn *et al.* 2016). However, it should be noted that these units do have some disadvantages associated with their use and may not be ideal for every general practice.

2.2 Function

Oxygen concentrators typically work via a pressure swing adsorption mechanism that separates oxygen from the principal component of air, nitrogen (Dobson 2001; Dorsch and Dorsch 2008; Rao *et al.* 2014). First, an air compressor serves to drive ambient air through a series of particulate filters to remove contaminants such as bacteria, through a heat exchanger and into a reservoir, where it is compressed in order to improve the efficiency of adsorption (Figure 2.1; Friesen 1992; Dobson 2001; Dorsch and Dorsch 2008).

Following compression, air then passes through a series of valves designed to balance flow through several sieve beds. These sieves contain an adsorbent, typically a silica and/or aluminum-based zeolite, which binds the gas components in the air. Adsorption depends both on the nature of the adsorbent and the gas properties, such as molecular size, polarity and electrochemical properties (Friesen 1992; Rao *et al.* 2014). Typical adsorbents bind most strongly with nitrogen, carbon dioxide, water vapor and other gases with a strong dipole moment, and weakly with oxygen and mono-atomic gases (Friesen 1992; Dorsch and Dorsch 2008). Oxygen concentrators use at least two sieve columns to provide continuous delivery of product gas, since once the adsorbent is fully occupied by nitrogen, gas must be bled off to allow further binding. This may be accomplished by flushing with product gas or by the application of brief negative pressure to the column. These columns must be slightly out of phase with each other in order to assure continuous generation of oxygen. More rapid cycling may be useful in increasing the rate of oxygen generation, but presents a more challenging engineering problem (Friesen 1992; Rao *et al.* 2014).

Following adsorption, the product gas is then passed through an oxygen analyzer to confirm the output of an adequate product (Dorsch and Dorsch 2008; International Organization for Standardization [ISO] 2016). It is then typically shunted into a storage vessel of varying volume. Depending on the size of this vessel, it may simply be used to reduce any pressure and flow fluctuations generated by the cycling of the sieve columns, or may act as a higher-pressure reservoir tank, allowing for storage of gas for situations where demand exceeds the supply capacity of the unit or during interruptions in power supply (Ezi-Ashi *et al.* 1983).

2.3 Product Gas

The USP standard for compressed oxygen gas requires 99% or greater purity in the final product (The United States Pharmacopeial Convention, Inc., 1990).

Veterinary Anesthetic and Monitoring Equipment, First Edition. Edited by Kristen G. Cooley and Rebecca A. Johnson.
© 2018 John Wiley & Sons, Inc. Published 2018 by John Wiley & Sons, Inc.

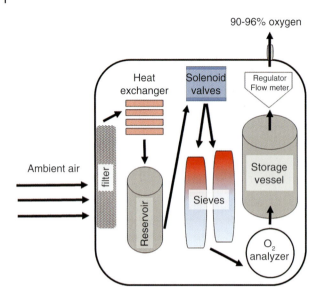

90-96% oxygen

Heat exchanger

Solenoid valves

Regulator
Flow meter

Ambient air

filter

Reservoir

Sieves

Storage vessel

O₂ analyzer

Figure 2.1 Schematic representing components of an oxygen concentrator. Ambient air is taken into the unit, heated and compressed before passing through adsorbing sieves. The oxygen concentration is analyzed (~90–96%) and stored for patient use.

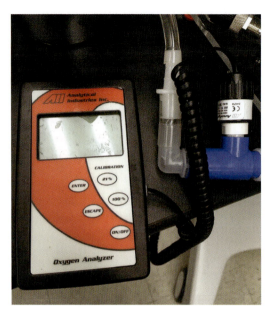

Figure 2.2 A simple, inexpensive oxygen analyzer that can be used in the patient's breathing circuit to ensure sufficient delivered oxygen concentrations. It requires prior calibration and the sensor (blue) can be placed anywhere in the breathing circuit, preferably in the inspiratory limb.

Due to inefficiencies in the adsorption process, units for medical use do not typically meet this standard. The current standard for oxygen concentrators is that the product gas will contain between 90 and 96% oxygen, and may be referred to as Oxygen 93% USP, Oxygen 90+, or oxygen-enriched air (ISO 2016). The remaining gas in this mixture is typically a mixture of nitrogen and argon, and has been shown to affect neither patient outcome nor equipment function (Friesen 1992). This composition may fluctuate somewhat during the course of a given anesthetic, but should not fall below this standard, providing that oxygen flow rates do not exceed the maximum rated flow rate for the unit. At higher oxygen flow rates, it is expected that oxygen composition of the product gas will decrease significantly, which may be of clinical concern, especially in an already hypoxemic patient or for those patients predisposed to hypoxemia (Carter *et al.* 1985). As with all anesthetic events, monitoring of inspired oxygen fraction is highly recommended with the use of an oxygen concentrator (Figure 2.2). Other factors that may reduce the output of an oxygen concentrator, include high altitude (Bunel *et al.* 2016) and high ambient humidity (Friesen 1992).

During closed-circuit anesthesia, argon has been noted to accumulate in the anesthetic circuit. While this is unlikely to cause clinical harm to patients, it may present a concern due to displacement of oxygen, especially if techniques incorporating an inspired oxygen fraction of less than 50% are used. As such, it is not recommended to use fresh gas flows of less than 0.5 L/min when an oxygen concentrator is being used (Parker and Snowdon 1988; Dorsch and Dorsch 2008). However, the produced argon does not interfere with conventional gas monitoring techniques or the function of modern vaporizers or precision flowmeters (Friesen 1992).

Notably, in North America, equipment designated for veterinary use only is not required to adhere to FDA standards, although many manufacturers will elect to do so. Clinicians and hospital administrators seeking to purchase equipment should consult with the manufacturer to determine what safety equipment is present, the expected output including recommended flow rates, and any other notable limitations particular to a certain product.

2.4 Clinical Use

The typical clinical use of oxygen concentrators is to supply continuous oxygen flow for use during procedures requiring either supplemental oxygen or inhalant anesthesia in place of that supplied by oxygen tanks (Burn *et al.* 2016). However, in large animal anesthesia, most oxygen concentrators are incapable of supplying oxygen at the rates needed in order to provide even low-flow anesthesia. As such, oxygen concentrators are not typically used for the provision of inhalant anesthetics in that setting. However, they have been evaluated in larger species for provision of supplemental oxygen during chemical immobilization or total intravenous anesthesia, either via continuous supplementation or pulsed delivery during inhalation. For example, they have been successfully used in a variety of species, including brown bears (Fahlman *et al.* 2014a), white-tailed deer (Fahlman *et al.* 2014b), horses (Coutu *et al.* 2015) and a variety of other wildlife species (Fahlman *et al.* 2012). Significant improvements were made in arterial oxygen tension with the provision of even low flows of 0.5–1 L/min, which are well within the capabilities of currently available oxygen concentrators.

Oxygen concentrators come in different configurations from multiple manufacturers. For example, there are large units that generate oxygen and store it in a very large bulk tank for in-hospital use (Figure 2.3; OxGen OnSite Oxygen Generator, Patterson Veterinary Supply, Columbus, OH). In addition, smaller units with the capability to store a moderate amount of oxygen are also available (e.g. Vetroson® Oxy-Gen™ Systems, Summit Hill Laboratories, Patterson Veterinary Supply, Columbus, OH; OG-20 Oxygen Generating System, OGSI, Vetamac, Rossville, IN). Devices that are more portable are also available (from many manufacturers) for remote use or for use in multiple areas of the hospital (Figure 2.4; e.g. OGS-20 Oxygen Generating System, OGSI, Vetamac, Rossville, IN; E2 Oxygen Concentrator, Patterson Veterinary Supply, Columbus, OH; Pureline® Series, Supera Anesthesia Innovations, Clackamas, OR). Readers are encouraged to contact each manufacturer in their area for exact product specifications and limitations that may affect delivery in certain situations.

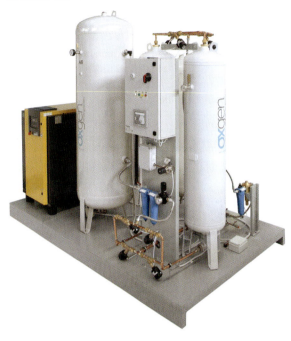

Figure 2.3 An example of a large oxygen concentrator that stores oxygen in a bulk tank for use within a veterinary hospital (photograph courtesy of Patterson Veterinary Supply, Columbus, OH).

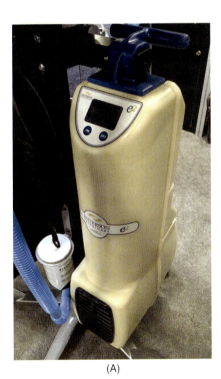

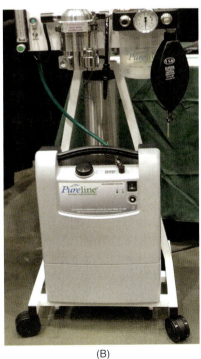

(A) (B)

Figure 2.4 Examples of portable oxygen concentrators for use in remote locations or on portable anesthesia machines. (A) E2 Oxygen Concentrator, Patterson Veterinary Supply, Columbus, OH. (B) Pureline® Series, Supera Anesthesia Innovations, Clackamas, OR.

2.5 Advantages

2.5.1 Cost

Aside from the initial up-front costs for an oxygen concentrator, there is little ongoing cost associated with their use, beyond replacement or cleaning of filters. Because of this, it has been recommended that such units be used in underserviced or remote areas (Friesen 1992; Shrestha *et al.* 2002; Bradley *et al.* 2015). Significant monetary savings may be realized by reduction in need for oxygen tanks, especially in areas where shipment is impractical or expensive (Dobson 2001; Enarson *et al.* 2008). Many repairs, when needed, can be performed inexpensively and by personnel without advanced training (Dobson *et al.* 1996; Bradley *et al.* 2015).

2.5.2 Reliability

Most FDA-approved oxygen concentrators have been noted to perform consistently for long periods, with little changes in output, except in extremes of humidity and altitude (Dorsch and Dorsch 2008; Bunel *et al.* 2016). In a field trial in a low-resource area of Egypt, of 22 machines, only 2 had developed mechanical problems within 1 year, one of which was repairable by local technicians (Dobson *et al.* 1996), with the machines outputting an average of 89% oxygen over 3712 hours.

2.5.3 Contaminant Filtration

The zeolite adsorption mechanism used to concentrate oxygen has been shown to be effective at filtering out contaminant gases. It should be noted, however, that many pollutants may bind irreversibly to the filter columns and as such will shorten the lifespan of oxygen concentrating units if used in heavily contaminated areas (Evans *et al.* 1983; Friesen 1992).

2.5.4 Portability

Oxygen concentrators with minimal storage capacity are highly portable and have been used in field situations to provide supplemental oxygen (Fahlman *et al.* 2014b). In small animal practice, anesthesia machines have been developed to incorporate small oxygen concentrators into the base of the unit.

2.6 Disadvantages

2.6.1 Low Gas Pressure

Many oxygen concentrators may be unable to generate sufficient pressure to supply gas-driven ventilators, which require a pipeline pressure of approximately 50 psig. However, Piston-driven ventilators do not have this requirement (Carter *et al.* 1985; Dobson 1992).

2.6.2 Maintenance Needs

Regular service is required, which may include replacement or cleaning of filters. However, this is generally not technically challenging (Bradley *et al.* 2015). In heavily contaminated areas, the zeolite adsorbent may become degraded over time, necessitating replacement (Evans *et al.* 1983).

2.6.3 Argon Accumulation

As discussed above, a significant portion of gas output by oxygen concentrators is ambient argon gas. Care should be taken to ensure that adequate oxygen is being supplied to patients, including inspired oxygen monitoring (Parker and Snowdon 1988).

2.6.4 Limited Flow Rates

Few available oxygen concentrators are capable of supplying flow rates greater than 5 L/min, with many smaller units having maximum flow rates significantly less than this. Particularly large patients, especially those on non-rebreathing circuits, may require oxygen flow rates greater than a unit is capable of supplying (Carter *et al.* 1985). Practitioners should be familiar with the capabilities of any oxygen concentrator units in use.

2.6.5 Limited Reserves

Smaller units may have a limited reserve capacity, which may become exhausted quickly should the unit fail to operate or if the electricity supply is interrupted. Reserve oxygen, a battery back-up and/or a back-up unit, as needed, should be readily available in such an event in order to ensure adequate oxygen delivery, especially during inhalant anesthesia (Dobson 1992). In these situations, pulsed delivery of oxygen may be used if applicable to the situation.

2.7 Hazards

2.7.1 Flame or Explosion

The primary hazards associated with the use of an oxygen concentrator are related to the product gas. Oxygen concentrators must be kept away from any sources of heat or open flame to prevent fire associated with inadvertent leakage of the product gas. This is especially important if a concentrator with a storage tank is used, which compounds the danger with that of a high pressure gas source, greater or equal to 350 psig (2400 kPa; Ezi-Ashi *et al.* 1983). Refer to Chapters 1 and 9 for further information on cylinder hazards.

2.7.2 Low Output

Environmental contamination, especially in high humidity areas, may reduce the concentration of oxygen output and may necessitate early replacement of the adsorbent. Oxygen monitoring should be used with these devices to ensure that adequate oxygen is being supplied to the patient (Evans *et al.* 1983; Dobson 1992).

2.7.3 Device Failure

The devices are mechanically simple and not overly prone to failure; however, care should be taken to ensure that back-up sources of oxygen are available in the event

of malfunction (Dobson *et al.* 1996; Enarson *et al.* 2008). Smaller units may only have a reserve volume sufficient to provide oxygen flow for a few minutes in the event of failure (Dobson 1992). Restriction of airflow to the device or blockage of filters may increase the risk of device overheating and shutdown and, as such, the location of the device should allow for adequate airflow and little overt contamination, and filters should be inspected routinely (Dorsch and Dorsch, 2008).

2.8 Summary

In summary, although there are some disadvantages to using oxygen concentrators (e.g. <100% oxygen delivery, low continuous supply, etc.), they may be economical and used to supply carrier gas to an anesthetic vaporizer or for supplemental oxygen delivery in some situations.

References

Bradley, B.D., Chow, S., Nyassi, E., Cheng, Y-L., Peel, D. and Howie, S.R. (2015) A retrospective analysis of oxygen concentrator maintenance needs and costs in a low-resource setting: experience from The Gambia. *Health Technol*, 4, 319–328.

Bunel, V., Shoukri, A., Choin, F., Roblin, S., Smith, C., *et al.* (2016) Bench evaluation of four portable oxygen concentrators under different conditions representing altitudes of 2438, 4200, and 8000 m. *High Alt Med Biol*, 17, 370–374.

Burn, J., Caulkett, N.A., Gunn, M., Cooney, C, Kuts, S.J. and Boysen, S.R. (2016) Evaluation of a portable oxygen concentrator to provide fresh gas flow to dogs undergoing anesthesia. *Can Vet J*, 57, 614–618.

Carter, J.A., Baskett P.J.F. and Simpson, P.J. (1985) The "Permox" oxygen concentrator. *Anaesthesia*, 40, 560–565.

Coutu, P., Caulkett, N., Pang, D. and Boysen, S. (2015) Efficacy of a portable oxygen concentrator with pulsed delivery for treatment of hypoxemia during equine field anesthesia. *Vet Anaesth Analg*, 42, 518–526.

Dobson, M.B. (1992) Oxygen concentrators for the smaller hospital – A review. *Trop Doct*, 22, 56–58.

Dobson, M.B. (2001) Oxygen concentrators and cylinders [Oxygen therapy in children]. *Int J Tuberc Lung Dis*, 5, 520–523.

Dobson, M.B., Peel, D. and Khallaf, N. (1996) Field trial of oxygen concentrators in upper Egypt. *Lancet*, 347, 1597–1599.

Dorsch, J.A. and Dorsch, S.E. (2008) Oxygen concentrators. In: *Understanding Anesthesia Equipment*, 5th ed. Philadelphia, PA: Lippincott Williams & Wilkins, pp. 76–80.

Enarson, P., La Vincente, S., Gie, R., Maganga, E. and Chokani, C. (2008) Implementation of an oxygen concentrator system in district hospital paediatric wards throughout Malawi. *Bull World Health Organ*, 86, 344–348.

Evans, T.W., Waterhouse, J. and Howard, P. (1983) Clinical experience with the oxygen concentrator. *British Medical Journal* (Clinical research ed.), 287, 459–461.

Ezi-Ashi, T.I., Papworth, D.P. and Nunn, J.F. (1983) Inhalational anaesthesia in developing countries. *Anaesthesia*, 38, 736–747.

Fahlman, Å., Caulkett, N., Arnemo, J.M., Neuhaus, P. and Ruckstuhl, K.E. (2012) Efficacy of a portable oxygen concentrator with pulsed delivery for treatment of hypoxemia during anesthesia of wildlife. *J Zoo Wildl Med*, 43, 67–76.

Fahlman, Å., Arnemo, J.M., Pringle, J. and Nyman, G. (2014a) Oxygen supplementation in anesthetized brown bears (*Ursus arctos*) – How low can you go? *J Wildl Dis*, 50, 574–581.

Fahlman, Å., Caulkett, N., Woodbury, M., Dike-Novakovski, T. and Wourms, V. (2014b) Low flow oxygen therapy from a portable oxygen concentrator or an oxygen cylinder effectively treats hypoxemia in anesthetized white-tailed deer (*Odocoileus virginianus*). *J Zoo Wildl Med*, 45, 272–277.

Friesen, R.M. (1992) Oxygen concentrators and the practice of anaesthesia. *Can J Anaesth*, 39, R80.

International Organization for Standardization [ISO] (2016) Medical gas pipeline systems – Part 1: Pipeline systems for compressed medical gases and vacuum. (ISO Standard No. 7396–7391).

Parker, C.J.R. and Snowdon, S.L. (1988) Predicted and measured oxygen concentrations in the circle system using low fresh gas flows with oxygen supplied by an oxygen concentrator. *Br J Anaesth*, 61, 397–402.

Rao, V.R., Kothare, M.V. and Sircar, S. (2014) Novel design and performance of a medical oxygen concentrator using a rapid pressure swing adsorption concept. *AIChE J*, 60, 3330–3335.

Shrestha, B.M., Singh, B.B., Gautam, M.P. and Chand, M.B. (2002) The oxygen concentrator is a suitable alternative to oxygen cylinders in Nepal. *Can J Anesth*, 49, 8.

The United States Pharmacopeial Convention, Inc. (1990) The National Formulary – USP XXII NF XVII, pp. 991–992

3

Small Animal Anesthetic Machines and Equipment

Craig Mosley[1] and Amanda Shelby[2]

[1] Specialty Medicine, VCA Canada, Calgary, AB, Canada
[2] Jurox Animal Health, Kansas City, Missouri, USA

3.1 Introduction

Safe anesthetic delivery and maintenance has become increasingly dependent upon mechanical and electrical equipment. It is necessary for the anesthetist to understand thoroughly equipment function and potential patient and personnel risks before adaptation for routine patient care. Anesthetic equipment includes various airway support products, oxygen delivery devices, anesthetic machines, scavenging systems, ventilators and many configurations of patient monitors and other support products. The anesthetic machines available to the veterinary anesthetist include nearly any human anesthetic machine, regularly produced machines specifically for the veterinary market and many limited-production and/or custom machines. As such, it is nearly impossible to describe all of the anesthetic machines used in small animal anesthesia. This chapter provides the reader with the operating principles and a practical working overview of a generic small animal anesthetic machine and its components.

3.2 Safety and Design

Since 1989 and 2000 respectively, human anesthetic breathing circuits (i.e. circle system) and machines sold in North America must meet minimum design and safety standards established by organizations such as the American Society for Testing and Materials (ASTM) and the Canadian Standards Association (CSA). The standards were updated in 2005 (ASTM F1850; Standard Specification for Particular Requirements for Anesthesia Workstations and Their Components). Anesthetic machines designed for veterinary use are not required to meet any specific design or safety standards beyond those associated with basic hazards to the operator

(i.e. electrical safety requirements). Safety features are often added on an *ad hoc* basis and there are no requirements for demonstrating equipment efficacy. Ideally, some safety features, such as airway pressure alarms and pressure release valves, should be integral into the design of the anesthetic machine. The inclusion of some of these safety systems on anesthetic machines may help eliminate preventable anesthetic accidents. However, until safety and design standards are adopted by the manufacturers of veterinary anesthetic equipment, there will remain numerous equipment options of varying quality, efficacy and safety available for delivering inhalant anesthetics to veterinary patients. Ancillary and support equipment for veterinary patients, including patient monitors and ventilators, are similarly devoid of required efficacy and safety testing. Fortunately, most reputable manufacturers and distributers readily provide the specifications, accuracy and any testing for efficacy of their designs. Regardless of the presence of standards, it will always be incumbent upon the veterinary anesthetist to understand thoroughly the function, principles of operation, use and routine maintenance of all anesthetic-related pieces of equipment and to ensure that the machine or piece of equipment is designed suitably well to accomplish its function safely.

3.3 The Basic Veterinary Anesthetic Machine

Inhalant anesthesia forms the basis of modern anesthetic protocols in veterinary medicine. The administration of potent inhaled anesthetics requires specific delivery techniques. The anesthetic machine enables the delivery of a precise yet variable combination of inhalant anesthetic and carrier gas or gases (i.e. oxygen, medical grade air, nitrous oxide). The basic components and functions

Veterinary Anesthetic and Monitoring Equipment, First Edition. Edited by Kristen G. Cooley and Rebecca A. Johnson.
© 2018 John Wiley & Sons, Inc. Published 2018 by John Wiley & Sons, Inc.

of all anesthetic machines are similar, but significant design differences exist among them.

Machines can be very simple, such as those used for mobile applications, to very complex anesthetic workstations with built-in ventilators, monitors and safety systems (Figure 3.1). Regardless of the design complexity, all anesthetic machines share common components: an oxygen source, oxygen regulator (which may be part of the gas supply system), oxygen flowmeter, and an inhalant vaporizer. If additional gases are used (i.e. nitrous oxide or medical grade air), there will also be a separate gas source, regulator and flowmeter for each gas that generally parallels the path of oxygen with some exceptions (i.e. oxygen flush valve). The basic anesthetic machine is used in conjunction with a breathing circuit and anesthetic waste gas scavenging system to safely deliver inhalant anesthetics and support breathing.

3.3.1 High-, Intermediate- and Low-Pressure Systems

Perhaps the simplest way to describe an anesthetic machine is to describe the components in order of the flow of gas through the machine, from source to patient. However, prior to describing these components, it is important to recognize that the gas pressure varies at different locations in an anesthesia machine, such that there are high, intermediate and low-pressure areas. With pressures of up to 2200 psi, the high-pressure area accepts gases directly from a source and subsequently reduces and regulates these pressures. This area includes gas cylinders, hanger yokes, yoke blocks, high-pressure hoses, pressure gauges, and regulators.

The intermediate-pressure area accepts gases from the central pipeline or from the regulators on the anesthesia machine and conducts them to the flush valve and flowmeters. This area includes pipeline inlets, outlets for ventilators, conduits from pipeline inlets to flowmeters, conduits from regulators to flowmeters, the flowmeter assembly, and the oxygen flush apparatus. The pressure usually ranges from 40–55 psi. The low-pressure area consists of the conduits and components between the flowmeter and the common gas outlet. This area includes vaporizers, piping from the flowmeters to the vaporizer, conduit from the vaporizer to the common gas outlet, and the breathing system. The pressure in the low-pressure area

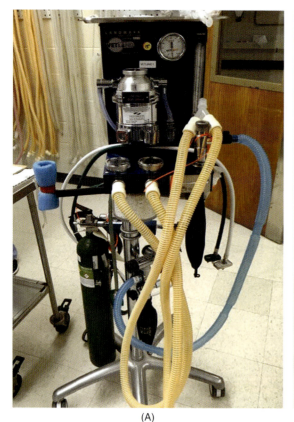 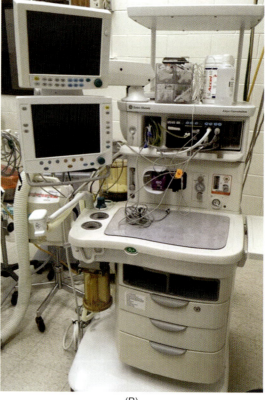

(A) (B)

Figure 3.1 Anesthetic machines for veterinary use can vary considerably in their complexity and sophistication. (A) Example of a portable anesthetic system and (B) a complete human anesthetic workstation available for use in veterinary medicine. Both systems provide all the components necessary for the controlled delivery of inhalant anesthetics.

is close to ambient pressure, but can vary depending upon how the system is being used (i.e. positive pressure ventilation vs. spontaneous ventilation), but should generally never exceed 30 cmH$_2$O (1 cmH$_2$O = ~0.014 psi), as these pressures are transmitted directly to the patient's lungs.

3.3.2 Gas Supply and Flow

Occasionally in veterinary medicine, multiple medical gases (i.e. oxygen, air and nitrous oxide) are used with the anesthetic machine. However, 100% oxygen is commonly used to deliver anesthesia and power anesthetic equipment (i.e. ventilators) in veterinary medicine. Indications for and contraindications to delivering multiple carrier gases must be well-known by the anesthetists and the anesthetic equipment must be properly designed and monitored to prevent the possibility of delivering a hypoxic gas mixture to the patient. All human machines have a proportioning system associated with the oxygen flow and oxygen concentration monitors to ensure a hypoxic gas mixture cannot be delivered. This is not generally the case with veterinary anesthesia machines. It is recommended when using multiple carrier gases, a gas analyzer or minimally an oxygen concentration monitor in the patient circuit is employed.

Gas flow within an anesthetic machine may take multiple routes once it enters the intermediate-pressure area. Minimally, gas must be delivered to the flowmeter, where it is then directed to the vaporizer and subsequently to the patient. However, in addition to this route of movement, there may be several more routes available for gas distribution in the anesthesia machine. Normally, on most anesthesia machines, intermediate-pressure gas is also diverted to a fresh gas flush valve that bypasses the flowmeter and vaporizer and delivers fresh gas directly to the breathing circuit. There are circumstances where flush valves may not be present or unavailable on veterinary anesthesia machines. Additionally, gas from the intermediate-pressure area may be diverted to one or more auxiliary oxygen outlets that may be used as the driving gas for a built-in or external ventilator or an external oxygen flowmeter.

3.3.3 Medical Gas Supply

Anesthetic machines ideally have two gas supplies, one from small, high-pressure tanks attached directly to the machine and a second source often originating from a hospital's central pipeline supply (see Chapter 1 for more details). The small tanks mounted directly onto the anesthesia machine are intended to be used as back up or a reserve gas source, should the pipeline malfunction or while working in an area without access to the pipeline. The most commonly used medical gas during veterinary anesthesia is 100% oxygen. Nitrous oxide, in conjunction with oxygen, as an adjunct carrier gas for the inhalants, is used less frequently due to low potency of nitrous oxide in veterinary medicine and the high abuse potential. Most medical gases are normally stored under high pressure in cylinders of various sizes or in low-pressure insulated cryogenic liquid bulk tanks. The characteristics (i.e. working pressure) and capacity of the gas cylinders varies with the type of gas they contain (see Chapter 1).

Alternatively, oxygen concentrators (see Chapter 2) can be used to supply a hospital with its oxygen requirements in circumstances where obtaining and storage of tanks is inconvenient, impossible or prohibitively expensive (i.e. remote communities). Most oxygen concentrators use a system of absorbing nitrogen from air to produce gas, resulting in an oxygen concentration of between 90 and 96%. Recently, small, integrated single machine oxygen concentrating units have been made available in the veterinary market (e.g. Pureline^{TM,} Supera Anesthesia Innovations, Clackamas, OR).

Most modern veterinary facilities will have some form of central gas supply and pipeline distribution system delivering medical gases to various work sites. The complexity of these systems can vary significantly; from a small bank of large (G or H) cylinders and a regulator, to more complex systems consisting of multiple large liquid oxygen tanks (Figure 3.2A), automatic manifolds, regulators, alarms and banks of large high-pressure cylinders for back up (Figure 3.2B). The size and complexity of the gas distribution system will depend upon the gas needs, the area of required gas distribution and the number of work sites required. Proper installation of large gas distribution systems is essential for safety and efficacy. All gas installations should be installed and properly evaluated prior to use by those with expertise in this area.

3.3.3.1 Medical Gas Safety

There are several international (ASTM), national and local documents related to the safe use, transport and storage of pressurized gases (see Chapters 1 and 9 for more details). There are also standards surrounding the installation of medical gas piping systems and some of these provisions have been incorporated into hospital accreditation requirements in veterinary medicine. However, the specific guidelines can vary significantly among jurisdictions and regions. There have been several well-documented medical accidents related to the inappropriate use of medical gases in humans, but the incidence of such accidents seems to be decreasing (Caplan *et al.* 1997; Mehta *et al.* 2013). The reduction of such accidents is likely in large part due to better monitoring, maintenance of gas delivery systems and the development of safety systems to help reduce and eliminate these problems. For example, all anesthetic equipment

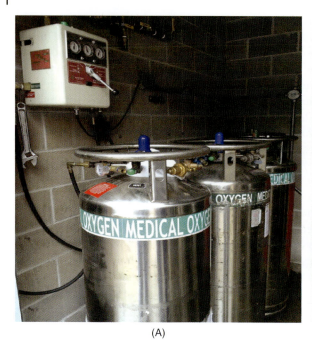
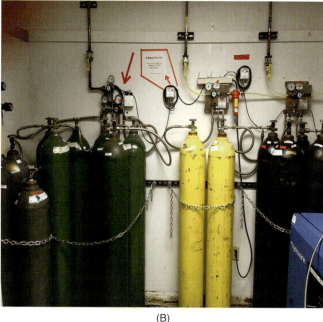

(A) (B)

Figure 3.2 Bulk oxygen requirements for larger hospitals are frequently met using large liquid oxygen tanks (A) or banks of compressed gas tanks (B). Both of these systems are normally designed with a backup supply, should the main supply fail or become depleted.

has a gas-specific non-interchangeable connector that is part of the base unit (anesthetic machine, ventilator). These connectors include the diameter index safety system, pin index safety system and quick connector. Color coding and labels describing content characteristics have also helped avoid mistakes (Table 3.1).

Color Coding Gas cylinders and gas lines are commonly colored coded to avoid improper use, but color-coding systems can vary among countries. For example, oxygen is colored white in Canada and green in the United States. In addition to color coding, all tanks have a labeling scheme consisting of various shaped labels, key words and colors that are all used to identify hazards associated with the gas they contain. Most tanks

Table 3.1 Color coding and labels describing content characteristics.

Common Medical Gas	Pin Index System	US color	International color
Oxygen (O_2)	2, 5	Green	White
Nitrous Oxide (N_2O)	3, 5	Blue	Blue
Medical Grade Air	1, 5	Yellow	White/black
Nitrogen (N_2)	1, 4	Black	Black
Carbon Dioxide (CO_2)	1, 6	Gray	Gray

originating from gas supply facilities normally have perforated tags (full, in use, empty) to track the cylinder's use status.

Cylinder Labels It is important to note that labeling requirements not only vary among countries but even within countries and can be regulated by multiple agencies and organizations. Labels typically give vital information regarding the cylinder's contents, chemical properties and danger potential.

Diameter Index Safety System The diameter index safety system (DISS) is a non-interchangeable gas-specific threaded connection system with unique colors (Figure 3.3). DISS is the gas connection used almost universally by all equipment and cylinder manufactures for the connection of medical gases.

Pin Index Safety System The pin index safety system (PISS) uses gas specific pin patterns that only allow connections between the appropriate cylinder yokes and small gas cylinders (E size). The PISS is commonly found on the yokes mounted on anesthesia machines and some cylinder specific regulator/flowmeters (Figure 3.4).

Quick Connectors There are many proprietary (manufacturer specific) quick connect systems that have been developed. These are standardized within a manufacturer but are not generally compatible with the quick connect

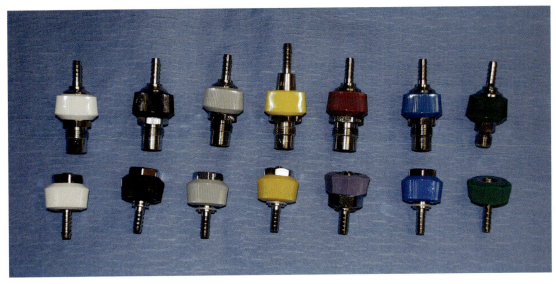

Figure 3.3 The diameter index safety system (DISS) uses a gas-specific non-interchangeable thread pattern to avoid incorrect gas delivery. Gases are also color coded as apparent in the figure (photograph courtesy of Thomas Riebold, College of Veterinary Medicine, Oregon State University).

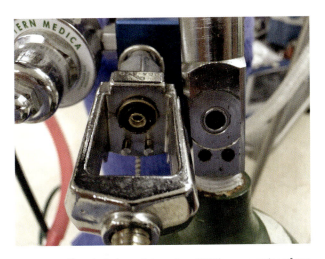

Figure 3.4 The pin index safety system (PISS) uses a series of gas specific pin positions on the yolk that correspond to similarly positioned pin receiver ports on the tank.

systems of another manufacturer (Figure 3.5). These systems facilitate rapid connecting and disconnecting of gas hoses and may be useful in situations where frequent connects and disconnects are required (i.e. multipurpose work areas).

3.3.4 Pressure Reducing Valve

The pressure reducing valve (or regulator) is a key component required to bring the high pressures of gas cylinders down to a more reasonable and safe working pressure (i.e. 45–50 psi). Regulators also reduce or prevent fluctuations in pressure as the tank empties. Regulators are normally found wherever a high-pressure

gas cylinder is in use (i.e. gas pipelines, cylinder connected directly to machine) (Figure 3.6). The regulators used for gas supply sources (i.e. pipelines or large oxygen cylinders) are normally adjustable, whereas those on most anesthetic machines are set by the manufacturer. The ASTM standard requires that regulators on anesthetic machines be set to preferentially use pipeline gases before using gas from the backup cylinder on the anesthesia machine. However, since neither pipeline systems nor veterinary anesthesia machines are required to meet ASTM standards, it is not uncommon for machines to draw from the reserve or backup tank preferentially rather than the pipeline. This problem can be avoided by ensuring that the pipeline pressure is set approximately 5 psi higher than the anesthetic machine's regulator for the reserve oxygen cylinder. Additionally, check valves can be installed to prevent pipeline gas from entering gas cylinders.

3.3.5 Pressure Gauges/Manometers

Pressure gauges are commonly used to measure cylinder pressures, pipeline pressures, anesthetic machine working pressures, and pressures within the breathing system. The most common type is the Bourdon tube gauge, which uses the principle that a flattened tube tends to straighten out or uncoil when pressurized, thus moving a pointer to the correct pressure. Cylinder, pipeline and anesthetic machine working pressures are normally expressed in pounds per square inch (psi) or kiloPascals (kPa), whereas the pressures within the breathing system of the anesthetic machine are normally expressed in centimeters of water (cmH_2O) (Figures 3.7 A and B). The gauge measuring the

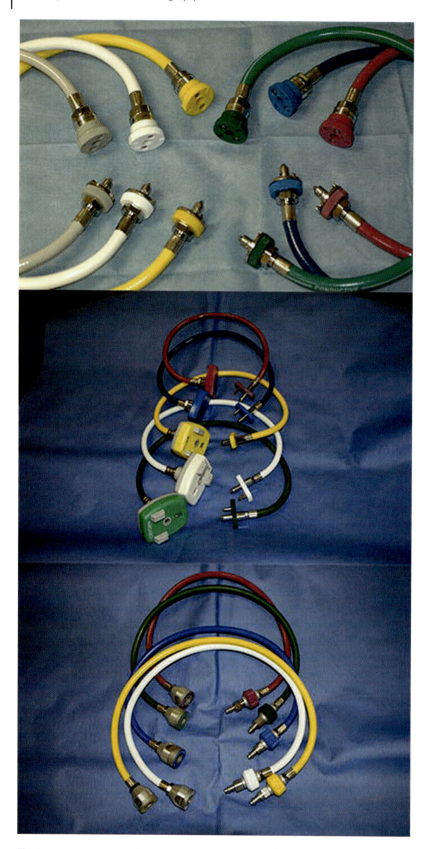

Figure 3.5 Proprietary quick connect gas couplings are available to ease frequent connecting and disconnecting of gas lines. These systems, such as the Ohmeda®-style system (multiple suppliers, e.g. Precision Medical, Northampton, PA), are manufacturer specific and are incompatible among various manufacturers (photograph courtesy of Thomas Riebold, College of Veterinary Medicine, Oregon State University).

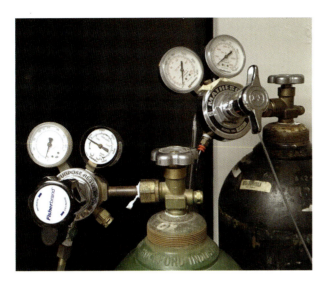

Figure 3.6 Pressure reducing valves/regulators are used to decrease the pressure of the gas in a compressed gas cylinder down to a lower pressure, sometimes referred to as the working pressure, normally 45–55 PSI. These valves maintain a constant pressure delivery from the gas supply and help prevent fluctuations associated with gas depletion and use.

pressure of the breathing system is often referred to as a pressure manometer. The information provided by these gauges is vital for safe operation of anesthesia equipment and clinical use in patients. Frequently, the patient manometer has positive and negative values on either side of zero. The positive values are beneficial for quantifying the pressure generated when manually or mechanically ventilating patients. The needle on a manometer

may move minimally into the negative value range when a patient takes a spontaneous breath, but this value should be very small, less than 2–3 cmH$_2$O; larger values suggest excessive resistance within the anesthetic machine and the cause should be investigated. However, it is important to recognize that negative deflections are influenced by the size of the patient's breath, rate of inspiration and the mechanics of the anesthetic machine (i.e. resistance to inspiration associated with the breathing circuit). Unless gas within the breathing circuit is restricted (i.e. by occluding the reservoir bag), only very small negative fluctuations should be seen.

3.3.5.1 Manometer Malfunction
Attention should be paid to the orientation of the needle on a patient manometer before the machine is in use and prior to any pre-use pressure checking. The needle should rest at zero and avoid touching the surface face of the manometer. If the needle is not resting at zero, the face can usually be removed from the manometer and a small screw can be turned to adjust the resting orientation of the needle. Once the needle is zeroed, the face of the manometer should be replaced before the machine is used. If the needle moves while the face plate is being reapplied, the entire manometer should be replaced as the needle is likely bent and will make contact with the face plate during use, thus causing inaccuracies when assessing the pressure generated within the breathing circuit. Frequently cracks will occur in plastic face plates of the manometer when alcohol is used to clean the unit; alcohol as a disinfectant should be avoided on all plastic surfaces of anesthesia equipment.

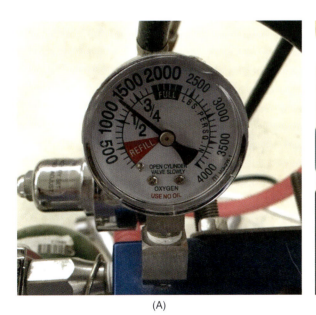

(A)

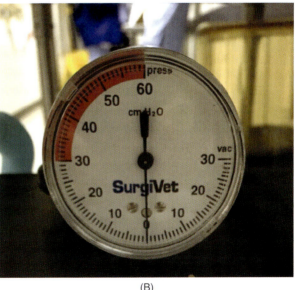

(B)

Figure 3.7 Pressure gauges are used to measure pressure in gas cylinders, anesthetic machines and breathing systems (A). Pressure gauges can be associated with a compressed gas tank, measured in pounds per square inch (PSI). Pressure gauges are found commonly on most anesthetic breathing circuits. (B) Note that the pressure in the breathing circuit is measured in cmH$_2$O.

3.3.6 Flowmeters

Flowmeters control the rate of gas delivery to the low-pressure area of the anesthetic machine and determine the fresh gas flow (FGF) to the anesthetic circuit. There must be a separate flowmeter for each gas type used with the anesthetic machine (Figure 3.8).

The breathing system type and volume, and the patient size, are all factors that influence selection of the rate of FGF. Several flowmeter designs are available, but most are based on a tapered gas tube with a moveable float (Thorpe tube). The gas normally flows in the bottom of the tube and out the top. The tube is narrower at the bottom and wider at the top, so as the float moves up the tube, more gas can flow around the float producing higher flow rates (Figure 3.9). Flowmeters can consist of either single or double tubes to improve accuracy.

A flow-control knob that adjusts a needle valve controls the amount of gas entering the tube. A float indicates the gas flow on a calibrated scale. On some flowmeters, the location on the float where the gas flow should be read is indicated (i.e. top, middle, etc.). Gas flow rates are expressed in mL/min or L/min. The spatial distance between vertical markings on the flowmeter does not necessarily correspond to equal changes in flow rate. For example, the distance between 0 and 1000 mL, as measured vertically on the flowmeter, may not be the same as the vertical distance between 1000 and 2000 mL. This is similar to the spatial separation of the percentages found on many vaporizers, where there is a greater spatial allocation on the dial for normal working percentages than for those rarely used. Some anesthetic machines may also have two flowmeters for the same gas placed in series, allowing even greater precision at lower gas flow rates (Figure 3.9).

Flowmeters are gas specific and calibrated at 760 mmHg and 20 °C. Accuracy may be affected if used under conditions significantly different from calibration, although this is rarely significant for routine clinical use. Flowmeters are also calibrated as a unit (flow tube, scale and float) and therefore, if any one of these fail, it is best to replace the whole unit. On the other hand, gasket, flow-control dial or knob and/or washer replacement or repair are unlikely to affect accuracy, but should only be performed by individuals familiar with flowmeter design and operation. The flow-control knob on contemporary human anesthesia machines must conform to ASTM standards. For example, the oxygen flow-control knob must be uniquely shaped and it must be on the right-most side of the flowmeter bank downstream of all other gases. These design considerations are important to minimize the accidental delivery of hypoxic gas mixtures.

3.3.6.1 Flowmeter Malfunction

The anesthetist should check flowmeter integrity at the time of initial positive pressure leak checking of the anesthesia equipment. By using the flowmeter to pressurize the closed system during the positive pressure leak test, the anesthetist can check the float for proper rotation. This indicates proper gas flow, smooth float acceleration and decline when the needle valve control knob is adjusted, and absence of any drift while in use. These issues can indicate fluctuating gas flow from an inconsistently regulated gas source, a defect in the O-ring seals on the needle valve cartridge, or debris in the flowmeter assembly. While a rare occurrence, construction on house gas piping and incorrect installation of needle valves can contribute to these issues. Additionally, care should be taken to avoid over-tightening the needle valve control knob when discontinuing use of the gas.

3.3.7 Vaporizers

Vaporizers change liquid anesthetic into vapor and meter the amount of vapor leaving the vaporizer. Most modern vaporizers are agent specific, concentration-calibrated, variable-bypass, flow-over the wick, out of the circuit vaporizers, and high resistance (or plenum) that are compensated for by temperature, flow and back pressure. Non-precision, low-resistance, in the circuit vaporizers continue to be found in veterinary medicine due to their lower cost, but without proper inspired inhalant gas monitoring, these vaporizers would seem to pose unnecessary risks during anesthesia, therefore their use should be discouraged unless used in conjunction with anesthetic agent monitors. Vaporizers are discussed in more detail in Chapter 5.

3.3.8 Oxygen Flush Valve

Oxygen flush valves are found on most, but not all, veterinary anesthetic machines; although their use clinically is rarely required, their misuse can result in significant patient harm. There is no convention regarding location, size or design of the flush valve in veterinary medicine and they vary dramatically (e.g. button, toggle or switch) (Figures 3.10 A and B).

Flush valves on human anesthetic machines must be a recessed button and easily accessible on the front of the machine, but these regulations are not routinely applied nor enforced for veterinary medicine. Flush valves are designed to rapidly deliver large volumes of non-anesthetic containing gas to the patient breathing circuit in emergencies. The flow originates downstream of the regulator within the intermediate-pressure area of the anesthetic machine (~50 psi) and bypasses the flowmeter and vaporizer, delivering gas at rates ranging between 35 and 75 L/min to the patient circuit. To avoid over-pressuring the patient circuit, the flush valve should be used very cautiously with non-rebreathing circuits, circuits attached to

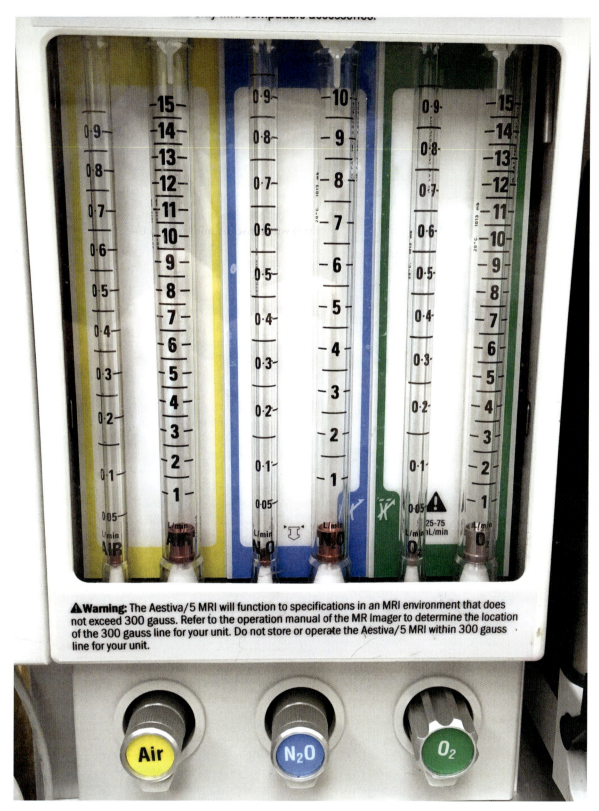

Figure 3.8 An example of multiple flowmeters arranged in series on a single anesthetic machine. Medical grade air (yellow) is on the left, nitrous oxide (blue) is in the center and oxygen (green) is on the right. Flowmeters on human anesthesia machines must conform to specific positioning (i.e. oxygen right-most flowmeter) and control-knob dimension (i.e. oxygen is furled and protrudes further). This is not always the case for flowmeters on anesthetic machines designed solely for veterinary use. These flowmeters are dual-stage flowmeters, allowing for increased precision of gas delivery.

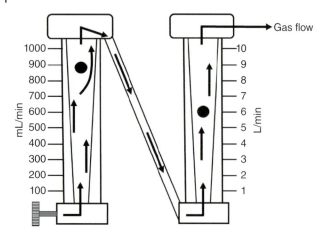

Figure 3.9 Diagram of flowmeter illustrating gas flow from bottom to top through a double tapered Thorpe tube. As the flow indicator (bobbin, ball or spindle) rises, flow increases because the orifice size increases. The double taper allows increased accuracy at the lower end of the tube while accurately metering higher flows from the top.

mechanical ventilators, and circuits with very low volumes (i.e. pediatric circle systems), as pressures within the breathing circuit may temporarily rise, creating dangerously high airway pressures. The adjustable pressure limiting (APL) valve should be fully open at all times to help prevent over-pressurizing the breathing circuit.

3.3.9 Common Gas Outlet

The common gas outlet leads from the anesthetic machine to the breathing circuit (Figures 3.11 A, B and C). Gas reaching the common gas outlet has traveled from the gas supply (cylinder or pipeline), through the regulator, flow-meter and vaporizer. The gas flowing from the common gas outlet delivers the anesthetic and carrier gas(s) to the patient circuit at the concentration and flow rate determined by the vaporizer setting and flowmeter flow rate. However, the concentration of inhalant gas from the common gas outlet is not usually equivalent to the gas concentration inhaled by the patient when using rebreathing circuits, particularly when using low flow rates, due to dilution of incoming gases with those already in the patient circuit. The exact configuration of the common gas outlet varies among manufacturers, but it is normally a taper 15 mm I.D. port. Human anesthesia machines must have a locking mechanism in place to prevent inadvertent disconnection from the machine (Figure 3.11 C); however, this is not a requirement in veterinary medicine. At least one company designs their fresh gas outlet with a quick connect system to prevent inadvertent disconnections.

3.3.9.1 Common Gas Outlet Malfunction

Leaks can occur at the common gas outlet where the anesthetist may repeatedly connect and disconnect patient breathing circuits (i.e. circle or non-rebreathing systems). Additionally, if the patient circuit becomes disconnected from the common gas outlet during an anesthetic procedure, the patient will not receive fresh gas (i.e. oxygen and inhalant). If left unnoticed, the patient may experience hypoxemia or lightening plane of anesthesia, leading to awareness. This may be identified by loss of volume in the patient reservoir bag or the unanticipated smell of anesthetic gas. Simple reconnection of the fresh gas connection resolves these concerns. Occasionally, leaks in the tubing connecting the fresh gas to the breathing circuit will occur, especially if alcohol is used to clean the tubing. Routine positive pressure

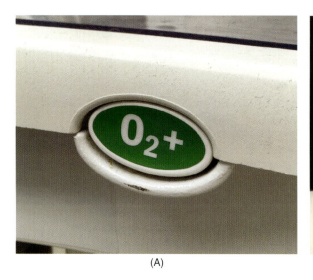

(A)

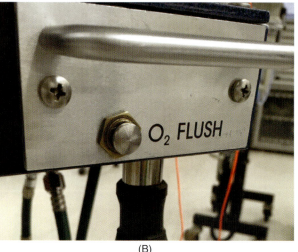

(B)

Figure 3.10 Examples of various flush valve buttons on anesthetic machines. On some machines, the oxygen flush button is recessed in a protective collar to prevent inadvertent activation if bumped (A).

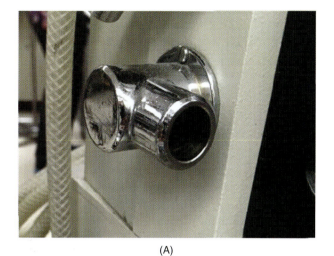

(A)

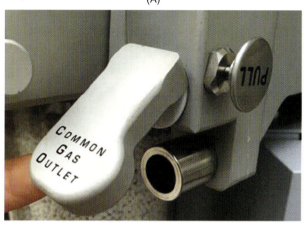

(B)

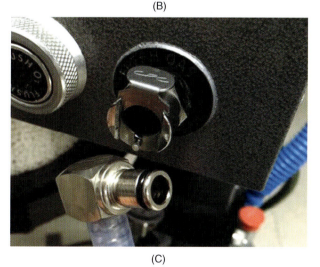

(C)

Figure 3.11 Common gas outlets deliver gas from the anesthetic machine to the patient breathing circuit. Push type taper connections are common in veterinary medicine and may be covered for additional safety (A, B). A quick connect/disconnect system can also prevent inadvertent disconnection of the gas supply between the patient circuit and anesthesia machine. Locking common gas outlets are standard on human anesthesia machines (C).

checking of the anesthesia equipment will help identify these leaks and provide an opportunity for any defect to be repaired or replaced.

3.4 Breathing Systems

The breathing system provides a conduit connecting the anesthetic machine to the patient. There are two principle categories of breathing systems described; non-rebreathing (Mapleson systems) and rebreathing (circle) systems. These systems are described in more detail in Chapters 9 to 11.

3.5 Waste Gas Scavenge Systems

The scavenge system directs waste gases from the anesthetic breathing circuit out of the immediate workspace and into the atmosphere. Scavenging systems are broadly classified as either active or passive and use a variety of methods with varying success for achieving efficient waste gas removal. The systems used and their components are probably one of the most misunderstood and under-appreciated elements used in association with the anesthetic machine. These systems are described in Chapter 8.

3.6 Routine Anesthesia Machine Checkout Procedures

Routine evaluation of the anesthetic machine and associated systems prior to, and throughout the anesthetic period, should be part of every anesthetist's standard operating procedure (SOP) and are detailed in Chapter 27. Historically, equipment failures appear to have been a relatively common cause of anesthetic related morbidity and mortality (Dorsch and Dorsch 2008). However, with improvements in technology, monitoring and the adoption of universal safety standards for human anesthetic equipment, complications related to equipment malfunctions have been reduced. Pre-anesthetic equipment checkout recommendations for human anesthetic equipment have been developed in conjunction with regulatory, industry and anesthesia personnel, and published in many countries. Unfortunately, there is no generally recognized standard for pre-anesthetic checkout recommendations in veterinary medicine. However, there are excellent checklists proposed for veterinary anesthetists, based on the Food and Drug Administration's Center for Devices and Radiological Health (see Chapter 27) (Hartsfield 2007, 2008).

3.6.1 Leak Testing

The two most commonly performed leak tests are the Positive Pressure Leak Test and the Negative Pressure

Leak Test. Briefly, the Positive Pressure Leak Test is completed prior to any anesthetic event and after any components of the machine or breathing circuit is changed or manipulated. To perform this test, the anesthetists should first assemble the machine with the appropriate breathing circuit and patient reservoir bag. The APL valve is closed and the patient end of the breathing circuit is completely occluded (i.e. using thumb, palm or rubber stopper). Using the oxygen flowmeter (or oxygen flush valve), fresh gas should enter the circuit until a pressure of approximately 30 cmH$_2$O is obtained. Once this pressure is reached on the manometer, the oxygen flow is turned off. If no leaks are present, the manometer needle should remain steady at the inflated pressure for 10 seconds. If the needle increases, oxygen is still entering the patient circuit. If the needle decreases, there is a leak present under positive pressure. The degree of a leak can be determined before releasing pressure from the circuit by increasing the oxygen flow rate until the manometer needle no longer decreases. According to ASTM standards in human medicine, a leak of 0.35 L/min at 30 cmH$_2$O is acceptable (Dorsch and Dorsch 2008). Common locations for leaks are at connections of the breathing circuit, in the patient reservoir bag, around the carbon dioxide absorbent canister, or an old conduit tubing (i.e. from the oxygen flowmeter to vaporizer or fresh gas outlet tubing). It is important that pressure from the positive leak test be released by opening the APL valve. This will test the integrity of the APL valve, as well as minimize the risk of inadvertent patient barotrauma resulting from a closed APL valve. Additional positive pressure leak tests for non-rebreathing circuits are described in Chapter 27.

The Negative Leak Test should be performed by the service technician during routine preventative maintenance and servicing. Also referred to as the Universal Leak Test, it is accomplished by fitting a suction bulb to a 15-mm I.D. connector (i.e. endotracheal tube adapter) on the common gas outlet or by attaching the bulb

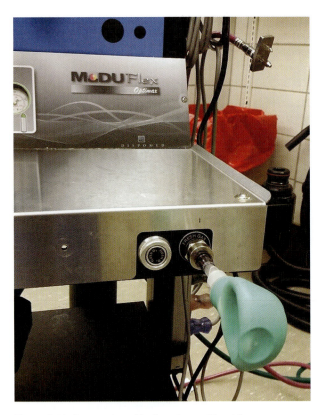

Figure 3.12 A compressed bulb syringe with a 15-mm endotracheal tube connector is placed at the common gas outlet during performance of the negative pressure leak test. The bulb syringe should remain deflated if no leak is present.

syringe directly to the fresh gas outlet tubing depending on the manufacturer's configuration of the machine. With the flowmeter in an "off" position, the anesthetist connects a depressed bulb syringe with the 15-mm endotracheal tube connector to the common gas outlet (Figure 3.12). When released, the bulb should remain depressed. If the bulb fills, there is a low-pressure leak. This test specifically helps identify and differentiate small leaks within the machine itself, by excluding aspects of the breathing circuit and reservoir bag.

References

Caplan, R., Vistica, M. and Posner, K. (1997) Adverse anesthetic outcomes arising from gas delivery equipment: a closed claims analysis. *Anesthesiology*, 87, 741–748.

Dorsch, J.A. and Dorsch, S.E. (2008) The anesthesia machine. In: *Understanding Anaesthesia Equipment*, 5th ed. Philadelphia, PA: Lippincott Williams & Wilkins, pp. 83–120.

Hartsfield, S.M. (2007) Anesthetic machines and breathing systems. In: Tranquilli, W.J., Thurmon, J.C. and Grimm,

K.A. (eds). *Lumb and Jones' Veterinary Anesthesia and Analgesia*, 4th ed. Ames, IA: Blackwell Publishing, pp. 453–494.

Hartsfield, S.M. (2008) Anesthesia Equipment. In: Carroll, G.L. (ed.). *Small Animal Anesthesia and Analgesia*. Ames, IA: Blackwell Publishing, pp. 3–24.

Mehta, S., Eisenkraft, J. and Posner, K. (2013) Patient injuries from anesthesia gas delivery equipment: a close claims update. *Anesthesiology*, 119, 788–795.

4

Large Animal Anesthesia Machines and Equipment

Amanda Shelby

Jurox Animal Health, Kansas City, Missouri, USA

4.1 History of the Large Animal Anesthesia Machine

The large animal anesthesia machinery has developed exponentially over the past half century. While similar to small animal and even human counterparts, routine use of ventilators has lagged behind. As early as 1854, George Dodd described an inhalation technique with a combination of chloric ether and chloroform in the horse, with improved safety for the patient and surgeon during minor procedures (Dodd 1854). In 1875, a description of intravenous chloral hydrate was administered to equine species as adjunctive to local and inhalation techniques (Wright 1958). Although these techniques were described, the large animal veterinary community hesitated to routinely implement their use, due to unpredictable side effects that included death. Further improvements were made with the introduction of halogenated agents and precision vaporizers.

In 1957, anesthesia equipment used for inhalation techniques specific to horses and cattle were described (Fisher 1957; Weaver 1960). With the invention of the Bird Mark 7 respirator in 1955, manufacturers realized adequate large animal ventilation was possible. Early large animal ventilators utilized a Bird Mark respirator with a "bag-in-a-barrel" bellows assembly. Beginning in the late 1970s and early 1980s, several companies emerged with a large animal anesthesia machine and ventilator control centers, which provides spontaneous or controlled ventilation.

Today, several options for large animal anesthesia control centers are commercially available to facilitate the delivery of inhalation anesthesia with spontaneous, patient initiated/assisted or controlled ventilation. Horses have a mortality rate of 1% (Johnston *et al.* 2002) during anesthesia, compared to small animal rates of 0.05% (canine) to 0.11% (feline) (Brodbelt *et al.* 2008). Therefore, the American College of Veterinary Anesthesia and Analgesia's

(ACVAA) established guidelines for anesthesia in the horse and a thorough understanding and correct implementation of machines, ventilators and accessory tools that are needed to optimally perform anesthetic episodes with minimal complications (Martinez *et al.* 1995).

4.2 Purpose

The purpose of an anesthesia machine is to facilitate the delivery of fresh gases to a patient. These gases at minimum include oxygen but can also include medical grade air, ambient air, nitrous oxide and inhalant anesthetics. The goal of implementing the use of an anesthetic machine and breathing circuit is to provide a controlled, reversible anesthetic episode, during which adequate oxygenation and ventilation is maintained.

4.3 Standards

In human medicine, strict standards exist for equipment relating to the delivery of inhalation anesthetics and ventilation (ASTM 2005). Unfortunately, in veterinary medicine these standards are not enforced or regulated. It is left to the individual manufacturer to adhere to any safety standards. Many manufactures will advertise their compliance with various agencies, such as the American Society for Testing and Material (ASTM 2005).

4.4 Similarity to Small Animal Machines

Anesthesia machines, independent of their intention for veterinary or human use, while varying in appearance, rarely differ significantly in their design or components.

Veterinary Anesthetic and Monitoring Equipment, First Edition. Edited by Kristen G. Cooley and Rebecca A. Johnson.
© 2018 John Wiley & Sons, Inc. Published 2018 by John Wiley & Sons, Inc.

With a thorough working knowledge of any anesthesia machine and its components, those designed for large animal use should not be intimidating. Simply they differ in size and commonly are accompanied by a ventilator. Description of the small animal anesthesia machine can be found in Chapter 3. In the following section, attention will be paid to specific differences that large animal anesthetic systems utilize as well as equipment beneficial for large animal anesthesia.

4.5 Components of the Anesthesia Machine

When learning the components of an anesthesia machine, two methods of approach are traditionally applied; flow of oxygen through the system or grouping of the components via pressure systems (i.e. high, intermediate, low pressure). Variations exist in the positioning of components, for example reservoir bag location compared to inspiratory and expiratory valves and carbon dioxide absorbent canister, between manufacturers.

Generally, the common pattern of gas flow through a circle system is from oxygen source, flowmeter, through the vaporizer, fresh gas inlet, inspiratory one-way valve, inspiratory breathing hoses, patient, expiratory breathing hoses, expiratory one-way valve, adjustable pressure-limiting (APL or pop-off) valve, reservoir bag, and carbon dioxide absorbent canister. In the circle system, depending on the manufacturer's configuration and selected fresh gas flow rate, excessive gas within the circuit is recycled or exits through the APL valve and is scavenged via an active or passive scavenger system.

4.5.1 High-Pressure System

The high-pressure system contains the gas source(s), yoke blocks if present, pressure hoses, regulators and the pressure gauge. Pressure within this area of the system can be as high as 2200 psi, the pressure of a full H or E cylinder.

4.5.1.1 Gas Source

The most common gas source for a large animal anesthesia machine is a house oxygen supply system, or "G" or "H" cylinders. Oxygen concentrators are commercially available but their practicality and functional ability for use in large animal anesthesia is limited. While most oxygen concentrators produce between 90 and 96% oxygen, their maximum oxygen flow rate is around 6 liters per minute (LPM) (Mosley 2015). This flow rate is sufficient for maintenance in adult large animals but insufficient for induction or insufflations during recovery (Mason *et al.* 1987). Regulations surrounding medical

gas safety on national and local levels are well established (ASTM 2005). Standards exist for installation of piping systems and frequently incorporated into hospital accreditation requirements.

Yoke Blocks or Hanger Yokes Most large animal machines do not have yoke hangers; however, if present and not in use, they should be blocked with a yoke plug. Oxygen cylinders have the pin index safety system (PISS), which discourages but does not completely prevent connection of the incorrect cylinder to the yoke block (Dorsch and Dorsch 2008a).

High-Pressure Hoses High-pressure hoses use the diameter index safety system (DISS). These connections are gas specific with non-interchangeable threaded connections. Veterinary manufacturers adhere to their use.

Pressure Gauges Pressure gauges within the high-pressure system are used to measure gas cylinder contents, pipeline pressures or anesthetic machine working pressures. These pressures are routinely expressed as pounds per square inch (psi) or kilopascals (kPa). A full oxygen tank (H or E) is roughly 2200 psi. Equations are available to estimate the volume remaining within these tanks. It is important to realize that these gauges only accurately report for cylinders with gas contents and not for those with liquid gases (i.e. nitrous oxide).

If a machine is equipped with a yoke block and house pipeline source, the house line should be set slightly higher than the regulator for the cylinder to preferentially select the gas source of higher pressure. This is to avoid depleting the oxygen cylinder intended for emergency use or transportation. Additionally, machines equipped with house gas source and cylinders frequently have check valves installed to prevent back flow or accidental depletion of the oxygen cylinder. The anesthesia machine working pressure is found on several large animal machines to ensure adequate pressure is entering the machine to drive the ventilator sufficiently (Figure 4.1).

Regulators Regulators are gas specific and are color coded and/or labeled for their respective gases. It is recommended to use medical grade regulators, although frequently in large animal anesthesia industrial regulators are utilized (Figure 4.2). The purpose of the regulator is to decrease the high pressure of gas cylinders to a safe working pressure for equipment (40–55 psi). Additionally, they function to prevent fluctuation in pressure as the tank empties. Adjustable and fixed regulators are available.

In the context of large animal anesthesia, adjustable regulators are desirable as higher outputs are sometimes necessary to adequately generate inspiratory flows high enough to operate some models of ventilators and for

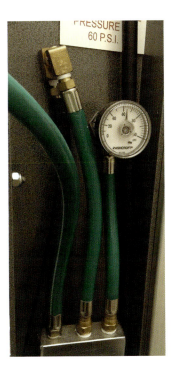

Figure 4.1 Pressure gauge shows operating pressure of gas source supplying the anesthesia machine and ventilator. Also note, one oxygen source is split to supply the flowmeter, drive gas for the ventilator and oxygen flush valve.

optimal use of demand valves (Riebold *et al.* 1980). The manufacturer often incorporates fixed regulators into the anesthesia machine.

4.5.2 Intermediate-Pressure System

The intermediate-pressure system includes pipeline inlets leaving the regulator to the flowmeter assembly,

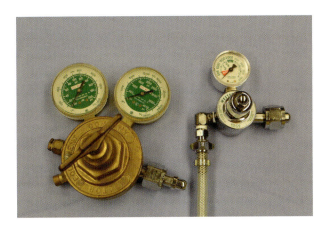

Figure 4.2 Industrial adjustable oxygen regulator (left). Two gauges are present to show the contents of the cylinder and the pressure the operator selects. Fixed medical grade oxygen regulator (right). One gauge is present to show remaining contents of the cylinder (photograph courtesy of Anderson da Cunha, Louisiana State University Baton Rouge, LA).

diversions for pipeline outlet connections of ventilators, and the oxygen flush valve. The pressure in this system is 40–60 psi, depending on the regulator of the machine or oxygen source.

4.5.2.1 Diversion for Pipeline Connections to Drive the Ventilator

While stand-alone machines do exist, most large animal anesthesia machines are commercially produced with ventilators built into their assembly. Splicing a house pipeline oxygen source before the flowmeter to drive the ventilator is common practice by the manufacturers (Figure 4.1).

4.5.2.2 Oxygen Flush Valve

The oxygen flush valve is typically clearly labeled with a green oxygen chemical symbol (O_2). Its location is downstream of the regulator from the oxygen source. It bypasses the flowmeter and vaporizer to deliver 35–75 LPM of oxygen to the patient circuit (Mosley 2015). It is routinely used to quickly fill the volume in the circuit and bellows assembly when performing pre-use operational pressure checks of the anesthesia equipment. When used to fill the bellows or reservoir bag during an anesthetic episode, the anesthetic concentration within the patient circuit will be diluted.

4.5.3 Low-Pressure Systems

The low-pressure system includes the flowmeter, vaporizer, conduit to the fresh gas outlet, fresh gas outlet to the breathing circuit, the breathing circuit, APL valve, carbon dioxide canister and scavenge assembly. Pressure in this system is measured frequently in centimeters of water (cmH_2O). Pressures in this system are common airway pressures and rarely exceed 60 cmH_2O, although some ventilation techniques for large animal patients exceed this threshold (Hopster *et al.* 2011).

4.5.3.1 Flowmeters

Most veterinary anesthesia machines have a single gas option of oxygen; however, several manufacturers offer additional gas options. If more than one gas is present on an anesthesia machine, ASTM standards require oxygen to be on the right-most side (ASTM 2005). Flowmeters are gas specific, calibrated as a unit and should clearly indicate which gas they regulate. Flowmeters on large animal machines should have capable flow rates of 10–15 LPM. Typical total fresh gas flow rates in adult horses, for maintenance anesthesia, are 2–5 LPM (Hubbell 2007). Higher fresh gas flow rates are necessary to minimize the turnover time for changes in anesthetic concentration within the large volume circuit of these machines.

4.5.3.2 Vaporizers

The common anesthesia circuit in use positions the vaporizer out of the circuit (VOC). There are several benefits to this configuration that can be found in Chapter 3; therefore, this is the only type of vaporizer that will be discussed at length in this chapter. Other vaporizers are discussed in Chapter 5.

A vaporizer's purpose is to control the concentration of volatile inhalant delivered to the patient. VOC are precision vaporizers that are agent specific, concentration-calibrated, with variable bypasses that compensate for temperature, flow and back pressure. Considering these features, vaporizers have limits to which output remains consistent. Most vaporizers function acceptably between 0.5 and 10 LPM fresh gas flow rate, at 15–35 °C (59–95 °F), and routine pressures associated with positive pressure ventilation and oxygen flush use. However, for use on large animal machines, where high peak inspiratory pressures, fresh gas flow rates, oxygen flush valve rates and back pressure are extreme, it is important to assure the output is acceptable.

Typically, high fresh gas flow rates slightly decrease output when compared to low fresh gas flow rates. Back pressure from the oxygen flush valve or during periods of high peak inspiratory pressures or positive end expiratory pressures, usually slightly increases output. Additionally, variations in the carrier gas (e.g. nitrous oxide, medical grade air or oxygen) can influence vaporizer output (Dorsch and Dorsch 2008b). Units are available which can test the output of vaporizers on site; however, routine maintenance is required, and recommendations on frequency vary among manufacturers. A monitor with a gas analyzer is beneficial in assisting the anesthetist in monitoring vaporizer output.

4.5.3.3 Common Gas Outlet

The common gas outlet supplies all fresh gases (gases originating from cylinder or pipeline, gases leaving the flowmeters and agents from the vaporizers) to the breathing system. This is a common place for a leak to occur in small animal machines, where the anesthetist switches between non-rebreathing and rebreathing circuits. However, in large animal machines, rarely is there cause to disconnect the fresh gas outlet from the circuit due to the rebreathing circuit's exclusive use.

4.5.3.4 Adjustable Pressure Limiting (APL) Valve

Commonly referred to as the "pop-off", the APL valve feature of the anesthesia machine allows excessive gas in the system to escape via a scavenge system or is used to facilitate positive pressure ventilation. Typically, pressure within the patient circuit will reach 1–3 cmH$_2$O before gas will escape via the APL valve if completely open (Mosley 2015). This provides slight positive end expiratory pressure (PEEP); however, this pressure is insignificant in large animal patients. The APL valve is ideally left fully open for spontaneous ventilation. More frequently, with the use of large animal anesthesia machines and ventilators, the APL valve is left closed and the patient is mechanically ventilated or allowed to spontaneously ventilate via the bellows assembly, which has a spill/dump valve that replaces the APL valve, if so designed.

4.5.3.5 Patient Breathing Circuit

The purpose of the breathing circuit is to direct all fresh gas to the patient; this includes gases leaving flowmeters and the vaporizer, and to remove expired gases. In use with the anesthesia machine, the breathing circuit provides a means to ventilate patients.

Circle systems are used in large animal anesthesia. These circuits have two limbs, one for inspiratory gases and another for expiratory. Unidirectional valves control the direction of gas flow in the limbs of the circle system. Carbon dioxide canisters filled with absorbent are present to remove carbon dioxide exhaled from the patient. Historically, circle systems were referred to as rebreathing circuits and further described as open, closed and semi-closed; however, the degree of "rebreathing" is dependent on the fresh gas flow rate. High fresh gas flow rates produce little rebreathing, while low fresh gas flow rates have a higher degree. In large animal anesthesia with the recommended maintenance fresh gas flow rates of 2–5 L/min for an average equine patient (500 kg), "closed" rebreathing circuits are utilized most frequently (Hubbell 2007). Full or closed rebreathing circuits utilize flow rates near metabolic oxygen consumptions (3–14 mL/kg/min; Mosley 2015).

Standard hosing for large animal rebreathing circuits is not regulated; however, most manufactures produce 5 cm or 2 inch hosing (Figure 4.3). Breathing circuits

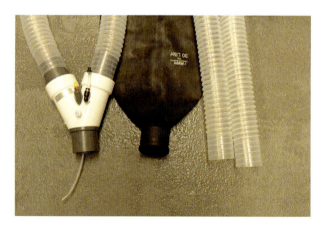

Figure 4.3 30-L reservoir bag, standard 5-cm or 2-inch circle system breathing circuit with wye piece, which has built-in capnograph port.

should be disinfected between patients. A properly dilute chlorhexidine solution is sufficient following complete rinse and drying of the circuit before re-use (Dorsch and Dorsch 2008b).

4.5.3.6 Reservoir Bag

The reservoir bag is commonly called the rebreathing or breathing bag, as its purpose is to provide a reservoir or volume of excess gas for the patient. The reservoir bag will move with the patient's expiration and inspiration, allowing quantification of the respiratory rate. The location of the reservoir bag within the circle system can vary from machine to machine; however, the most common location following the flow of gases through the circuit is between the exhalation unidirectional valve and the carbon dioxide absorbent canister.

The recommended size should be 5–10 times a patient's tidal volume (10–20 mL/kg; Mosley 2015). Routine sizes for large animal use are 15 and 30 L (Figure 4.3). Depending on the anesthesia machine in use, the ventilator bellows allow spontaneous ventilation and replace the need for the reservoir bag. The size of the reservoir bag or bellows influences the volume of the circuit and thus the time it takes to change anesthetic concentrations within the circuit and patient. The reservoir bag also allows the anesthetist to manually assist ventilation. A breath can be given to a patient by closing the APL valve, compressing the reservoir bag to a desired pressure on the patient manometer, then opening the APL valve. The standard large animal reservoir bag fitting is 5 cm or 2 inches. Cleaning the reservoir bag between patients is recommended. A chemical disinfection can be used followed by rinsing and complete drying, but over time can contribute to decreased lifetime of the reservoir bag (Dorsch and Dorsch 2008b). Alcohol should be avoided.

4.5.3.7 Carbon Dioxide Canister and Absorbent

The carbon dioxide canister contains a chemical absorbent to remove carbon dioxide from exhaled gases. Canisters should rest on screens to avoid granules of the chemical absorbent from entering the circuit. In large animal systems where high peak flows of gases are common, the screen will not prevent 100% of the dust or granules entering aspects of the anesthesia circuit or anesthesia machine (Lauria 1975; Davis 1979). Carbon dioxide absorbing materials have been shown to discourage large reservoirs of bacterial growth that could lead to respiratory infections; however, it is ideal to wipe clean the canisters when changing the absorber (Murphy *et al.* 1991; Leijten *et al.* 1992).

Recommendations on when to change the absorbent vary between manufacturers, because absorptive capacities differ (Higuchi *et al.* 2001). The use of a capnograph

is ideal to maximize use of the carbon dioxide absorbent. When inspired carbon dioxide presents itself, the absorber should be changed (Ohrn *et al.* 1991). However, other causes of inspired carbon dioxide are possible; for example, displaced or cracked of unidirectional valve or excessive dead space. The granules should be checked in the canister before use. Unused granules will crumble easily, whereas exhausted granules will not due to the chemical reaction they undergo when exposed to carbon dioxide.

Absorbent should likely be changed when 50% of the granules of the canister have visibly changed color, when the granules no longer crumble easily, when there is no presence of heat or moisture forming during use, or when absorbent is exposed to the environment for longer than two weeks. The screens should be checked for obstructive granules and all residual dust should be removed from where the canister rests on the machine, as this dust can warp seals and create a source for leaks (Dorsch and Dorsch 2008b). The machine should be leak tested following this routine maintenance.

4.5.3.8 Manometer

The manometer gauge is usually graduated in cmH_2O. This gauge corresponds with pressure generated in the patient breathing circuit. Attention is paid to this gauge when leak checking the anesthesia machine before use and during manual or mechanical ventilation. At rest, the needle on the gauge should be at zero. The highest number routinely corresponds to the peak inspiratory pressure reached at the end of the inspiratory plateau. The gauge should return to zero at the beginning of the expiratory phase, unless positive end expiratory pressure (PEEP) is utilized.

Often the gauge has negative values as well (Figure 4.4). When a patient is spontaneously breathing, the needle

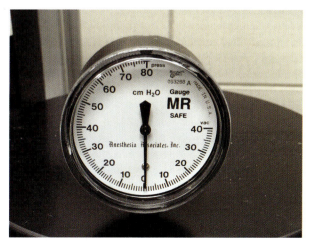

Figure 4.4 Patient manometer demonstrating positive and negative values to reflect positive pressure (controlled) breath or spontaneous breathes respectively.

will move into the negative values. It is important to recognize that the pressure is not usually equivalent to pressure generated in the airway, as there is some elasticity in the breathing circuit (Cote *et al.* 1983).

4.5.4 Scavenge or Evacuation System

Scavenge systems are responsible for removing excessive waste gas from the anesthesia circuit. There are two basic types of systems: active and passive. Both collect and scavenge excess waste gas leaving the breathing circuit to avoid or minimize exposure to the environment and personnel. Active systems have been shown to minimize waste gas exposure more effectively than passive systems (Armstrong *et al.* 1977; Gardner 1989). The ASTM standard for scavenge fittings is 19 and 30 mm male; however, in human medicine, 19 mm is being phased out (Dorsch and Dorsch 2008b).

4.5.4.1 Active Scavenge Systems

An active scavenge system utilizes vacuum or suction to remove waste gas. Ideally, this system would include, at minimum, an interface and reservoir collection system. The interface can be open or closed. If using an open interface, it is vital that the reservoir has sufficient capacity to accommodate the volume of waste gas leaving the anesthetic system. This is difficult to accomplish during anesthesia of large animals and thus the use of an open interface increases the risk of waste anesthetics entering the work environment and exposing personnel.

A closed interface used with an active system ideally would have a positive and a negative pressure relief valve as well as an APL valve. The positive pressure relief valve will open and allow waste anesthetic to escape when gases leaving the anesthetic system exceed the capacity of the scavenge reservoir. The negative pressure relief valve is a safety feature where ambient air will be pulled into the scavenge interface if the suction/vacuum exceeds the volume entering from the patient circuit, thus avoiding removal of fresh gas from the patient. The APL valve allows the degree of vacuum or suction to be adjusted accordingly.

Considering the flow rates utilized in large animal anesthesia, the APL valve on the scavenge interface is usually left completely open. When the scavenge APL valve is closed, back pressure on the patient circuit can be experienced, especially if the scavenge system lacks a negative pressure relief valve. When a positive pressure relief valve is in place, over pressurization of the patient circuit is avoided.

Unfortunately, the positive pressure relief valve can vent waste gas into the room, increasing risk of exposure. Adjustment to the APL valve should be made when the scavenge reservoir bags are full or completely deflated. Often large animal active scavenge systems require multiple large volume (3 L) scavenge reservoir bags to accommodate the high fresh gas flows and large tidal volumes leaving the patient circuit.

4.5.4.2 Passive Scavenge Systems

Passive waste gas elimination systems do not use negative pressure via vacuum or suction. These systems can be very simple in construction. Appropriate size tubing (19 or 30 mm) can be attached to the back of the APL valve on the anesthesia machine and positioned away from the work environment. This tubing should not be kinked or excessive in length, as this could cause an increase in the resting circuit pressure. Alternatively, commercial activate charcoal canisters, which absorb waste anesthetics, can be placed on this tubing (Figure 4.5). These canisters have limited absorption abilities. The manufacturers' recommendations for weighing and discarding the canisters at their point of exhaustion should be followed to minimize waste gas exposure. More complex passive systems contain a positive pressure relief valve. The positive pressure relief valve functions in the same capacity as in the active scavenge system. It relieves excessive pressure into the room if an obstruction in the passive system occurs or its capacity is maximized.

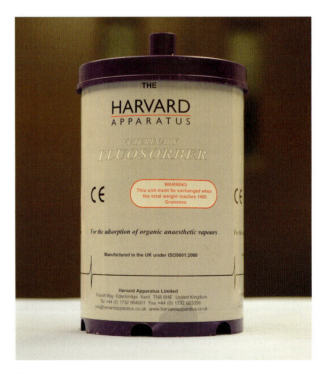

Figure 4.5 Charcoal canister for absorbing waste anesthetics as a passive scavenge source for large volume capacity anesthetic systems.

4.6 Large Animal Anesthesia Workstations

The ACVAA recommends that supplemental oxygen and the means to ventilate should be available when anesthetizing horses (Martinez *et al.* 1995). Large animal anesthesia machines fulfill these guidelines by providing supplemental oxygen, a means to deliver volatile anesthetics and facilitate assisted or controlled ventilation. Stand-alone anesthesia machines are commercially available; however, most manufactures produce complete anesthesia workstations, and machines with built-in ventilators, to simplify the transition between spontaneous, assisted and controlled ventilation modes.

When inhalation anesthetics are utilized, ventilators have a strong foothold in large animal anesthesia. On inhalation anesthetic, horses frequently hypoventilate and develop hypoxemia (Steffey *et al.* 1977; Hodgson *et al.* 1986; Grandy *et al.* 1987). While the use of 100% oxygen and controlled ventilation does not always correct hypoxemia, immediate implementation of controlled ventilation maximizes partial pressure of oxygen in arterial blood (PaO_2) (Steffey *et al.* 1977; Hodgson *et al.* 1986; Day *et al.* 1995; Wolff and Moens 2010).

4.6.1 Anesthesia Machines

Several stand-alone anesthesia machines are or have been commercially available (Figure 4.6). These options will reliably deliver oxygen and inhalation anesthetics to patients in a similar fashion to the small animal counterpart. A reservoir bag and circle breathing circuit is required. Pre-use procedures involve pressure checking the circuit for leaks and ensuring all parts are functioning properly as recommended before each use.

4.6.2 Ventilators

Ventilators function to replace the patient reservoir bag with a bellows or piston and the APL valve with a spill valve. The ventilator's purpose is to provide assisted or controlled ventilation. Large animals can significantly benefit from implementation of positive pressure ventilation with 100% oxygen (Day *et al.* 1995; Wolff and Moens 2010). Stand-alone ventilators are commercially available and can be attached to an anesthesia machine by replacing the reservoir bag with the hose from the ventilator. However, most ventilators are sold assembled within an anesthesia workstation.

4.6.2.1 Ventilator Classification

There are a variety of ways to describe or classify ventilators. The most common include their control variable, power source, drive and cycling mechanisms and type of

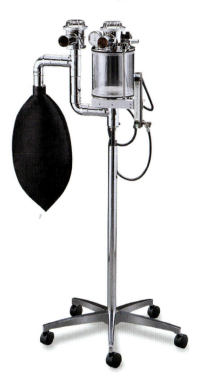

Figure 4.6 Matrix VML® Large Animal Anesthesia Machine (photograph courtesy of Midmark Corporation, Dayton, OH).

bellows. These are discussed in further detail elsewhere (Chapter 6); however, these terms will be used to describe the common commercially available large animal anesthesia ventilators within this chapter.

4.7 Common Commercially Available Machines

This section describes currently available anesthesia workstations as well as discontinued units that can frequently be found in use. Descriptions of the units rely heavily on the operations manuals and information provided by the manufacturer. Before purchase or operation of a ventilator or anesthesia workstation, the user should be familiar with the operations manual and follow the manufacturer's pre-use check out and maintenance schedule. Table 4.1 compares specifications regarding the large animal ventilators described below.

4.7.1 Mallard Rachel Model 2800 A, B and C Series

The Mallard Rachel Model 2800 includes the A, B and C series (AB Medical, Redding, CA, USA). Although Model A and B are still widely in service, Model C is the only model now currently available. Minor differences in function exist between models. Early models had stacking

Table 4.1 Specifications of commercially available large animal anesthesia ventilators.

	Classification	Bellows	VT limit (L)	I.T.	Inspiratory Flow (LPM)	RR (BPM)	Modes of Ventilation	Pressure relief safety valve	O₂ Flush (LPM)	Absorber Volume (L)	Options
Mallard Model Rachel 2800 C	Dual circuit, Microprocessor based, electronic, time cycled, pressure limited,	Standing	18	0.1–3 sec	10–650	2–80 BPM	Controlled Spontaneous (through bellows or bag) Assist (with manual button)	Adjustable, Preset 80 cmH₂O		6	MRI conditional, Small animal ventilator/circuit assembly
SurgiVet DHV 1000	Dual circuit, Electronically controlled, pneumatically driven, time cycled, volume limited	Hanging	15	Variable	Variable	0–15	Controlled Spontaneous (via bellows or bag) Assisted (with manual button)	Adjustable, 10–60 ±5 cmH₂O	10–15	5	MRI conditional with 3T and less up to 720G
Tafonius	Microprocessor controlled, piston driven, single circuit, electronically timed, volume cycled, pressure limited	Piston	20	0.5–4 sec	Up to 900	1–30	Spontaneous, controlled	Adjustable 10–80 cmH₂O	60–70		"Wind God" has multiparameter vitals monitor and gas analyzer
Dräger AVE	Dual circuit, electronically controlled, time cycled, volume limited	Hanging	15	Variable		1–99	Spontaneous(via bag), controlled		50		
JD Medical (Bird Mark 7) LAVC-2000-D-2	Dual circuit, pneumatically controlled, time cycled, pressure limited	Hanging	20	Variable	0–450+	4–30 BPM	Assisted, patient initiated, Controlled, spontaneous	Pressure limited ventilator, set by operator	85	6.5	Customizable

VT, tidal volume; I.T., inspiratory time; LPM, liters per minute; RR, respiratory rate; BPM, breaths per minute

unidirectional valves, a different carbon dioxide absorber assembly, and a 21-L ascending or standing bellows.

Model C's bellows are reduced to 18 L, which allows for faster change in anesthetic gas concentration within the circuit. As with any standing bellows, PEEP produced by the standing bellows is not detrimental during anesthesia of a large animal patient and may demonstrate variable benefit (Swanson and Muir 1988; Wilson and Soma 1990; Wilson and McFeely 1991; Moens *et al.* 1998).

The spill valves located at the top of the bellows are depressed once the bellows have fully ascended and 4–6 cmH$_2$O pressure is applied, resulting in PEEP. The Model C has a pneumatic vacuum pump, which allows the operator to eliminate this PEEP if desired. Additionally, Model C can be purchased as MRI conditional. The controller of the MRI conditional unit is pneumatic with minor differences in controls, but is void of electronics and ferrous metals for MRI compatibility (Figure 4.7). The manufacturer recommends placing the unit as far as possible from the MRI unit.

4.7.1.1 Classification

Mallard series ventilators are microprocessor-based with an electronic control system. They are dual circuit ventilators, meaning there is a physical separation between the drive gas and patient circuit gas. They are time cycled and pressure limiting, with an ascending (standing) bellows. The Model C MRI conditional unit is pneumatically controlled and driven, void of electronic and ferrous materials.

4.7.1.2 Controls for Model C

Drive Gas Control Knob The drive gas control knob is a large black knob located on the left side of the control box. Turning this knob changes the drive gas flow rate, inspiratory flow rate, or rate at which the bellows will descend, and will be noted as low, medium or high on the corresponding gauge to the left of the knob. To change the desired drive gas flow, pull the knob out prior to adjusting and push it back in to set. This flow rate will ultimately be limited by the gas supply line pressure, which can be identified by a gauge on the back of the machine. While the machine's recommended inlet line pressure is 60 psi, it can function between 50 and 120 psi of medical grade air or oxygen. Higher inlet gas supply pressure produces higher inspiratory flows. This machine can produce inspiratory flows that range from 10–650 LPM.

On/Off/Standby The mechanical ventilator will deliver positive pressure breaths when placed in the "on" mode. Once connected to a patient's breathing circuit with no

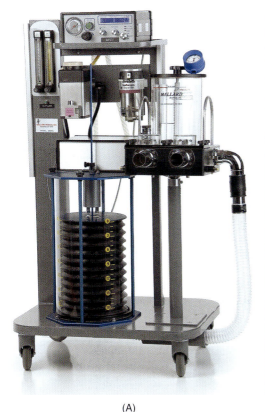
(A)

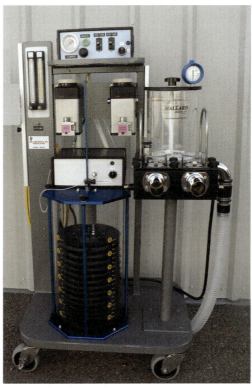
(B)

Figure 4.7 Mallard Rachel 2800C (a), Rachel 2800C-MRI conditional (b), (photograph courtesy of Ken Brown, AB Medical Technologies, Inc., Redding, CA).

leaks, placing in "off" or "standby" mode will allow for spontaneous ventilation. "Standby" mode allows the anesthetist to make selections to the ventilator settings without initiating positive pressure ventilation (PPV). "Standby" mode is not present on the MRI compatible pneumatic controller.

Inspiratory Time Inspiratory time is represented in the LED display and controlled by the corresponding knob below. Inspiratory time range is from 0.1–3 seconds.

Respiratory Rate or Expiratory Time Depending on the model in use, the labeling for this control is respiratory rate or expiratory time. Both will influence the inspiratory to expiratory (I:E) ratio. For the standard electronic controller, the respiratory rate range is 2–80 breaths per minute.

Manual Button When the operator depresses the manual button, the bellows will compress to deliver a breath until the button is released. This feature is utilized when electrical power fails or to give a breath during spontaneous ventilation when the bellows is being used as the patient's "reservoir bag".

4.7.1.3 Safety Features
Safety Pressure Relief Valve Located on the back of the machine, the safety pressure relief valve is an adjustable valve preset at 80 cmH$_2$O. Its intent is to prevent over-pressurization of the patient's lungs and minimize barotrauma.

Failure to Cycle The failure to cycle light illuminates when the machine is placed in "standby" for more than 30 seconds. An audible alarm will sound when the machine is in "on" mode and fails to deliver a breath.

Low Gas Pressure The low gas pressure light will illuminate and an audible alarm will sound when the inlet supply gas line drops below 30 psi. Ideal inlet supply gas pressure is 60 psi.

4.7.1.4 Performance Verification Procedures
Performance verification procedures outlined in the operations manual are to be completed and recorded by in-house personnel on a routine basis. Traditional positive pressure leak testing is difficult to perform in these models when utilizing the bellows. The spill valves located at the top of the bellows assembly open at 4–6 cmH$_2$O. Under a positive pressure hold or pause, the bellows assembly will not hold pressure above this threshold. Depression of the manual breath button will pressurize the circuit until the operator releases the button. Large leaks within the ventilator assembly can be appreciated in this manner, but due to the lack of ability to hold an "inspiratory pause", slow

leaks that present themselves under positive-pressure ventilation are difficult to appreciate before use.

Passive leak testing should be performed before each anesthetic case. This involves connecting the breathing circuit and ventilator hose correctly. Create a closed system by obstructing the patient end of the breathing circuit and releasing the bellows' hold from the guide rod that exits the top of the bellows assembly. No passive leaks are present if the bellows remain standing at the top of the bellows assembly. Care should be taken to avoid bending the rod that extends out of the top of the bellows assembly.

Servicing and Warranty An authorized Mallard service representative should perform servicing of the machine. The machine typically comes with a one-year warranty from date of purchase. An operator familiar with the machine and operations manual can replace rubber components such as O-rings and seals in house.

Cleaning, Disinfecting and Sterilization Ultimately, agents compatible with plastics and serving as standard medical detergents can be used to clean the exterior of the machine. The manufacturer recommends one part white vinegar to three parts water or a dilution of 2% glutaraldehyde for routine cleaning of bellows. Disassembly of the bellows is not recommended. A nasogastric tube and pump can facilitate placing the vinegar solution into the ventilator hose and bellows. Alcohol should not be used on any part of the machine. The spill valves will occasionally require disassembly, balancing and cleaning. The manufacture provides directions for this procedure as well as replacing the bellows assembly.

4.7.1.5 Mallard Specialty Machine
Mallard developed a modified version of the Model C series to assist with anesthetizing an elephant (Figure 4.8). It was designed for use in patients up to 18 000 pounds with tidal volume ranging from 25–125 L. Its unique design facilitates inspiratory flow rates of up to 1100 LPM. The ventilator control is the same as that which controls the Model C series. It is capable of providing a respiratory rate of 2–12 BPM with an inspiratory time of 0.2–8 seconds.

4.7.2 SurgiVet Complete Large Animal System

The SurgiVet Complete Large Animal System with LDS 3000 and DHV1000 (Smiths Medical, Norwell, MA, USA) is a complete workstation that includes the LDS 3000 large animal anesthesia machine, with the DHV 1000 large animal ventilator assembled neatly in a mobile cart with monitoring shelf (Figure 4.9). The DHV ventilator can be purchased separately and is compatible with other stand-alone large animal anesthesia machines.

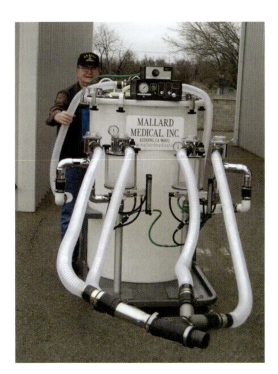

Figure 4.8 Mallard specialty ventilator designed for an elephant (photograph courtesy of Ken Brown, AB Medical Technologies, Inc., Redding, CA).

The DHV ventilator was designed for spontaneous, controlled or assisted ventilation of patients over 250 pounds. It is equipped with a descending or hanging bellows, which do not add PEEP to the patient circuit and can be more challenging to determine leaks when compared to an ascending or standing bellows. For optimal function, oxygen or medical gas source should be set at 55–60 psi. Beyond 65 psi could damage the unit. MRI compatibility is available as conditional with a 3 Tesla or less MRI at the 720 gauss line.

4.7.2.1 Classification

The DHV 1000 is classified as an electronically controlled, pneumatically driven, time cycled, dual circuit ventilator. The bellows assembly is a hanging or descending configuration.

4.7.2.2 Controls for the DHV 1000 Ventilator

On/Off Toggle Switch   The on/off toggle switch can be moved to the "on" position to give individual breaths or remain in the "on" position to control ventilation.

Tidal Volume Wheel   The volume wheel is rotated to predetermine maximum tidal volume desired by the operator. The operator should recognize that the volume selected does not accurately represent patient tidal volume, as some volume will be lost in the compliancy of the breathing circuit. Maximum tidal volume is 15 L.

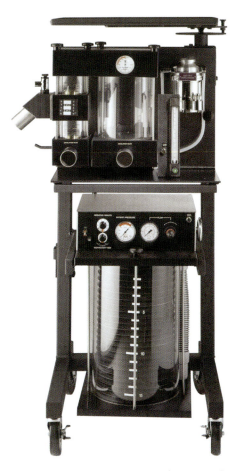

Figure 4.9 SurgiVet® LDS 3000 and DHV 1000 large animal anesthesia machine (Smiths Medical ASD Inc., Minneapolis, MN).

Limiting the tidal volume decreases circuit volume, allowing faster changes in anesthetic concentration.

Respiratory Rate   The operator rotates a dial to select a respiratory rate of between 2–15 breaths per minute.

Inspiratory Time   The inspiratory knob adjusts the length of inspiration. Routine inspiratory times for large animals are between 1 and 3 seconds.

Inspiratory Flow Control   The inspiratory flow knob controls the force at which the breath will be given over the selected inspiratory time. Adjustment to inspiratory time or flow can change the delivered volume. It is important to closely observe the patient manometer and bellows to determine if adequate breaths are delivered. A gauge is positioned directly next to the flow control knob. Under most circumstances, the needle on this gauge will usually reside at between 40 and 50 psi and should never drop below 38 psi.

Manual Breath Button   The operator can facilitate a manual breath by depressing the manual breath button.

The machine does not have to be "on" for this feature to function. It is independent of electrical power as it is pneumatically controlled.

Oxygen Flush Valve   The oxygen flush valve allows for delivery of oxygen, which bypasses the flowmeter. Typical rates of delivery are between 10 and 15 LPM according to the operations manual, which is relatively low compared to human standards of 35–75 LPM (Dorsch and Dorsch 2008b).

4.7.2.3 Safety Features
Patient Circuit Relief Valve   The patient circuit relief valve functions as an adjustable pressure relief valve. It is located on the back of the ventilator. By rotating the knob, pressure within the circuit can be relieved between 10 and 60 cmH_2O. It should be noted that under usual circumstances, while ventilating large animal patients, the valve should be left closed at 60 cmH_2O ± 5 cmH_2O or above 40 cmH_2O, as these pressures are frequently experienced during adequate ventilation.

4.7.2.4 Performance Verification Procedures
The manufacturer recommends pressure testing of the anesthesia machine and ventilator for leaks before each use. Specific guidelines are provided in the operations manual.

Leak Testing the Bellows   Leak testing of the bellows is a passive leak test. With the bellows set at 5 L, obstruct where the reservoir bag or ventilator hose attaches. When slack is allowed in the bellows by increasing the tidal volume, the bellows should not fall. If the bellows do not hold at the original 5 L, a leak in the bellows is present. The bellows requires repair or replacement.

Leak Testing the Ventilator   Leak testing of the ventilator is a positive pressure leak test. With the ventilator hose connected in the location of the reservoir bag and APL valve closed, turn on the ventilator to pressurize the circuit. The ventilator should cycle to 60 cmH_2O or the pressure set on the patient circuit relief valve. The bellows will compress slightly during the ventilator's cycle then return to its originating volume. A leak is present if the bellows compresses and does not return to complete dissention.

4.7.2.5 Servicing and Warranty
Standard advertised warranties, depending on the part, range from 90 days–2 years. The machine itself is warranted for 2 years. Smiths Medical ASD, Inc. provides a 24-hour technical support hotline.

4.7.2.6 Cleaning, Disinfecting and Sterilization
The manufacturer recommends leak testing the ventilator daily. Within the operations manual, routine maintenance is clearly defined. Clean the exterior of the machine with a soft cloth and mild detergent in water. Dilute chorhexidine solutions can be used to disinfect the ventilator hose and bellows. Do not use alcohol.

4.7.3 JD Medical LAVC 2000, 3000 Series

The JD Medical LAVC 2000, 3000 Series (JD Medical Dist. Co., Inc. Phoenix, AZ) offers custom configured large animal anesthesia workstations (Figure 4.10). Their ventilators typically utilize Bird Mark 7 respirators. Originally, the Bird respirator was developed around the end of the Second World War to transport wounded soldiers in aircrafts. It was one of the first respirators to be used in both small and large animal ventilators. Without incorporating a bellows assembly necessary for large animal ventilation, the Bird is a single circuit ventilator. When it is used with the bellows assembly, it operates as a dual circuit ventilator. The ventilator functions to give a breath by pressurizing the space between bellows and bellows housing to force the bellows upward.

The LAVC series anesthesia ventilators can provide spontaneous, controlled or patient initiated/assisted ventilation. It limits tidal volume based on pressure, making it unique among its competitors. Spontaneous ventilation is possible with the LAVC 2000 and 2000-D models by removing a gray cap located on the bottom left corner of the machine's base. Removing this cap breaks the seal between the bellows and the respirator. Placing a hand or temporarily covering this hole will

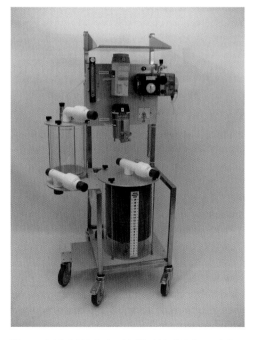

Figure 4.10 2000-D-2 with Bird Mark 7 Servo (photograph courtesy of JD Medical Distribution Company, Phoenix, AZ).

initiate a controlled or "demand" breath. Otherwise, with the cap off, the patient is capable of spontaneous/passive breathing.

The bellows will move with patient respirations in this spontaneous ventilation mode. For controlled ventilation, the cap must be in place to create a dual circuit. On the LAVC 2000-D-2 model, spontaneous ventilation is accomplished with the use of the reservoir bag and connecting hosing from the bottom of the carbon dioxide absorbent canister to the "T" of the reservoir and patient circuit. The patient circle hosing will attach to the front of the "T" for the reservoir bag and the connection at the top of the carbon dioxide assembly.

For controlled ventilation, reconfigure the hose to connect the outlet at the bottom of the carbon dioxide canister with back portion of the "T" on top of the bellows assembly. The patient circle hosing will attach to the top of the carbon dioxide canister and the top of the bellows assembly.

Standard options for the addition of nitrous oxide, hanger yokes for "E" tanks, monitoring selves, and multiple vaporizers are available. The LAVC 2000-D-2 model is equipped with a selector switch when multiple vaporizers are installed. It is the responsibility of the operator to select the appropriate agent and ensure only that agent is being delivered to the patient. While designed to prevent accidental overdose by allowing oxygen to flow through one vaporizer at a time, it is possible for the patient to not receive inhalant when the selector switch is positioned for agent A and the operator turns on the dial for agent B. Model LAV 3000 is a stand-alone ventilator compatible with any stand-alone large animal anesthesia machine.

4.7.3.1 Classification

It is classified as dual circuit, pneumatically driven and controlled, time cycled and pressure limited. Because this ventilator is pneumatically driven and controlled, it does not require electrical power. Fifty psi is the recommended inlet pressure for optimal function. It is important in pneumatically controlled ventilators to maintain adequate inlet drive pressure to ensure optimal operation.

4.7.3.2 Controls

Inspiratory Flow Knob The inspiratory flow knob control directly affects inspiratory time and how quickly the inspiratory pressure will be achieved. This can be increased or decreased by turning this black knob. Inspiratory flow range is zero to over 450 liters per minute.

Inspiratory Pressure Control The inspiratory pressure control is located on the right side of the Mark 7 respirator. The manometer to the left of the inspiratory flow knob is graduated in cmH_2O and mmHg. Adjustments to the inspiratory pressure control will correspond to increase or decrease in the limiting pressure delivered during inspiration.

Sensitivity The sensitivity control is located on the left side of the respirator and determines the amount of patient effort required to trigger an assisted breath. By manipulating this control, the operator decides if patient initiated or controlled ventilation is desired. Increasing the sensitivity control to the highest setting facilitates controlled ventilation. The lowest setting could cause the ventilator to fire at a rapid rate. If patient initiated ventilation is desired, the sensitivity control should be adjusted so the patient must generate negative 2–3 cmH_2O before the machine will cycle a breath. The range on the inspiratory sensitivity is negative 0.5 to negative 8 cmH_2O.

Expiratory Time or Apnea Control The expiratory time or apnea control determines the respiratory rate. The range is 2–30 breaths per minutes or 5–15 seconds. If the operator desires to allow the patient to initiate breaths with assistance, this control should be adjusted to the minimum number of breaths necessary for effective/safe ventilation. In this mode, if the patient becomes apneic and fails to initiate a breath, the ventilator will still provide a safe minimum respiratory rate. When the operator has moved the sensitivity control to its maximum setting facilitating controlled ventilation, the expiratory timer or apnea control knob selects the desired respiratory rate.

Hand Timer The hand timer control is commonly referred to as the "red pin" and is located in the center of the sensitivity control. As the ventilator cycles, this pin will move in and out. By compressing this pin, the operator can trigger a manual breath. A breath will be given to the selected pressure on the inspiratory pressure control.

Adjustable PEEP Valve An adjustable PEEP valve can be installed near the APL valve on top of the bellows assembly. Adjusting this valve and the oxygen flowmeter will create PEEP. The operator should pay attention to the patient manometer to determine if the desired PEEP is obtained.

4.7.3.3 Performance Verification Tests

In performance verification tests, leak testing is a positive pressure test where first the operator inflates the bellows. The highest desired pressure is selected on the inspiratory pressure control knob. The operator creates a closed system by covering the patient end of the y-piece with a hand or reservoir bag. By pushing in on the hand timer or "red pin", the machine delivers a "manual" breath to the preset pressure. The unit will cycle off when pressure is reached and bellows should return to initial position. If the ventilator fails to cycle off or if flow continues to cycle for an extended period, a leak is present. When a leak is present, often the bellows will fail to completely return to the full hanging position.

4.7.3.4   Servicing and Warranty

The manufacturer provides guidance to recommended yearly preventative maintenance. The manufacturer, approved distributor or service provider can complete this. It includes thorough cleaning, calibrating and performance verification tests of the machine. The manufacturer provides an exchange or cleaning and calibration of the servo ventilator controller when damaged or not working properly.

4.7.3.5   Cleaning, Disinfecting and Sterilization

A sensing valve is located in the center of the bottom plate of the bellows assembly. It is activated when the bellows completely descends and is responsible for opening the exhalation valve at the top of the bellows. This valve requires regular evaluation to ensure proper function and may require replacement. Over time, this valve can bend or tilt. If the ventilator fails to cycle off of inspiration and a leak cannot be identified, this must be checked for correct installation and alignment. The ventilator will not operate properly with this valve misaligned. A specialized tool is required and is provided by the manufacturer. Removing and cleaning the bellows should be completed on a regular basis, depending on the use of the unit. A dilute chlorhexidine solution is sufficient. The bellows should be reassembled after being thoroughly rinsed and dried. The operator should perform the pressure check following reassembly.

4.7.4   Tafonius

The Tafonius (Hallowell EMC, Pittsfield, MA, USA) is the newest generation of large animal anesthesia machines (Figure 4.11). It features a unique design, in that it utilizes a piston which allows an adjustable "virtual reservoir bag" in place of a bellows assembly, an Airway Pressure Servo System (APSS) that functions to remove the patients' "work of breathing", and an initialization process which checks for leaks and compensates for compliance within the patient circuit.

The machine can facilitate spontaneous, patient initiated/volume assisted or controlled ventilation. The piston is used in place of a traditional reservoir bag and moves as the patient breathes. If the anesthetist desires visualization of respirations, a reservoir bag can be

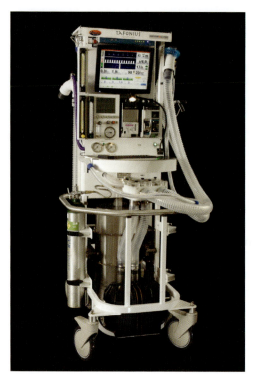

Figure 4.11 Tafonius "Wind God" (photograph courtesy of W. Stetson Hallowell, Hallowell EMC, Pittsfield, MA).

placed on the standard circuit hose connected to the drain port at the bottom of the absorber canister. The operator should consider the additional volume added to the circuit by including the reservoir bag and the impact this has on the time it takes to turn over inhalant concentrations in the larger volume circuit.

The Tafonius is provided with a battery backup, which can provide ventilation to a patient in the event of lost power for roughly 6 to 8 hours, depending on electrical demand. The Tafonius "Wind God" and Tafonius Junior both feature a piston ventilator. The "Wind God" version comes with a touch screen multi-parameter monitor and the ability to save all data collected. The vitals monitor includes blood pressure, invasive and non-invasive, electrocardiogram, pulse oximetry, capnography, airway pressure, temperature, and gas analysis.

4.7.4.1   Classification

It is classified as microprocessor-controlled, piston driven, single circuit, electronically timed, volume cycled and pressure limited, with a piston drive mechanism that acts as an adjustable volume "virtual reservoir bag".

4.7.4.2   Controls

The Tafonius has several controls that are characterized by independent and dependent variables. Independent variables are controllable by the operator (e.g. tidal volume, inspiratory time, respiratory rate, maximum working pressure limit, continuous positive airway pressure [CPAP]/PEEP and inspiratory pause).

The primary independent controls will change in spontaneous mode to reflect the patient's respiratory rate, inspiratory time and tidal volume; however, when ventilate mode is selected, the ventilator will deliver to the operator's selected independent controls. Dependent variables such as inspiratory flow, expiratory time, minute volume and the inspiratory to expiratory (I:E) ratio, are dependent upon the operator's selections of the aforementioned variables.

Tidal Volume   The capable tidal volume range is 0.05–20 L. This allows for use in a large range of patient sizes on a circle system. Adaptors are provided to convert to a standard (22 mm) small animal circle breathing circuit and endotracheal tube connection (15 mm). When the operator performs the leak and compliancy portion of the performance verification process, the Tafonius compensates for circuit compliancy, ensuring the tidal volume selected by the operator is the tidal volume delivered to the patient.

Respiratory Rate and Inspiratory Time   The respiratory rate and inspiratory time can be set from 1–30 breaths per minute and 0.5–4 seconds, respectively.

Inspiratory Pause   The inspiratory phase feature is unique to the Tafonius. By utilizing a pause at the peak of the inspiratory phase, the operator assists in providing more time for equilibrium of gas exchange within the alveoli. This is done with the hope of minimizing ventilation to perfusion (V/Q) mismatch. However, as everything has a consequence, prolonged inspiratory pauses can reduce venous return and cardiac output and ultimately blood pressure. This feature's adjustable limit is up to 40% of inspiratory time.

Maximum Working Pressure Limit   The operator may select a maximum working pressure limit. The adjustable range is 10–80 cmH$_2$O. When the maximum working pressure is reached, the ventilator immediately discontinues the inspiratory phase, sounds an alarm and switches to the expiratory phase.

CPAP/PEEP   The operator has the ability to select a positive pressure to be held throughout the respiratory cycle. In principle, this assists to maintain open alveoli or is used in conjunction with recruitment techniques (Moens *et al.* 1998; Mosing *et al.* 2013). However, CPAP and PEEP can cause decrease in venous return, cardiac output and blood pressure (Swanson and Muir 1988; Wilson and Soma 1990). In spontaneous mode, CPAP is used. When ventilate mode is selected, the CPAP automatically becomes PEEP. The maximum setting for CPAP/PEEP is 20 cmH$_2$O.

Fresh Gas Flow (FGF)   The operator can adjust variable fresh gas flow mixtures of ambient air and oxygen. Theoretically, by utilizing a lower fraction of inspired oxygen (FiO$_2$), there is a decrease in absorption atelectasis; however, this has not proven to be consistently beneficial in the horse (Nyman and Hedenstierna 1989; Hubbell *et al.* 2011; Crumley *et al.* 2013). First, the operator must enable the FiO$_2$ control. The operator selects the desired fresh gas flow and FiO$_2$. The machine pulls ambient air and computes the amount of oxygen required to create the selected FiO$_2$ and FGF. The oxygen flowmeter remains in the *off* position during use of this feature. Fresh gas mixture will travel through the vaporizer and deliver volatile anesthetics. It is ideal to utilize this feature in ventilation mode or in patients who have adequate spontaneous ventilation. This feature is designed to be utilized with only oxygen and ambient air as carrier gases, and therefore it is inappropriate to use with nitrous oxide.

Buffer Volume   The buffer volume button allows the operator to change the size of the "virtual reservoir". Reducing the total volume of the circuit decreases the time it takes for the patient to accurately reflect the set anesthetic concentration (i.e. faster changes in anesthetic depth). The buffer volume limit is 0–20 L.

Assist Mode   When the operator selects the inspiratory flow button, an assist option will appear. The operator selects an inspiratory flow rate represented in LPM. This feature converts the machine to a "flow-triggered" system from a pressure-triggered one. When the patient generates the selected inspiratory flow, the machine will "assist" to deliver the operator's selected tidal volume. If the patient does not generate adequate inspiratory flow, or has a period of apnea, the machine will deliver the set tidal volume. This feature is only available when the machine is placed in "ventilation mode".

Dependent Variables   The dependent variables include inspiratory flow, minute volume, expiratory time, and inspiratory to expiratory (I:E) ratio. These variables are influenced and automatically updated when the operator selects values for the respiratory rate, tidal volume and inspiratory time. While dependent, they should not be ignored. They are important to ensure that a complete and adequate respiratory cycle occurs from the operator's selections. The operator may also calculate or determine these figures; however, the Tafonius "Wind God" unit completes this task for convenience.

4.7.4.3 Performance Verification Procedures

The Tafonius computer undergoes an initialization procedure where the software confirms proper function of the entire system. This first step occurs once the unit has been turned on and requires nothing additional from the operator. The final steps of the performance verification procedure include initialization of the piston, pressure checking for leaks, and establishing compliancy within the circuit.

Initialize Piston The initialize piston operation is directed to ensure the patient circuit is not connected to a patient or obstructed. By selecting the initialize piston, the machine will establish the piston's "zero" position. Ventilation mode cannot be used until the piston has been initialized.

Leak and Compliance Test Once the piston is initialized, the operator is instructed to obstruct the patient end of the Y-piece. The machine moves the piston to generate a positive pressure hold test up to 20 cmH$_2$O and a compliance test with PEEP. Specific values identifying the leak in mL/min at 20 cmH$_2$O and compliancy are displayed for the operator to determine if acceptable. If the operator selects finish, the machine is ready for use.

Leaks occur in similar places on the Tafonius models as on other machines. Attention should be paid to the carbon dioxide absorbent canister, unidirectional valve assembly and patient breathing circuit.

4.7.4.4 Servicing and Warranty

Online support is available by connecting the Tafonius units to the internet via an Ethernet cable. This allows a service technician to access your machine and help identify areas of concern or error messages. Additionally, this allows for software updates and observation of the machine while in use. Yearly maintenance contracts are available.

4.7.4.5 Cleaning, Disinfecting and Sterilization

Alcohol should not be used to clean the exterior of the unit. The piston can be rinsed out with clean water and left open to dry. The plugs at the bottom of the piston below the carbon dioxide absorbent canister should be removed when the machine is not in use, to allow condensation to empty and completely dry. The piston rests in a fully ascended position to allow it to dry. It is recommended to open the unidirectional valves and remove the disks so they may dry as well.

4.7.5 Dräger AVE

Sold as a component of Narkovet-E Large Animal Anesthesia Machine, the Dräger AVE model is no longer manufactured but can still be found in use. The LAS-4000

(VETLAND Louisville, KY) and Titan XL (DRE Louisville, KY) offer a large animal anesthesia workstation with a reconditioned Dräger AVE ventilator (Figure 4.12). Minor variations in controls may exist between models and manufacturers. These anesthesia workstations can facilitate spontaneous or controlled ventilation.

To spontaneously ventilate a patient, an appropriately sized reservoir bag is connected to the reservoir arm. A standard 5-cm hose is connected to the top of the reservoir arm and a port on the back of the carbon dioxide absorbent canister. The APL valve has 3 cmH$_2$O resistance when completely open, for spontaneous ventilation.

For controlled ventilation, the hose will connect from the carbon dioxide absorbent canister outlet to the top of the ventilator. The APL valve must be closed completely for the ventilator to function. The ventilator is designed with the option for the drive gas to be oxygen and air. Within the currently available anesthesia workstations, the ventilator has the ability to utilize a mixture of ambient room air at 67%, and oxygen at 33% as a drive gas. The inlet gas pressure should be 50 psi. At 42 psi, the ventilator will fail to function.

4.7.5.1 Classification

The Dräger AVE is a dual circuit, electronically controlled, time cycled, volume limiting and pneumatically driven with a descending/hanging bellows.

4.7.5.2 Controls

On/Off Switch In order to utilize the ventilator portion of the anesthesia workstation, the operator must turn the

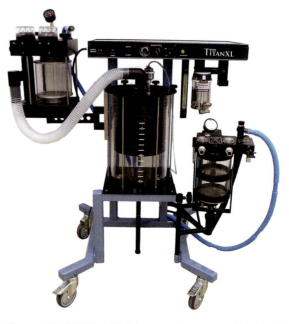

Figure 4.12 DRE Titan XL (photograph courtesy of Nathan C. Claypool, DRE, Louisville, KY).

switch to the "on" position. During spontaneous ventilation, the switch will remain in the "off" position and the use of a reservoir bag is employed.

Tidal Volume   A rocker switch that the operator presses to move the bottom plate within the bellows assembly controls tidal volume. This limits the maximum size breath delivered to the patient. The tidal volume range is 0.5–15 L.

I:E Ratio and Respiratory Rate   The I:E ratio can be set from 1:1–1:8 and the respiratory rate from 1–99 breaths per minute.

Inspiratory Flow   A knob labeled inspiratory flow to the right of the inspiratory flow gauge allows the operator to change the rate or force at which a breath will be given over the inspiratory time. The operator does not directly select inspiratory time. It is determined by the selected I:E ratio and respiratory rate. This adjustable inspiratory flow can produce working pressures of 25 ± 5 cmH$_2$O–100 cmH$_2$O ± 10 cmH$_2$O.

Manual Breath Button   During ventilation mode, a manual breath can be given via depression of the manual breath button.

4.7.5.3   Performance Verification Procedures
The manufacturers recommend daily performed and recorded performance verification tests to ensure proper function of the anesthesia workstation. The operations manuals clearly outline the tests to be performed. When assembled for spontaneous ventilation, a positive pressure hold test can be performed similar to that in small animal machines to identify leaks. First, the APL valve must be closed and the patient end of the Y-piece obstructed. The operator pressurizes the system utilizing the oxygen flush valve until a maximum pressure is reached, usually 30–40 cmH$_2$O for routine large animal patients. This pressure will hold when no leaks are present. A positive pressure test can be performed on the ventilator portion of the anesthesia workstation; however, slow leaks are difficult to appreciate, as this test method does not have a pressure holding phase.

4.7.5.4   Servicing and Warranty
In the operations manual, the manufactures recommend service inspections every 6 months by a qualified technician. The standard advertised warranty is 3 years. The machine is routinely sold with the Dräger Vapor 19.1 vaporizer, which comes with a standard 10-year warranty and does not require regular servicing outside of routinely checking output. Other vaporizers will have variable warranties and service recommendations. A 24-hour technician support hotline is available.

4.7.5.5   Cleaning, Disinfection and Sterilization
It is recommended that the interior of the bellows be cleaned with a liquid disinfectant. It is important to ensure the bellows is thoroughly rinsed and completely dry before being placed back into the bellows housing. Disassembly of the unidirectional valves is recommended routinely as is cleaning. The exterior of the machine can be wiped down with disinfectant.

4.8   General Cautions

Manufacturer's guidelines and operations manuals should always be thoroughly reviewed before the use of any equipment. Proper performance verification tests should all be performed prior to equipment use.

Oily or greasy substances should never be used on anesthesia equipment, as this could produce an explosion when combined with oxygen. Oxygen compatible lubricants are available.

4.9   Miscellaneous Equipment for Large Animal Anesthesia

4.9.1   Surgical Tables, Padding and Positioning

Several commercial surgical tables are specifically designed for large animal use. Some accommodate a variety of positions, such as dorsal and lateral, have the ability to lift, and/or tilt, and are mobile on sturdy casters. Desirable features require review of the operator's needs and hospital arrangements. Tilt tables can be used to secure a patient while standing and assist in positioning on a surgical table or restraint of a patient (Figure 4.13). Pads specifically made for large animals are used on surgical tables to assist in minimizing the occurrence of neuropathies and myopathies (Figure 4.14). When large animals are positioned in lateral recumbency, the front dependent limb should be pulled forward to relieve pressure on the radial nerve.

4.9.2   Recovery Aids and Stalls

Following general anesthesia, appropriately padded stalls are routinely used for equine recoveries. Ropes, helmets, halters, and dimly-lit rooms in padded stalls with secure footing are all components which individuals routinely use to recover equine patients (Figure 4.15). Some facilities utilized slings, inflatable floors and pools to assist recovery. Other large animal species may require specialized equipment to improve the quality of recover.

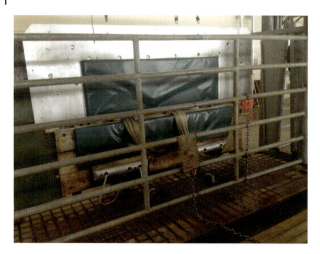

Figure 4.13 Tilt table positioned in tandem with cattle shoot (photograph courtesy of Chance Armstrong, Auburn University, Auburn, AL).

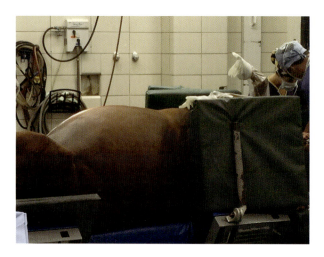

Figure 4.14 Equine patient positioned in dorsal recumbency with adequate padding to reduce risks of neuropathy or myopathy.

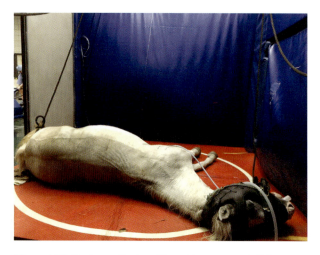

Figure 4.15 Equine patient positioned in recovery stall for a rope assisted recovery with padded walls, secure footing and helmet.

4.9.3 Demand Valves

Demand valves are used to deliver manual breaths by depressing a button valve when connected to compressed oxygen source (Figure 4.16). The valves are designed to allow passive expiration; however, due to large animals' expiratory volume, this valve may be restrictive and is often removed to allow for complete expiration. Additionally, the operator should ensure the demand valve has a high inspiratory flow capacity desirable for large animals. While most have maximum flow rate limits of 160 LPM at 50 psi, valves with high flows are described for use in horses delivering 200 LPM at 50 psi and 275 LPM at 80 psi (Riebold *et al.* 1980; Mosley 2015). Adaptors may be required to utilize the demand valve on a large animal endotracheal tube.

4.9.4 Oxygen Insufflation

During recovery, insufflation of oxygen has been determined as helpful to optimize PaO_2. Adult horses require a minimum of 15 LPM O_2 to improve PaO_2, while foals or smaller ruminants may require 5 LPM (Mason *et al.* 1987; Crumley *et al.* 2012).

4.9.5 Intubation

4.9.5.1 Oral and Nasotracheal Tubes

Like small animal endotracheal and nasotracheal tubes, large animal tubes are commonly referenced by the internal diameter in millimeters (mmID). Routinely used are Murphy style cuffed endotracheal tubes. The outer diameter of the endotracheal or nasotracheal tube can vary between manufacturers.

Most endotracheal tubes intended for large animal use are made of silicone. Routine sizes for adult horses and large ruminants are 24–30 mmID. Ruminants typically require slightly smaller than a horse of equal size. Foals

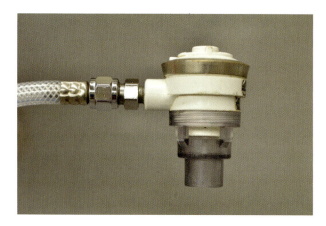

Figure 4.16 Demand valve (photograph courtesy of Anderson da Cunha, Louisiana State University Baton Rouge, LA).

and small ruminants will utilize a large variety of endotracheal or nasotracheal tubes, depending on patient size and species.

Some consider it common practice to remove the oral tracheal tube and replace with a nasotracheal tube for equine recoveries. Ideally, nasotracheal tubes should be made of silicone and have thin walls to maximize internal diameter size to reduce resistance. Many commercially available large animal endotracheal and nasotracheal tubes come with a funnel-shaped adaptor, which attaches to a standard 5-mm large animal circle system wye piece. Some elect to remove this funnel and use 22-mm adaptors, which often facilitate a gas sampling port (Figure 4.17).

4.9.5.2 Devices to Assist Intubation
Mouth gags, long laryngoscope blades and stylets are helpful for various large animal species (Figure 4.17). Often intubation in large animal species is blind. Active suction may be helpful to remove gastric secretions in ruminants and pigs during the intubation process.

4.9.6 Monitoring

While no monitor can replace a dedicated anesthetist who is knowledgeable about the equipment in use and anesthetic considerations specific to that species, gas

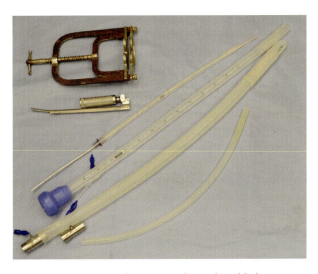

Figure 4.17 Intubation devices. Mouth gag, long blade laryngoscope, endotracheal tube with stylet, large animal endotracheal tube with funnel adaptor, endotracheal tube with 22-mm adaptor with capnograph connection port, nasotracheal tubing and 22-mm connector with capnograph connection port (top to bottom) (photograph courtesy of Anderson da Cunha, Louisiana State University, Baton Rouge, LA).

analyzers with capnography, blood gas analysis and invasive blood pressure are essential to minimize complications, morbidity and mortality in extended large animal procedures, as well as monitoring routine vitals.

References

Armstrong, R.F., Kershaw, E.J. and Bourne, S.P. (1977) Anaesthetic waste gas scavenging systems. *Br Med J*, 1, 941–943.

ASTM F1850-00 (2005) Standard Specification for Particular Requirements for Anesthesia Workstations and Their Components (Withdrawn 2014), ASTM International, West Conshohocken, PA, www.astm.org

Brodbelt, D., Blissitt, K., Hammond, R., Neath, P., Young, L.E. *et al.* (2008) The risk of death: the confidential enquiry into perioperative small animal fatalities. *Vet Anaesth Analg.* 35, 365–373.

Cote, C.J., Petkau, A.J. and Ryan, J.F. (1983) Wasted ventilation measured *in vitro* with eight anesthetic circuits with and without inline humidification. *Anesthesiology*, 59, 442–446.

Crumley, M.N., Hodgson, D.S. and Kreider, S.E. (2012) Effects of tidal volume, ventilatory frequency, and oxygen insufflation flow on the fraction of inspired oxygen in cadaveric horse heads attached to a lung model. *Am J Vet Res*, 73, 134–139.

Crumley, M.N., McMurphy, R.M., Hodgson, D.S. and Kreider, S.E. (2013) Effects of inspired oxygen concentration of ventilation, ventilatory rhythm, and gas exchange in isoflurane-anesthetized horses. *Am J Vet Res*, 74, 183–190.

Davis, R. (1979) Soda lime dust. *Anaesth Intens Care*, 8, 390.

Day, T.K., Gaynor, J.S., Muir, W.W., Bednarski, R.M. and Mason, D.E. (1995) Blood gas values during intermittent positive pressure ventilation and spontaneous ventilation in 160 anesthetized horses position in lateral or dorsal recumbency. *Vet Anesth*, 24, 266–276.

Dodd, G.H. (1854) *Modern Horse Doctor*. Boston, MA, J.P. Jewett.

Dorsch, J.A. and Dorsch, S.E. (2008a) Medical gas cylinders and containers. In: *Understanding Anesthesia Equipment*, 5th ed. Baltimore, MD: Williams & Wilkins, p. 7.

Dorsch, J.A. and Dorsch, S.E. (2008b) The anesthesia machine. In: *Understanding Anesthesia Equipment*, 5th ed. Philadelphia, PA, Lippincott Williams & Wilkins, pp. 83–120.

Fisher, E.W. (1957) A closed circuit anaesthesia apparatus for adult cattle and for horses. *Vet Rec*, 69, 769–771.

Gardner, R.J. (1989) Inhalation anaesthetics – exposure and control: a statistical comparison of personal exposures in operating theatres with and without anaesthetic gas scavenging. *Ann Occup Hyg*, 33, 159–173.

Grandy, J.L., Steffey, E.P. and Miller, M. (1987) Arterial blood PO$_2$ and PCO$_2$ in horses during early halothane-oxygen anaesthesia. *Equine Vet J*, 19, 314–318.

Higuchi, H., Adach, A., Arimura, S. and Al, E. (2001) The carbon dioxide absorption capacity of Amsorb is half that of soda lime. *Anesth Analg*, 93, 221–225.

Hodgson, D.S., Steffey, E.P., Grandy, J.L. and Woliner, M.J. (1986) Effects of spontaneous, assisted, and controlled ventilator modes in halothane-anesthetized geldings. *Am J Vet Res*, 47, 992–996.

Hopster, K., Kastner, S.B., Rohn, K. and Ohnesorge, B. (2011) Intermittent positive pressure ventilation with constant positive end-expiratory pressure and alveolar recruitment manoeuvre during inhalation anaesthesia in horses undergoing surgery for colic, and it influence on the early recovery period. *Vet Anaesth Analg*, 38, 169–177.

Hubbell, J.A.E. (2007) Horses. In: Tranquilli, W.J. and Grimm, K.A. (eds). *Lumb and Jones' Veterinary Anesthesia and Analgesia*, 4th ed. Ames, IA: Blackwell Publishing, pp. 717–730.

Hubbell, J.A.E., Aarnes, T.K., Bednarski, R.M., Lerche, P. and Muir, W.W. (2011) Effect of 50% and maximal inspired oxygen concentrations on respiratory variables in isoflurane-anesthetized horses. *BMC Vet Res*, 7, 23.

Johnston, G.M., East, J.K., Wood, J.L.N. and Taylor, P.M. (2002) The confidential enquiry into perioperative equine fatalities (CEPEF): mortality results of phases 1 and 2. *Vet Anaesth Analg*, 29, 159–170.

Lauria, J.I. (1975) Soda-lime dust contamination of breathing circuits. *Anesthesiology*, 42, 628–629.

Leijten, D.T.M., Rejger, V.S. and Mouton, R.P. (1992) Bacterial contamination and the effect of filters in anaesthetic circuits in a simulated patient model. *J Hosp Infect*, 21, 51–60.

Mallard Ventilator Operational Instructions and Routine Maintenance Model 2800B/2800C/2800C-P/28PBA Large Animal Ventilator System (2014) Redding, CA, AB Medical Technologies, Inc.

Martinez, E.A., Wagner, A.E., Driessen, B. and Trim, C. (1995) The American College of Veterinary Anesthesiologists guidelines of anesthetic monitoring. *J Am Med Vet Assoc*, 206, 936–937.

Mason, D.E., Muir, W.W. and Wade, W. (1987) Arterial blood gas tensions in horses during recovery from anesthesia. *J Am Med Vet Assoc*, 190, 989–994.

Moens, Y., Lagerweij, E., Gootjes, P. and Poortman, J. (1998) Influence of tidal volume and positive end-expiratory pressure on inspiratory gas distribution and gas exchange during mechanical ventilation in horses position in lateral recumbency. *Am J Vet Res*, 59, 307–312.

Mosing, M., Rysnik, M., Bardell, D., Cripps, P.J. and Macfarlane, P. (2013) Use of continuous positive airway pressure (CPAP) to optimise oxygenation in anaesthetised horses – a clinical study. *Equine Vet J*, 45, 414–418.

Mosley, C.A. (2015) Anesthesia equipment. In: Grimm, K.A., Tranquilli, W.J., Greene, S.A. and Robertson, S.A. (eds). *Veterinary Anesthesia and Analgesia: The Fifth Edition of Lumb and Jones*. Ames, IA: John Wiley & Sons, Inc., pp. 23–85.

Murphy, P.M., Fitzgeorge, R.B. and Barrett, R.F. (1991) Viability and distribution of bacteria after passage through a circle anaesthetic breathing system. *Br J Anaesth*, 66, 300–304.

Nyman, G. and Hedenstierna, G. (1989) Ventilation-perfusion relationships in the anaesthetized horse. *Equine Vet J*, 21, 274–281.

Ohrn, M., Gravenstein, N. and Good, M.L. (1991) Duration of carbon dioxide absorption by soda lime at low rates of fresh gas flow. *J Clin Anaesth*, 3, 104–107.

Riebold, T.W., Evans, A.T. and Robinson, N.E. (1980) Evaluation of the demand valve for resuscitation of horses. *J Am Med Vet Assoc*, 176, 623–626.

Steffey, E.P., Wheat, J.D., Meagher, D.M., Norrie, R.D., McKee, J. et al. (1977) Body position and mode of ventilation influences arterial pH, oxygen, and carbon dioxide tension in halothane-anesthetized horses. *Am J Vet Res*, 38, 379–382.

SurgiVet DHV 1000 Large Animal Ventilator Model V7275 Operations Manual (2007) [Available from Surgivet.com], St Paul, MN: Smiths Medical ASD, Inc.

SurgiVet LDS 3000 Large Animal Anesthesia Machine V7025/V7025 MR Conditional Operations Manual, St Paul, MN, Smiths Medical ASD, Inc.

Swanson, C.R. and Muir, W.W. (1988) Hemodynamic and respiratory responses in halothane-anesthetized horses exposed to positive end-expiratory pressure alone and with dobutamine. *Am J Vet Res*, 49, 539–542.

Weaver, B.M.Q. (1960) An apparatus for inhalation anaesthesia in large animals. *Vet Rec*, 72, 1121–1125.

Wilson, D.V. and McFeely, A.M. (1991) Positive end-expiratory pressure during colic surgery in horses: 74 cases (1986–1988). *J Am Med Vet Assoc*, 199, 917–921.

Wilson, D.V. and Soma, L.R. (1990) Cardiopulmonary effects of positive end-expiratory pressure in anesthetized, mechanically ventilated ponies. *Am J Vet Res*, 51, 734–739.

Wolff, K. and Moens, Y. (2010) Gas exchange during inhalation anaesthesia of horses: a comparison between immediate versus delayed start of intermittent positive pressure ventilation – a clinical study. *Pferdeheikunde*, 26, 706–711.

Wright, J.G. (1958) Anaesthesia and narcosis in the horse. *Vet Rec*, 70, 329–336.

5

Anesthetic Vaporizers

Sharon Fornes[1], Kristen G. Cooley[2], and Rebecca A. Johnson[2]

[1] *Veterinary Centers of America (VCA) Bay Area Specialists, San Leandro, California, USA*
[2] *School of Veterinary Medicine, University of Wisconsin, Madison, Wisconsin, USA*

5.1 Introduction

Modern anesthetic vaporizers are designed to deliver controlled amounts of volatile anesthetics in the presence of a carrier gas (e.g. oxygen, nitrous oxide, etc.). The percentage of an agent that is delivered when allowed to passively vaporize without the use of a vaporizer is frequently higher than that necessary to provide a safe anesthetic plane. Thus, vaporizers are required to provide safe, controllable anesthetic levels (Hartsfield 2007). Current, safer vaporizers have evolved from older, non-calibrated units, whose output varied and depended on temperature and gas flow.

5.2 Vaporizer Physics

5.2.1 Saturated Vapor Pressure

All materials have a critical temperature above which they cannot be liquefied (are present in only the gaseous phase), despite how much the pressure is increased (Davis and Kenny 2007a). At or below the critical temperature, a substance can exist in both liquid and gaseous forms; the gaseous form is termed a "vapor" (Boumphrey and Marshall 2011). All liquids can evaporate at room temperature (~20–25°C) and atmospheric pressure (~760 mmHg or 101.3 kPa). That is, molecules of liquid with enough kinetic energy, which are near the surface and traveling in the correct direction, can overcome the pull of intermolecular forces to vaporize. For example, liquid anesthetic within a closed container at a constant temperature will vaporize and come into equilibrium with the gaseous phase above it. The pressure exerted by the gas at dynamic equilibrium with the liquid anesthetic (equal number of molecules leaving the liquid and re-entering it) is the agent's saturated vapor pressure (Figure 5.1; Dorsch and

Dorsch 2008). If the closed container of liquid anesthetic is heated, the equilibrium shifts to increase the amount of anesthetic vapor in the gas phase and subsequently the vapor pressure increases. Barometric pressure does not affect anesthetic vapor pressures *per se*, as the vapor pressure is dependent on the chemical properties of the specific liquid agent and the environmental temperature. Thus, at a specific temperature, each substance will have a known saturated vapor pressure that decreases non-linearly with decreasing temperature and vice versa (Boumphrey and Marshall 2011).

5.2.2 Latent Heat of Vaporization

The heat of vaporization of any liquid is the number of calories needed to change one gram of a liquid into a vapor (Davis and Kenny 2007b; Dorsch and Dorsch 2008). The temperature of the liquid decreases as vaporization ensues, because heat flows from the surroundings down a gradient. Equilibrium is eventually established in this way.

5.2.3 Boiling Point

Energy is required for vaporization from the liquid to the gas phase. Molecules near the surface of a liquid are easily vaporized, while molecules deep within the liquid require more energy. The most common way to add energy to initiate a phase transition from liquid to vapor is to add heat. Under conditions of constant pressure, the temperature at which a liquid enters the vapor phase is called the boiling point, where bubbles of saturated vapor rise to the surface and leave (Dorsch and Dorsch 2008). The boiling point remains constant until the phase transition from liquid to gas is complete. Therefore, the boiling point of a liquid is the temperature at which its saturated vapor pressure is equal to the atmospheric

Veterinary Anesthetic and Monitoring Equipment, First Edition. Edited by Kristen G. Cooley and Rebecca A. Johnson.
© 2018 John Wiley & Sons, Inc. Published 2018 by John Wiley & Sons, Inc.

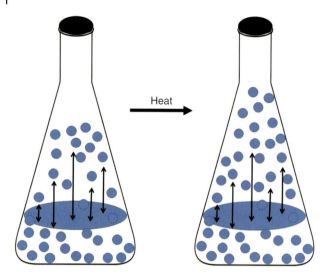

Figure 5.1 An agent's saturated vapor pressure is the pressure exerted by the gas when the number of molecules are leaving and entering the liquid anesthetic phase. Heat will shift this equilibrium and cause more molecules to enter the vapor, increasing the saturated vapor pressure (illustration courtesy of Dr Rebecca Johnson, University of Wisconsin-Madison, WI).

pressure and thus, boiling point varies with deviations in atmospheric pressure.

5.2.4 Partial Pressure

Partial pressure is a portion of the total pressure from any single gas in a mixture. For example, $P_{total} = P_1 + P_2 + P_3$ ..., where P represents pressure (Dorsch and Dorsch 2008). Partial pressures depend only on the temperature of the agent and are unaffected by the total pressure above the liquid. The highest partial pressure that can be exerted by a gas at a certain temperature is its vapor pressure.

5.2.5 Volume Percent

Volume percent is defined as the volume of anesthetic vapor per 100 volumes of total gas (Dorsch and Dorsch 2008). The relationship between volume percent and partial pressure is governed by Dalton's Law, which states that in a mixture of non-reacting gases, the total pressure is equal to the sum of the partial pressures of each gas. Therefore, volume percent = partial pressure/total pressure × 100. Volume percent reflects ratios of gas molecules in a mixture, whereas partial pressure reflects the absolute amount. Anesthetic potency is directly related to partial pressure, but only indirectly to volume percent.

5.2.6 Specific Heat and Thermal Conductivity

The specific heat is the amount of heat needed to raise the temperature of 1 g of a substance by 1°C (Dorsch and

Dorsch 2008). Kelvin may also be used here, as the change from one degree to another degree is the same in Celsius and Kelvin. For example, °K = °C + 273, so °K1 – °K2 = °C1 + 273 – °C2 + 273 = °C1 – °C2. Substances with high specific heat require more energy to raise the temperature of a certain quantity of the substance. An agent's specific heat is taken into account when designing the vaporizer, to avoid heat conduction to the liquid anesthetic. Substances with both a high specific heat and high thermal conductivity are advantageous in vaporizer construction. Thermal conductivity is the measure of the speed with which heat flows through a substance. Thermal conductivity is highest in copper, aluminum (MRI compatible vaporizers), brass and steel (in that order), and hence are used in vaporizer fabrication.

5.3 Vaporizer Classification

Vaporizers are classified by many factors, including output regulation, method of vaporization, type of temperature compensation, circuit location, resistance to flow, and agent specificity (Hartsfield 2007).

5.3.1 Regulation of Vaporizer Output

Inhalational anesthesia was first attempted by using the "soporific sponge (sleep sponge)" soaked in "medicinal elixirs", such as opium, mandragora (mandrake), hemlock juice, and other substances, by the Salerno (Italy) school of medicine in the late twelfth century and by Ugo Borgognoni (Hugh of Lucca) in Italy in the thirteenth century (www.discoveriesinmedicine.com/A-An/anesthetics). The actual use of vaporizable substances came in 1846, when dentist William T.G. Morgan used his "Letheon" inhaler in a publicly attended ether-anesthetized surgery (Ford 1946). The amount of liquid anesthetic used was typically measured by how the patient responded or did not respond during anesthesia. The use of ether, and later chloroform, led to the evolution of various devices used for the vaporization of these liquids.

Current anesthetic vaporizers deliver reliable amounts of anesthetic gas factoring in the agent's vapor pressure, atmospheric pressure and changes in temperatures. Since most current inhalant agents have high saturated vapor pressures and can vaporize to clinically unsafe levels (e.g. sevoflurane at 20°C at atmospheric pressure of 760 mmHg with water vapor subtracted out is ~160 mmHg/(760–47) mmHg × 100 = ~22%). Current vaporizers are used to reduce this percentage to useful levels, by adjusting the gas that flows through a vaporization chamber (variable-bypass) or by adding a set amount of vapor directly to fresh gas flows (measured-flow) (Dorsch and Dorsch 2008).

5.3.1.1 Variable-Bypass

Most currently used mechanical (Tec-type, Dräger Vapor 19.1, etc.; multiple manufacturers) and electrical, central processor unit (CPU) controlled (Aladin Cassette, GE Healthcare, Madison, WI; Vetland EX3000 Electronic Veterinary Anesthesia Machine, Vetland Medical Sales and Services, LLC, Louisville, KY) vaporizers are variable-bypass, with a fully saturating vaporizing chamber. These vaporizers split the fresh, carrier gas entering the vaporizer into two streams. For example, as gas enters the vaporizer, a specific amount is directed over the vaporizing chamber to pick up vaporized inhalant. This mixture then re-combines with a subset of carrier gas that travels through the bypass chamber that avoids the vaporizing chamber, thus reducing the amount of inhalant delivered to the patient to safer levels (Figure 5.2). In mechanical vaporizers, the splitting ratio is adjusted manually, whereas in electrically driven systems, a CPU changes the ratio and alarms may be added. Changing the carrier gas flow rate through the vaporizer does not change the splitting ratio and does not change the final volume percent.

When the vaporizer dial is in the "off" position, the carrier gas only flows through the bypass chamber and does not enter the vaporizing chamber. A locking mechanism is frequently found on the dial control to ensure that the anesthetic chamber does not accidently get turned on if the dial is bumped (Figure 5.3). Once this safety mechanism is disengaged, the dial is readily turned to any setting on the vaporizer. Once it is turned to "off",

and the safety lock is engaged, the locking mechanism will need to be unlocked to turn the vaporizer on to deliver anesthesia through the vaporizer chamber.

5.3.1.2 Measured Flow

While variable-bypass systems split the fresh carrier gas flow, a measured flow system adds a separate stream of saturated vapor directly to the carrier gas flow (Figure 5.4). Early anesthetic vaporizers, such as the Copper Kettle (Figure 5.5) and other measured vaporizing systems (e.g. Verni-Trol), were used along with two separate flowmeters and calculations or pre-made charts (Figure 5.6); the modern Tec 6 evolved from these models.

The Verni-Trol and Copper Kettle are no longer manufactured and are not covered by the American Society for Testing and Materials (ASTM) guidelines (see below). In these vaporizers, the percentage of anesthetic delivered was determined by the temperature of the anesthetic agent (non-temperature compensated), the fresh gas flow (FGF), as well as the number on the vaporizer dial. As described by Guy-Lussac's Law, the pressure of a gas with fixed mass and volume is directly proportional to the gas's absolute temperature. Because of this, measured-flow vaporizer settings on these older units had to be adjusted if there was any change in the temperature of the constituent gases. This was necessary to maintain a constant and predictable rate of delivery. Additionally, as anesthetic agent vaporization occurred in these older systems, temperature decreased due to evaporation of liquid. Thereby, these vaporizers were

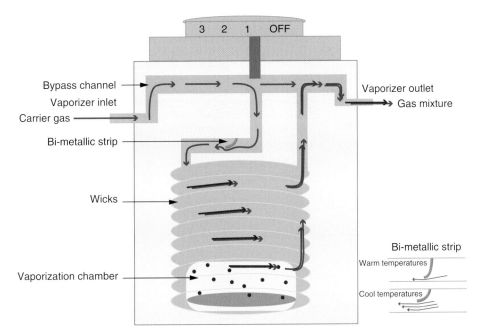

Figure 5.2 Schematic of a variable-bypass vaporizer. The carrier gas is split into two streams, one entering the bypass chamber and one diverted over into the vaporization chamber. This splitting ratio varies, depending on the dial setting. The bi-metallic strip also adjusts this ratio, depending on location and temperature. In this example, the bimetallic strip is located at the entrance to the vaporization chamber.

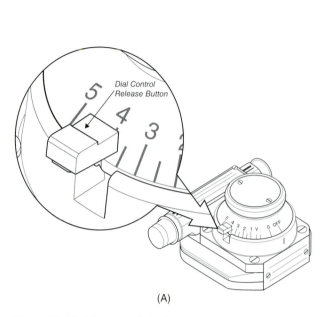

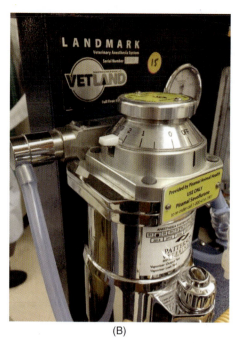

(A)
(B)

Figure 5.3 (A) Schematic of a locking mechanism on the vaporizer dial control (photograph courtesy of Midmark Corporation, Dayton, OH). (B) The locking mechanism (white knob) on a Tec-type sevoflurane vaporizer. The lock is upward, preventing the dial from turning in this position.

constructed of metal with high specific heat and thermal conductivity to help maintain the temperature in the vaporizer (e.g. copper for Copper Kettle or silicon bronze for Verni-Trol; Mosley 2015). For more detailed instructions in using these vaporizers, readers are directed to older textbooks and other reviews (Hartsfield 2007; Dorsch and Dorsch 2008; Dhulkhed *et al.* 2013).

One modern measured flow vaporizer is the Tec 6/Tec 6 Plus vaporizer for desflurane (Figure 5.7). It measures and adjusts the fresh carrier gas flow rate automatically. Since desflurane has an extremely high vapor pressure (~669 mmHg) and a low boiling point (23.5°C) at room temperature, it will periodically boil, which will greatly alter delivery. For example, while it is boiling, inhalant delivery will be increased; as it cools, vapor pressure decreases due to loss of latent heat of vaporization, which reduces desflu-

rane delivery (Boumphrey and Marshall 2011). The Tec 6 electrically heats desflurane to 39°C to stabilize temperature-dependent vaporization. The carrier gas is completely separate, the desflurane vapor is directly added to the fresh gas flow so that clinically useful, and economical flows can be used (Boumphrey and Marshall 2011).

5.3.2 Vaporization Method

The vaporization method includes the Flow-over, Bubble-through or Injection Vaporization methods.

5.3.2.1 Flow-Over Vaporizers
Flow-over methods utilize carrier gas to pass over the liquid anesthetic, which is subsequently vaporized (Dorsch and Dorsch 2008). This stream is completely diverted

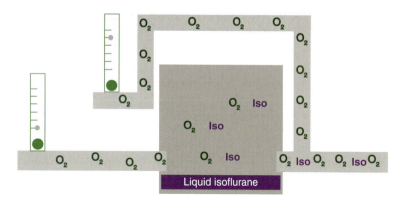

Figure 5.4 Schematic of a measured-flow vaporizer such as a Copper Kettle or Verni-Trol. Two separate flowmeters are used for the carrier gas stream and the stream passing over the liquid anesthetic which, in this example, is isoflurane (purple). The isoflurane vapor should be fully saturated and should combine with the carrier gas at the outlet.

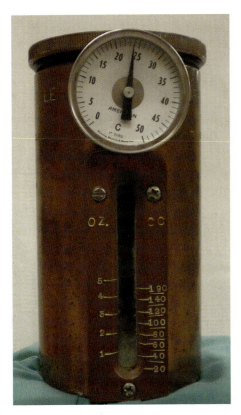

Figure 5.5 A Copper Kettle vaporizer with temperature gauge used to calculate the measured flows directed through the vaporizer.

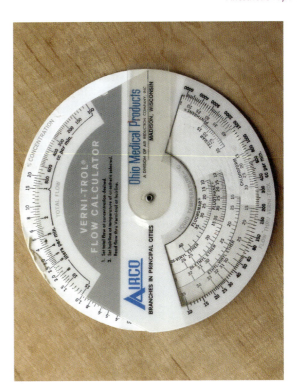

Figure 5.6 Example of a chart supplied by the manufacturer of a measured-flow vaporizer (Verni-Trol). The pressure, temperature and desired concentration are all considered when using these devices (photograph courtesy of Dr Rebecca Johnson, University of Wisconsin-Madison, WI).

through the vaporizing chamber (e.g. Ohio 8 Bottle) or is split to eventually combine with fresh gas to create the desired amount of anesthetic (e.g. Tec-type, Vapor 19.1, etc.). Usually, a wick is used to increase the surface area contacted by the carrier gas, thus improving the efficiency of vaporization (Figure 5.8). Wicks are constructed of cloth, Teflon or metal, consist of different shapes, and increase the surface area of the agent exposed to fresh gas. The flow-over technique is one of the most widely used vaporization methods in modern anesthesia.

5.3.2.2 Bubble-Through Vaporizers
Some vaporizers (e.g. Copper Kettle) use small bubbles as a way to increase the surface area of the liquid anesthetic. Instead of utilizing wicks, some of the fresh gas flow is bubbled through a porous disk of sintered material. The disc is submerged into the anesthetic agent and bubbles form when fresh gas is sent through the tiny holes. The tiny bubbles greatly improve the efficiency of the vaporizer, because of their large total surface area.

5.3.2.3 Injection Vaporizers
The injection method of vaporization distributes a known amount of liquid anesthetic or vapor into a known volume of fresh gas. to supply a precise concentration of

anesthesia to the patient (Dorsch and Dorsch 2008). For example, the Tec 6 vaporizer adds desflurane vapor directly to the fresh gas flow (Figures 5.7 and 5.9). A differential pressure transducer controls a variable resistance at the vaporizing chamber outflow to adjust concentration. In addition, the vaporizer dial provides a second variable resistance to precisely control output (Boumphrey and Marshall 2011).

Although somewhat different mechanistically, the Somnosuite® (Somnosuite® Low Flow Anesthesia System, Kent Scientific Corporation, Torrington, CT), a vaporizer specifically made for smaller mammals, also employs the technique of directly injecting liquid inhalant into the fresh gas flow; this allows use of minimal amounts of carrier gas and inhalant and reduces waste gas exposure (Figure 5.10).

5.3.3 Temperature Compensation

Vaporizers compensate for temperature fluctuations in two ways: either with automatic thermocompensation or through supplied heat (Dorsch and Dorsch 2008). Most commonly used vaporizers use metal jackets with high specific heat and thermal conductivity to provide a "heat sink", thereby allowing heat to move more rapidly

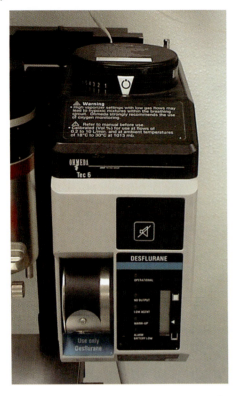

Figure 5.7 The Tec 6 vaporizer used with desflurane. It measures and adjusts the fresh gas flows automatically to deliver a clinically useful desflurane concentration (since its saturated vapor pressure is very high). It requires an electrically heated source to ensure steady levels of desflurane due to its low boiling point (photograph used with permission from Darci Palmer, Southeastern Veterinary Surgery Center, Columbus, GA,).

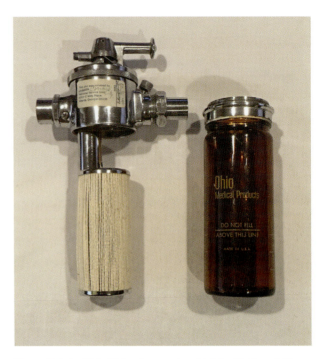

Figure 5.8 An Ohio #8 Bottle vaporizer (right) with the wicking mechanism removed (left). Wicks were used in these flow-over vaporizers to increase the surface area of vaporization in agents with low vapor pressures.

between the vaporizing chamber and environment (Hartsfield 2007). If the vaporizer contains a wick, it is important that the wick is in contact with the metal so that heat lost from vaporization can be replaced quickly. In addition, current vaporizers also compensate by automatic adjustment of the splitting ratio of the carrier gas. For example, the use of rods, cones or fluid-filled aneroid bellows provide thermocompensation by altering the bypass chamber output. As the temperature decreases, metal contracts and the bellows change shape, resulting in more resistance at the bypass channel or less resist-

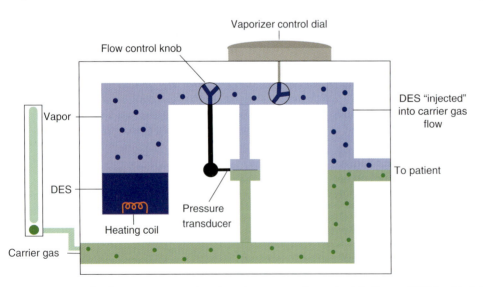

Figure 5.9 Example of an injection vaporizer. A precise amount of vaporized desflurane (DES) is added directly to the fresh gas flow, which is separate from the vaporizing chamber.

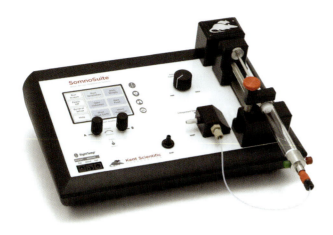

Figure 5.10 The Somnosuite® is specifically designed for small patients and is used to reduce the amount of fresh gas usage, inhalant and waste gas flows (photograph courtesy of Kent Scientific Corporation, Torrington, CT).

ance at the vaporizing chamber, thereby directing more carrier gas through the vaporizing chamber itself.

Tec-type vaporizers also use the bi-metallic strip (e.g. brass, steel) to change the splitting ratio. A bi-metallic strip consists of two metals with very different degrees of thermal expansion (the amount of heat needed to expand the metal). The metals are adhered together. When the temperature drops, one metal contracts far more than the other and the unit bends in one direction. In a vaporizer, the bi-metallic strip offers resistance to flow, although the placement within the vaporizer varies between types. For example, if it is located at the entrance to the vaporizing chamber (a common place in modern vaporizers), when the temperature of the vaporizing chamber drops, the strip bends and moves away. This reduces the resistance to flow and allows more gas into the vaporizing chamber (Figure 5.2).

The Tec 6/desflurane vaporizer uses supplied heat to provide thermocompensation (as discussed above) and the Aladin vaporizer has an electronically controlled heat source. As a result, they require a power source to function. Conversely, older vaporizers such as the Copper Kettle are manually adjusted for changes in temperature; these calculations are specified on their associated charts (Figure 5.6).

5.3.4 Circuit Placement and Agent Specificity

5.3.4.1 Vaporizer in Circuit (VIC)
Non-precision VICs, such as the Ohio #8 Bottle, were once commonly used in veterinary medicine. Because these vaporizers are jars with dials ± wicks, they were recommended for use with low potency anesthetics or anesthetic gases that have a low vapor pressure. They could be drained and cleaned for use with multiple inhalants. However, use of isoflurane or sevoflurane (with the potential to vaporize to concentrations >20% at room air and temperature) could lead to very high inhalant levels delivered to the patient if used with a VIC, especially if the wick is present to increase vaporization surface area.

VICs (Figure 5.11) are not thermocompensated or concentration-calibrated; their output changes directly with respiratory minute volume, positive pressure ventilation and room or vaporizer temperature and indirectly with fresh gas flow rate. The unpredictability of anesthetic output is difficult to gauge without the use of monitors for anesthetic concentration. Being able to respond to the change in anesthetic levels is important when monitoring patients on a VIC (Hartsfield 2007). Additional information pertaining to the use of these older vaporizers can be found in other textbooks (Hartsfield 2007).

5.3.4.2 Vaporizers Out of Circuit (VOC)
VOCs are located outside of the patient breathing circuit (Figure 5.12) and are commonly used in practice. They are thermocompensated, concentration-calibrated and are specific to a particular anesthetic agent. Although inhalants may have similar vapor pressures (enflurane

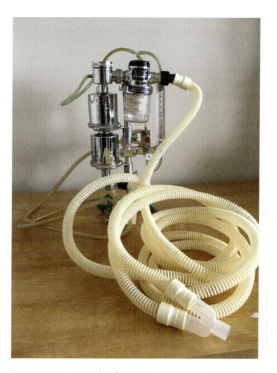

Figure 5.11 Example of an anesthetic machine (Stephens Anesthetic Machine, Eickemeyer, Stratford, Ontario, Canada) with a VIC (blue labels). The VIC sits between the inspiratory valve and the inspiratory limb of the Y-piece in this instance (photograph courtesy of Dr Rebecca Johnson, University of Wisconsin-Madison, WI).

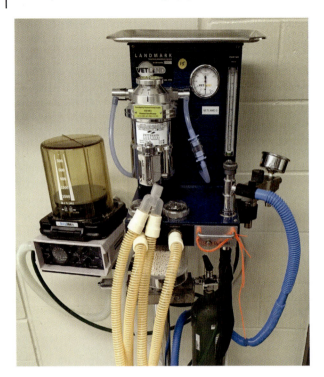

Figure 5.12 Example of an anesthetic machine with a VOC completely removed from the breathing system (photograph courtesy of Dr Rebecca Johnson, University of Wisconsin-Madison, WI).

and sevoflurane), these vaporizers must be drained and re-calibrated before inter-changing inhalants.

5.3.5 Flow Resistance

5.3.5.1 Draw-Over Vaporizers
The draw-over vaporizer is usually found within the breathing circuit and is uncommon in modern clinical practice. In these vaporizers, the patient's respiration is used to draw carrier gas through the vaporizer and as such, may be used in places where pressurized gas may not be attainable (e.g. field techniques). Their disadvantages have been discussed above (see VIC).

5.3.5.2 Plenum Vaporizers
Plenum vaporizers (also known as concentration-calibrated) rely on pressurized gas to flow through the vaporizer and carry the inhalant. As such, they have high internal resistance and must have a continuous supply of carrier gas. As described above, the proportion of carrier gas that is diverted through the vaporizing chamber determines the amount of inhalant delivered to the patient and relies on the vaporizer dial setting (Hartsfield 1999). The higher the vaporizer dial setting, the more carrier gas passes through the vaporizing chamber and the higher the percentage achieved at the vaporizer output. These include the Tec-type, Copper Kettle and Aladin vaporizers.

5.4 Other Factors Affecting Vaporizers

5.4.1 Carrier Gas Flow Rate

The fresh carrier gas flow rate can alter vaporizer output, especially in draw-over vaporizers. This is particularly seen at lower (<250 mL/min) and higher (>15 L/min) flow rates. At lower flow rates, the resistance of the splitting valve in some variable-bypass vaporizers directs more gas through the bypass chamber, decreasing the output. Similarly, at exceedingly high flow rates, full saturation at the vaporizer chamber is difficult to reach. Thus, vaporizers are less accurate at fresh gas flow extremes. However, at clinically useful flow rates, all modern vaporizers are more accurate.

5.4.2 Carrier Gas Type

The use of carrier gases, except when at 100%, slightly alter vaporizer output. For example, air and nitrous oxide are less viscous than 100% oxygen and differ in their densities. This affects the turbulence of carrier gas and may unequally change the resistance through the bypass and vaporization chambers, altering the splitting ratio and the vaporizer output (Palayiwa *et al.* 1983). For example, the splitting valve in variable-bypass and Tec 6 vaporizers decreases the gas flowing through the vaporizing chamber, resulting in decreased vaporizer output; this effect is likely not clinically significant (Graham 1994; Boumphrey and Marshall 2011).

5.4.3 Multiple Vaporizer Use

Vaporizers in series should have locking mechanisms that prevent more than one anesthetic vaporizer with different agents to be used simultaneously. If there is not a locking mechanism, the vaporizers should be placed in order of lowest to highest vapor pressure and potency to reduce chances of over-anesthetizing the patient. For example, if the vaporizer with the most volatile agent is downstream, this will reduce the risk of high concentrations of a volatile agent contaminating a vaporizer designed for an agent with a lower vapor pressure. Thus, the suggested order of placement would be methoxyflurane, sevoflurane, isoflurane and halothane. In addition, vaporizer outputs are additive and can lead to high inspired levels if more than one is engaged; if more than one vaporizer is turned on, vaporizer order is inconsequential.

5.4.4 Back-Pressure Compensation

Modern vaporizers utilize back-pressure compensation mechanisms, such as the Pumping Effect or the Pressurizing

Effect, to prevent increased or decreased anesthetic gas uptake. The "Pumping Effect", also known as the "Hill and Lowe Effect", especially occurs when there is less agent in the vaporizing chamber, at low carrier gas flows, when there is use of the oxygen flush valve, or during positive pressure ventilation when positive pressure is retrogradely transmitted to the outlet of the vaporizing chamber (Dorsch and Dorsch 2008). Two problems can occur:

1) carrier gas can be resaturated if the vaporizer is inefficient and did not result in 100% saturation during the first pass through; and
2) saturated gas is forced through the bypass inlet, resulting in increased inhalant levels (Boumphrey and Marshall 2011).

Mechanisms used to reduce this effect include increasing the length in the vaporizer inlet, one-way check valves near the vaporizer outlet (Keet *et al.* 1963), and a large bypass chamber compared to the size of vaporizing chamber (Dhulkhed *et al.* 2013).

The "Pressurizing Effect" mainly happens at high flows and low vaporizer settings and is due to compression of fresh gas in the vaporizing chamber (Dorsch and Dorsch 2008). The increased pressure at the vaporizer outlet will compress the carrier gas so there are more molecules per mL. However, the saturated vapor pressure does not change and the number of inhalant molecules does not increase. This results in inhalant dilution in the vaporizing chamber and reduced output concentration (Dhulkhed *et al.* 2013).

5.4.5 Barometric Pressure Changes with Altitude (Boumphrey and Marshall 2011)

Most vaporizers are calibrated at sea level (Gorelov 2005). Barometric pressure changes when the vaporizer is used at high altitude or in a hyperbaric chamber, which can affect performance. For example, although the effect of altitude minimally affects anesthetic potency as determined by the agent's partial pressure (Schreiber 1975), in those vaporizers where gas flow splitting occurs at the entrance to the vaporizing chamber, altitude may affect the output in terms of volume percent (Dhulkhed *et al.* 2013). Newer vaporizers, where the splitting occurs at the outlet of the vaporizing chamber, are less affected by barometric pressure. Specifically, an agent's saturated vapor pressure is unchanged by barometric pressure *per se* and the vaporizer output is also unaffected. However, the agent concentration (in volume percent) will change. As an example (Boumphrey and Marshall 2011), the change in agent concentration in the delivered fresh gas flow can be calculated by the following equation:

$$\%^{del} = \%^{cal} \times \left(P^{cal} / P^{atm} \right) \tag{5.1}$$

where $\%^{del}$ is the agent (in volume percent) actually delivered by the vaporizer; $\%^{cal}$ is the agent percent of vaporizer at the atmospheric pressure where the vaporizer was calibrated; P^{cal} is the agent's partial pressure where the vaporizer was calibrated; and P^{atm} is the partial pressure at the new altitude.

If the vaporizer is set to 3% at atmospheric pressure where the vaporizer was calibrated (101.3 kPa), then the agent's partial pressure = 3% of 101.3 kPa = 3.039 kPa.

If the vaporizer is kept at 3% but the altitude is increased and the atmospheric pressure decreases to 75 kPa, then

$$\%^{del} = 3 \times 101.3 / 75 = 4.052\% \tag{5.2}$$

The agent's partial pressure is still 4.052% of 75 kPa = 3.039 kPa.

Thus, within a hyperbaric chamber (high pressure), the percentage of agent delivered decreases. At high altitude (low pressure), the percentage of the agent delivered increases.

Altitude also decreases the temperature, an effect that varies with moisture content. This is termed the "lapse rate" (Boumphrey and Marshall 2011) and is 6.49°C per 1000 m from sea level until 11 000 m. Although this changes an agent's saturated vapor pressure, most vaporizers are temperature compensated and can be used in most conditions. Barometric pressure also alters the viscosity and density of carrier gases, which affects vaporizer output (Dorsch and Dorsch 2008).

An exception to these factors is the Tec 6 injection vaporizer that is not pressure compensated and the concentration delivered is constant in the fresh gas flow. Thus, the vaporizer setting must be increased to maintain the partial pressure of the agent at high altitude (Boumphrey and Marshall 2011).

5.4.6 Inhalants

Vaporizers are currently manufactured to be agent specific. The unique vapor pressures of each particular anesthetic agent require uniquely calibrated vaporizers; vaporizers cannot be used interchangeably. If a vaporizer meant for an agent with lower vapor pressure (sevoflurane) is mistakenly filled with an agent with higher vapor pressure (isoflurane), the vaporizer output will be higher than anticipated from the dial setting (Rose and McLarney 2014). Conversely, if an agent lower vapor pressure (sevoflurane) is placed into a vaporizer meant for an agent with higher vapor pressure (isoflurane), lower than expected concentrations will occur. When halothane was more readily available, isoflurane and halothane were frequently used in the same vaporizer due to their similarities in vapor pressure. However, halothane placed in an isoflurane vaporizer may produce less output, and isoflurane in a halothane vaporizer may produce more output than expected (Steffey *et al.* 1983; Dorsch and Dorsch 1994; Mosley 2015). Thus, manufacturers recommend against this practice, unless vaporizers are serviced and re-calibrated between agent use (Mosley 2015). Color coding of vaporizers is used as a safety feature to help ensure the incorrect agent is not used in a specific vaporizer. For example, in the US, halothane vaporizers are marked with red labels, isoflurane vaporizers have purple markings, and sevoflurane vaporizers have yellow signage.

5.5 Maintenance and Repair

Manufacturer's recommendations should always be followed for vaporizer care. Daily vaporizer care includes cleaning the external surfaces and re-filling with the appropriate anesthetic to be ready for the next procedure. When older agents such as methoxyflurane and halothane were being used, vaporizers were frequently drained and cleaned to reduce preservative build up. This may require servicing from a trained repair person. Consult the vaporizer equipment manual to learn proper removal and drainage methods for each specific vaporizer.

It is recommended that vaporizers be serviced approximately every 6 months to 1 year to replace worn parts and recalibrate if required; signage should be used to indicate the last servicing date. Some companies recommend less frequent servicing. Recalibration includes ensuring correct temperature compensation and potentially replacing the wicks in the unit (Hartsfield 1999).

5.5.1 Filling

Most vaporizers contain a window to view the amount of anesthetic within the unit and a fill line to indicate the appropriate fill amount. Care should be made to make sure that the vaporizer is not overfilled and that it is at least half-full at all times. Overfilling the vaporizer can result in anesthetic gas leaking into the system. This is less common in modern vaporizers, as they are designed to stop or minimize overfilling (Rose and McLarney 2014). A vaporizer that is more than half-empty could result in delivery of less gas to the patient (Hartsfield 2007).

Vaporizers have a filling port consisting of a screw cap funnel, a keyed filler port or a cassette sump (Hartsfield 2007). The screw cap funnel system is opened and the anesthetic liquid is poured into the vaporizer. Bottle adapters (Figure 5.13A) can be used to reduce the spillage of the liquid and to reduce the amount of waste anesthetic gas (WAG) that is vaporized into the environment and thereby the exposure to veterinary healthcare professionals (Hartsfield 2007).

The keyed filler port is useful to fill the vaporizer with the correct anesthetic gas and reduce waste anesthetic gases in the environment. The keyed adapter only fits into the vaporizer that is specific for that adapter and inadvertent filling with the incorrect agent is avoided (Figure 5.13A, B). Because the keyed filler port system is

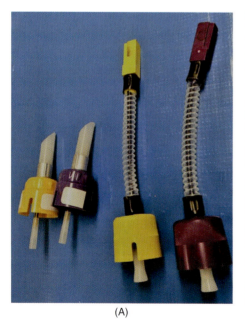
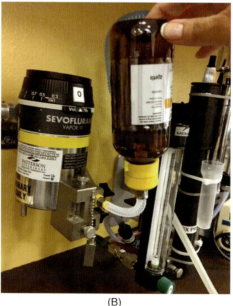

(A) (B)

Figure 5.13 (A) Bottle pour adapters and keyed adapters used to reduce waste gas exposure when vaporizers are filled. (B) Example of how keyed adapters only fit into the filler port specifically made for the agent in use.

completely enclosed, there is little to no WAGs contaminating the environment.

Cassette sumps are used on Aladin electric vaporizers for enflurane, halothane, isoflurane, sevoflurane or desflurane (Figure 5.14). Electricity warms or cools the liquid to maximize the vaporization point (desflurane is not heated), measures the liquid level. and the vaporizer or anesthetic machine provides an alarm when the liquid is low. Cassette sumps are easily placed into the anesthetic machine and reduce the WAGs to the environment (Eger and Weiskopf 2003).

Care should be taken when filling or moving most conventional vaporizers. If the vaporizer is overfilled or tipped, this could result in anesthetic agent in the bypass chamber and high concentrations of anesthesia the next time the machine is turned on. If overfilling or tipping occurs, it is recommended to drain the vaporizer, turn the vaporizer on and flush with a high flow of oxygen until no agent is in the machine. This can be confirmed with an anesthetic gas monitor if available (Rose and McLarney 2014).

5.6 Current Vaporizer Standards

An international standard covers human vaporizers (International Standards Organization 2004) and the American Society for Testing and Materials (ASTM 2000) has standard specifications for human anesthesia workstations (Dorsch and Dorsch 2008). No standards exist for veterinary institutions. However, these suggestions likely should be followed and include:

1) The variable effects in ambient temperature and pressure, tilting, back pressure, and input flow rate and gas mixture composition on output must be stated in the manufacturer's documents.

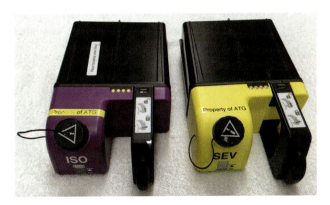

Figure 5.14 Cassette sumps/Aladin vaporizers used for isoflurane and sevoflurane (although they are made for many other agents as well). These vaporizers are electrically heated and are easily placed into the GE Aisys CS machine (photograph courtesy of Dr Rebecca Johnson, University of Wisconsin-Madison, WI).

2) The average delivered concentration shall not deviate from the set value by greater than ±20% or ±5% of the maximum setting, whichever is greater, without back pressure.

3) The average concentration delivered shall not deviate from the set value by more than +30% or −20%, or by more than +7.5% or −5% of the maximum setting, whichever is greater. Pressure fluctuations at the common gas outlet should be 2 kPa with a total gas flow of 2 L/min or 5 kPa with a total gas flow of 8 L/min.

4) A system that prevents gas from passing through the vaporizing chamber of one vaporizer and then through another must be present.

5) The vaporizer output shall be less than 0.05% if in the "OFF" or "zero" position.

6) All vaporizer control knobs must open counter clockwise.

7) Either the maximum/minimum filling levels or the actual useable volume and capacity shall be displayed.

8) The vaporizer must be designed so that it cannot be overfilled when in the normal operating position.

9) VOCs must have non-interchangeable proprietary or 23-mm fittings (15-mm and 22-mm fittings cannot be used). With 23-mm fittings, the inlet must be male and the outlet female. The direction of gas flow must be marked.

10) VICs must have standard 22-mm fittings or screw-threaded weight-bearing fittings with the inlet female and outlet male. The direction of gas flow must be indicated and the vaporizer marked "for use in the breathing system".

5.7 The Modern Vaporizer

The "ideal" vaporizer should have the following characteristics: output does not change with fresh gas flow, temperature and pressure, low internal resistance, lightweight, easy to use, economical, and corrosion-resistant. Current vaporizers have many properties, such as concentration-calibration, dial controlled, flow-over or injection, temperature compensated, agent specific, and out of circuit. In addition, many current vaporizers appear similar; however, they differ between manufacturers in structure, such as vaporization chamber size and mounting options. Readers are referred to their websites for precise details concerning each. Although many vaporizer properties have been discussed above, details associated with examples of specific vaporizer types are presented here. This list is not meant to be exhaustive, as other commercially available vaporizers may also be available.

5.8 Specific Vaporizers

5.8.1 Simple Vaporizers

Simple vaporizers include Ohio 8 Bottle, Stephen's Universal Vaporizer, etc. These vaporizers are constructed quite simply and were originally designed for agents with low vapor pressure for safety. They consist of a glass jar as a vaporizing chamber and a non-precision dial that controls the amount of carrier gas diverted to the vaporizing chamber (Figure 5.8). Some have wicks that aid in vaporization. With the recommended agents (low vapor pressures), carrier gas is rarely fully saturated when leaving the chamber. They are draw-over, non-temperature compensated and not concentration-calibrated. Because of their low internal resistance, they are used as VICs. Their main advantage is their low cost and potential use with multiple anesthetics; however, care must be used with agents with high vapor pressures.

5.8.2 Copper Kettle

The Copper Kettle vaporizer is a measured-flow, bubble-through, temperature compensated (manually), VOC and multipurpose vaporizer (Mosley 2015; Figure 5.5). It was the first precision vaporizer (1952) and was the basis for the modern Tec 6 vaporizer design (Morris 1952). The flow through the vaporizing chamber and the flow through the bypass chamber are measured and controlled separately; charts are used to calculate flows based on conditions and desired inhalant levels. It can accurately deliver methoxyflurane, halothane, isoflurane or sevoflurane. For more information concerning Copper Kettle or Verni-Trol vaporizers, the reader is referred to other sources (Hartsfield 2007; Dorsch and Dorsch 2008).

5.8.3 Tec 2

The Tec 2 (Ohmeda) halothane vaporizer (Dhulkhed *et al.* 2013) was the first agent-specific, precision vaporizer (Figure 5.15). It was of the variable bypass, flow-over with a wick, VOC, temperature compensated, plenum type, and the concentration was poorly calibrated. It had concentric wicks, and the dial, which had to be pulled out to turn, was located at the front. Unfortunately, its bi-metallic strip was located on the outlet side of the vaporizing chamber and the presence of the preservative thymol in halothane frequently caused the bi-metallic strip to stick. It also produced inaccurate concentrations at low flows (<4 L/min) and low dial settings.

5.8.4 Tec 3

The Tec 3 vaporizer was introduced in the 1960s, due to the problems with the Tec 2 with regards to thymol and

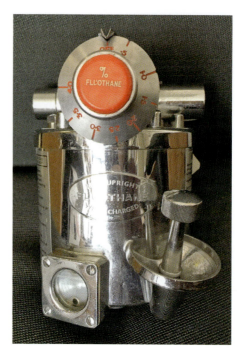

Figure 5.15 Tec 2 halothane vaporizer. These are rarely used in modern veterinary medicine. The dial is on the front of the vaporizer that requires the user to pull to turn (photograph courtesy of Dr Rebecca Johnson, University of Wisconsin-Madison, WI).

inaccurate inhalant delivery (Dhulkhed *et al.* 2013). It is agent-specific, precision, flow-over with wick, variable-bypass, temperature compensated, and VOC (Mosley 2015; Figure 5.16). The dial is on the top with a locking device. Its long carrier gas channel reduces the issues associated with back pressure. The bi-metallic strip is located concentrically within the vaporizing chamber, so is in close contact with the inhalant temperature, and the polytetrafluoroethylene coating helps to protect from direct contact with the thymol. In addition to reduced sensitivity to back pressure, this vaporizer is more accurate at low dial settings than the Tec 2. However, tipping to 180 degrees can alter output.

5.8.5 Tec 4

The Tec 4, designed in 1983 (Dhulkhed *et al.* 2013) for isoflurane only, is also agent-specific, precision, flow-over with wick, variable-bypass, temperature compensated, and VOC (Mosley 2015; Figure 5.17). The dial is on top and it has a safety interlocking mechanism with a release button. It was designed to attach to a back bar (Selectatec system), where different vaporizers could be selected for use and the carrier gas can bypass the "off" vaporizers directly through the Selectatec mount. In this vaporizer, tipping has minimal effect on output due to addition of a baffle system.

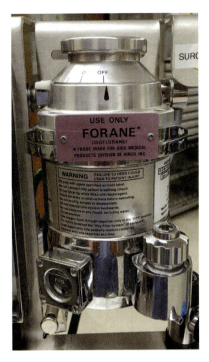

Figure 5.16 Tec 3 isoflurane vaporizer. It replaced the Tec 2 to improve output accuracy (photograph courtesy of Dr Rebecca Johnson, University of Wisconsin-Madison, WI).

5.8.6 Tec 5

The Tec 5 is a relatively common vaporizer in current veterinary medicine. It is also agent-specific, precision, flow-over, variable-bypass, temperature compensated, and VOC (Mosley 2015; Figure 5.18). It is made for many inhalants, including enflurane, halothane, isoflurane and sevoflurane. The control dial is on top and the release lever is on the back, with a safety interlock system so two vaporizers cannot be turned on at once. This vaporizer also uses the Selectatec system for carrier gas bypass (no gas enters the vaporizer in the "0" position) and is key or funnel filled. There is an internal baffle system, the bi-metallic strip is at the bottom in a separate bypass chamber (as temperature decreases, less gas goes through the bypass channel), and it has a spiral wick. However, it is more prone to the "Pumping Effect" than the Tec 4 and tilting can result in chamber overfilling.

5.8.7 Tec 6/Tec 6 Plus

The Tec 6/Tec 6 Plus vaporizer is uniquely suited for desflurane and is classified as measured-flow, electrical thermocompensated, agent-specific and back-pressure compensated (Mosley 2015). It also has an LCD display

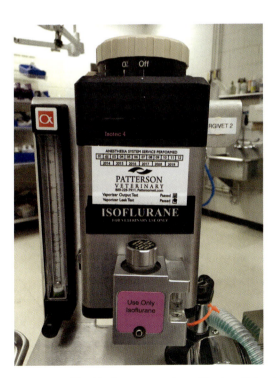

Figure 5.17 Tec 4 isoflurane vaporizer with a top dial and filler port/drain on the front. Note the use of signage detailing the last service date (photograph courtesy of Dr Rebecca Johnson, University of Wisconsin-Madison, WI).

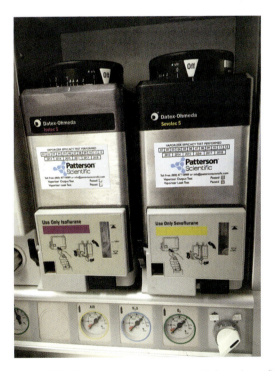

Figure 5.18 Side-by-side Tec 5 isoflurane (left) and sevoflurane (right) vaporizers. The dials are on the top and these examples are filled using a keyed system. When one is in use (the isoflurane vaporizer in this case), care should be taken that the second is turned off. The locking devices are white buttons on the dial labelled "off" (photograph courtesy of Dr Rebecca Johnson, University of Wisconsin-Madison, WI).

and requires electricity (with a battery backup), and the vaporizer will not turn on until internal checks are passed. It is a referred to as a "gas/vapor blender", because it injects desflurane vapor into the fresh gas flow (Figure 5.7). The fresh gas flow does not enter the vaporizing chamber, but the desflurane is introduced directly into the fresh gas. Because desflurane has a very high vapor pressure and boiling point (which is near room temperature), high fresh gas flows are required to dilute the vapor to a useable concentration and heat must constantly be supplied for steady output. Two mechanisms govern the release of desflurane into the gas flow, as mentioned above: i) the vaporizer setting; and ii) a valve and pressure transducer within the vaporizer. When the vaporizer is turned on, desflurane vapor moves to a pressure regulator to reduce the pressure to usable levels (10–20 cmH$_2$O; Mosley 2015). The vapor then travels to a restrictor controlled by the dial setting, where it joins the carrier gas (Mosley 2015). Its unique design also prevents desflurane from spilling into the fresh gas flow if tipped. The Tec 6 Plus has an LED screen and a large capacity (425 mL) to extend the use between refills.

5.8.8 Tec 7

The Tec 7 is the newest member of the Tec series (Figure 5.19). It is similar to the Tec 5 (agent-specific, precision, plenum type, variable-bypass, temperature compensated, and VOC). The concentration dial is on the top with

a rear locking mechanism and dial release lever. It is easy to operate and fill, and has fine dial calibrations and a spill-proof mechanism.

5.8.9 Dräger Vapor 19.1

The Dräger Vapor 19.1 vaporizer is similar to newer Tec types and is agent-specific, precision, flow-over, variable-bypass, temperature compensated, and VOC (Figure 5.20). It has a larger vaporizing chamber than the Tec 3 and Tec 4, so is frequently used in the large animal clinic (Mosley 2015). It is made for enflurane, halothane, isoflurane and sevoflurane. It employs a cone system controlled by the vaporizer dial to regulate vaporizer output. It does not have an outlet check valve, but relies on a tortuous inlet to protect from the "Pumping Effect". It should not be tipped by more than 45 degrees. Dräger also manufactures the D Vapor and the DIVA, which are measured-flow desflurane vaporizers, similar to the Tec 6 (Mosley 2015).

5.8.10 Penlon Sigma Delta

The Penlon Sigma Delta vaporizer is unique as the manufacturer (Penlon Limited, Ablingdon, UK) claims there is limited need for preventative maintenance (~10 years for non-halothane vaporizers). It is agent-specific, precision, flow-over with wick, variable-bypass, temperature

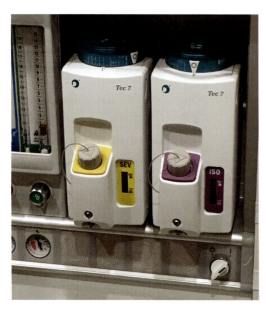

Figure 5.19 Side-by-side Tec 7 sevoflurane (left) and isoflurane (right) vaporizers on an MRI-compatible anesthetic machine. They are similar to the Tec 5 and easy to use (photograph courtesy of Dr Rebecca Johnson, University of Wisconsin-Madison, WI).

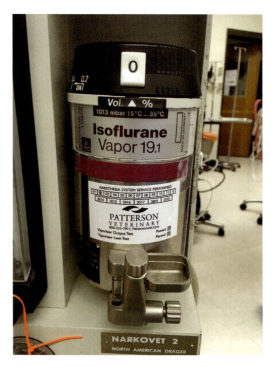

Figure 5.20 Dräger Vapor 19.1 isoflurane vaporizer (photograph courtesy of Dr Rebecca Johnson, University of Wisconsin-Madison, WI).

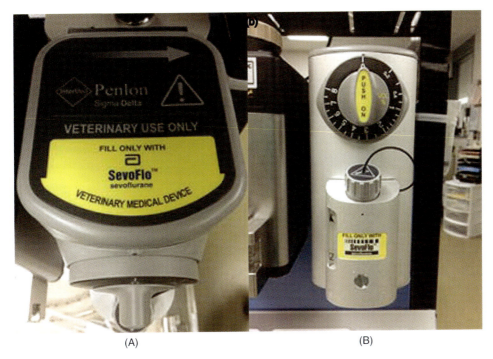

(A)   (B)

Figure 5.21 The top (A) and mounted (B) Sigma Delta vaporizer. The manufacturer suggests maintenance only every 10 years (non-halothane) or 5 years (if halothane is used) (photograph courtesy of Dr Erin Wendt-Hornickle, University of Minnesota, St Paul, MN).

compensated, and VOC (Mosley 2015) and can be made for enflurane, halothane, isoflurane and sevoflurane. The temperature-compensating element changes slowly, taking 1–2 hours to compensate for changes in room temperature (Mosley 2015). It is also lightweight with multiple mounting mechanisms and filling options available (Figure 5.21). Penlon also produces the Sigma Alpha vaporizer for desflurane.

5.8.11 Matrx™ VIP 3000®

The vaporizer MatrxTM VIP 3000® is similar to other modern vaporizers (agent specific, precision, plenum type, variable-bypass, temperature compensated, and VOC; Figure 5.22). They are commonly used in veterinary medicine and can be found through many distributors.

5.8.12 Ohio Calibrated Vaporizer

The Ohio Calibrated vaporizer was used for many years in veterinary medicine and can still be found in use (Figure 5.23). It is agent-specific, precision, flow-over with wick, variable-bypass, temperature-compensated, and VOC (Mosley 2015). It can be made for use with halothane, isoflurane and sevoflurane. The dial is on the top and tipping may increase output (Mosley 2015).

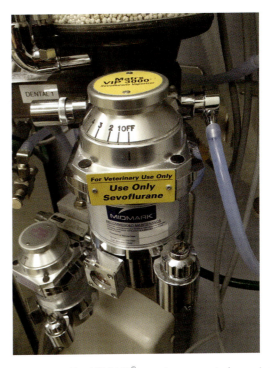

Figure 5.22 Two VIP 3000® vaporizers mounted on a single anesthetic machine. Either the isoflurane or sevoflurane vaporizer can be placed within the circuit using quick-connect adapters on the inlet and outlet; however, both cannot be connected simultaneously (photograph courtesy of Dr Rebecca Johnson, University of Wisconsin-Madison, WI).

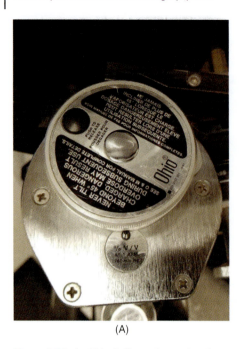
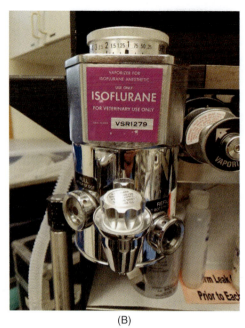

(A) (B)

Figure 5.23 An Ohio Calibrated vaporizer for use with isoflurane. The dial is located on the top (A) and has two viewing ports for the inhalant level within the vaporization chamber (B) (photograph courtesy of Dr Rebecca Johnson, University of Wisconsin-Madison, WI).

5.8.13 Aladin Cassette

The Aladin Cassette is a unique vaporizer made for use in newer GE Healthcare machines (Aisys CS, GE Healthcare, Madison, WI; Figure 5.14). It contains an anesthetic-specific vaporizing chamber and a central processing unit (CPU). Each cassette is magnetically coded for its agent to allow the machine to recognize which agent is in use. It incorporates both a variable-bypass and measured flow techniques. A throttle valve controls the flow through the vaporizing chamber and saturation occurs through metal plates/lamellae used as wicks. The CPU measures temperature and pressure and adjusts the amount of agent added to the bypass. Inhalants are poured directly into cassettes, which are placed into slots within the anesthetic machine; tipping these is not an issue.

5.8.14 Vetland EX3000 Electronic Veterinary Anesthesia Machine and Harmony 5

The vaporizer in the Vetland EX3000 (Vetland Medical Sales and Services, LLC, Louisville, KY), used in this electronically driven machine, displays its output on a color touchscreen and incorporates internal monitors and alarms. It is a precision vaporizer, with temperature and pressure compensation and a flow range of 25 mL–4 L per minute. Both isoflurane and sevoflurane vaporizers are internally incorporated into the machine and it has backup battery power (Figure 5.24). The manufacturer states the vaporizers are calibrated for life, but still recommends

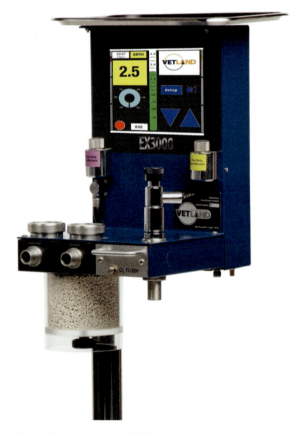

Figure 5.24 The Vetland XC300 Electronic Small Animal Anesthesia System. All parts, including the vaporizers, are electrically driven. Multiple safety features and alarms are incorporated into the machine. The newly introduced Harmony 5 also has pulse oximetry and capnography capabilities (photograph courtesy of Vetland Medical Sales & Services, LLC, Louisville, KY).

verification of output periodically. In addition, the Harmony 5 Anesthetic Machine is similar to the EX3000, but also incorporates capnometry and pulse oximetry.

5.9 Summary

Modern vaporizers have many advantages over older devices, such as precise agent delivery and compensation for changes in temperature and pressure. Although vaporizer design has progressed over the last few years, the newest vaporizers (Tec 6, Tec 7, Aladin, EX3000) are remarkably easy to use and have advanced anesthetic delivery systems.

References

Boumphrey, S. and Marshall, N. (2011) Understanding vaporizers. *Contin Ed Anesth Crit Care Pain*, 11, 199–203.

Davis, P.D. and Kenny, G.N.C. (2007a) The gas laws. In: *Basic Physics and Measurement in Anaesthesia*, 5th ed. Edinburgh, UK: Butterworth Heinemann, pp. 47, 109.

Davis, P.D. and Kenny, G.N.C. (2007b) Heat capacity and latent heat. In: *Basic Physics and Measurement in Anaesthesia*, 5th ed. Edinburgh, UK: Butterworth Heinemann, pp. 109.

Dhulkhed, V., Shetti, A., Naik, S. and Dhulkhed, P. (2013) Vapourisers: physical principles and classification. *Indian J Anaesth*, 57, 455–463.

Dorsch, J.A. and Dorsch, S.E. (1994) The anesthesia machine. In: *Understanding Anesthesia Equipment: Construction, Care, and Complications*, 3rd ed. Baltimore: Williams & Wilkins.

Dorsch, J.A. and Dorsch, S.E. (2008) Vaporizers (anesthetic agent delivery devices). In: *Understanding Anesthesia Equipment*, 5th ed. Philadelphia, PA: Williams & Wilkins, pp. 121–181.

Eger, E. and Weiskopf, R.B. (2003) Vaporization and delivery of potent inhaled anesthetics. In: Eger, E.I. II, Eisenkraft, J.B., Weiskopf, R.B. (eds). *The Pharmacology of Inhaled Anesthetics*. New Providence, NJ: Baxter Healthcare Corporation, pp. 204–208.

Ford, W.W. (1946) Ether inhalers in early use. *N Engl J Med*, 234, 713–726.

Gorelov, V. (2005) Calibration of vapourisers. *Anaesthesia*, 60, 420.

Graham, S.G. (1994) The desflurane Tec 6 vaporizer. *Br J Anaesth*, 72, 470–473.

Hartsfield, S.M. (1999) Anesthesia equipment. In: Paddleford, R.R. (ed.). *Manual of Small Animal Anesthesia*, 2nd ed. Philadelphia, PA: W.B. Saunders Company, pp. 92–97.

Hartsfield, S.M. (2007) Anesthetic machines and breathing systems. In: Tranquilli, T.G., Thurmon, J.C., Grimm, K.A. (eds) *Lumb and Jones' Veterinary Anesthesia*, 4th ed. IA: Blackwell Publishing, pp. 462–475.

Keet, J.E, Valentine, G.W. and Riccio, J.S. (1963) An arrangement to prevent pressure effect on the vernitrol vapourizer. *Anesthesiology*, 24, 734–737.

Morris, L.E. (1952) A new vapourizer for liquid anesthetic agents. *Anesthesiology*, 13, 587–593.

Mosley, C.A. (2015) Anesthesia equipment. In: Grimm, K.A., Lamont, L.A., Tranquilli, W..J, Greene and S.A., Robertson, S.A. (eds) *Veterinary Anesthesia and Analgesia: The Fifth Edition of Lumb and Jones*. Ames, IA: Wiley-Blackwell, pp. 44–51.

Palayiwa, E., Sanderson, M.H. and Hahn, C.E. (1983) Effects of carrier gas composition on the output of six anaesthetic vaporizers. *Br J Anaesth*, 55, 1025–1038.

Rose, G. and McLarney, J.T. (2014) Vaporizers. In: *Anesthesia Equipment Simplified*. New York: McGraw Hill Education, pp. 45–60.

Schreiber, P.J. (1975) Effects of barometric pressure on anesthetic equipment. *Audio Digest (Anesthesiol)*, 17, 14.

Steffey, E.P, Woliner, M.J. and Howland, D. (1983) Accuracy of isoflurane delivery by halothane specific vaporizers. *Am J Vet Res*, 44: 1072–1078.

6

Anesthetic Ventilators

Katrina Lafferty

Wisconsin National Primate Research Center, University of Wisconsin, Madison, Wisconsin, USA

6.1 Introduction

In order to successfully and appropriately ventilate veterinary patients, physiological and anatomical parameters need to be understood. There are many texts discussing the physiological and anatomical components of ventilation; this chapter will focus on the physical components of mechanical ventilation. It is not standard to have small animal ventilators outside academic veterinary institutions or veterinary specialty hospitals, but with the continuing decrease in cost and further demands from clients for better-quality patient care, many veterinary practices are adding mechanical ventilators to their equipment list.

6.2 Ventilator Function in the Breathing Circuit

The mechanical ventilator serves as an automated substitute for the reservoir bag in the breathing system, with its own advantages and disadvantages (Table 6.1). The usage of a mechanical ventilator can allow for a better regulation of respiration and administration of inhalant gases. The ventilator will deliver a set number of breaths, of a set volume and pressure. The ventilator can free up the anesthetist, allowing for more time to be spent dealing with other aspects of anesthetic care (Amaranth and Botros 1980). As positive as that all seems, mechanical ventilation does come with a few warnings. Use of a mechanical ventilator removes a level of contact between patient and anesthetist. The "squeeze" of the reservoir bag is no longer utilized as a subjective way to consider alterations in lung compliance or monitor respiratory actions via bag movement. The ventilator is often seen as a "set it and forget it" piece of equipment and vigilance in

monitoring respirations may be decreased (Marks *et al.* 1989).

The vast majority of commercially available ventilators use a bellows-in-a-box design. The bellows, which resemble an accordion and replaces the reservoir bag during mechanical ventilation, sit inside a box that is attached to an electrical unit with dials for setting various respiratory parameters (Figures 6.1 and 6.2).

The breath delivered by the ventilator has four stages:

1) inspiratory flow;
2) inspiratory pause;
3) expiratory flow; and
4) expiratory pause.

Gases only move into and out of the patient during the stages of flow; there is no movement during the stages of pause. During inspiration, driving gas fills the housing and compresses the bellows, forcing anesthetic gases through the breathing system and into the patient. While in expiration, the interior of the bellows fill with expired and fresh gases and re-inflate (Del Valle and Hecker 1995).

6.3 Tidal Volume Delivery

Tidal volume is the amount of air that moves in and out of the respiratory system during a full breath (inhalation and exhalation). Standard values for small animal anesthetic patients are between 7 and 15 mL/kg. When setting tidal volumes on a mechanical ventilator, recommended settings are up to 20 mL/kg (Johnson 2007). During mechanical ventilation, there are a number of elements that can affect the actual delivered tidal volume, such as changes in fresh gas flows and system and equipment leaks.

Veterinary Anesthetic and Monitoring Equipment, First Edition. Edited by Kristen G. Cooley and Rebecca A. Johnson.
© 2018 John Wiley & Sons, Inc. Published 2018 by John Wiley & Sons, Inc.

Table 6.1 Advantages and disadvantages of mechanical ventilation.

Advantages	Disadvantages
Frees hands of anesthetist for other monitoring	Loss of physical contact between patient and anesthetist
Decreases "fatigue" from continuous manual breaths	May be difficult to recognize ventilator malfunctions
Delivers more consistent inhalant anesthetic gases	Requires expensive specialized equipment and training
Delivers more even respiratory rate and volume	Changes in venous return and potential hypotension
	Possibility for barotrauma, volutrauma, atelectrama, etc.
	May be difficult to clean

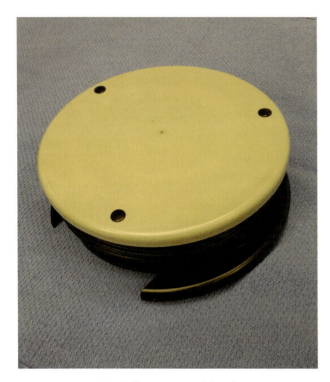

Figure 6.1 Ascending bellows, separated from housing unit. During expiration, they will rise; however, when not connected to a patient, they are collapsed.

6.3.1 Fresh Gas Flow

In some older model ventilators, turning up the fresh gas flow may cause a subsequent increase in tidal volume delivered and an increase in delivered system pressure during inspiration. The increase in volume and pressure delivered is particularly relevant in neonatal, pediatric, or very small patients managed with a mechanical ventilator. Newer model ventilators utilize designs with fresh gas compensation to prevent delivery of excess volume and/or pressure (Gravenstein *et al.* 1987).

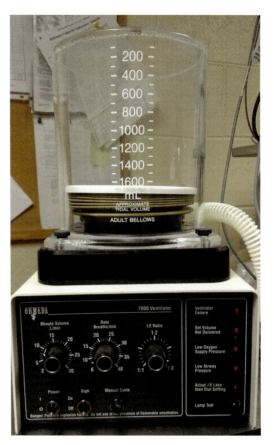

Figure 6.2 Ascending bellows within housing unit. They are collapsed and not attached to a patient.

6.3.2 System and Equipment Leaks

Leaks within the breathing system can lead to a decrease in tidal volume delivered. Common sites for tidal volume loss include:

- inappropriately sized, underinflated or leaking endotracheal tube cuff;
- use of laryngeal mask airway (LMA) with a mechanical ventilator;
- a hole or incomplete connection in breathing hoses;
- open adjustable pressure limiting (APL) valve;
- a crack or hole in sidestream capnometer sampling line; and
- use of sidestream capnometer with pediatric or very small patient (Gravenstein *et al.* 1987)

6.4 Driving Gas

The driving source for the mechanical ventilator can be electrically powered, pneumatically powered, or pneumatically powered with electric control. Currently available ventilators tend to fall into the last category. Electrically powered mechanical ventilators will require a wall outlet or battery pack to provide power to the internal motor that drives the unit. Electrically powered ventilators do not require a separate gas source to drive the bellows; however, in the event of an electrical failure, the ventilator will not run without a battery pack. Pneumatically powered ventilators rely on a high-pressure gas source to complete the bellows action. The driving gas can be oxygen, compressed medical air, or a mixture of the two. From an economic standpoint, it is less expensive to use medical air or a mixture as the driving gas. Pneumatically driven ventilators utilize an internal pressure-reducing valve to downgrade compressed gas pressures from a typical 50-psi gas source (Kacmarek *et al.* 2016).

6.5 Bellows Construction

As previously mentioned, bellows are frequently an accordion style device that can collapse on inspiration or expiration, depending on the style of construction. The bellows will attach either to the top or the bottom of the housing unit. There are three types of bellows: ascending, descending and piston.

6.5.1 Ascending Bellows

Most ventilators designed post-1985 have an ascending bellows style. Ascending bellows are also referred to as floating bellows, upright bellows or standing bellows. Ascending describes the way the bellows are moving during expiration. The bellows move upward during the expiratory phase of the breathing cycle. The bellows attach to the bottom of the housing unit; compression occurs during inspiration and expansion occurs during expiration (Figure 6.3). Ascending bellows style units allow for easier detection of system leaks or disconnection; any leak within the ventilator or breathing system will appear as an inability of the bellows to rise to the top of the housing unit (Grogono and Travis 1993). Ascending bellows will completely collapse during complete disconnection; the ventilator will continue to deliver small tidal volumes, even with disconnection (Gravenstein and Nederstigt 1990).

6.5.2 Descending Bellows

In a descending bellows unit, the bellows are attached to the top of the housing unit. The bellows will descend, or fall toward the bottom during expiration. Descending bellows are also called hanging bellows. Descending bellows have fallen out of favor in the last few decades owing to some safety issues. With hanging bellows style ventilators, it can be difficult to detect leaks or disconnections.

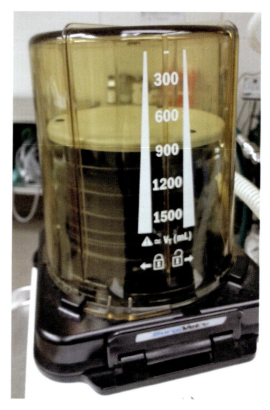

Figure 6.3 Ascending bellows at mid-point of expiration. When the patient fully expires, the bellows will be at the top of the housing unit.

The bellows will continue to fill with driving gas, and gravity will pull in room air with incomplete disconnections. Descending bellows also collect humidity within the bellows that adds weight to the system and may lessen tidal volume delivered to the patient (Sinclair and van Bergen 1992) (Figures 6.4 and 6.5).

6.5.3 Piston-Driven

Piston-driven ventilators are the least common of the three styles of ventilator bellows, but are taking up increasing market space. Piston ventilators use an electric motor to fire the piston and drive a precisely set tidal volume to the patient. The piston itself is of a fixed size; the distance the piston moves determines the volume delivered to the patient (Figure 6.6). All the pieces in the ventilator are rigid and the ventilator delivers an exact volume each time. The piston-driven ventilators tend to be quiet; the piston motion is electrically powered so there is no need for a driving gas source. Many models have a piston that is hidden from view that takes away the comfort in seeing the bellows moving. It can be difficult to hear the cycling sound made by the piston-driven ventilators and harder to detect auditory

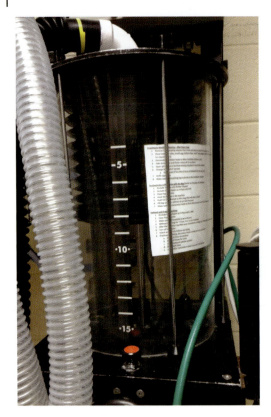

Figure 6.4 Dräger large animal ventilator with descending bellows. Bellows are hanging at approximately 8 L.

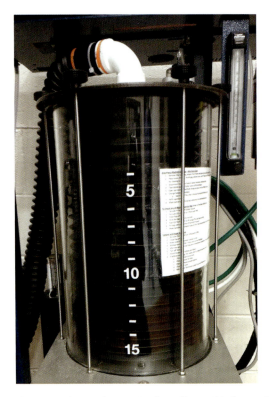

Figure 6.5 Dräger large animal ventilator with descending bellows. Bellows are completely distended.

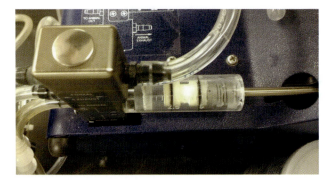

Figure 6.6 Harvard 683 piston driven small animal ventilator (Harvard Apparatus, Holliston, MA).

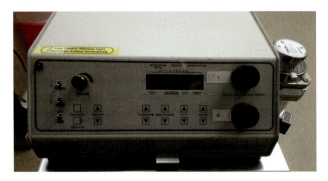

Figure 6.7 Engler ADS1000 piston driven small animal ventilator (Vetland Medical Sales and Services, Louisville, KY).

indicators of a disconnection or patient-ventilator asynchrony. The anesthetist must rely more heavily on patient cues and anesthetic monitors to notice machine malfunctions (Bachiller *et al.* 2008) (Figure 6.7).

6.6 Pressure Limiting Controls

Ventilators have a design structure created to modulate inspiratory pressure. As with anesthetic machines, driving gas flow entering the ventilator unit is at a pressure well above safety standards. Without regulation, too high an inspiratory flow may cause barotrauma. The pressure-limiting mechanisms have many names: pressure-limiting valve, driving gas pressure-relief valve, inspiratory pressure limit, adjustable pressure relief valve, etc. (Figure 6.8). The names will vary depending on the model, but most mechanisms will have "pressure-limiting" or "pressure-relief" in the descriptive title. The mechanisms are adjustable and may be a source for human error. When setting the pressure limiting controls, a pressure volume set too low will lead to inadequate ventilator drive. A volume set too high may lead to damaging airway pressure (Pan and van der Aa 1995).

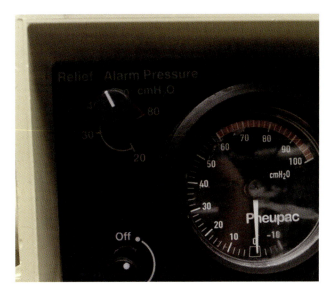

Figure 6.8 Pressure limiting valve on a Surgivet Pneupac ventilator (Smiths Medical, Dublin, OH), which is a safety device to alert personnel to high pressures within the system.

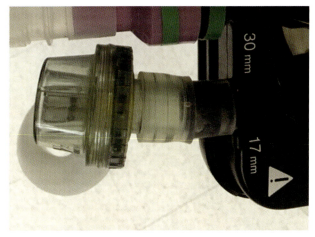

Figure 6.9 Exhaust valve on a Surgivet portable monitor (Smiths Medical, Dublin, OH) that vents the driving gas.

6.7 Gas Pressure Alarm

Some higher-end ventilators come equipped with a gas pressure alarm, also called a low-pressure alarm. This alarm is designed to alert the anesthetist if the driving system pressure has dropped below a sufficient force to move the bellows. The required function pressure will vary, depending on the ventilator type, with a typical minimum pressure requirement of 35 psi (Lawrence 1988). The required functional pressure may limit the use of additional equipment such as an oxygen concentrator or in-circuit humidifier, as the driving pressure may not be adequate for the function.

6.8 Exhaust Valve

The exhaust valve (also called the exhalation valve, ventilator relief valve, or bellows control valve) is a component of bellows-driven ventilators. It is located outside the ventilator-housing unit, but opens into the bellows unit (Figure 6.9). The exhaust valve closes during inspiration to allow for correct system pressure. During expiration the bellows refill and expand, pushing the driving gas through the now open exhaust valve and into the atmosphere. The function of the exhaust valve in mechanical ventilation is essentially the opposite of venting during manual ventilation. During mechanical ventilation, excess pressure and gas is vented during expiration; during manual ventilation, excess pressure

and gas is vented during inspiration (through the APL-valve) (Rajnish and Srinivasan 2013).

6.9 Spill Valve

During mechanical ventilation, the APL-valve is separated from the breathing system. A spill valve (also called vent valve, dump valve, or ventilator relief valve) exists to move excess respiratory system gases through to the scavenging system and essentially takes the function of the APL-valve (Figure 6.10). Specifically in ascending bellows design, the spill valve has a minimal opening pressure of 2–4 cmH$_2$O. This is designed to allow bellows to fill during expiration without venting through the spill valve. However, the translation is that ascending-style ventilators have 2–4 cmH$_2$O of positive-end expiratory pressure (PEEP) inherent within the system (Andrews 1989).

6.10 Ventilator Hose Connection or Ventilator Hose Switch

All bellows-driven ventilators require a way to switch the positive-pressure reservoir source from the reservoir bag to the bellows unit. Older and more economical models usually have a hose that connects the ventilator to the reservoir bag port (Figure 6.11). The hose is a standard 22-mm male conical fitting that is universal. Newer or more high-end ventilator models may have internal connections between ventilator and breathing system (Figure 6.12). Switching between the two is as simple as flipping a switch or lever to initiate or terminate mechanical ventilation (Caplan *et al.* 1997).

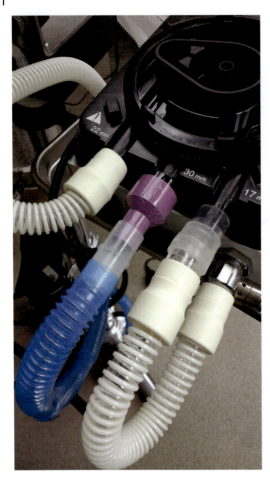

Figure 6.10 Spill valve on a Surgivet SAV 2500 (Smiths Medical, Dublin, OH). The spill valve is identifiable by the purple connector and blue scavenge hose, and vents gas within the breathing system.

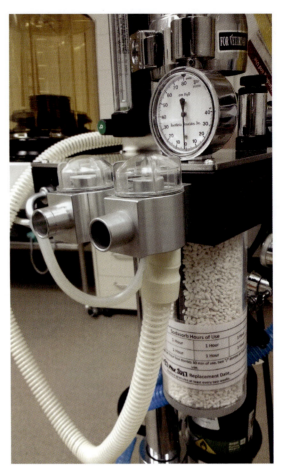

Figure 6.11 Ventilator hose connected to rebreathing bag connector to supply mechanical ventilation to the breathing system.

6.11 Ventilation Modes

Some ventilator models offer a variety of ventilatory modes. Modes can be divided into two primary categories: controlled or assisted. The most common modes are volume-controlled ventilation (VCV), pressure-controlled ventilation (PCV), synchronized intermittent mandatory ventilation (SIMV), and pressure-support ventilation (PSV). Volume-driven ventilation is available on all commercial ventilators, and pressure-driven ventilation is common. Intermittent- and supportive-ventilation modes are more common in high-end or critical care ventilators.

6.11.1 Volume-Controlled Ventilation (VCV)

Volume-controlled ventilation (VCV) is also described as tidal volume preset, volume preset or volume constant. This is the most commonly used ventilator mode and is available on essentially every bellows-driven

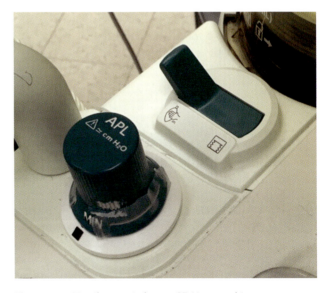

Figure 6.12 Ventilator switch on a GE Aisys machine (GE Healthcare, Madison, WI), which switches between manual and mechanical ventilation techniques.

mechanical ventilator. In VCV, the tidal volume is selected, or the minute volume and respiratory rate are set to be delivered to the patient (Gravenstein and Nederstigt 1990). Volume driven ventilation delivers a constant flow until the set volume is reached, independent of patient drive. The end airway pressure resulting from the delivered volume is dependent on the compliance and resistance of the breathing system as well as the patient. Using the pressure-limiting control prevents excessive inspiratory pressure and resultant barotrauma (Pan and van der Aa 1995).

6.11.2 Pressure-Controlled Ventilation (PCV)

Pressure-Controlled ventilation (PCV) is also called pressure-limited or lung-protective. This type of ventilation delivers a variable volume determined by the preset pressure limit. The tidal volume will change with each breath, dependent on patient resistance/compliance or a patient "bucking" the ventilator (patient-ventilator asynchrony) (Tung and Morgan 2002). Inspiratory pressure is set to avoid atelectasis or barotrauma and is often the mode of choice for critical patients (Cadi *et al.* 2008). Flow is delivered in a "decelerating flow pattern". Inspiratory flow is highest at the beginning of inspiration. When resistance is met, flow will decrease slightly and be maintained through the rest of the inspiratory period. Anesthesia ventilators using PCV use a preset I:E ratio (inspiratory:expiratory relationship); increase in respiratory rate leads to a decrease tidal volume (Tung and Morgan 2002). PCV is useful for situations where there is an airway leak or when utilizing a laryngeal mask airway (LMA). It can only be applied to situations with small leaks; larger leaks will prevent the ventilator from reaching the preset pressure and will lead to an excessive inspiratory time (Ward *et al.* 2016).

6.11.3 Synchronized Intermittent Mandatory Ventilation (SIMV)

Synchronized intermittent mandatory ventilation (SIMV) delivers automated breaths at a set rate, but also allows spontaneous patient ventilation that occurs interspersed between mechanical breaths. The spontaneous breaths draw gas from a secondary source to allow for controlled inhalant inspiration. The secondary source is derived either from a continual gas flow within the ventilator circuit, or a separate demand valve allowing gas to enter from a reservoir. The continual flow method does not change the effort of patient ventilation, but does utilize a much higher volume of fresh gas (Wood *et al.* 2017). The demand valve is the reverse, when fresh gas flow usage is more economical but inspiratory work is greatly increased. SIMV is often used as a method to wean a patient from the

mechanical ventilator, allowing for a low number of mechanical breaths (Ramos-Navarro *et al.* 2016).

6.11.4 Pressure-Support Ventilation (PSV)

The pressure-support ventilation (PSV) is also known as pressure-assisted or assisted spontaneous ventilation. This ventilation mode is a support system for patients that are spontaneously ventilating, just not in a fully sustainable way. When a patient initiates a breath, PSV will respond by supplementing with a positive pressure breath. This method of ventilation will only work with patients exhibiting a regular respiratory pattern. If a patient becomes apneic, PSV will not initiate any supportive breaths. Some ventilators are equipped with a "back up" rate and will shift to a controlled form of ventilation in the face of an apneic patient. In using PSV, a spontaneous breath baseline pressure is preset and once that pressure is reached the ventilator will initiate. The inspiratory trigger pressure is usually set between 5 and 10 cmH$_2$O and is set so that it will respond to inspiratory pressure with appropriate expectations for each patient. Tidal volume is calculated by considering the amount of pressure support, lung compliance and patient ability/effort. PSV can ultimately decrease the respiratory work and effort by the patient and is often useful in a critical care setting (Nicholson *et al.* 2017).

6.12 Cleaning and Sterilization

Overall, the ventilator unit can be disassembled and sanitized as needed, following cases where contamination is a concern. Each ventilator will have different requirements for steam autoclavability and gas sterilization. It is advisable to consult the individual equipment manual in preparation for sanitization.

6.13 Pressure Checking

Before each case, the anesthetic ventilator should go through a full machine check, just as an anesthesia machine should be checked completely before each use. The following are generally applicable notes for pressure checking of ascending and descending bellows ventilators. Please refer to the manufacturer's manual for additional information.

6.13.1 Pressure Check for Ascending Bellows Ventilator:

- Switch the machine over to the ventilator per the specific machine requirements.

- Attach rebreathing hoses.
- Occlude Y-piece.
- Turn on oxygen flow until bellows have completely filled and are touching the top of the bellows housing.
- Turn off the oxygen flow while maintaining complete occlusion of the Y-piece.
- If the system is complete and free from leaks, the bellows will remain upright.
- If the bellows begin to fall, there is a leak in the system.

6.13.2 Pressure Check for Descending Bellows Ventilator:

- Switch the machine over to the ventilator per the specific machine requirements.
- Attach rebreathing hoses.
- Plug in ventilator if required.
- Turn on the ventilator and allow it to fire once.
- IMMEDIATELY after the ventilator has fired, completely occlude the Y-piece.
- The bellows should be hanging; if they begin to fall, it means there is a leak in the system.

6.13.3 Areas of Common Leaks:

- Check hose connections.
- Check hoses for holes/tears.
- Confirm APL is closed (if this is required of the unit).
- Check anesthesia machine for leaks (inspiratory/expiratory valves, carbon-dioxide absorbent canister).
- Check that bellows housing unit is assembled correctly and closed.

6.14 General Concerns and Troubleshooting

As with any piece of anesthesia equipment, mechanical failure is a real concern. The most common issues with a mechanical ventilator include hypoventilation, hyperventilation, excessive airway pressure, loss of electrical power, and alarm failure. Once comfortable, ventilators are easy to use, but can lead to a false sense of patient security.

6.14.1 Breathing Circuit Disconnections

Breathing circuit disconnection is consistently one of the most common causes of a critical situation during anesthesia (Cooper *et al.* 1984). Ventilators have many fail-safe mechanisms to alert the anesthetist to a disconnection. Pneumatic and electric pressure monitors exist in newer model machines to alert to a decrease in system pressure and/or volume (Slee and Pavlin 1988).

6.14.2 Hypoventilation

6.14.2.1 Ventilator Failure

The ventilator is an inanimate, electronic device that is subject to failure. Loss of power can occur and is more of an issue if battery backup is not available. As with all electronics, there is also a risk of internal dysfunction. There have been reports of very high fresh gas flows causing the bellows to freeze (Wong and Li 2005). The anesthetist should remain aware when turning the ventilator on or off. In situations where the ventilator has been turned off for a moment during circuit disconnection, etc. the anesthetist should remain mindful and turn it on again. Cessation of the ventilator will result in hypoventilation in patients completely dependent on mechanical ventilation. Incorrectly seated or assembled bellows can lead to a leak in the ventilator system. Disconnections or misaligned bellows housings can occur during cleaning and reassembly or during transport and inadvertent impact (Feeley and Bancroft 1982).

6.14.2.2 Incorrect Ventilator Settings

It is easy enough to set a respiratory rate too low on the ventilator, or have a machine bumped during surgery or transit. Machine trouble-shooting should always include a rechecking of programmed ventilation parameters.

6.14.3 Hyperventilation

6.14.3.1 Rebreathing System and Ventilator Concerns

Incorrectly assembled bellows housing or a moderately size rent in the bellows material can lead to loss of driving gas. Driving gas escapes into the bellows housing and can cause excessive pressure during inspiration (Lampotang *et al.* 2005).

6.14.4 Incorrect Ventilator Settings

As noted under the hypoventilation section, if the ventilator is firing too often, include a check of ventilator settings as part of the trouble-shooting process.

6.14.5 Excessive Airway Pressure

Usage of the oxygen flush is generally discouraged when a patient is connected to the anesthesia circuit. During mechanical ventilation, airway pressure build-up can easily occur if care is not taken. The spill valve is designed to close during inspiration and with the APL valve closed as well, immediate and significant barotrauma from use of the flush valve is a real concern (Andrews 1989).

6.14.6 Alarm Failure

As with all machines, the ventilator is only as good as the anesthetist operating the machinery. Alarms exist to provide an early alert of impending problems and modern ventilator alarms are more sophisticated than ever before. However, alarms can fail or be confused by readings that range outside programmed algorithms. This is more common when using a non-veterinary specific ventilator on a veterinary patient.

6.15 Pediatric Ventilation

Pediatric ventilation is possible with the right type of ventilator and correct adapters. Historically, the concern with pediatric ventilation was regarding the large volume within the ventilator system and the potential for delivery of an excessive tidal volume and/or increased airway pressure. Many modern ventilators come with programmed settings that are suitable for very young patients (Figure 6.13) and many have pediatric-sized bellows available.

For very small or exotic patients, it is possible to ventilate through a non-rebreathing modified Mapleson-D

(Bain) circuit (Park *et al.* 1998). In order to ventilate using a non-rebreathing circuit, it is necessary to have a universal control arm to facilitate the mechanical ventilation (Figures 6.14 and 6.15).

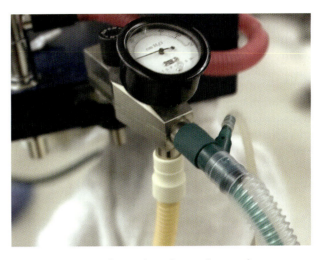

Figure 6.14 Universal control arm for attachment of a non-rebreathing system.

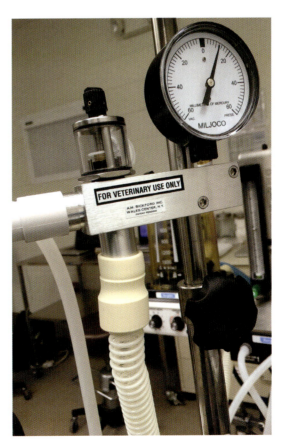

Figure 6.15 Universal control arm with a mechanical ventilator hose attached.

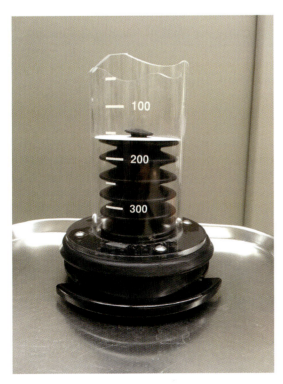

Figure 6.13 Pediatric bellows for use in small patients.

6.16 Basic Ventilator-Patient Set-up

Available ventilator settings will vary greatly between types of ventilators. However, there are a few basic tips to setting up a ventilator for a patient. In a perfect world, the anesthetist will be able to anticipate the likelihood of a patient requiring mechanical ventilation and can set up the ventilator beforehand. One method is to attach an appropriately-sized rebreathing bag to the end of the Y-pieces and set the ventilator to allow for reasonable inflation of the bag. Test lungs also exist that serve to function more closely to patient lungs. This method is not a foolproof method. Each patient will have differing pulmonary pathology and lung compliance. It is also reasonable to preset the ventilator using conservative settings and adjust based on the end-tidal carbon dioxide readings or blood gas analysis once the patient is connected.

6.17 Small Animal Mechanical Ventilators

There exists a wide variety of small animal ventilators available for use in veterinary medicine. What follows is a listing and description of the most common small animal ventilators on the market at the time of publishing. This list is not exhaustive but provides a good starting point for the practitioner looking to improve patient care with mechanical ventilation.

6.17.1 Hallowell EMC 2000 and 2002, Matrx 3000

The three listed ventilators are nearly interchangeable in description and the manufacturer's guide for the Hallowell EMC 2000 and Matrx 3000 are identical. In fact, the Matrx 3000 is the Hallowell EMC 2000, produced and sold by Matrx (Midmark Corporation, Dayton, OH). The Hallowell EMC 2002 is the replacement for the 2000. The 2000 is no longer produced, but is still prevalent in veterinary practice. The primary change in the Hallowell EMC 2002 is the addition of an inspiratory flow control. The inspiratory flow control allows finer tuning of the patient tidal volume. Features of the Hallowell EMC and Matrx ventilators include (Figure 6.16):

- time-cycled;
- ascending bellows;
- pneumatically driven, electronically controlled;
- pre-set I:E ratio of 1:2;
- 3 sets of varying sized bellows (0–300 mL, 300–1600 mL, 1600–3000 mL); and
- ability to deliver tidal volumes between 20 mL and 3 L.

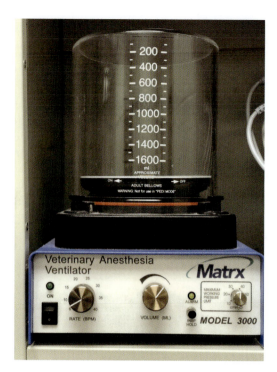

Figure 6.16 Matrx 3000 ventilator (Midmark Corporation, Dayton, OH). Only the tidal volume and respiratory rate can be manually changed; tidal volume is calculated based on those settings.

The control panel includes:

- on/off switch;
- respiratory rate dial;
- volume control dial (labeled inspiratory flow on the 2002);
- inspiratory hold button;
- maximum working pressure limit; and
- optional adjustable I:E ratio.

6.17.2 Surgivet SAV 2500

The Surgivet SAV 2500 (Smiths Medical, Dublin, OH) is a fairly accessible and easy-to-use ventilator. It has minimal controls but is satisfactory for most anesthetic cases (Figure 6.17). Features of the SAV 2500 ventilator include:

- time-cycled;
- ascending bellows;
- pneumatically driven, electronically controlled;
- 3 different sized bellows available (pediatric, adult, foal);
- manual breath button:
  - this feature is pneumatically controlled for power loss situations;
- optional universal ventilator mount to allow for portability.

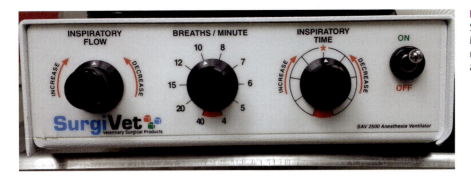

Figure 6.17 Control panel of a Surgivet 2500 ventilator (Smiths Medical, Dublin, OH). Inspiratory flow, respiratory rate and inspiratory time are dialed in.

The control panel includes:

- on/off switch;
- inspiratory flow;
- breaths/minute; and
- inspiratory time.

6.17.3 Surgivet 2550, Surgivet PneuPAC (VentiPAC, ParaPAC)

The Surgivet 2550 (Smiths Medical, Dublin, OH) is a small portable ventilator, similar to the SAV 2500 (Figure 6.18). The 2550 has the addition of a pressure manometer and additional controls to allow for more fine-tuning of the ventilator settings. This model can be used for short-term ICU ventilation when appropriate. Features of the Surgivet 2550 ventilator include:

- time-cycled;
- ascending bellows;
- pneumatically driven;
- optional universal ventilator mount to allow for portability;
- pressure manometer to display inflation pressures;
- pediatric and adult bellows;
- MRI conditional; and
- air mixture control:
  - allows for mixing of air as a driving gas to conserve oxygen supply.

The control panel includes:

- on/off switch;
- inspiratory time, adjustable from 0.5–3 seconds;
- expiratory time, adjustable from 0.5–6 seconds;
- flow control;
- pressure manometer;
- relief pressure control; and
- air mixture control.

6.17.4 DRE Bonair Mechanical Ventilator

Features of the DRE Bonair Mechanical Ventilator (DRE Veterinary, Avante Health Solutions, Deerfield, IL) include:

- time-cycled;
- ascending bellows;
- electronic;
- optional mount to allow for portability;
- adult and pediatric bellows; and
- pressure manometer to display inflation pressures.

The control panel includes:

- on/off switch;
- inspiratory time;
- expiratory time;
- flow control; and
- adjustable high and low pressure alarms.

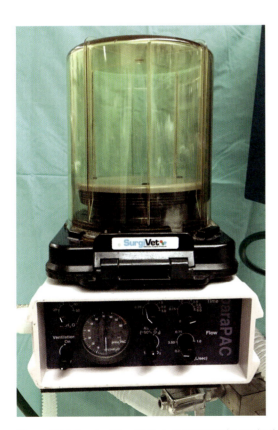

Figure 6.18 Surgivet ParaPAC ventilator (Smiths Medical, Dublin, OH). It has an ascending bellows and many adjustment knobs.

6.17.5   DRE Puma Mechanical Ventilator

Features of the DRE Puma Mechanical Ventilator (DRE Veterinary, Avante Health Solutions, Deerfield, IL) include:

- ascending bellows;
- electronically controlled pressure and volume;
- respiratory rates up to 120 breaths/minute;
- tidal volumes from 50 ml–1500 ml;
- adjustable I:E ratio from 10:1–1:10; and
- adult and pediatric bellows.

The control panel includes:

- LCD screen;
- breaths/minute;
- I:E ratio;
- pressure max/minimum;
- alarm silence; and
- ventilation modes.

6.17.6   DRE Ohio V5A Ventilator

The Ohio anesthesia ventilator (DRE Veterinary, Avante Health Solutions, Deerfield, IL) is an antiquated model that is no longer produced, nor is available commercially or as a refurbished product. However, this ventilator is still used in practice. Features of the Ohio anesthesia ventilator include:

- descending bellows;
- time-cycled;
- manual breath button; and
- tidal volume up to 1500 mL.

The control panel includes:

- on/off switch;
- low pressure alarm;
- expiratory flow rate;
- inspiratory flow dial;
- expiratory time;
- manual inspiration button;
- inspiratory pressure; and
- inspiratory pressure trigger.

6.17.7   GE Datex-Ohmeda Aisys Carestation

The GE Aisys (GE Healthcare, Madison, WI) is a combination of an Aisys workstation with an Ohmeda 7900 mechanical ventilator (Figure 6.19). The unit is largely digital, including ventilator controls, vaporizer settings and gas flow. The display includes spirometry and can give feedback on flow, volume and pressure loops. Features of the Aisys Mechanical Ventilator include:

- includes volume control, pressure control, SIMV and manual ventilation;

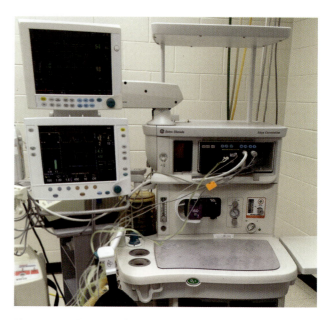

Figure 6.19 GE Datex Ohmeda Aisys Carestation (GE Healthcare, Madison, WI). The ventilator and physiologic monitoring systems are integrated into the machine.

- ascending bellows;
- electronically controlled pressure and volume;
- respiratory rates up to 100 breaths/minute;
- tidal volume of 20 ml–1500 ml; and
- adjustable inspiratory time from 2:1–1:8.

6.17.8   Datascope Anestar

The Datascope Anestar (Mindray North America, Redmond, WA) is another workstation with an anesthesia machine and integrated ventilator (Figure 6.20). This is the only small animal anesthesia machine that utilizes descending, or hanging, bellows. The Anestar control unit has an LCD screen with controls below the on-screen indicators. Features of the Datascope Anestar Ventilator include:

- descending bellows;
- electronically controlled pressure and volume;
- respiratory rates up to 60 breaths/minute;
- tidal volumes from 40 mL–1400 mL;
- adjustable I:E ratio from 4:1–1:5;
- adjustable PEEP from 3–15 cmH$_2$O;
- multiple ventilation modes including pressure, volume and SIMV;
- battery back-up with 30 minutes' use; and
- heated breathing circuit (97 °F).

The control panel includes:

- LCD screen;
- tidal volume;
- respiratory rate;

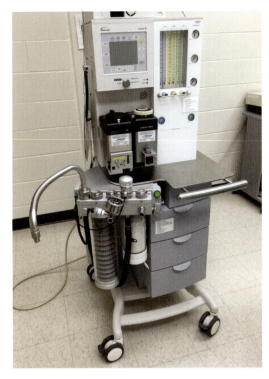

Figure 6.20 Datascope Anestar anesthesia machine and ventilator with descending bellows (Mindray North America, Redmond, WA).

- I:E ratio;
- PEEP;
- ventilator mode;
- peak pressure;
- mean pressure;
- minute volume;
- alarm silence; and
- ventilation modes.

6.17.9 Harvard Model 683 Small Animal Ventilator

The Harvard 683 ventilator (Harvard Apparatus, Holliston, MA) is a mainstay ventilator in research and exotic animal practices (Figure 6.21). The ventilator is piston driven and delivers exact tidal volumes of between 0.5 mL and 30 mL. Features of the Harvard Model 683 Small Animal Ventilator include:

- piston driven;
- two piston/cylinder assemblies, one for 0.5–3 ml tidal volumes, one for 3–30ml tidal volumes;
- able to ventilate patients as small as 0.25 kg;
- respiratory rates from 30–150 breaths/minute;
- electronic;
- optional mount to allow for portability;
- adult and pediatric bellows; and
- pressure manometer to display inflation pressures.

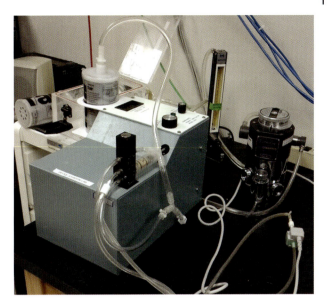

Figure 6.21 Harvard Small Animal Ventilator for use in rodents (Harvard Apparatus, Holliston, MA).

6.17.10 Engler ADS 1000/2000 Piston Ventilator

The Engler ADS (Vetland Medical Sales and Services, Louisville, KY) is a piston-driven microprocessor controlled ventilator (Figures 6.7 and 6.22). It can be used as a ventilation-only unit or have an anesthetic vaporizer mounted to create an anesthetic ventilator. Features of the Engler ADS 1000/2000 Piston Ventilator include:

- electronically controlled;
- internal battery back-up with up to 12 hours of operation; and
- toggle switch to allow for either "lab mode" ventilation of lab animal patients of less than 1 kg or "normal mode" ventilation of patients from 1–68 kgs.

The control panel includes:

- LCD screen;
- on/off switch;
- inspiratory and expiratory ports;
- volume control;
- weight button;
- flow rate buttons;
- breaths/min buttons;
- peak inspiratory pressure buttons; and
- assist buttons.

6.18 Large Animal Mechanical Ventilators

What follows is a listing and description of the most common large animal ventilators on the market at the time of publishing. There are not nearly as many large

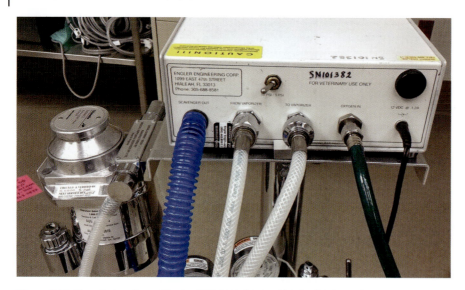

Figure 6.22 Rear-facing view of Engler ADS 1000 (Vetland Medical Sales and Services, Louisville, KY), showing connections and pressure toggle switch.

animal ventilators as small animal ventilators. It does not include every commercially available ventilator, but does have a wide sampling and can be used as a reference.

6.18.1 Vetland LAS 4000

The Vetland LAS 4000 (Vetland Medical Sales and Services, Louisville, KY) is the most current model of Vetland ventilator, but is similar to previously produced models (Figure 6.23). Features of the Vetland LAS 4000 include:

- descending bellows;
- volume preset and time-cycled;
- respiratory rates up to 99 breaths/minute;
- tidal volumes from 1 L–15 L; and
- adjustable I:E ratio from 1:1–1:8.

The control panel includes:

- on/off switch;
- tidal volume increase/decrease rocker switch;
- respiratory rate;
- I:E ratio;
- inspiratory flow gauge;
- inspiratory flow control dial; and
- oxygen flush valve.

6.18.2 Mallard Large Animal Ventilators

There are several models of the Mallard large animal ventilators (Mallard Medical, Redding, CA), the 2800, 2800B, 2800C and 800C-P (Figures 6.24 and 6.25). The models are similar in design and any differences should be

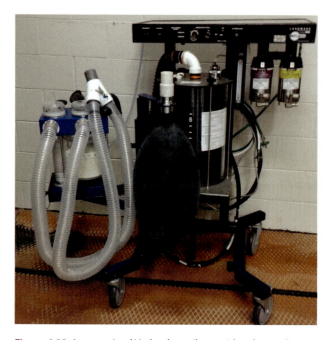

Figure 6.23 Large animal Vetland ventilator with a descending bellows (Vetland Medical Sales and Services, Louisville, KY).

explained in the specific model owner's guide. Features of the Mallard large animal ventilators include:

- ascending bellows;
- adjustable inspiratory flow 10–600 L/min;
- electronically controlled;
- electronically and pneumatically powered;
- 18–21 L bellows capacity;
- time-cycled;

- respiratory rate from 2–15 breaths/minute; and
- manual breath button.

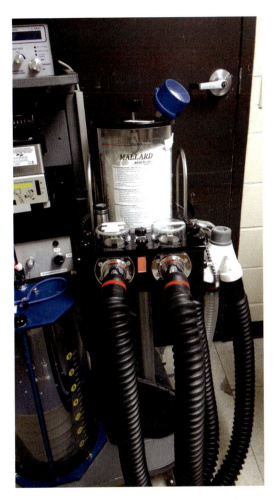

Figure 6.24 Bellows and vaporizer unit on a Mallard large animal ventilator (Mallard Medical, Redding, CA) with an ascending bellows.

The control panel includes:

- on/standby/off switch;
- respiratory rate;
- inspiratory flow control dial; and
- oxygen flush valve.

6.18.3 Dräger Ventilator

The Dräger large animal ventilator AV and AV-E are not currently in production but are still widely in use (Figure 6.26). Features of the Dräger large animal ventilators include:

- descending bellows;
- adjustable inspiratory flow 10–600 L/min;
- electronically controlled;
- electronically and pneumatically powered;
- manually altered tidal volume 4–16 L;
- time-cycled; and
- respiratory rate from 1–99 breaths/minute.

The control panel includes:

- on/off switch;
- respiratory rate dial;
- inspiratory flow dial;
- inspiratory flow gauge;
- I:E ratio dial; and
- oxygen flush valve.

6.18.4 Tafonius

The Tafonius (Hallowell EMC, Pittsfield, MA), nicknamed the "wind god", is a Hallowell EMC ventilator (Figures 6.27 and 6.28). It is the only available large

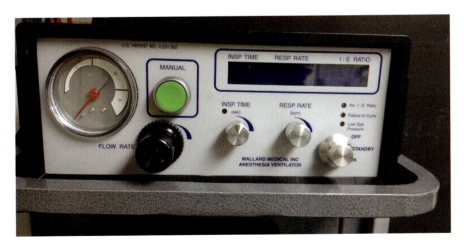

Figure 6.25 Close up of the control panel for the Mallard large animal ventilator (Mallard Medical, Redding, CA). Flow, inspiratory time and respiratory rate can be manually adjusted.

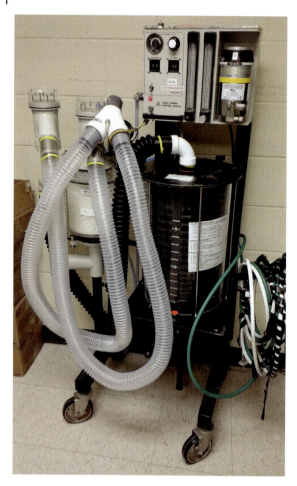

Figure 6.26 Dräger large animal ventilator. It is not currently manufactured, but many are still in use.

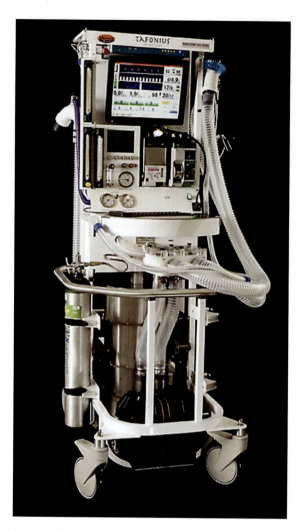

Figure 6.28 Tafonius large animal ventilator complete workstation (photograph courtesy of W. Stetson Hallowell, Hallowell EMC, Pittsfield, MA).

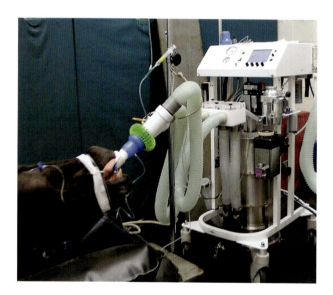

Figure 6.27 Tafonius Junior large animal ventilator that does not incorporate a multiparameter monitoring system used in an anesthetized horse (photograph courtesy of W. Stetson Hallowell, Hallowell EMC, Pittsfield, MA).

animal piston driven ventilator. The piston is driven by a linear actuator, similar to a hydraulic piston and is nearly silent when functioning. It does not require any driving gas. Features of the Tafonius large animal ventilator include:

- servomotor driven piston;
- adjustable inspiratory flow up to 1200 L/min;
- peak airway pressure of 80 cmH$_2$O; and
- tidal volume of 50 mL–20 L; and
- computer controlled ventilatory parameters.

6.18.5 Surgivet DHV 1000

Features of the Surgivet DHV 1000 large animal ventilator include (Smiths Medical, Dublin, OH include:

- descending bellows;
- adjustable inspiratory flow 10–600 L/min;
- pneumatically driven;
- electronically controlled;
- manually altered tidal volume 4–16 L;
- time-cycled; and
- manually adjustable tidal volume.

The control panel includes:

- on/off switch;
- respiratory rate dial;
- inspiratory flow dial;
- inspiratory flow gauge;
- inspiratory time dial; and
- manual breath button.

6.19 Conclusion

Adding a ventilator to a practice, or upgrading older model ventilators, is often a next step in the growing business trying to improve patient care. Mechanical ventilators on the surface can seem intimidating; there are so many switches, levers, hoses and buttons. However, with continued exposure and practice, an anesthetist can start to see the pattern of parts in all ventilators and can learn to use any ventilator with which they are faced. Their key is continued use of the ventilator and continuing attention to the assembly of the individual ventilator. While it is not currently an expectation for a practice to have a mechanical ventilator, a ventilator has the ability to act as a workhorse in terms of improving the quality of patient care and setting a practice above competitors.

References

Amaranth, L. and Botros, A.R. (1980) Circle absorber and soda lime contamination. *Anesth Analg*, 59, 711–712.

Andrews, J.J. (1989) Understanding your anaesthesia machine and ventilator. In: *Review Course and Lectures.* Cleveland, OH: International Anaesthesia Research Society, p. 59.

Bachiller, P.R., McDonough, J.M. and Feldman, J.M. (2008) Do new anesthesia ventilators deliver small tidal volumes accurately during volume-controlled ventilation? *Anesth Analg*, 1065, 1392–1400.

Cadi, P., Guenoun, T., Journois, D., Chevallier, J.M., Diehl, J.L. and Safran, D. (2008) Pressure-controlled ventilation improves oxygenation during laparoscopic obesity surgery compared with volume-controlled ventilation. *Br J Anaesth*, 100, 709–716.

Caplan, R.A., Vistica, M.F., Posner, K.L. and Cheney, F.W. (1997) Adverse anesthetic outcomes arising from gas delivery equipment: a closed claims analysis. *Anesthesiology*, 87, 741–748.

Cooper, J.B., Newbower, R.S. and Kitz, R.J. (1984) An analysis of major errors and equipment failures in anesthesia management: considerations for prevention and detection. *Anesthesiology*, 60, 34–42.

Del Valle, R.M. and Hecker, R.B. (1995) A review of ventilator modalities used in the intensive care unit. *Am J Anesth*, 22, 23–30.

Feeley, T.W. and Bancroft, M.L. (1982) Problems with mechanical ventilators. *Int Anesthesiol Clin*, 20, 83–93.

Gravenstein, J.S. and Nederstigt, J.A. (1990) Monitoring for disconnection: ventilators with bellows rising on expiration can deliver tidal volumes after disconnection. *J Clin Monit*, 6, 207–210.

Gravenstein, N., Banner, M.J. and McLaughlin, G. (1987) Tidal volume changes due to the interaction of anesthesia machine and anesthesia ventilator. *J Clin Monit*, 3, 187–190.

Grogono, A.W. and Travis, J.T. (1993) Anesthesia ventilators. In: *Anesthesia Equipment: Principle and Applications*, 3rd ed. St Louis, MO: Mosby, pp. 140–147.

Johnson, L.R. (2007) Respiratory physiology, diagnostics, and disease. *Vet Clin North Am*, 37, 829–1012.

Kacmarek, J.K., Robert, M. and Stoller, A. (2016) *In: Egan's Fundamentals of Respiratory Care, E-Book,* 1st ed. St Louis, MO: Heuer Elsevier Health Sciences, pp. 987–1015.

Lampotang, S., Sanchez, J.C., Chen, B. and Gravenstein, N. (2005) The effect of a bellows leak in an Ohmeda 7810 ventilator on room contamination, inspired oxygen, airway pressure, and tidal volume. *Anesth Analg*, 101, 151–154.

Lawrence, J.C. (1988) Breathing system gas pressure monitoring and venting, ventilator monitors and alarms. *Anaesth Intens Care*, 16, 38–40.

Marks, J.D., Schapera, A., Kraemer, R.W. and Katz, J.A. (1989) Pressure and flow limitations of anesthesia ventilators. *Anesthesiology*, 71, 403–408.

Nicholson, T.T., Smith, S.B., Siddique, T., Sufit, R., Ajroud-Driss, S. *et al.* (2017) Respiratory pattern and tidal volumes differ for pressure support and volume-assured pressure support in amyotrophic lateral sclerosis. *Ann Am Thorac Soc*, 14, 1139–1146.

Pan, P.H. and van der Aa, J.J. (1995) Positive end-expiratory pressure: effect on delivered tidal volume. *J Clin Anesth*, 7, 443–444.

Park, J.W., Chung, S.H., Choe, Y.K., Kim, Y.K., Shin, C.M. and Park, J.Y. (1998) Predictable normocapnia in controlled ventilation of infants with Jackson Rees or Bain system. *Anaesthesia*, 53, 1180–1184.

Rajnish, K.J. and Srinivasan, S. (201) Anaesthesia ventilators. *Indian J Anaesth*, 157, 525–532.

Ramos-Navarro, C., Sanchez-Luna, M., Sanz-López, E., Maderuelo-Rodrigues, E. and Zamora-Flores, E. (2016) Effectiveness of synchronized non-invasive ventilation to prevent intubation in preterm infants. *AJP Rep*, 6, 264–271.

Sinclair, A. and van Bergen, J. (1992) Flow resistance of coaxial breathing systems: Investigation of a circuit disconnect. *Can J Anaesth*, 39, 90–94.

Slee, T.A. and Pavlin, E.G. (1988) Failure of low pressure alarm associated with the use of a humidifier. *Anesthesiology*, 69, 791–793.

Tung, A. and Morgan, S.E. (2002) Modeling the effect of progressive endotracheal tube occlusion on tidal volume in pressure-control mode. *Anesth Analg*, 95, 192–197.

Ward, S.L., Quinn, C.M., Valentine, S.L., Sapru, A., Curley, M.A. *et al.* (2016) Poor adherence to lung-protective mechanical ventilation in pediatric acute respiratory distress syndrome. *Pediatr Crit Care Med*, 17, 917–923.

Wong, D.T. and Li, A.Q. (2005) Ventilator bellow standstill. *Can J Anaesth*, 52, 774–775.

Wood, S.M., Thurman, T.L., Holt, S.J., Bai, S., Heulitt, M.J. and Courtney, S.E. (2017) Effect of ventilator mode on patient-ventilator synchrony and work of breathing in neonatal pigs. *Pediatr Pulmonol*, 52, 922–928.

7

Humidification and Positive Pressure Equipment

Stephanie Keating[1] and Stuart Clark-Price[2]

[1] College of Veterinary Medicine, University of Illinois, Urbana, Illinois, USA
[2] College of Veterinary Medicine, Auburn University, Auburn, Alabama, USA

7.1 Humidification

7.1.1 Terminology and General Concepts

Humidity refers to the amount of water vapor present in gas and can be more specifically described in the following terms:

- *Absolute humidity*: The total mass of water vapor present in a given volume gas, typically expressed in mg H_2O/L or g H_2O/m^3.
- *Maximum humidity*: Also referred to as the *humidity at saturation*. The maximum mass of water vapor that can be present within a given volume of gas. This value is dependent on temperature; warmer temperatures increase the water-holding capacity of gas, and colder temperatures decrease it. Thus, gases saturated with water vapor at differing temperatures will differ in absolute humidity.
- *Relative humidity*: The percent ratio of water vapor in a given volume of gas in relation to the maximum water vapor capacity of the gas at a given temperature. It is the percentage of saturation.
- *Saturated vapor pressure*: The partial pressure exerted by water vapor in a gas mixture at the maximum humidity, expressed in mmHg.
- *Isothermic saturation boundary*: The location in the airway at which inspired gases reach core body temperature and become fully saturated with water vapor (100% relative humidity).

Examples of temperature effects on humidity levels are shown in Tables 7.1 and 7.2.

7.1.2 Physiologic Considerations

7.1.2.1 Anatomic Sites of Moisture Exchange

The nose and upper airways play a major role in heating and humidifying inspired gases. Mammalian nasal passages are tortuous, creating turbulent gas flow and increasing contact time with a large surface area of well-vascularized mucosa where heat and moisture exchange occurs. Passage of room air through the nose and nasopharynx increases the temperature from 22–32 °C and raises relative humidity from 30–100% (Rouadi *et al.* 1999). The bronchi and bronchioles play a lesser role in gas conditioning during regular ventilation (McFadden *et al.* 1985), but become increasingly important when nasopharyngeal heating and humidification mechanisms are bypassed with the placement of an endotracheal tube or supraglottic airway device (Dias *et al.* 2005).

7.1.2.2 Heat and Moisture Balance During Respiration

As unconditioned medical gas passes through the respiratory tract during inspiration, heat and moisture is absorbed from the mucosal surface of the airways, increasing the temperature and absolute humidity of the gas, while cooling and drying the respiratory mucosa. This process continues as inspired gas travels distally in the airways, until the gas composition stabilizes at core body temperature and becomes fully saturated with water vapor (100% relative humidity). This point is the isothermic saturation boundary (ISB). This gradient and the location of the ISB is dynamic, shifting over the course of a breath and with changes in fresh gas flow, tidal volume, inspired gas temperature and humidity, and different airway management techniques (Ingelstedt 1956; Déry 1973; McFadden *et al.* 1985; Dias *et al.* 2005). Delivering inspired gas between 32 and 34°C and 100% relative humidity has been recommended to maintain the ISB at an optimal location (Sottiaux 2006).

During expiration, the temperature of warm and humidified gas decreases as it moves back into the proximal airways. As the gas cools, the water content exceeds its holding capacity and condensation occurs, depositing water on to the surface of the airways. Condensation continues until a new equilibrium is reached, with the

Veterinary Anesthetic and Monitoring Equipment, First Edition. Edited by Kristen G. Cooley and Rebecca A. Johnson.
© 2018 John Wiley & Sons, Inc. Published 2018 by John Wiley & Sons, Inc.

Table 7.1 Saturated water vapor pressure (mmHg) and absolute humidity (mg H_2O/L) in water-saturated gas at different temperatures.

Temperature (°C)	Saturated vapor pressure (mmHg)	Absolute humidity (mg H_2O/L)
0	4.6	4.8
10	9.2	9.4
20	17.5	17.3
30	31.8	30.3
31	33.7	32.0
32	35.7	33.8
33	37.7	35.6
34	39.9	37.5
35	42.2	39.6
36	44.6	41.5
37	47.1	43.9
38	49.7	46.2
39	52.4	48.6
40	55.3	51.3

Table 7.2 Temperature and absolute humidity of gases during inhalation.

Location	Temperature (°C)	Absolute humidity (mg H_2O/L)
Room air	22	10
Larynx	31-33	26-32
Trachea	34	34-38
Main bronchi	37	44

Modified from Williams *et al.* 1996

expired gas remaining at 100% relative humidity, but with lower absolute humidity at a lower temperature. While this partially rehydrates the respiratory mucosa and minimizes water loss, expired gases contain more heat and moisture than inspired gases, resulting in a net loss for the patient (Cole 1953). In contrast, inspiring saturated gases warmer than body temperature would result in a decrease in gas temperature within the respiratory tract, causing water condensation within the airways during inspiration, with a net increase in airway temperature and moisture.

7.1.3   Clinical Implications of Inspired Gas Composition

7.1.3.1   Effects of Unconditioned Gases
Medical gases accessed through hospital pipelines are delivered at approximately room temperature (23°C)

and contain little moisture, with the relative humidity of medical air and oxygen at approximately 5.4 and 2.1%, respectively (Dawson *et al.* 2014). Dry gases maintain the integrity of the anesthesia machine, preventing the accumulation of water and corrosion of regulators and valves, and allow the delivery of high-inspired concentrations of the carrier gas; however, they also have the potential to disrupt physiologic functions. The effects of dry gas inhalation are greater when endotracheal tube or supraglottic airway devices are in place, a result of bypassing nasopharyngeal heating and humidification mechanisms (Dias *et al.* 2005).

Disruption of Respiratory Function   Changes in respiratory function begin rapidly, with an increase in mucus viscosity and a decrease in mucociliary clearance beginning after 10 minutes of breathing unconditioned medical gases (Sottiaux 2006). The onset and extent of physiological dysfunction depends on the temperature and humidity of the inspired gas, the character of ventilation, and duration of exposure (Noguchi *et al.* 1973; Fonkalsrud *et al.* 1975; Jiang *et al.* 2015). The adverse respiratory effects of unconditioned gases include:

- ciliary dyskinesia and complete paralysis of the muco-ciliary elevator (Hirsch *et al.* 1975);
- sloughing of the respiratory epithelium (Hirsch *et al.* 1975);
- increased mucus viscosity and mucus pooling, causing inspissation of small airways or endotracheal tube obstruction (Marfatia *et al.* 1975);
- increased surface tension and decreased surfactant production (Fonkalsrud *et al.* 1975);
- decreased pulmonary compliance and functional residual capacity (Noguchi *et al.* 1973);
- increased work of breathing (Rashad *et al.* 1967);
- bronchospasm (Fontanari *et al.* 1985); and
- inflammation (Jiang *et al.* 2015)

The resolution of these changes is variable and depends on the duration of exposure to non-humidified gases. While pulmonary mechanics return to normal within 24 hours of re-introducing humidified gases, inflammation worsens within 3 hours and damage to the respiratory epithelium, mucous glands and basement membrane may persist for weeks (Fonkalsrud *et al.* 1975; Hirsch *et al.* 1975; Marfatia *et al.* 1975).

Loss of Body Heat   Mucosal heat and moisture required to bring unconditioned inspired gases to body temperature and 100% relative humidity are partially lost during expiration. These must be replaced from systemic reserves, resulting in a progressive decrease in body temperature. Inhalation of warmed and humidified gases decreases the rate and extent of heat loss in experimental animals (Marfatia *et al.* 1975) and preserves body heat in human neonates and patients undergoing liver transplantation (Han *et al.* 2013; Meyer *et al.* 2015).

Loss of Body Water Body water is also lost during inspiration of unconditioned gases. For example, inhalation of dry gas for 6 hours resulted in a 2% decrease in body weight in rabbits during general anesthesia, reflecting evaporative fluid losses. This same loss was not observed when administered gases were fully humidified (Marfatia *et al.* 1975).

Desiccation of CO_2 Absorbent Administration of high flows of dry medical gases or use of a heat and moisture exchanger (HME) keep the moisture levels in the anesthesia machine low, contributing to the desiccation of CO_2 absorbent.

7.1.3.2 Effects of Excess Humidification
The prevention of heat and evaporative losses improves patient care. However, excessive heat and/or over-humidification can result in significant clinical adverse effects, similar to the administration of non-conditioned gases.

Disruption of Respiratory Function Inspiring warmed and over-humidified gases is as non-physiological as inspiring unconditioned medical gas. As warmed gas saturated with water vapor contacts the cooler surface of the respiratory mucosa, water condenses causing "rain out" within the respiratory tract. This increases the volume of respiratory secretions, causes ciliary damage and altered function, and results in the following sequelae:

- increased airway resistance (Cheney and Butler 1968);
- decreased functional residual capacity (Noguchi *et al.* 1973);
- altered surfactant function (Tsuda *et al.* 1977);
- atelectasis and increased intrapulmonary shunt fraction (Noguchi *et al.* 1973);
- arterial hypoxemia (Noguchi *et al.* 1973); and
- positive water balance (Lellouche *et al.* 2006).

Heat Gain If inspired gases are heated above body temperature and fully saturated with water vapor, evaporative cooling cannot take place within the respiratory tract (Walker *et al.* 1961). If other sources of heat loss are also reduced, overheating of patients may occur. This is possible with active humidification devices, but does not occur with passive methods of humidification (Hofmeister *et al.* 2011).

Dysfunction of the Anesthesia Circuit This increase in airway and circuit humidity can also have a negative impact on the function of the anesthesia machine. Condensation can cause incompetence of one-way valves, leading to the inspiration of expired gases. Condensed water can also accumulate within dependent parts of the breathing hoses, causing a reduction in the internal diameter of the hosing and increased resistance to airflow. Airway pressure and flow sensors may also be obstructed with condensed water, resulting in ventilator dysfunction.

Effects on Capnography Increased humidity can result in condensation on the infrared (IR) transmitting windows within a capnograph, increasing IR absorption. Condensation can also accumulate within the sampling lines of sidestream capnographs, reducing the partial pressure of water in sampled gases (Fletcher *et al.* 1983). Both of these changes will result in false elevations in CO_2 measurements. Additionally, sidestream sampling lines may become occluded with condensed water, preventing the sampling of patient gases.

7.1.4 Methods of Humidification

Humidification of the patient airway and breathing circuit can be performed either by passive or active methods. Passive methods work by reducing the rate of loss of airway water during anesthesia, whereas active methods work by introducing water into the breathing circuit or airway.

7.1.4.1 Passive Humidification
Heat and Moisture Exchangers Heat and moistures exchangers (HMEs) are the most frequently used humidification devices. The HME has a 15 mm and 22 mm connection port and is placed between the patient interface and the anesthesia circuit, acting as an "artificial nose" to passively heat and humidify patient gases. Each disposable unit is comprised of plastic housing surrounding an insert that captures and condenses water vapor. During exhalation, humidified gas from the patient condenses within the HME and is released back to the patient during inspiration, preserving moisture without the risk of over-humidification. Different materials have been used to act as the condensation element, including paper, cellulose and metalized polyurethane foam, as well as aluminum, ceramic or stainless steel fibers. Because the efficacy of humidification is dependent on the absolute humidity of expired gases and flow rates, HMEs are less effective in hypothermic patients, patients with large tidal volumes, and when leaks are present within the breathing system (Chikata *et al.* 2013). HMEs can be classified as either hydrophobic or hygroscopic (Figures 7.1 and 7.2), depending on the composition of the moisture retaining membrane.

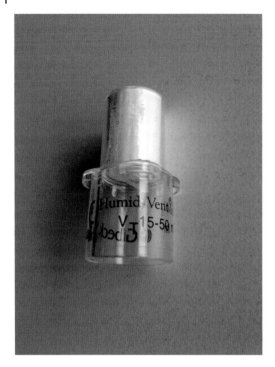

Figure 7.1 Hygroscopic and bacteriostatic heat and moisture exchanger (HME).

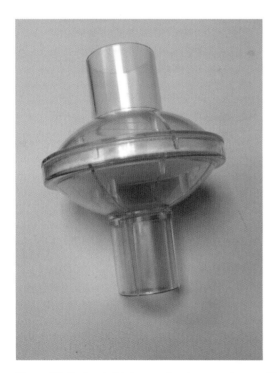

Figure 7.2 Hydrophobic heat and moisture exchanger (HME) with electrostatic bacterial and viral filter.

Hydrophobic membrane HMEs contain a water repellant condensing membrane to conserve water (Figure 7.1). The membrane is pleated to maximize sur-face area and contains small pores resulting in more effective viral and bacterial filtration than electrostatic filters (Wilkes *et al.* 2000), with 100% removal efficiency of mycobacterium (Vezina *et al.* 2004). While performance differs among hydrophobic HME models, generally they cause greater resistance to ventilation than hygroscopic HMEs, particularly when saturated (Lucato *et al.* 2005).

Hygroscopic membrane HMEs contain condensation materials such as wool, foam or paper-like material impregnated with hygroscopic salts, such as calcium chloride or lithium chloride, that have a chemical affinity for water and increase water retention (Figure 7.2). Additionally, bactericides may also be applied to the material. Filters can also be added to the HME, to create a heat and moisture exchanging filter (HMEF). Filter mechanisms may be similar to hydrophobic membrane HMEs that employ mechanical filtration with pleated sheets of densely arranged fibers, or may be electrostatic, using electrostatic charges with less densely arranged fibers. The advantages and disadvantages of HMEs are listed in Table 7.3.

Fresh CO₂ Absorbent Fresh CO_2 absorbent granules not only contain moisture, but also produce heat and water during the exothermic reaction that occurs when it is exposed to CO_2. As the CO_2 absorbent becomes exhausted, humidity within the system decreases (Strum and Eger 1994), and can be replenished by replacing the absorbent.

Low Fresh Gas Flow Rates The rate of fresh gas flow determines the amount of rebreathing and thus the amount of heat and moisture conserved from expired gases and CO_2 absorbent. The combination of low fresh

Table 7.3 Advantages and disadvantages of HMEs.

Advantages	Disadvantages
Inexpensive	Increases circuit dead space
Small and lightweight	Creates an additional site for circuit disconnection
Easy to use	Increases resistance and work of breathing when wet
Disposable	Potential for obstruction with fluids and secretions
Silent	Less effective humidification than active devices
Does not require a power source	Minimal preservation of heat
Filters bacterial and viral contaminants	Places weight on the endotracheal tube and circuit in small patients
Eliminates risk of over-humidification	
Prevents unwanted condensation within the anesthesia machine	Contributes to desiccation of CO_2 absorbent

gas flows with an HME increases the humidification efficacy of the HME further (Bicalho *et al.* 2014).

Coaxial Circuits The use of coaxial circuits theoretically preserves heat and moisture by allowing the inspired fresh gas to be exposed to the heat from expired gases in the surrounding expiratory limb. While coaxial circuits do not increase core temperature compared to conventional circle circuits, inspired gas is warmer and more humidified, resulting in better mucociliary function (Mizrak *et al.* 2011).

7.1.4.2 Active Humidification

A number of active humidification devices are available for use with standard human anesthesia equipment, but are not routinely used in veterinary patients. This lack of use is likely due to cost, lack of perceived benefit, and a paucity of supportive literature in veterinary patients. Furthermore, these devices are not compatible with large animal anesthesia circuits without adaptation. However, active humidification devices are frequently used in the veterinary intensive care unit for supplemental oxygen administration. Guidelines for active humidification have been created by the American Association for Respiratory Care, which recommend delivering gas between 34 and 41°C with 100% relative humidity, corresponding to an absolute humidity range of 33–44 mg H_2O/L (Restrepo and Walsh 2012). Active humidification devices can be classified as humidifiers that produce water vapor, or nebulizers that produce water vapor and droplets.

Humidifiers Humidifiers may be unheated or heated. Unheated humidifiers humidify gases by passage through a room temperature water reservoir, while heated humidifiers contain a humidification chamber with an electrically heated water reservoir. The devices are placed on the proximal end of the inspiratory limb of the circuit. Gas from heated humidifiers will cool along the length of the circuit, causing water to condense within the hosing. The inspiratory limb may be heated to prevent condensation or contain water traps to prevent the aspiration of water. Heated humidifiers provide the most effective humidification, delivering fully saturated gases at or above 37°C, but carry the risk of over-humidification and corresponding complications (see above), as well as electrical shock, hyperthermia, thermal injury to the airway and aspiration of water. To regulate humidifier output and increase safety of these devices, all heated humidifiers have alarms, as well as thermal sensors at the humidifier outlet and at the level of the wye piece; these are connected in a feedback loop to maintain appropriate temperature control. In addition to being heated or

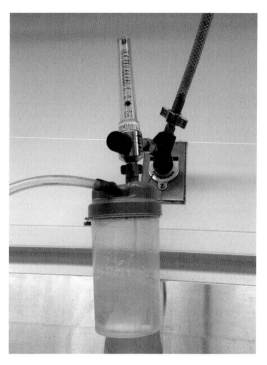

Figure 7.3 Bubble humidifier used for flow-by or nasal oxygen in the ICU or peri-operative setting.

unheated, humidifiers are further classified as either bubble, passover, counter flow or inline humidifiers, based on the method of humidification:

- *Bubble Humidifiers*: Bubble, or cascade, humidifiers direct gas flow through tubing or a capillary system into the base of a water reservoir (Figures 7.3 and 7.4). Water vapor content increases in the gas bubbles as they pass through the reservoir. Greater humidity results from a larger surface area (a greater number of smaller bubbles) and more equilibration time (lower flow rates). While it is not routinely used during veterinary anesthesia, this is the most common system of active humidification utilized in veterinary medicine for flow-by or nasal oxygen administration, with bubble humidifiers connected to wall-mounted oxygen delivery systems.

- *Passover Humidifiers*: With pass-over humidifiers, gas travels over a heated water reservoir to collect water vapor before administration to the patient. Wicks may be used within the reservoir to increase surface area for water transfer to further increase the absolute humidity of the gas (Figure 7.4).

- *Counter Flow Humidifiers*: Counter flow humidifiers provide effective humidification with less resistance than other active and passive humidification devices. With these devices, heated water enters the humidification chamber through small pores and travels down the chamber over a large surface area, while gas travels

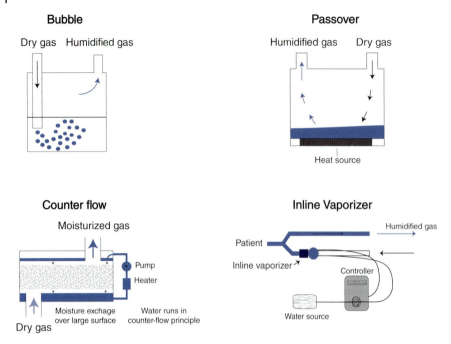

Figure 7.4 Illustrations depicting multiple types of humidifiers/vaporizers used in clinical patients.

in the opposite direction to maximizing humidification (Schumann *et al.* 2007; Figure 7.4).

- *Inline Vaporizers*: The more recently developed inline vaporizer injects water vapor into the circuit just proximal of the wye piece, essentially eliminating condensation within the circuit. There is a heating element at the site of vapor injection, and controls to adjust the heat and humidity delivered to the patient (Tiffin *et al.* 2011; Figure 7.4).

Nebulizers Nebulizers (also called atomizers or aerosolizers) produce microdroplets and water vapor. The size of the droplets varies among nebulizers, with droplet size determining the site of deposition within the respiratory tract (Phipps and Gonda 1990). The main types of nebulizers are pneumatic, ultrasonic and mechanical. Pneumatic nebulizers use a stream of forced gas to break the water into droplets, which can be further reduced in size by striking a baffle or anvil before release from the nebulizer. Ultrasonic nebulizers use a transmitter to apply ultrasonic frequencies (1–2.5 MHz) to water to produce small droplets (Flament *et al.* 2001). Mechanical nebulizers force a stream of water through a rapidly rotating disc to generate the water droplets.

The use of nebulizers is typically limited to the perioperative period in veterinary medicine; however, the incorporation of a nebulizer into an anesthetic circuit has been successfully used to humidify inspired gases during rodent

anesthesia, with small reductions in inspired anesthetic concentrations (Martenson *et al.* 2005).

Heated Breathing Circuits Heated breathing circuits without an additional humidification unit are available for veterinary and human patients. The inspiratory limb is heated with a wire coiled around the length of the hosing, an electronic temperature display and thermal sensors. Although heated breathing circuits did not have a significant effect on body temperature in human burn patients that underwent general anesthesia, the humidity and temperature of inspired gases was significantly higher than with conventional circuits, providing respiratory benefits (Kwak *et al.* 2013).

Addition of Water to the Circuit Rinsing the anesthesia breathing hoses and reservoir bag with distilled water and draining the excess before use can increase the absolute humidity of inspired gases (Chase *et al.* 1962).

7.2 Positive Pressure Equipment

7.2.1 Terminology and General Concepts

- *Positive end-expiratory pressure (PEEP)*: The pressure above atmospheric pressure that remains in the alveoli at the end of expiration and during the expiratory pause, expressed in cmH_2O. *Applied (extrinsic)* PEEP results from the application of a mechanical device that prevents full exhalation. *Auto (intrinsic)* PEEP is an accumulation of air within the lungs that results from insufficient exhalation before the next inhalation.

- *Continuous positive airway pressure (CPAP)*: The pressure applied to the airway continuously throughout the respiratory cycle in spontaneously breathing patients, expressed in cmH_2O.

7.2.2 Physiologic Considerations

7.2.2.1 Advantages of Positive Airway Pressure
Maintenance of positive pressure in the airways minimizes alveolar collapse that can occur due to the change in expiratory flow from endotracheal tube insertion bypassing the glottis, compressive forces, resorption atelectasis or pulmonary pathology. Maintaining alveolar expansion using PEEP or CPAP reduces ventilation/perfusion mismatch, improves oxygenation, and prevents mechanical trauma and inflammation from continuously re-opening collapsing pulmonary units during mechanical ventilation (Michelet *et al.* 2006; Briganti *et al.* 2010; Staffieri *et al.* 2010).

7.2.2.2 Disadvantages of Positive Airway Pressure
Positive intrathoracic pressure from using PEEP and CPAP techniques can decrease venous return, with subsequent reductions in cardiac output and arterial blood pressure. Because of this, airway pressure should be minimized in patients with elevated intracranial pressure, hypovolemia or hypotension. If significant PEEP is applied without an appropriate tidal volume, volutrauma and barotrauma can occur, resulting in pulmonary over-distension, compromise to the epithelial–endothelial barrier and pulmonary edema (Kerr and McDonell 2009).

7.2.3 Methods of Positive Pressure Application

Positive end-expiratory pressure valves maintain positive pressure in the anesthesia system through a valve held in the closed position with a spring holding a specific pressure against it (Figures 7.5–7.8). Once the force of expiratory gas exceeds the pressure from the spring, expired gases can move through the circuit. PEEP devices are available as fixed pressure valves, or adjustable valves controlled by a dial, often up to 20 cmH_2O, that have connections for an anesthesia machine or manual resuscitator (bag valve mask, self-inflating bag, Ambu bag). The PEEP valve must be applied in the correct orientation or it will function as a closed pop-off valve and obstruct circuit gas flow.

Newer veterinary ventilators designed for anesthetic use have electronically controlled PEEP and CPAP settings, preventing the need for external devices. All ventilators with ascending bellows impart a degree of PEEP (2–8 cmH_2O) to allow the bellows to fill during expiration.

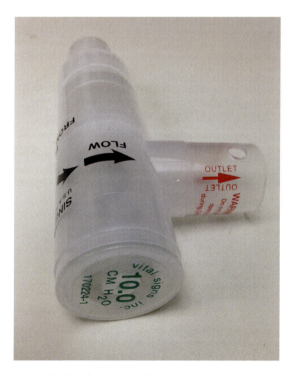

Figure 7.5 Fixed pressure PEEP valve imparting 10 cmH_2O.

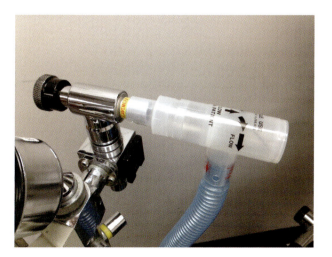

Figure 7.6 Fixed pressure PEEP valve placed distally to the pop-off valve on an anesthesia machine.

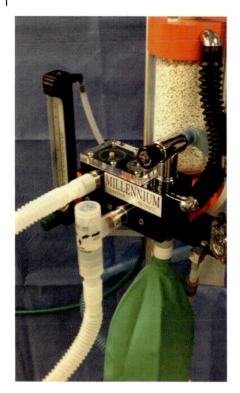

Figure 7.7 Fixed pressure PEEP valve placed on the expiratory limb of the breathing circuit between the hosing and the unidirectional expiratory valve.

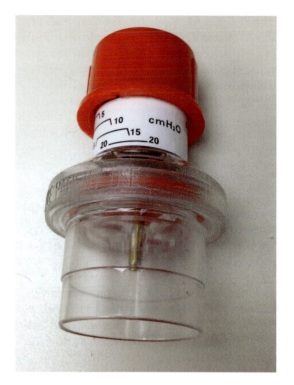

Figure 7.8 Adjustable PEEP valve for use with a manual resuscitator.

References

Bicalho, G.P., Braz, L.G., de Jesus, L.S., Pedigone, C.M., de Carvalho, L.R. *et al.* (2014) The humidity in a Dräger Primus anesthesia workstation using low or high fresh gas flow and with or without a heat and moisture exchanger in pediatric patients. *Anesth Analg*, 119, 926–931.

Briganti, A., Melanie, P., Portela, D., Breghi, G. and Mama, K. (2010) Continuous positive airway pressure administered via face mask in tranquilized dogs. *J Vet Emerg Crit Care (San Antonio)*, 20, 503–508.

Chase, H.F., Trotta, R. and Kilmore, M.A. (1962) Simple methods for humidifying non-rebreathing anesthesia gas systems. *Anesth Analg*, 41, 249–256.

Cheney, F.W. Jr. and Butler, J. (1968) The effects of ultrasonically-produced aerosols on airway resistance in man. *Anesthesiology*, 29, 1099–1106.

Chikata, Y., Oto, J., Onodera, M. and Nishimura, M. (2013) Humidification performance of humidifying devices for tracheostomized patients with spontaneous breathing: a bench study. *Respir Care*, 58, 1442–1448.

Cole, P. (1953) Further observations on the conditioning of respiratory air. *J Laryngol Otol*, 67, 669–681.

Dawson, J.A., Owen, L.S., Middleburgh, R. and Davis, P.G. (2014) Quantifying temperature and relative humidity of medical gases used for newborn resuscitation. *J Paediatr Child Health*, 50, 24–26.

Déry, R. (1973) The evolution of heat and moisture in the respiratory tract during anaesthesia with a non-rebreathing system. *Can Anaesth Soc J*, 20, 296–309.

Dias, N.H., Martins, R.H., Braz, J.R. and Carvalho, L.R. (2005) Larynx and cervical trachea in humidification and heating of inhaled gases. *An Otol Rhinol Laryngol*, 114, 411–415.

Flament, M.P., Leterme, P. and Gayot, A. (2001) Study of the technological parameters of ultrasonic nebulization. *Drug Dev Ind Pharm*, 27, 643–649.

Fletcher, R., Werner, O., Nordström, L. and Jonson, B. (1983) Sources of error and their correction in the measurement of carbon dioxide elimination using the Siemens-Elema CO_2 Analyzer. *Br J Anaesth*, 55, 177–185.

Fonkalsrud, E.W., Sanchez, M., Higashijima, I. and Arima, E. (1975) A comparative study of the effects of dry vs. humidified ventilation on canine lungs. *Surgery*, 78, 373–380.

Fontanari, P., Burnet, H., Zattara-Hartmann, M.C. and Jammes, Y. (1985) Changes in airway resistance induced by nasal inhalation of cold dry, dry, or moist air in normal individuals. *J Appl Physiol*, 81, 1739–1743.

Han, S.B., Gwak, M.S., Choi, S.J., Kim, M.H., Ko, J.S. *et al.* (2013) Effect of active airway warming on body core temperature during adult liver transplantation. *Transplant Proc*, 45, 251–254.

Hirsch, J.A., Tokayer, J.L., Robinson, M.J. and Sackner, M.A. (1975) Effects of dry air and subsequent humidification on tracheal mucous velocity in dogs. *J Appl Physiol*, 39, 242–246.

Hofmeister, E.H., Brainard, B.M., Braun, C. and Figueiredo, J.P. (2011) Effect of a heat and moisture exchanger on heat loss in isoflurane-anesthetized dogs undergoing single-limb orthopedic procedures. *J Am Vet Med Assoc*, 239, 1561–1565.

Ingelstedt, S. (1956) Studies on the conditioning of air in the respiratory tract. *Acta Oto-Laryngol Suppl*, 131, 1–80.

Jiang, M., Song, J.-J., Guo, X.-L., Tang, Y.-L. and Li, H.-B. (2015) Airway humidification reduces the inflammatory response during mechanical ventilation. *Respir Care*, 60, 1720–1728.

Kerr, C.L. and McDonell, W.N. (2009) Oxygen supplementation and ventilatory support. In: Muir, W.W. and Hubbell, J.A.E. (eds). *Equine Anesthesia*, 2nd ed. St Louis, MO: Saunders Elsevier, pp. 341–342.

Kwak, I.S., Choi, D.Y., Lee, T.H., Bae, J.Y., Lim, T.W. and Kim, K.W. (2013) The effect of heated breathing circuit on body temperature and humidity of anesthetic gas in major burns. *Korean J Anesthesiol*, 64, 6–11.

Lellouche, F., Qader, S., Taille, S., Lyazidi, A. and Brochard, L. (2006) Under-humidification and over-humidification during moderate induced hypothermia with usual devices. *Intensive Care Med*, 32, 1015–1021.

Lucato, J.J., Tucci, M.R., Schettino, G.P., Adams, A.B., Fu, C. *et al.* (2005) Evaluation of resistance in 8 different heat-and-moisture exchangers: effects of saturation and flow rate/profile. *Respir Care*, 50, 636–643.

Marfatia, S., Donahoe, P.K. and Hendren, W.H. (1975) Effect of dry and humidified gases on the respiratory epithelium of rabbits. *J Pediatr Surg*, 10, 583–592.

Martenson, M., Houts, J., Heinricher, M. and Ogden, B. (2005) A simple device for humidification of inspired gases during volatile anesthesia in rats. *Contemp Top Lab Anim Sci*, 44, 46–48.

McFadden, E.R., Pichurko, B.M., Bowman, H.F., Ingenito, E., Burns, S. *et al.* (1985) Thermal mapping of the airways in humans. *J Appl Physiol*, 58, 564–570.

Meyer, M.P., Hou, D., Ishrar, N.N., Dito, I. and te Pas, A.B. (2015) Initial respiratory support with cold, dry gas versus heated humidified gas and admission temperature of preterm infants. *J Pediatr*, 166, 245–250.

Michelet, P., D'Journo, X.B., Roch, A., Doddoli, C., Marin, V. *et al.* (2006) Protective ventilation influences systemic inflammation after esophagectomy: a randomized controlled study. *Anesthesiology*, 105, 911–919.

Mizrak, A., Bilgi, M., Koruk, S., Ganidagli, S., Karatas, E. *et al.* (2011) Comparison of the coaxial circle circuit with the conventional circle circuit. *Eurasian J Med*, 43, 92–98.

Noguchi, H., Takumi, Y. and Aochi, O. (1973) A study of humidification in tracheostomized dogs. *Br J Anaesth*, 45, 844–848.

Phipps, P.R. and Gonda, I. (1990) Droplets produced by medical nebulizers. Some factors affecting their size and solute concentration. *Chest*, 97, 1327–1332.

Rashad, K., Wilson, K., Hurt, H.H. Jr., Graff, T.D. and Benson, D.W. (1967) Humidification of anesthetic gases on static compliance. *Anesth Analg*, 46, 127–133.

Restrepo, R.D. and Walsh, B.K. (2012) Humidification during invasive and noninvasive mechanical ventilation. *Respir Care*, 57, 782–788.

Rouadi, P., Baroody, F.M., Abbott, D., Naureckas, E., Solway, J. and Naclerio, R.M. (1999) A technique to measure the ability of the human nose to warm and humidify air. *J Appl Physiol*, 87, 400–406.

Schumann, S., Stahl, C.A., Möller, K., Priebe, H.-J. and Guttmann, J. (2007) Moisturizing and mechanical characteristics of a new counter-flow type heated humidifier. *Br J Anaesth*, 98, 531–538.

Sottiaux, T.M. (2006) Consequences of under- and over-humidification. *Respir Care Clin N Am*, 12, 233–252.

Staffieri, F., Driessenk B., Monte, V.D., Grasso, S. and Crovace, A. (2010) Effects of positive end-expiratory pressure on anesthesia-induced atelectasis and gas exchange in anesthetized and mechanically ventilated sheep. *Am J Vet Res*, 71, 867–874.

Strum, D.P. and Eger, E.I. (1994) The degradation, absorption, and solubility of volatile anesthetics in soda lime depend on water content. *Anesth Analg*, 78, 340–348.

Tiffin, N.H., Short, K.A., Jones, S.W. and Cairns, B.A. (2011) Comparison of three humidifiers during high-frequency percussive ventilation using the VDR-4 Fail-safe breathing circuit hub. *J Burn Care Res*, 32, e45–50.

Tsuda, T., Noguchi, H., Takumi, Y. and Aochi, O. (1977) Optimum humidification of air administered to a tracheostomy in dogs. Scanning electron microscopy and surfactant studies. *Br J Anaesth*, 49, 965–977.

Vezina, D.P., Trépanier, C.A., Lessard, M.R., Gourdeau, M., Tremblay, C. and Guidoin, R. (2004) An *in vivo* evaluation of the mycobacterial filtration efficacy of three breathing filters used in anesthesia. *Anesthesiology*, 101, 104–109.

Walker, J.E., Wells, R.E. Jr. and Merrill, E.W. (1961) Heat and water exchange in the respiratory tract. *Am J Med*, 30, 259–267.

Wilkes, A.R., Benbough, J.E., Speight, S.E. and Harmer, M. (2000) The bacterial and viral filtration performance of breathing system filters. *Anaesthesia*, 55, 458–465.

Williams, R., Rankin, N., Smith, T., Galler, D. and Seakins P. (1996) Relationship between the humidity and temperature of inspired gas and the function of the airway mucosa. *Crit Care Med*, 24, 1920–1929.

8

Waste Anesthetic Gas Collection and Consequences

Heidi Reuss-Lamky

Oakland Veterinary Referral Services, Bloomfield Hills, Michigan, USA

8.1 Introduction

Waste anesthetic gases (WAGs) can be defined as all fugitive anesthetic gases and vapors, including isoflurane, sevoflurane, desflurane, and enflurane, oxygen, nitrous oxide, carbon dioxide, nitrogen, helium or any other agent or gas, which can escape from the anesthetic circuit or be exhaled by the patient and released into anesthetizing areas and recovery rooms. WAG management intuitively seems prudent, but because occult exposure is difficult to detect without special monitoring, ignorance and/or a cavalier attitude about them may result in devastating consequences (AANA 2013).

Also known as fluranes, modern halogenated ethers such as isoflurane, sevoflurane and desflurane, are extremely volatile liquids that evaporate rapidly at room temperature. They are also clear, colorless and odorless at trace levels. Physiologic advantages of fluranes include rapid onset of effects, a low probability of irritation and low frequency of side effects. Fluranes are often used in a closed system in combination with oxygen (± nitrous oxide) to induce and maintain general anesthesia (Saber and Hougaard 2009).

Fluranes are delivered with an anesthetic machine to allow for mixtures of oxygen, halogenated anesthetic gases, nitrous oxide and ambient room air to be administered to the patient. In a rebreathing system, recirculation of anesthetic gases occurs within the anesthetic machine, once carbon dioxide has been removed. Carbon dioxide is usually removed by either a strong base carbon dioxide absorbent such as soda lime (Sodasorb®, Sodasorb® LF, W.R. Grace and Company, Midmark Corporation, Versailles, OH), barium hydroxide lime (Baralyme®, Chemetron Medical Division, Allied Healthcare Products, St Louis, Missouri) or by calcium hydroxide (Amsorb®, Armstrong Ltd, Coleraine, Northern Ireland), which does not contain a strong base and is not associated with compound A or carbon monoxide formation (Kharasch and Powers 2002; Saber and Hougaard 2009).

8.2 Occupational WAG Exposure

Occupational exposure to WAGs has been studied since 1967. Occupational exposure may be associated with operating rooms at hospitals, inside the practices of specialists and recovery rooms, and within dental and veterinary facilities (McKelvey and Hollingshead 2000b). The most common causes of WAG pollution include leaks from around the patient's airway (e.g. mask or endotracheal tube), anesthetic machine and breathing circuit, ventilator, active scavenger pumps, scavenging devices and connection tubing. Leaks may also be due to an accidental spill of liquid inhalant and the continued exhalation of gases after the conclusion of the anesthetic procedure (NIOSH 2007). The main route of occupational WAG exposure for healthcare workers is via inhalation (Saber and Hougaard 2009). In addition, WAG exposure may occur in trace amounts. Trace anesthetic gas concentrations are expressed in parts per million (ppm), and represent a volume-to-volume relationship. For example, 100% of any gas is 1 million ppm, and 1% is equivalent to 10 000 ppm (AANA 2013).

There are two categories for health implications associated with WAG exposure in humans, short and long term. Neurologic symptoms are most frequently associated with short-term (acute) exposure, usually occurring immediately or shortly after contact. Short-term symptoms may include fatigue, headaches, drowsiness, nausea, depression and irritability (Muir *et al.* 2000; Saber and Hougaard 2009).

Long-term or chronic implications become evident days, weeks, or even years after the exposure. Historical examples of conditions associated with long-term WAG exposure include genotoxicity, reproductive disorders,

Veterinary Anesthetic and Monitoring Equipment, First Edition. Edited by Kristen G. Cooley and Rebecca A. Johnson.
© 2018 John Wiley & Sons, Inc. Published 2018 by John Wiley & Sons, Inc.

liver and kidney damage, neoplasia, hematopoietic changes, pruritus and chronic nervous system dysfunction associated with neuronal apoptosis and alterations in dendritic and glial morphology (Muir *et al.* 2000; NIOSH 2007; Saber and Hougaard 2009; Colon *et al.* 2017). Organ toxicity caused by long-term exposure to inhalants is most likely due to biodegradation of metabolic by-products. Individuals who may be immunocompromised, suffering from pre-existing liver or kidney damage, or in the first trimester of pregnancy are most prone to the adverse effects of environmental WAG exposure (Muir *et al.* 2000; NIOSH 2007). Interestingly, long-term exposure to trace levels of WAGs has recently been implicated in increased drug and alcohol addiction (Gold *et al.* 2004). In addition, more than 35 days of continuous isoflurane exposure (set at 150 ppm lowest observed adverse effect level [LOAEL] overall) also caused decreased body weight gain in mice (Saber and Hougaard 2009).

8.3 Physical Properties and Elimination

8.3.1 Methoxyflurane and Halothane

Patients receiving methoxyflurane, one of the oldest halogenated gases, retained 50–80% of metabolites in body fat, which were then metabolized by the liver and excreted by the kidneys. Primary MOF metabolites included fluoride ions, dichloroacetic acid, methoxyfluroacetic acid and carbon dioxide (Muir *et al.* 2000). However, MOF is no longer commercially available in the US (McGlothlin and Moenning 2013).

Similarly, halothane recipients metabolized 20–40%, after being mobilized from fat; it is subsequently excreted by the kidneys. Major halothane metabolites included triflouracetic acid, and fluoride, chloride and bromide ions (Muir *et al.* 2000). These metabolites may persist for many days in the liver. Similar to methoxyflurane, halothane is no longer commercially available in the US.

8.3.2 Isoflurane, Enflurane, Sevoflurane and Desflurane

Comparatively, contemporary inhalants such as isoflurane and desflurane require metabolism of a mere 0.2%–0.02%, respectively, and do not result in a significant increase in serum fluoride ions when used in routine clinical cases. Isoflurane is considered the most potent flurane, as 50% of human patients exposed to a painful stimulus will remain immobile after inhaling 12 000 ppm (minimum alveolar concentration or MAC), while MAC values for sevoflurane and desflurane are

21 000 and 60 000 ppm, respectively (Saber and Hougaard 2009; AANA 2013).

Approximately 2.5–3% of enflurane (seldom used) and sevoflurane are metabolized and do result in increased fluoride ion concentrations; however, they are rarely associated with nephrotoxicity in the clinical situation. Because sevoflurane is partially degraded by the strong bases present in carbon dioxide absorbents, it is also associated with fluoromethyl 2,2-difluoro-1-(trifluoromethyl)-vinyl ether (FDVE), known as compound A (Saber and Hougaard 2009).

Desflurane boils near room temperature and rapidly dissipates. As per the manufacturer's Material Safety Data Sheet (MSDS), both enflurane and desflurane are identified by the Environmental Protection Agency (EPA) as hazardous waste (code number D022). This is due to the presence of trace amounts of chloroform. Isoflurane does not contain chloroform and is not considered a hazardous waste under EPA regulations (AANA 2013).

8.4 Pharmacodynamics

Many hematopoietic, cellular and animal studies, as well as behavioral assessments have been conducted surrounding exposure to anesthetic agents on fertility, carcinogenicity, teratogenicity and reproduction (AANA 2013). Obviously, the health implications can vary drastically, depending upon the agent used. Unfortunately, much of the following information is riddled with contradictions. Some reports indicate no definitive cause-and-effect relationship between exposure to WAGs and disease, while other reports seem irrefutable. Complicating matters is the sheer number of potential hazards encountered in a typical healthcare setting (i.e. antineoplastic [chemotherapy] and antiviral drugs, sterilizing and disinfecting agents, X-rays [ionizing radiation] and anesthetic gases) so as to make interpretation of research data muddy and inconclusive (Lawson *et al.* 2012). These caveats must be considered when discussing the issues below; this chapter is not meant to be an exhaustive compilation of physiology, but a brief overview of effects.

8.4.1 Airway and Dermal Irritation

Desflurane and isoflurane may be associated with airway irritation, but personnel are not expected to develop issues with occupational exposure levels; sevoflurane is associated with the least amount of airway irritation. Furthermore, contact dermatitis, occupational asthma or allergies to isoflurane or sevoflurane have been rarely described (Saber and Hougaard 2009).

8.4.2 Reproductive Effects

Since 1971, multiple epidemiological studies have been performed to determine the risk of spontaneous abortion, birth defects, and other reproductive issues such as decreased fertility after occupational exposure to WAGs (Boivin 1997; AANA 2013; McGlothlin and Moenning 2013). WAGs were initially implicated in the risk of spontaneous abortions in dental and veterinary personnel, where anesthetic gases were not scavenged in their facility; however, this correlation was not substantiated in further studies. Confounding factors included sample size, consistency of exposure levels, and facility type or size. For example, many hospital operating rooms were designed with appropriate engineering controls in mind, while smaller medical facilities, retrofitted inside strip malls and office buildings, were not. In addition, challenges associated with patient compliance and cooperation may factor in, since pediatric and/or veterinary patients may resent restraint and may try to remove anesthesia masks frequently until fully subdued (Lawson *et al.* 2012).

In an American Society of Anesthesiologists survey, the risk of spontaneous abortions was 1.3–2 times the general population among female physician anesthesiologists and nurse anesthetists. Similarly, working hospital anesthetists had spontaneous abortion rates of approximately 18.2% versus 14.7% in a control group. In addition, 12% of working anesthetists were infertile, much higher than 6% within the control group (McKelvey and Hollingshead 2000b). Indeed, 16% of the children of practicing nurse anesthetists developed birth defects, versus a 6% incidence in a control group (McKelvey and Hollingshead 2000b). However, these studies are difficult to interpret, as agents and exposure amounts varied. Additionally, atmospheric measurements of WAG exposure were not performed, control measures were inconsistent, and it was possible that nitrous oxide may have been partially responsible for some of the reproductive hazards (Boivin 1997; McKelvey and Hollingshead 2000b).

8.4.3 Hepatic and Renal Effects

Many halogenated organic compounds can cause depression of hepatic function and hepatocellular damage. An increased risk (1.5–1.6-fold) of developing liver disease was found in operating room personnel exposed to WAGs (Paddleford 1999). However, it is difficult to determine whether WAGs or some other occupational hazards are causative. Halothane is associated with "halothane hepatitis", which is defined as massive hepatic necrosis that is a result of the production of toxic by-products with an immune-mediated response in some patients (McKelvey and Hollingshead 2000a). This condition is considered rare. Methoxyflurane has also been implicated as being potentially hepatotoxic, whereas enflurane, isoflurane and nitrous oxide do not appear to be hepatotoxic (Paddleford 1999). A significant increase in renal disease was reported in female operating room personnel (1.2-1.4-fold) and dental assistants (1.2-1.7-fold) compared to the normal population. Again, it is unclear whether the increase was the result of exposure to methoxyflurane, nitrous oxide, other anesthetic agent(s), or other occupational factor(s) (McKelvey and Hollingshead 2000b).

8.4.4 Neurologic and Oncogenic Effects

Headaches, nausea, fatigue and irritability are associated with WAG exposure. Other short-term effects reported included depression, lethargy and ataxia. Long-term effects reported myoneuropathies, impaired short-term memory, neuron destruction and learning disabilities/cognitive disorders (Paddleford 1999; Saber and Hougaard 2009; NIOSH 2007; Colon *et al.* 2017). It has been postulated that these cognitive effects may be a contributing factor for higher medical error rates made by nursing personnel in the ICU, emergency and operating rooms (McGlothlin and Moenning, 2013). In general, none of the commonly-used veterinary anesthetic agents or nitrous oxide appear to be carcinogenic, but valid studies to support this hypothesis do not yet exist (Saber and Hougaard 2009).

8.4.5 Nitrous Oxide Effects

Nitrous oxide has been implicated as a known health hazard. Prolonged nitrous oxide anesthesia is associated with audiovisual impairment, difficulty with concentration and equilibrium, bone marrow depression (primary granulocytopenia), and pernicious anemia (McGlothlin and Moenning 2013). It is not metabolized *in vivo* (0.0004%), but undergoes a physiochemical reaction with vitamin B_{12} that results in bone marrow changes and neurologic disease. It also indirectly inhibits deoxyribonucleic acid (DNA) synthesis, which can result in reproductive disorders such as increased risk of infertility, spontaneous abortion, congenital abnormalities and premature births (Muir *et al.* 2000; McGlothlin and Moenning 2013).

While biologic effects of fluranes are debatable, there is little doubt that long-term, low-level exposure to nitrous oxide (N_2O) should be avoided, especially during pregnancy (McGlothlin and Moenning 2013). Female personnel, as well as female spouses of male personnel exposed to many hours of N_2O per week, have higher levels of spontaneous abortions and are less fertile than the general population. Rats exposed to high levels of

N$_2$O demonstrated abnormalities in sperm morphology, reduced ovulation and retarded fetal development (McKelvey and Hollingshead 2000b). In addition, an increased risk of neurologic, renal and kidney dysfunction, and an increased risk of cervical cancer have been found in exposed personnel (Paddleford 1999; McKelvey and Hollingshead 2000b). Nitrous oxide usage has declined significantly over the years due to potential for abuse, rising nitrous oxide gas costs and the development of newer inhalants with superior induction and recovery performances (McKelvey and Hollingshead 2000b).

8.5 History of Governmental Regulations and Trace (Waste) Gas Exposure

The Occupational Safety and Health Act of 1970 underscored the importance of implementing standards that would protect workers from potential hazards associated with health and safety in the workplace. In 1977, the National Institute for Occupational Safety and Health (NIOSH), working alongside the US Department of Health Education and Welfare, first published criteria for a "Recommended Standard for Occupational Exposure to Waste Anesthetic Gases and Vapors". This document encouraged the development of standards for minimizing the risk of elevated trace gas exposure in operating room personnel and continues to serve as valuable resource today (AANA 2013).

In 1988, NIOSH published an updated version, *Guidelines for Health Care Workers* (publication #88-1190), which prompted the American Dental Association, the American Hospital Association, and the American Society of Anesthesiologists to published expanded guidelines and recommendations for managing waste anesthetic gases.

A 1991 survey undertaken by the American Association of Nurse Anesthetists (AANA) determined that more than half of the respondents were "very concerned" about chronic exposure to WAGs, which reinforced the need for further education, training and exposure surveillance. Subsequently, OSHA made revisions to the recommendations regarding WAG management in 1992, and again in 2000. Today, the US Department of Labor works under OSHA's authority to continue educating healthcare workers about the potential risks (AANA 2013).

In 1994, the US's NIOSH published a warning that nitrous oxide may have harmful effects on health, while the Occupational Health and Safety Act of Quebec, Canada, gave pregnant women the right to be reassigned or leave their place of employment if working conditions were deemed hazardous to them or their unborn child (Boivin 1997). Subsequently, most authorities agree that exposure to excessive levels of WAGs should be avoided and controls to reduce exposure should be implemented.

8.6 WAG Exposure Level Recommendations

The American College of Veterinary Anesthesia and Analgesia (ACVAA) recommends that veterinary hospitals institute and maintain protocols for controlling WAGs, based on the possibility that small amounts may adversely affect human health. Official federal government standards and prior research to support definitive data surrounding WAG exposure recommendations is lacking. Instead, a responsible and practical approach was adopted, which dictates that waste and trace exposure levels should be kept as low as possible, while utilizing good practices and procedures (AANA 2013).

The National Institute for Occupational Safety and Health recommends that the workplace environmental concentration of halogenated agents should not exceed 2 parts per million (ppm) over an 8-hour period of time. Workplace environmental exposure to inhalants combined with N$_2$O should not exceed 0.5 ppm, while the N$_2$O level should not exceed 25 ppm over the same 8-hour period (AANA 2013). These levels are time-weighted averages (TWA) over the course of a typical 8-hour day of surgical procedure(s). It has been widely accepted that these levels dictate a safe working environment for employees, including pregnant women. Regardless, pregnant women should follow the advice of their healthcare provider.

Other countries have also established occupational exposure standards for trace gas exposure, ranging from 25 ppm (Netherlands) to 100 ppm (Italy, Sweden, Norway, Denmark, Great Britain); nonetheless, all unanimously agree that WAGs should be scavenged (McGlothlin and Moenning 2013).

8.7 Reducing Environmental WAG Exposure

Many factors impact environmental WAG levels, but when utilizing good work practices, the presence and efficacy of a gas scavenging system is paramount. In fact, gas scavenging is the single-most important step to regulating WAG pollution for healthcare personnel, and is endorsed by every professional organization and government agency (McGlothlin and Moenning 2013). One 1982 survey of veterinary hospitals demonstrated that gas scavenging reduced the indoor environmental concentration of waste halothane by 64–94% (McKelvey and Hollingshead 2000b; AANA 2013). Appropriate control measures must include collection and removal of WAGs, detection and correction of leaks, an effective ventilation system, and institution of good WAG management practices (AANA 2013).

8.7.1 Gas Scavenging Systems

Gas scavenging systems have become the *de facto* standard for anesthetic machines in the US since 1980, and function to collect WAGs from the anesthetic circuit and dispose of them to the outside atmosphere. Waste gas scavenging is required for every kind of anesthetic delivery system (ADS), because many users typically deliver more oxygen than the patient requires (Saber and Hougaard 2009; McGlothlin and Moenning 2013). These gas capturing systems consist of an adjustable pressure limiting (APL) or pop-off valve and scavenger hosing attached to either a non-rebreathing (open) or (semi-closed or closed) rebreathing circuit, waste gas interface (gas capture mechanism joining the disposal system), and a disposal/scavenging system to vent WAGs outside of the building. There are two types of scavenging systems available, active and passive.

8.7.1.1 Active Scavenging Systems

Active scavengers use mechanical methods to eliminate WAGs by using a vacuum pump or fan to suck gases into the scavenger (Figure 8.1). Local active scavenging units

are typically located adjacent to the ADS and require activation via manually flipping a switch. Central vacuum systems can facilitate WAG removal from multiple ADSs and are situated in one central location within the building, as long as each ADS is equipped with a waste gas interface (Figure 8.2).

As per the Food and Drug Administration's (FDA) Anesthesia Apparatus Checkout Recommendations of 1986 (revisions submitted 1992), gas flow through the waste gas interface valve must be adjusted during each procedure to compensate for a number of innate variations. Adjustments may be based on fresh gas flow use, such as during low flow or closed system techniques (~500 *in vivo* 1000 mL/min), when higher flows are required, or if the oxygen flush valve is activated. Even facility-wide demand on the vacuum supply system can necessitate adjustments (AANA 2013). Caution must be used with active scavenging systems, as it is possible to create a negative pressure within the anesthetic circuit if the suction is too strong. The negative pressure relief valve can negate this effect, but will draw room air into the system when activated (AANA 2013).

Utilizing either passive or active systems can create the potential for blockage and resistance to exhalation, resulting in excessive pressure within the anesthetic circuit. A positive pressure relief valve on the ADS or waste gas interface can prevent this from occurring (AANA 2013). Waste gas interface reservoir bags temporarily store WAGs from the manifold until they can be drawn into the scavenging system. The bag should not be allowed to over-inflate, but maintained somewhere between empty and half-filled. Over-distended waste gas

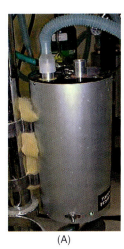
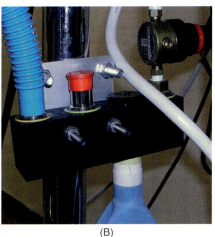
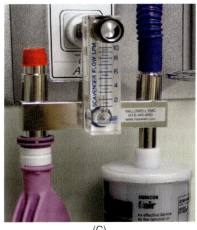

(A) (B) (C)

Figure 8.1 Active scavengers can be situated locally at the base of an anesthetic machine (A), or centrally, whereas the main vacuum is at one central location inside the facility. Pictured is an active scavenger interface (B). Central scavenging interfaces can also provide dual functionality, accommodating both active and passive scavenging methods (C). Dual scavenging functionality can be advantageous, especially during power outages when active scavenging systems will not work (photograph C courtesy of Stetson Hallowell from www.Hallowell.com).

- the function and performance of all components of the anesthesia delivery system(s);
- how the facility measures and monitors waste gases in the anesthetizing area(s);
- effective work practices and techniques commonly utilized to help reduce trace anesthetic gas exposure within the facility;
- potential adverse effects of chronic exposure to WAGs;
- governmental agencies and regulations surrounding WAG exposure;
- resources and recommendations from other professional organizations; and
- other OSHA guidelines for hospitals and healthcare facilities providing anesthesia include quarterly inspection (or as deemed necessary by the manufacturer) and testing of the anesthetic delivery system by a factory-trained service provider (AANA 2013).

8.8.1 The Anesthetic Delivery System

It is imperative to regularly inspect all anesthetic equipment, and service anesthetic machines on an annual basis. Maintenance logs should be kept for each anesthetic machine, vaporizer and ventilator. Leakage from anesthetic machines can be a significant source of WAGs. Leaks can occur from missing, worn or damaged "O" rings, washers or other seals, loose dome covers, poorly sealed carbon dioxide canisters, loose hose connections, holes in hoses or reservoir bags, or vaporizer caps not completely tightened (Coleman 2016). Damaged hoses, reservoir bags and endotracheal tubes should be discarded (NIOSH 2007). Leak test anesthetic machines on a routine basis, or whenever the integrity of the anesthetic machine has been compromised (as when changing the carbon dioxide canister or after performing repairs and/or maintenance). Leak testing should be performed using only oxygen (AANA 2013).

8.8.2 Perform an Anesthetic Machine Leak Test

Checking anesthetic machines for low pressure is simple and all anesthetists need to know how to perform this simple task (McKelvey and Hollingshead 2000b):

1) Place a Y-hose and reservoir bag on the machine.
2) Close the pop-off valve.
3) Occlude the end of the wye hose.
4) Fill the reservoir bag to a pressure of 30 cm of water.
5) Observe the needle on the pressure manometer. Pressure within the circuit should not decrease by more than 5 cm of water in 30 seconds. Leaks greater than 300 mL per minute should be located and corrected (McKelvey and Hollingshead 2000b).

Location of the leak can be determined by spraying an approved leak detection solution (e.g. 10% detergent solution has been used but is controversial due to explosion risk) onto suspect areas. These include the edges of the carbon dioxide canister, dome covers, inhalation and exhalation ports, at the base of the APL valve and manometer threads, nitrous oxide and oxygen connections, and male/female vaporizer caps (Paddleford 1999) (Figure 8.5). Once the circuit is pressurized, the presence of bubbles forming around any of the aforementioned areas warrants further scrutiny, investigation and possible repair. The most common locations for anesthetic machine leaks are usually associated with the seals around the carbon dioxide canister, vaporizer cap or holes around the neck of deteriorated reservoir bags. See below for additional troubleshooting tips.

Alternately, Freon detecting devices may be used to help locate leaks in the anesthetic machine and circuits. Generally called leak detectors, Freon detectors are used to "sniff" trace halogenated gas leaks as small as 5 mL. Unfortunately, leaks located inside of the vaporizer are only usually noticed by trained service technicians (Rasmussen and Thorud 2007).

The anesthetic machine should be disconnected from the oxygen and nitrous oxide at the end of each workday. Unplug wall outlet connections and close gas cylinder valves to prevent gas loss due to machine leaks or unintentional (accidental) gas flows (AANA 2013).

8.8.3 Other Environmental Control Strategies

Although scavenging WAGs is an important and key factor in WAG exposure, many other simple work practices can

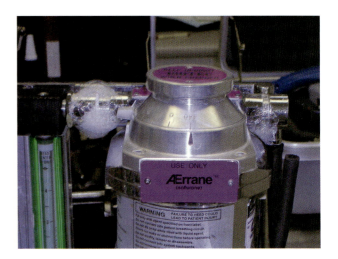

Figure 8.5 Detecting leaks associated with the inlet and outlet of this vaporizer is confirmed by the presence of bubbles at these connection points.

help mitigate occupational exposure in clinical practice (AANA 2013).

8.8.3.1 Anesthetic Induction Chambers

The primary goal of any anesthetic induction is rapid airway access. Use anesthetic induction chambers only when necessary and indicated (Paddleford 1999). When the anesthetic induction chamber is opened to retrieve the animal, large amounts of WAGs escape into the room. For best results, use the smallest chamber possible, ensure the chamber has a good seal, is not damaged, and is equipped with two outlets; one for delivery of the inhalant and one for scavenging. Once the patient is removed, quickly replace the lid and continue to run oxygen through the chamber for several minutes to help purge residual WAGs into the scavenger. Alternately, the Induction Chamber Evacuator (ICevac) system, currently under development by Safe Niche Products (www.safenichescience.com), may be preferred by some facilities, because it provides smoother inductions and reduces exposure to personnel by rapidly evacuating WAGs from a 10-gallon anesthetic induction chamber in less than 60 seconds (Figure 8.6).

It is important to note that patients induced in anesthetic chambers exit with fur that is contaminated with the inhalant agent, so use chambers in well-ventilated areas. Residual anesthetics can be removed from the chamber (as well as all anesthetic hoses and reservoir bags) after use, by thoroughly cleaning with soap and water (McKelvey and Hollingshead 2000b). As an alternative to the anesthetic induction chamber induction, many smaller patients will tolerate mask induction while

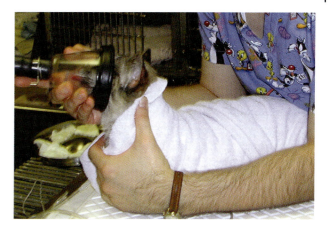

Figure 8.7 Ensure anesthetic masks are properly fitted and secured over the patient's face before turning on the inhalant.

wrapped "burrito"-style in a towel or placed in a cat bag (Reuss-Lamky 2006; Figure 8.7).

8.8.3.2 Anesthesia Masks

Avoid masks for maintaining anesthesia, as leakage around the mask diaphragm can be a source of WAG exposure. If masks must be used, ensure a snug diaphragm fit over the patient's face with an appropriately-sized mask (NIOSH 2007) (Figure 8.7). Start with oxygen first, and do not turn on the vaporizer until the mask is securely in place (NIOSH 2007; AANA 2013). When the procedure is finished, turn the vaporizer off first, and continue oxygen for several minutes to help purge WAGs from the circuit.

8.8.3.3 Endotracheal Tubes

Always use cuffed endotracheal tubes. Do not turn the vaporizer on until the endotracheal tube cuff has been inflated and attached to the anesthetic circuit (NIOSH 2007). Improperly inflated endotracheal tubes can be an overlooked source of WAG exposure. Check proper inflation by closing the APL valve and exerting gentle pressure on the reservoir bag. The cuff should be inflated to its "minimum no leak volume". To protect the patient's lungs, a leak should occur at slightly less than approximately 20 cm H_2O. Ensure the endotracheal tube and cuff is not damaged prior to use. Commercial products are available to help to verify proper cuff inflation (see Chapter 14) (NIOSH 2007).

8.8.3.4 Reservoir Bags, Y Hoses and WAG Bags

Holes in Y hoses, reservoir bags and WAG bags located at the base of the active scavenging interface can be a common source of WAGs. Damaged hoses and bags should be discarded and replaced immediately. It may be prudent to change WAG bags located on the active scavenger's interface on a regularly scheduled basis.

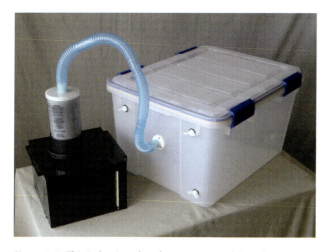

Figure 8.6 This induction chamber evacuation (ICevac) system prototype, currently under development by Safe Niche Products (www.safenicheproducts.com), is designed to evenly distribute incoming anesthetic gases during induction and incorporates a strong vacuum to rapidly remove residual WAGs before extracting the patient.

8.8.3.5 Oxygen Flow Rates

Use appropriate oxygen flow rates (<3 L/min) or low flow (closed system) anesthesia to minimize the amount of WAGs produced (McKelvey and Hollingshead 2000b; NIOSH 2007). There is no need to "charge" the anesthetic circuit with the inhalant gases prior to attaching it to the patient. Always run higher oxygen flow rates (2–3 L/min) for the first 3–5 minutes of anesthesia to remove room air from the circuit (that develops after a period of disuse) and to avoid dilution of the inhalant.

Low flow anesthesia entails decreasing the oxygen flow rate for maintenance of anesthesia to as low as 500 mL for patients weighing up to 100 pounds and adjusting the APL valve to maintain the reservoir bag to be approximately three-quarters full. It has been suggested that the oxygen flow rate required for meeting the oxygen demands of the anesthetized patient and for maintaining oxygen hemoglobin saturation (SpO_2) and the partial pressure of arterial oxygen saturation (PaO_2), is actually very low (Ko 2005). Since most vaporizers require a minimum flow rate of 350–500 mL, this lower flow rate should be sufficient for delivery of the inhalant while reducing costs (by reducing oxygen use and extending the life of charcoal canisters) and WAGs, as well as meeting the patient's oxygen demands (Ko 2005). Always verify minimum flow rate requirements with the vaporizer's manufacturer. If preferred, SpO_2 and blood gases can be assessed to ensure adequate oxygenation during low flow anesthesia. While using low flow anesthesia, higher oxygen flow rates will be indicated hourly or whenever rapid anesthetic plane changes are required. It is the author's opinion that patients receiving low flow anesthesia should be closely monitored at all times.

Oxygen flow rates exceeding 3L/min are associated with greater release of WAGs, especially if effective scavenging is unavailable (McKelvey and Hollingshead 2000b). Regardless of the anesthetic technique used, on completion of the procedure, turn off the vaporizer first while providing several minutes of oxygen flow to purge WAGs into the scavenging system (AANA 2013).

8.8.3.6 Nitrous Oxide Monitoring

Nitrous oxide monitoring may be accomplished with dosimetry badges, hand-held monitoring devices, and infrared spectrophotometry. Exposure levels exceeding 25 ppm of nitrous oxide, measured over an 8-hour TWA, are not permitted (AANA 2013). Advances in infrared videography enable visualization of nitrous oxide, making leak detection even easier (McGlothlin and Moenning 2013).

8.8.3.7 Low-Pressure System Leaks

Low-pressure leaks are usually associated with the patient circuit and components. Low-pressure system components may consist of the carbon dioxide absorber, APL valve, inhalation and exhalation valves, gas analyzer connections, the endotracheal tube or mask, plus any other additional points of connection such as PEEP valves and humidifiers. Leaks located between the fresh gas inlet (from the back of the machine) and the gas outlet (toward the carbon dioxide absorber) are usually due to inappropriate vaporizer installation (AANA 2013) (Figure 8.5).

8.8.3.8 High-Pressure System Leaks

High-pressure leaks are typically associated with cylinder gas supply system. Leaks may occur where the supply hose plugs into the wall outlet and to the anesthetic delivery system. Ensure that high-pressure gas supply hoses are of factory quality and protect them from kinks and excessive strain at the fittings (AANA 2013).

8.8.3.9 Breathing Circuit Disconnection

Avoid unnecessary breathing circuit disconnection (AANA 2013). Anesthetic circuit disconnects often associated with patient repositioning can be averted if the anesthetist loosens and twists only the Y hose connection near the endotracheal tube. Firmly grasp the endotracheal tube to ensure it does not move throughout the twisting motion.

If the patient must be disconnected from the breathing circuit, turn off the oxygen, halogenated agent and nitrous oxide first, and empty the reservoir bag into the scavenger before disconnecting the patient. Never expel the contents of the reservoir bag into the room (McKelvey and Hollingshead 2000b; AANA 2013).

Maintain the machine connection for several minutes after the cessation of anesthesia and allow the patient to breathe 100% oxygen at 2–3 times maintenance rates for a period of several minutes (NIOSH 2007). Periodically refill the circuit with fresh oxygen and expel previous gases into the scavenger to assist in WAG removal. Before final disconnect, turn the oxygen off and gently expel the remaining contents of the reservoir bag into the scavenging system (McKelvey and Hollingshead 2000b; AANA 2013; NIOSH 2007).

8.8.3.10 Non-rebreathing Circuits

Non-rebreathing circuits utilize higher (200–300 mL/kg/min) flow rates and can be a contributing factor of WAGs. Ensure that Bain or other non-rebreathing circuits are connected to the scavenging system before use (AANA 2013).

8.8.3.11 Ventilation and Evacuation Systems

Levels of WAGs can vary greatly, depending on the location in the hospital. Ensure that the ventilation system in the operating room performs at least 15–21 air changes per hour or more, and a minimum of 3 fresh air changes per hour. As such, periodic inspection and performance testing of the ventilation and air conditioning system is also advised (NIOSH 2007; AANA 2013).

The recovery room is considered the most contaminated area in the hospital. In 1996, the American Society of Peri-anesthesia Nurses (ASPAN) posed concern over WAG exposure in the post-anesthesia environment to nursing personnel, stating that better engineering controls, technologies and personal protective equipment (PPE) were needed to protect these workers (McGlothlin and Moenning 2013).

Prevention is accomplished by ensuring that all rooms used for induction, maintenance and recovery of anesthetized patients have at least 15–21 air changes per hour (AANA 2013). Finally, periodic inspection and performance testing of the central vacuum system is advised quarterly or in accordance with the manufacturer's instructions (AANA 2013). Because patients continue to exhale residual inhalants for a period post-operatively, remain at least 3 feet (0.914 m) away from the faces of these recovering anesthetic patients (McKelvey and Hollingshead 2000; AANA 2013).

8.8.3.12 Vaporizers

Vaporizer associated leaks are commonly due to inappropriate installation or misplacement onto the manifold, or a loose vaporizer fill cap (Figure 8.5). Vaporizer leaks can be detected during failure of a leak test.

Vaporizer Filling   Fill vaporizers beneath a ceiling-mounted hood with an evacuation fan, or ideally, outdoors (NIOSH 2007). If this is not possible, fill vaporizers at the end of the day, or when the least amount of staff is present. Liquid anesthetic can be absorbed through the skin, so it is imperative to wash hands immediately after filling the vaporizer, or wear plastic or vinyl gloves or other protective outerwear (gowns, respirators, etc.) (McKelvey and Hollingshead 2000b). Avoid overfilling the vaporizer. Install key-fill model vaporizers on all anesthetic delivery systems and utilize keyed agent fillers when possible (AANA 2013; McKelvey and Hollingshead 2000b) (Figure 8.8). Use specially designed anti-spill adapters (pour spouts) to reduce exposure from spills when filling non-key-fill vaporizers (Figure 8.9).

Sealed plastic bags are a safe place to store filling adapters when not in use. Remember to cap empty bottles before discarding them into ordinary trash (McKelvey and Hollingshead 2000b; AANA 2013).

Accidental Spills of Liquid Inhalants   Waste liquid inhalants may result from draining the vaporizer or due to accidental spills. Small volume spills of liquid inhalants evaporate readily in well-ventilated areas and usually dissipate before clean-up efforts can be initiated. The odor

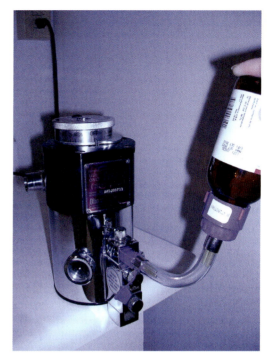

Figure 8.8 Key-fill vaporizers and keyed filling nozzles can help minimize liquid inhalant spills. Liquid inhalant bottles often contain color coded "lock and key" plastic rings that match agent-specific filling spouts to help prevent accidental pouring of the wrong liquid inhalant into the agent-specific vaporizer. Key-fill isoflurane vaporizer and filling adapter pictured.

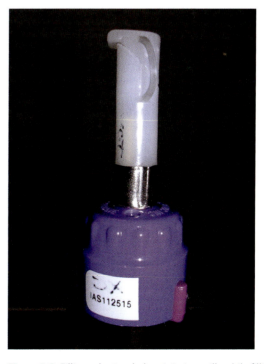

Figure 8.9 Filling adapters help minimize spills while filling the vaporizer. Isoflurane anti-spill adapter shown.

threshold for liquid anesthetics is approximately 50 ppm (which greatly exceeds NIOSH guidelines), so smelling anesthetic agents is never advised (McKelvey and Hollingshead 2000b; AANA 2013).

Accidental volume spills will require immediate action. Increase room ventilation by using fans and opening windows. Try to isolate the contaminated area by closing doors and pass-throughs and turn the central vacuum off to avoid the spread of the fumes to other areas. Absorbent materials (sorbents) such as vermiculite, carbon-based sorbents, chemical "spill pillows" or even kitty litter, can be used to clean up as much of the spill as possible before placing into a tightly sealed plastic bag or glass container. Clearly label the contents on the outside of the container (McKelvey and Hollingshead 2000b; AANA 2013).

Contaminated articles of clothing should be removed and placed in an airtight container outdoors, along with the contaminated absorbent material used to clean up the spill. Only staff wearing the proper protective vinyl or plastic clothing and gloves (not rubber or latex) and respirators should be allowed access to the contaminated area (McKelvey and Hollingshead 2000b). It is the responsibility of each healthcare facility to verify operating permits regarding incineration of anesthetic agents with a disposal service specific for chemical waste (AANA 2013).

Accidental large volume spills of liquid inhalants are considered a hazardous material situation and should not be taken lightly. For large spills or if the facility affected is not prepared to properly manage clean-up of the liquid anesthetic spill, the building should be immediately evacuated and the local fire department should be summoned (McKelvey and Hollingshead 2000b).

8.8.3.13 Carbon Dioxide Canisters

Use caution when reassembling the carbon dioxide canister, as dust particles can hamper a leak tight seal. Ensure the carbon dioxide canister is securely seated after changing the soda sorb (AANA 2013).

8.8.3.14 Carbon Dioxide Monitor Sampling

Some sidestream end-tidal carbon dioxide ($ETCO_2$) monitors utilize 120 mL (or more) per hour sample size to perform carbon dioxide analysis, while mainstream $ETCO_2$ scavenging monitors are not a significant source of WAGs. Therefore, anesthetic monitors utilizing sidestream $ETCO_2$ technology must employ a scavenging system. Contact the equipment manufacturer for more information (AANA 2013).

8.9 Monitoring WAG Exposure

Hospitals desiring monitoring of WAGs in their work environment have several options available. Badges or detector tubes can be purchased and worn for a period,

and then returned to the supplier for analysis. Ideally, quarterly testing should be performed in each anesthetizing location and cylinder storage area. Measurements shall be reported as a time-weighted average of over 8 hours (AANA 2013). Alternatively, consult an industrial hygienist for a more comprehensive facility evaluation, which can be located under the heading of "Occupational Safety".

8.9.1 Establish a Hazard Communication Program

Every facility should develop a safety and health plan that outlines exposure hazards as well as control methods. Implemented training programs will help workers recognize, understand and minimize unnecessary exposure to WAGs, while complying with OSHA's 1990 "right to know" requirement. Furthermore, OSHA regulations stipulate that each facility should create a mechanism to identify and record any injury or illness related to exposure (AANA 2013).

Anesthetic cylinders should be secured and clearly labeled and the MSDS made readily available. Schedule regular staff training as required by OSHA hazard communication standard (www.osha.gov, Section 29 CFR 1910.1200), and ensure that scavenging systems are installed and maintained properly, while exhausted away from windows, doors and air intake vents.

Develop a monitoring plan to quantitatively evaluate the efficacy of a WAG control system. This plan may also entail baseline and periodic liver and kidney testing for operating room personnel, as well as monitoring anesthetic gas concentrations near the breathing zones of the most heavily exposed workers. Environmental sampling records should be available to all workers exposed to occupational WAG levels (AANA 2013). NIOSH advises keeping detailed exposure records for 30 years, even once employment has ended. Other surveillance recommendations include maintaining medical records for occupational workers exposed to WAGs as well as the records of their families, especially the outcomes of pregnant females and wives of male workers (NIOSH 2007; AANA 2013).

8.10 Summary

Although there is not a specific cause-and-effect relationship, scientific literature to date supports the possible link between trace anesthetic gas exposure and potential adverse effects to healthcare workers. Until definitive information is available, it is prudent to assume that minimizing occupational exposure to WAGs is in the best interest of all workers. The responsibility for assuring a safe work environment is shared by employers, manufacturers and workers, as well as local and federal governments. Anesthesia professionals are obligated to limit their exposure levels by ensuring that scavenging systems are maintained and functioning properly, adjusted as needed, and that good work practices are utilized and enforced. Anesthesia professionals should also espouse EPA recommendations and requirements for operation, maintenance and disposal of all inhalant agents (AANA 2013).

References

American Association of Nurse Anesthetists (AANA) (2013) *Management of waste anesthetic gases.* Available from: https://www.aana.com/resources2/professionalpractice/Documents [accessed October 2017].

Boivin, J.F. (1997) Risk of spontaneous abortion in women occupationally exposed to anesthetic gases: a meta-analysis. *Occup Environ Med*, 54, 541–548.

Coleman, D. (2016) *Anesthesia machines: finding leaks.* Available from: Veterinary Team Brief, https://www.veterinaryteambrief.com/article/anesthesia-machines-finding-leaks [accessed October 2017].

Colon, E., Bittner, E.A., Kussman, B., McCann, M.E., Soriano, S. and Borsook, D. (2017) Anesthesia, brain changes, and behavior: insights from neural systems biology. *Prog Neurobiol*, 153, 121–160.

Gold, M.S., Byars, J. and Frost-Pineda, K. (2004) Occupational exposure and addictions for physicians: case studies and theoretical implications. *Psychiatr Clin N Am* 27, 745–753.

Kharasch, E. and Powers, K. (2002) Comparison of Amsorb, sodalime, and Baralyme degradation of volatile anesthetics and formation of carbon monoxide and compound A in swine *in vivo. Anesthesiology*, 96, 173–182.

Ko, J. (2005) *Oxygen flow rate in inhalant anesthesia. Proc Am Coll Vet Surg, San Diego, CA.* October, p. 542.

Lawson, C., Rocheleau, C. and Whelan, E. (2012) Occupational exposure among nurses and risk of spontaneous abortion. *Am J Obstet Gynecol*, 204, 327.

McGlothlin, J. and Moenning, J.E. (2013) Waste anesthetic gases (WAGs) among employees in the healthcare industry. *Clin Found.* Available from: www.clinicalfoundations.org, pp. 2–6.

McKelvey, D. and Hollingshead, K. (2000a) Anesthetic agents and techniques. In: *Small Animal Anesthesia and Analgesia,* 2nd ed. St Louis: Mosby, pp. 128–139

McKelvey, D. and Hollingshead, K. (2000b) Workplace safety. In: *Small Animal Anesthesia and Analgesia,* 2nd ed. St Louis: Mosby, pp. 191–209.

Muir, W., Hubbell, J., Skarda, R. and Bednarski, R. (2000) Anesthetic toxicity, oxygen toxicity, and drug interactions. In: *Handbook of Veterinary Anesthesia,* 3rd ed. St Louis: Mosby, pp. 198–200, 202.

National Institute for Occupational Safety and Health (NIOSH) (2007) *Waste anesthetic gases occupational hazards in hospitals.* Available from: https://www.cdc.gove/niosh/docs/2007-151/pdfs/2007-151.pdf [accessed October 2017].

Paddleford, R. (1999) *Anesthetic agents. In: Manual of Small Animal Anesthesia,* 2nd ed. Philadelphia, PA: W.B. Saunders, p. 74.

Rasmussen, H. and Thorud, S. (2007) Using refrigerant leak detector to monitor waste gases from halogenated anesthetics. *J Am Assoc Lab Anim Sci*, 46, 64–69.

Reuss-Lamky, H.L. (2006) *Waste anesthetic gases – The invisible threat.* National Association of Veterinary Technicians in America, Winter, 59–65.

Saber, A.T. and Hougaard, K.S. (2009) Isoflurane, sevoflurane and desflurane. *The Nordic Expert Group for Criteria Documentation of Health Risks from Chemicals,* 43, 3–4, 96.

Wolforth, J. and Dyson, M. (2011) Flushing induction chambers used for rodent anesthesia to reduce waste anesthetic gas. *Lab Anim*, 40, 76–83.

9

Hazards of the Anesthetic Delivery System and Operating Room Fires
Odette O

Canada West Veterinary Specialists, Vancouver, BC, Canada

9.1 Hazards of the Anesthetic Delivery System

Modern anesthetic machines are built with increasing complexity that can provide both added safety and hazard. Both anesthesia care provider errors and Anesthetic Delivery System (ADS) malfunctions have the potential to lead to an adverse anesthetic event, including patient death. Even though the modern electrical anesthetic workstations used for human anesthesia have many built-in self-checks and safety mechanisms, errors are still reported and include problems such as sensor errors, electrical failure, operator mistakes, etc. In an effort to increase the safety of anesthetic machines used in the field of human anesthesia, the American Society of Anesthesiologists (ASA) published guidelines in 2004 for determining anesthetic machine obsolescence (www.asahq.org). In addition, in an effort to collect and analyze data, share knowledge and improve anesthesia care, an Anesthesia Incident Reporting System (AIRS) that is maintained by the Anesthesia Quality Institute, a federally designated Patient Safety Organization (PSO), is available (www.aqihq.org 2016). This online system allows anesthesia care providers to submit adverse anesthetic event case information, with the option of confidentiality. Recently, a voluntary small animal anesthesia adverse event reporting system was tested with promising results published (McMillan and Darcy 2015).

Nonetheless, in the current field of veterinary anesthesia, it will still likely be a while before a tool such as this is launched and used broadly enough to collect useable data to guide everyday patient care decisions. As a result, an everyday challenge in veterinary medicine includes the common use of older, refurbished machines plus countless re-uses of breathing systems. In addition, there is a frequent requirement for patient transport, leading to disconnection and reconnection of the patient from the ADS, possibly in a number of different locations and between many different anesthetic machines. A thorough understanding of the gas supply system, anesthetic machine, breathing system, ventilator and scavenge (jointly referred to as the ADS), its functions, as well as regular system checks and maintenance servicing, is of paramount importance in the attempt to minimize anesthetic risk to the patient. A concrete knowledge base will make anesthesia safer by both decreasing equipment misuse (operator error) and facilitating early detection and troubleshooting of equipment failure. Since it is nearly impossible to create a single chapter detailing every possible malfunction in each piece of equipment, a general list is provided here with more comprehensive details of each portion of the ADS provided in other chapters of this book (see Chapters 1–6).

9.1.1 Gas Source

Depending on the size of the facility, oxygen (O_2) is most commonly provided, either by cylinders containing liquid or compressed gas. Liquid O_2 can cause burns if directly handled without proper safety precautions, since its boiling point at sea level (760 mmHg) is $-183\,°C/-297\,°F$. Cylinders themselves are highly pressurized items, especially when full, and should be properly stored and transported in order to prevent human injury or damage to the building and its contents (Figure 9.1). A fire hazard exists when opening a cylinder too quickly, especially in the presence of grease or dust. Adiabatic change occurs when the gas quickly expands without the ability to exchange heat into its surrounding environment. As a result, extreme heat may be produced with the possibility of igniting flammable gases including O_2 and nitrous oxide. In order to prevent the three elements of the fire triangle from being present – fuel, oxidizing agent and ignition – it is important to ensure that the cylinder valve is clean and to open a full tank slowly.

Veterinary Anesthetic and Monitoring Equipment, First Edition. Edited by Kristen G. Cooley and Rebecca A. Johnson.
© 2018 John Wiley & Sons, Inc. Published 2018 by John Wiley & Sons, Inc.

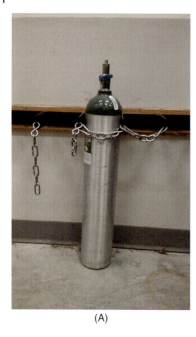
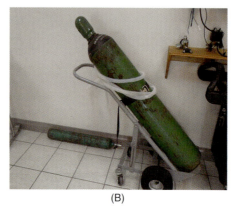
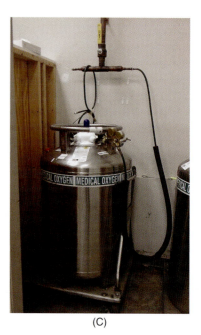

(A)   (B)   (C)

Figure 9.1 Stored tanks. (A) E tank properly stored and secured to a permanent wall with chains; (B) H tank properly secured on a transport trolley; (C) Liquid oxygen tank in use – notice the ice formation on top of cylinder.

Potential danger exists when the gas, especially O_2, is not connected to the source prior to use, disconnected from the source during operation, or runs out without the anesthesia care provider noticing. In addition, leaks or an obstruction at any location from the medical gas source through the medical gas supply pipeline and anywhere in the anesthetic machine or breathing circuit, may lead to the inability to provide an adequate amount of O_2 to the patient. Tools to help prevent this type of occurrence include the incorporation of O_2 fail-safe alarms on the hospital pipeline and the anesthetic machine, plus incorporating the routine use of a gas analyzer if available.

The diameter index safety system (DISS), pin index safety system (PISS), and safety keyed gas-specific quick connects, exist in order to help prevent accidental misconnections of incorrect medical gases; however, these systems are not infallible. For example, a case report involving a human patient unexpectedly receiving high levels of carbon dioxide (CO_2) instead of the intended nitrous oxide (N_2O) during an anesthetic event, despite use of a safety keyed quick-connects, was reported (Ellett *et al.* 2009). In addition, it is possible that the wrong type of medical gas is filled into a cylinder (Jawan and Lee 1990) or that the gas is contaminated with items such as metal, hydrocarbons, oils, water and/or cleaners. Errors like these may lead to the delivery of impure or hypoxemic mixtures of gases.

9.1.2 Pressure Regulators

After leaving its source, medical gases pass through a pressure regulator before entering the anesthetic machine. This device decreases source gas pressures to a safe operating level, usually approximately 50 psi. A malfunction in this part can cause abnormally high-pressured gases to be delivered to the anesthetic machine, potentially causing damage to the associated flowmeter. A second-stage O_2 pressure regulator is present just upstream of the flowmeter in some anesthetic machines (Figure 9.2). It permits constant and consistent flow of O_2 to the machine, even if pressure in the supply line decreases (Subrahmanyam and Mohan 2013). Failure of this pressure regulator may result in decreased or irregular O_2 delivery to the flowmeter.

9.1.3 Flowmeters

A color-coded, gas-specific flowmeter exists for each type of medical gas that an anesthetic machine is capable of delivering. Potential dangers of this portion of the ADS include:

- incorrect type of medical gas provided by the flowmeter via errors in medical gas source connection;
- a leak upstream of a flowmeter leading to the inability to provide enough gas flow.
- O_2 flowmeter not turned on, or accidentally turned off – older machines do not have a protective barrier around the O_2 flowmeter knob to prevent accidental knob turning;
- ball/bobbin stuck within the tube or an improperly-calibrated flowmeter, resulting in the incorrect display of the gas amount being delivered to the patient;

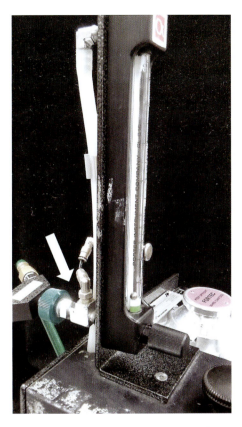

Figure 9.2 Second-stage O_2 pressure regulator (white arrow) located immediately upstream of the flowmeter permits consistent O_2 flow to machine, even in the event that the supply line pressure decreases.

- the wrong flowmeter turned on – more possible in older machines where O_2 and N_2O are not coupled; and
- flow of the medical gas too low or too high, leading to the possibility of delivering a hypoxemic gas mixture (i.e. $O_2 < 25\%$, $N_2O > 75\%$).

9.1.4   Oxygen Flush

The O_2 flush button provides 100% O_2 at a rate of 35–75 L/min directly into the patient breathing system at extremely high pressures. O_2 delivered at this rapid rate creates pressures equivalent to 1000–2500 cmH_2O, resulting in the risk of barotrauma, increased intrathoracic pressure, hypotension and possibly pneumothorax in the patient attached to the breathing system (Atlee 2006). Activation of the O_2 flush valve should *never* occur with a patient attached to the breathing system. Increasing O_2 flow using the flowmeter is a much safer, low-pressure alternative to increase gas flow to the system. The O_2 flush valve should not be activated to fill the rebreathing bag during a stable anesthetic plane, since it bypasses the vaporizer, delivering O_2 without inhalant. Anesthetic mishaps related to problems with the O_2

flush valve have been reported, including an inappropriately light anesthetic plane resulting from an internal leak in the O_2 flush due to a faulty O-ring (Mun and No 2013). In some cases, the O_2 flush valve is useful to quickly reduce the amount of inhalant in the system (i.e. patient excessively deep, cardiopulmonary arrest, etc.); however, the patient should always be disconnected first and the connection port plugged before flushing the system to ensure excess gas is removed via the scavenge.

9.1.5   Vaporizers

The most widely-used vaporizers in current veterinary medicine are concentration-calibrated, variable bypass types. It is likely that the most common adverse vaporizer events are related to operator error. A vaporizer setting that is too low or high may cause patient movement and consciousness, or conversely, excessive patient cardiovascular and respiratory depression. If a vaporizer is filled with the wrong type of inhalant, unpredictable and potentially unsafe output may result. In these instances, vaporizer output will be lower than expected if an agent with a lower saturated vapor pressure (SVP) is filled into the vaporizer, which was designed for an agent with a higher SVP and/or lower minimum alveolar concentration (MAC); for example, if sevoflurane was poured into an isoflurane vaporizer (Tobias 1998). On the other hand, vaporizer output will be greater than expected if an inhalant with greater SVP is filled into a vaporizer designed for an agent with lower SVP and/or higher MAC (i.e. isoflurane filled into a sevoflurane vaporizer).

Other sources of unpredictably high vaporizer output include:

- vaporizer overfilling or tipping (i.e. models such as Ohmeda Tec 3 and lower) (Scott 1991);
- more than one vaporizer in series is simultaneously turned on either in some older machines or via vaporizer interlock failure in newer ones;
- improperly placed vaporizers; e.g. if the vaporizer is placed between the anesthetic machine and breathing system, the potential for reverse gas flow and high output may occur (Dorsch and Dorsch 2011);
- the pumping effect; this phenomenon is seen in older vaporizers designed without an outlet check valve positioned upstream of the common gas outlet, to prevent bypass gas from entering the vaporizing chamber during mechanical ventilation and increasing output; seen especially with low fresh gas flow use; and
- vaporizers being used at altitude (hypobaric conditions).

Other reasons for low output include:

- empty, incorrectly seated or leaking vaporizer;

- the use of sevoflurane with a desiccated CO_2 absorber, resulting in anesthetic agent breakdown (Dorsch and Dorsch 2011); and
- vaporizers being used below sea level (hyperbaric conditions).

9.1.6 Fresh Gas Flow

Fresh gas flow from the common gas outlet can be affected by accidental disconnection, a leak or occlusion. In some anesthetic machines, the fresh gas tubing must be moved when transitioning from a rebreathing to non-rebreathing system, and this step is often forgotten or goes unnoticed until a pre-use machine check is performed (see Chapter 27) or a patient is placed on the machine and no gas flow in the system is noted.

9.1.7 The Breathing System

This portion of the anesthetic delivery system includes the breathing tubes, inspiratory:expiratory (I:E) unidirectional valves, reservoir bag, adjustable pressure limiting (APL) or pop-off valve, CO_2 absorbent and canister, and face mask or endotracheal tube (ETT).

Problems can occur in each component of the breathing system. For example, breathing tubes may become obstructed, disconnected or leak from either the patient or the machine end, or any distance in between. Improper selection of the breathing tube (ETT) size for the patient may lead to increased work of breathing and greater resistance to flow according to the Poiseuille law:

$$\Delta P = 8\mu LQ / \pi r^4 \qquad (9.1)$$

where ΔP = change in pressure, 8μ = dynamic viscosity, L = length, Q = volumetric flow rate, π = 3.14, and r = radius. Improper ETT choice may also lead to increased mechanical dead space being present in small patients, resulting in the rebreathing of CO_2. For coaxial systems, this can occur if the inner tube becomes displaced or kinked (e.g. Bain system, universal F circuit), potentially resulting in increased work of breathing, greater re-inspired CO_2 due to enormous dead space, and respiratory acidosis (Jellish *et al.* 2001). It is possible to place a universal F circuit onto the I:E limbs of the machine backwards, thereby losing the benefit of exhaled gases warming the inhaled ones in the coaxial system.

All associated valves represent another area for hazard. I:E unidirectional valve hazards include incompetent valves either via a leak or obstruction. An obstructed expiratory valve results in high inspired CO_2 from the inhalation of previously exhaled gases (Figure 9.3).

Positive End-Expiratory Pressure (PEEP) valves (see Chapter 7), used to add positive pressure to the system at the end of expiration, are intended to be placed on the expiratory limb of the breathing circuit. One-way (unidirectional) PEEP valves will completely obstruct the breathing system, leaving a patient unable to ventilate if placed backwards on either the inspiratory or expiratory limb. If this valve is placed on an expiratory limb during mechanical ventilation, the excessive positive pressure may lead to barotrauma in the patient. Bidirectional

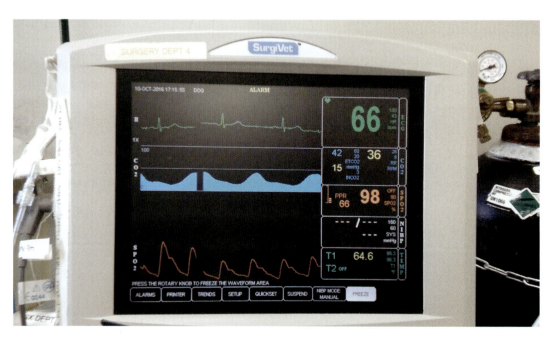

Figure 9.3 Capnograph waveform showing high levels of inspired CO_2 (15 mmHg shown in yellow). This may result from increased dead space, insufficient fresh O_2 flow in a non-rebreathing system, a faulty one-way valve in a rebreathing system, or exhausted CO_2 absorber.

PEEP valves will not inhibit gas flow if incorrectly set up, but PEEP will not be delivered to the patient (ERCI 1983). In addition, the use of PEEP valves may decrease the tidal volume delivered to the patient, an effect especially pronounced in patients with smaller tidal volumes and high compliance (Dorsch and Dorsch 2011).

The APL valve, also known as the pop-off, overflow or relief valve, is designed to permit excess gas to leave the circuit and prevent high pressure in the system. Although a mechanical malfunction of this part is possible, human error is most often the culprit of hazards related to this portion of the anesthetic machine. Neglecting to open the APL valve after a pre-use check, when manually delivering a breath or when disconnecting a mechanical ventilator, results in excessive positive pressure in the breathing system, and the potential for barotrauma, hypotension, pneumothorax and possible death of the patient (Ioannidis *et al.* 2015). The anesthesia care provider should always check that this valve is open prior to connecting every patient to the breathing system. New safety devices have been manufactured to avoid over pressurization of the system when placed in the breathing circuit, by allowing gas to escape when a set pressure is reached (~20 or 30 cmH$_2$O; EMD Safety Valve, Essential Medical Devices, LLC, www.essentialmedicaldevices.com). In addition, quick release occlusion valves can be used to prevent gas escaping from the APL valve when a button is depressed; however, upon release of the button, the valve opens and no physical closure of the actual APL valve is necessary (Figure 9.4; Pop-Off Occlusion Valve, Smiths Medical, Dublin, OH). One product is manufactured that combines both the quick release APL valve and a safety pressure relief valve (Figure 9.5; Safety Pressure Relief Valve, Supera Anesthesia Innovations, Clackamas, OR).

Reservoir bag hazards include omission of incorporating it in the setup, selecting the wrong bag size, a hole in bag or improper seating of the bag on the mount causing a leak, and the bag becoming twisted resulting in obstruction. These issues may lead to accidental environmental exposure to inhalant, difficulty with patient oxygenation and maintaining an appropriate anesthetic plane, as well as the inability to hand-ventilate the patient. The diligent implementation of the pre-use anesthetic machine check should help to detect and resolve these issues prior to each use of the machine.

9.1.8 Mechanical Ventilators

The use of mechanical ventilation to provide intermittent positive pressure ventilation (IPPV) in veterinary medicine is variable, with the likelihood of use increasing at referral hospitals where longer anesthetic episodes and procedures that necessitate its use may potentially be more common (see Chapter 6). Mechanical ventilation is associated with potential negative consequences; as

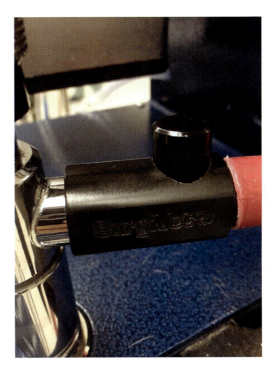

Figure 9.4 Example of a quick release occlusion valve that opens to the scavenge once the button is released. Only upon button depression is the valve closed.

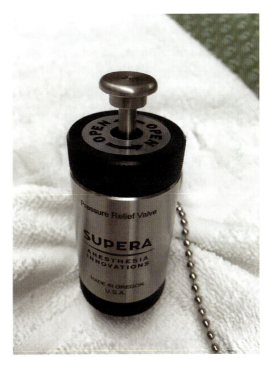

Figure 9.5 Example of a safety pressure valve in combination with a quick release occlusion valve. The internal valve opens when the system pressure reaches a set value.

with many medical decisions, its institution should be considered with a risk: benefit analysis to the patient. Since mechanical positive pressure into the thorax is employed, the expected increased venous return during negative pressure ventilation is not seen, resulting in decreased perfusion. This consideration may be of increased importance in patients who are at risk of or may not tolerate hypotension, especially those who are hypovolemic or in other states of shock. In recent years, the recognition of the importance of negative intrathoracic pressure has led to the use of intrathoracic pump devices to improve vital organ perfusion during states of hypotension and shock (Segal *et al.* 2013).

A primary concern of instituting IPPV in a patient is the possibility of creating injury. It is important to carefully calculate, adjust and monitor ventilator settings in order to avoid alveolar over-distension. IPPV-related damage to the lungs occurs via pressure (barotrauma) and volume (volutrauma). As the alveloli open and close during mechanical ventilation, increased shearing forces from pressure and volume changes may result in atelectrauma. Thus, pulmonary over-inflation can result in subcutaneous emphysema, pulmonary interstitial emphysema, pneumomediastinum, pneumopericardium, pneumoperitoneum, pneumothorax, hypoxemia, tachycardia and even cardiac arrest (Mitchell *et al.* 2000). In human medicine, the terms used for injuries associated with mechanical ventilation are ventilator-associated lung injury (VALI) or ventilator-induced lung injury (VILI); it is caused by high airway pressure and/or large volumes (Ioannidis *et al.* 2015). The main determining factor for barotrauma appears to be dynamic hyperinflation, with the main influential elements being transpulmonary pressure, tidal volume, and intrinsic positive end-expiratory pressure (PEEP).

There are multiple factors that may prevent proper functioning of a mechanical ventilator, so pre-use checks should be included anytime its use is anticipated. Leaks or an obstruction anywhere in the system (i.e. the housing, piston or bellows, fresh gas flow, spill valve, scavenge) may result in detrimental outcomes. A computer-driven ventilator may cease operation with power failure or a computer malfunction. Ventilators may be either electrically, compressed gas, or pneumatically driven. If either the electrical source or driving gas source is disconnected or runs out, the ventilator may stop functioning. Leaks in the bellows may predispose a patient to hypoventilation as the bellows may not be able to provide a large enough tidal volume. In addition, a lighter-than-expected anesthetic depth may result due to the dilutional effect of driving gas mixing into the patient fresh gas (see below). Barotrauma may also occur from the high-pressured driving gas, making its way into a large enough hole in the bellows.

There are many different types of ventilators available on the current market. Piston ventilators are not commonly used in veterinary medicine, but it is important to monitor them for leaks on the piston housing and diaphragm and maintain the motor in good working order to ensure proper function. Bellowed ventilators are more readily available to veterinary practitioners at this time. Hanging (descending) bellows are not preferred, since a leak may entrain room air and dilute inhalant levels being provided to the patient. Standing (ascending) bellows are preferred. A leak is more visible to the anesthesia care provider because the bellows do not fill properly during exhalation if a leak is present (Figure 9.6). An important part of decreasing hazards associated with mechanical ventilation is to perform regular checks prior to each use, to ensure proper settings for each patient, as well as close patient monitoring after institution of IPPV.

9.1.9 CO₂ Management

CO_2 exhaled by the patient into the breathing system needs to be removed in order to prevent excessive patient rebreathing (Figure 9.3). In the non-rebreathing systems (see Chapter 11), the O_2 flow rate is solely responsible for removing CO_2. Thus, if the O_2 flow is

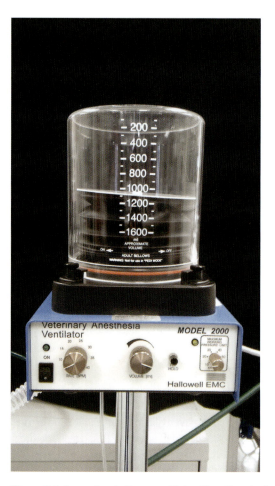

Figure 9.6 Ascending bellows ventilator. Note that the bellows are filled upward during exhalation.

too low, inappropriate buildup of CO_2 will occur in the system. For rebreathing systems (see Chapter 12), CO_2 absorbers such as soda lime are used to remove CO_2. CO_2 absorbers work by a chemical reaction and in a finite capacity. If the absorber is exhausted, excessive CO_2 will build up in the system. Strong alkalis used in some absorbers present additional hazards to both the anesthesia care provider and patient, including irritation and/or burns to eyes or skin with contact, and if inhaled into the respiratory tract, even the potential for pneumonitis. The CO_2 absorber canister is also a common place for leaks in the system.

Desiccated absorbent presents two serious potential hazards. First, CO_2 absorbers are known to produce carbon monoxide (CO) when exposed to volatile anesthetics. CO is produced more when inhalants and dry CO_2 absorber interact; for example, after prolonged use of absorbent without it being changed or after a flowmeter has inadvertently been left turned on over a weekend devoid of notice (hence issues are commonly seen during early Monday morning cases, ERCI 1998). Interestingly, different inhalants produced differing amounts of CO. Desflurane in the presence of desiccated absorber produces the greatest amount of CO, followed by enflurane, then isoflurane. Halothane and sevoflurane were not found to produce any notable amounts of CO (Fang *et al.* 1995). However, after the publication of clinical case reports of carboxyhemoglobin in pediatric anesthetic patients, a study found the production of CO with sevoflurane and dried soda lime in a clinical setting (Wissing *et al.* 2001).

The second risk of inhalant contact with desiccated CO_2 absorber is Compound A formation. Compound A (fluoromethyl-2,2-difluoro-1-[trifluoromethyl] vinyl ether) is a breakdown product of sevoflurane, which occurs when it is exposed to alkaline agents such as soda lime, especially at low O_2 flow rates. Compound A production increases with dry CO_2 absorber and has been linked to renal injury; Compound A production in swine anesthetized with sevoflurane was 5 to 10 times greater and associated with evidence of renal inflammation when desiccated absorber was used (Steffey *et al.* 1997).

Consequently, it is important to replace CO_2 absorber regularly to ensure proper CO_2 absorption, as well as to prevent use of desiccated product that may lead to CO and/or Compound A production. Monitoring devices are also an important tool in determining possible issues with CO_2 absorption. For example, assuming minimal dead space and the proper functioning of I:E unidirectional valves, the capnograph waveform will demonstrate unusually high inspired CO_2 if the O_2 flow is too low in a non-rebreathing system or the absorber is exhausted in a rebreathing system (Figure 9.3). While use of a standard pulse oximeter will not detect carboxyhemoglobinemia, a pulse co-oximeter will certainly increase safety in this

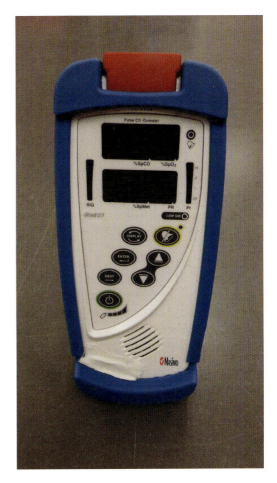

Figure 9.7 Masimo Rad 57 Co-Oximeter.

regard (Masimo Pulse Co-Oximetry, Masimo Corporation, Irvine, CA; Figure 9.7). Unfortunately, at this point, there is no clinically convenient way to detect Compound A formation during an anesthetic event.

9.1.10 Endotracheal Tube (ETT)

There are many dangers associated with the ETT. As discussed later in this chapter, airway fires are a potential hazard for the patient, since the ETT contains a flammable fuel source. Upper as well as lower airways can suffer thermal damage and burnt pieces pose an aspiration risk if left behind in the airway after the fire is extinguished. In addition, inhalation of broken pieces of the ETT is also possible when a patient awakens rapidly and begins to bite on the tube. ETT obstruction either by the patient biting down on the tube, mucous secretions, excessive application of lubricant, etc. is of concern, since ventilation is hindered under these circumstances. Care should be taken always to extubate a patient with the ETT pulled out rostrally instead of laterally. Incisor teeth are less likely to tear a tube with contact, whereas

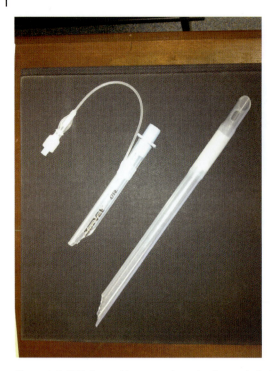

Figure 9.8 ETT sheared into two pieces by the teeth during improper extubation of a canine patient.

molars are able to shear through an ETT easily, creating risk for aspiration or ingestion of the distal portion of the tube (Figure 9.8).

Patients with difficult airways (e.g. unable to open mouth: temporomandibular joint issues, laryngeal mass, trauma, etc.) are also at risk, since it is sometimes challenging to obtain a patent airway and minimize trauma while doing so. Use of a stylet is sometimes necessary under these conditions, but it is important that this piece of equipment is used carefully, in order to prevent tracheal perforation or loss of the stylet into the trachea. Traumatic intubation may result in laryngeal edema and/ or possible spasm, potentially resulting in airway obstruction. Failure to obtain an airway through nasotracheal or orotracheal intubation may necessitate a surgical tracheostomy in some cases.

Proper ETT fit and placement along with appropriate cuff inflation is important to both patient and anesthesia care provider safety. Esophageal and endobronchial intubations are a preventable anesthetic mishap. Proper placement length of the ETT should be distal to the larynx but proximal to the thoracic inlet. Visual confirmation of tracheal intubation using a laryngoscope, use of anesthetic monitors including capnography and pulse oximetry, pre-measurement of tube length, and using the largest possible diameter ETT will help to minimize the frequency of these incidents. However, if they occur, early recognition and correction is of paramount importance. Use of an ETT of the largest possible diameter will

also decrease airway resistance and help prevent tube obstruction with respiratory secretions.

The tracheal mucosa in human subjects has a capillary perfusion pressure of 22 mmHg ($\approx$30 cmH$_2$O, 3.3 kPa) (Seegobin and van Hasselt 1984). Over-inflation of an ETT cuff to pressures above this value prevents proper perfusion and can cause ischemia and necrosis of the tracheal mucosa. Tracheal rupture, subcutaneous emphysema, pneumomediastinum or pneumothorax, dyspnea and death are potential immediate consequences, whereas tracheal stricture formation after healing may become a chronic problem. In a retrospective study of 20 cats, 70% of those developing tracheal rupture post-intubation had received dental prophylaxis; ETT cuff over-inflation, changes in patient position without protecting the airway, use of a stylet for intubation, removal of the ETT without cuff deflation, and type of ETT were potential risk factors (Mitchell *et al.* 2000).

The use of high-volume, low-pressure cuffed ETTs, along with selecting largest diameter ETTs possible, in order to minimally inflate the cuff for a proper seal, is recommended. Proper cuff inflation techniques and use of a cuff-pressure manometer (Posey Cufflator, Posey Company, Arcadia, CA; Figure 9.9) also increase patient safety. In addition to the above-mentioned consequences, ETT cuff over-inflation has been reported to critically obstruct the tube lumen in an intubated patient (Hofstetter *et al.* 2010). On the other hand, under-inflated ETT cuffs may permit the aspiration of gastric contents more readily than a properly inflated one. An under-inflated ETT may also lead to a leak in the breathing system, with the patient potentially unable to receive positive pressure ventilation and anesthetic gases entering the operating room instead of the waste scavenging system.

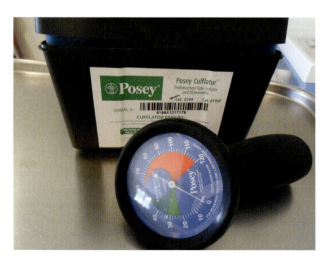

Figure 9.9 Posey Cufflator used to check ETT cuff inflation pressures.

9.1.11 Scavenge Systems

A properly functioning scavenge system used routinely is an integral part of anesthesia safety (see Chapter 8). The function of this system is to remove anesthetic waste gas from the work environment. The scavenge system may be active or passive, with either an interface that is either an open or closed reservoir (Dorsch and Dorsch 2011). In the closed-reservoir interface, valves are located between the patient breathing system and the facility vacuum or ventilation. Malfunction of these valves may pose a problem, especially if excessive vacuum creates negative pressure in the system and the negative pressure relief valve is ineffective. Conversely, weak vacuum can cause positive pressure buildup in the reservoir and excessive positive pressure in the system, especially if the pop-off valve does not open to vent gases into the room. Open-reservoir scavenging interface systems avoid potential positive and negative pressure buildup, since they are continuously open and valveless. However, it should be noted that accidental occlusion of these ports may prevent proper pressure relief. For example, an active scavenge system with an open interface developed excessive PEEP in a patient when the scavenging system transfer tubing became obstructed upstream of the interface (Elakkumanan *et al.* 2012).

Newer scavenging system connections consist of 19 or 30 mm outer diameter (O.D.) female connections, in order to prevent accidental misconnections with the breathing system. However, older fittings may be of 22 mm O.D., which may allow accidental misconnections of scavenge tubing with breathing tubes. Thus, caution should be exercised to prevent misconnections in any facility that continues to use outdated equipment. It is recommended that current anesthetic machine standards be incorporated into modern practices.

Equipment failures, such as an occlusion or leaks, can occur anywhere in the ADS, from the gas source to the ETT and anywhere in between. However, accidental equipment misuse incidents leading to anesthetic morbidity and mortality likely outnumber the actual failure of anesthetic equipment in modern veterinary medicine, especially if pre-use checkout protocols are routinely employed. Nonetheless, the possibility of either or both of these events occurring does still exist and may result in what could have been a preventable negative outcome. Increasingly, resources and guidelines are becoming more readily available, but successful use of these tools relies on the diligence of the anesthesia care provider.

9.2 Operating Room Fires

Peri-operative fires in modern veterinary medicine are rare. In human medicine, estimates of the occurrence of operating room fires range from 500–600 annually in the US (ECRI 2009). Currently, there is no literature available to quantify this disaster in veterinary medicine. Nonetheless, if it occurs, this preventable event may result in potentially dire consequences for the veterinary patient, personnel and the facility alike. Personnel safety in veterinary medicine often focuses on zoonotic agents and dangerous animals, but fire prevention and an emergency plan should also be in place and reviewed regularly in every veterinary facility. General fire prevention and safety guidelines are provided by a number of resources, including the Food and Drug Administration (FDA) and Occupational Health and Safety Administration (OSHA), whereas practice advisories regarding peri-operative fires are provided by groups such as the American Society of Anesthesiologists (ASA), Association of peri-operative Registered Nurses (AORN), and the Council on Surgical and Peri-operative Safety (CSPS) (www.FDA.gov).

The ASA has published an invaluable resource in its updated practice advisory on preventing and managing operating room fires from the perspective of anesthesiologists; this document is the main resource used for information provided in this part of this chapter (Apfelbaum *et al.* 2013). This ASA Advisory addresses surgical and/or airway fires during the anesthetic care period with the following purpose(s):

1) Identify situations conducive to fire.
2) Prevent the occurrence of operating room (OR) fires.
3) Reduce adverse outcomes associated with OR fires.
4) Identify the elements of a fire response protocol.

The traditional fire triangle containing an ignition source, fuel and an oxidizing agent is now more commonly referred to as the fire tetrahedron or fire pyramid (Figure 9.10). This concept involves the original three components of the triangle, along with a necessary chemical chain reaction. This exothermic process

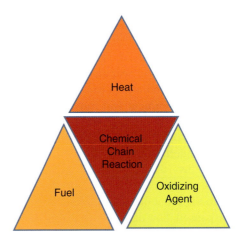

Figure 9.10 Fire Tetrahedron.

continues the fire until one or more of these elements are removed. There are four stages to a fire: incipient, growth, fully developed and decay. The fire tetrahedron creates the incipient stage, also known as ignition. Fires in the OR can be difficult to recognize early, since this stage may present itself with only a popping noise or very small flames, but fires are most easily extinguished at this stage. Growth is the shortest of the four stages, but occurs quickly, consuming combustible fuels until the fire is fully developed. This stage is the one with highest temperatures, where all combustible materials are on fire. The last stage, decay, is the longest but is still dangerous as a new fire can ignite.

Every veterinary procedure and operating area is potentially hazardous, because it provides all of the ingredients necessary for creating a fire! These areas are known as increased risk environments. An oxidizer is provided anytime O_2 is present at a greater concentration than room air (~20.9%). This risk increases with increasing levels of O_2 and when nitrous oxide is in use, because although not directly flammable, these oxidizing agents are required by a fuel in order for it to burn. This enriched oxidizer situation is present in patient breathing systems, regardless of whether it is supplied by face mask or endotracheal intubation. There are multiple ignition sources including electrocautery units, lasers, drills/burrs, fiber optic light cables found with endoscopes, and defibrillators. These items have the ability to create enough heat to potentially raise the temperature of a material to result in ignition. An exothermic reaction then occurs, allowing flammable materials to become fuel for the fire. Most objects in the operating area have the potential to be flammable. Possible fuel sources can come from either the patient, patient care equipment, or the room itself. Patient fuel sources include fur and gases produced in the gastrointestinal tract. Fuel sources from equipment used in patient care include blankets, bandages, gauzes, surgical drapes, and alcohol-based cleansing solutions. This category also contains components of the patient breathing system, including supplemental O_2 masks and ETTs.

In these high-risk environments, dangerous situations occur when the ignition source is near an oxidizer in the presence of fuel. Operating room fires can happen anywhere in the surgical environment and can involve the room, electrical equipment or the patient. *Surgical fires* specifically occur within or on a patient. These types of fires are specifically dangerous, because they may occur when caregivers have diverted attention, be difficult to immediately recognize, and involve an unconscious, immobile patient. In the event of a surgical fire, the procedure needs to be paused, flow of supplemental gases to the patient should be immediately discontinued, burning items should be removed from the patient, and the patient fire smothered using saline. This type of situation is particularly prevalent in surgeries of the head and neck, especially when the use of laser or electrocautery is employed.

Airway fires are defined as fires that happen in the airway of the patient; this is a subset of surgical fires. Since ETTs and breathing systems are both flammable fuel sources, airway fires are responsible for a few human deaths annually in the US. These types of fires are of particular concern, since supplemental gases must be discontinued in order to remove the oxidizer, and the patient must be extubated to put out the fire using saline in the airway (Hart *et al.* 2011). Once the fire has been extinguished, the patient should be assessed for injury, inspected for remnants of the burnt ETT left in the airway, then re-intubated as soon as possible along with the formulation of an overall patient care plan. If the initial attempt at extinguishing the fire is unsuccessful, it is advisable to use a CO_2 fire extinguisher (Figure 9.11). If this effort is not successful, activate the fire alarm and evacuate personnel along with the patient, if possible. It is also

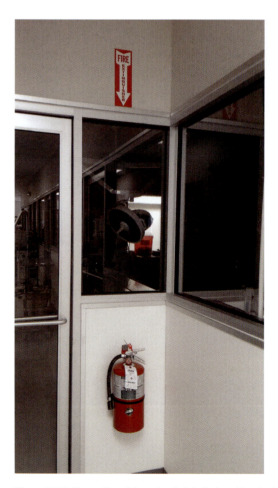

Figure 9.11 Fire extinguisher clearly labeled and located in an easily accessible area.

prudent to contain the fire by closing the door if automatic fire doors are not present and turn off the medical gas supply to the room. At this point, no attempts should be made to re-enter the room (Apfelbaum *et al.* 2013).

Few will argue with the fact that the safest manner in which to deal with a fire is to prevent its occurrence in the first place. The anesthesiologist and/or anesthetist have a vital role in communicating potential risks to the surgeon and surgical care team, as well as soliciting their involvement in fire prevention. Small steps such as allowing alcohol-based solutions to dry completely before initiating the use of electrocautery, draping to allow air circulation underneath a patient who is being supplemented with flow-by O_2 to prevent buildup of oxidizer, and unplugging and properly storing fiber optic lights when not in use, are simple ways to help reduce fire risk in the OR.

If a procedure creates a high-risk situation, the anesthesia care provider needs to inform the entire team of potential risk, provide ways to help minimize it, and review a safety plan in the event of a fire. For instance, the use of electrocautery or laser in an airway surgery with a patient inspiring more than 21% O_2 creates a high risk environment for airway fires and avoidance of the use of laser and electrocautery in airway surgery is advisable whenever possible. Electrosurgical equipment was involved in 68% of reported surgical fires, many of which involve supplemental use of O_2 (Dorsch and Dorsch 2011). For example, in 2016, a surgical fire ensued in a human patient receiving supplemental O_2 during eyelid surgery using electrocautery. This emphasizes the current and present dangers of this type of procedural setup; the supplemental O_2 is a powerful oxidizing agent, while the cautery provided a heat source, and eyelashes of the patient became the fuel (ASA 2016). Thus, the use of electrocautery or lasers in procedures of the head, neck and upper body should be performed with extreme caution and only if no other alternative is available.

However, if communication of fire risk is clear and use of this equipment is unavoidable, then optimal planning is necessary. If possible, provision of FIO_2 at less than 100% and use of cuffed ETTs for head, neck and upper thorax procedures is safer. Furthermore, for airway surgeries, packing of the local area around the ETT with saline-soaked gauze and ensuring that it remains moist, will help decrease the presence of oxidizer outside of the airway area. While there are no ETTs that are resistant to electrocautery heat, specific laser-safe ETTs are available when lasers are employed. However, an important note is that the cuff is still flammable in these ETTs. These tubes are more laser safe attributable to a protective coating and wrap (i.e. Teflon, foil), but it does not completely cover the ETT, still making them potentially laser-vulnerable (Green *et al.* 1992). Filling the ETT cuff with saline or water will make it less flammable if the cuff is punctured, and adding dye such as methylene blue may help the surgeon detect tube damage earlier. Potential heat sources causing ignition will be decreased by minimizing the time that lasers electrocautery are activated, as well as using the lowest settings possible.

As part of being thoroughly prepared, it is important for each facility to have a fire safety plan. Elements of a successful fire safety plan involve posting protocols in obvious areas with regular review by all members of the surgical and anesthesia team. *All* staff members need to be familiar with the plan, their specific assigned roles in case of a fire emergency, as well as the emergency phone number and the location of firefighting supplies. Fire extinguishing supplies may include sterile saline in the OR, CO_2 fire extinguishers, and fire blankets. OR fire awareness and prevention is clearly a team effort, requiring a fire plan be in place that is clearly communicated and understood by all staff members, recognizing potential hazards, working to minimize risk factors, and responding quickly in the event of an emergency.

References

American Society of Anesthesiologists (ASA) Committee on Equipment and Facilities. *Guidelines for Determining Anesthesia Machine Obsolescence.* Available from: http://www.asahq.org [accessed June 29, 2016].

Anesthesia Incident Reporting System. Available from: https://www.aqihq.org/airs [accessed June 23, 2016].

Apfelbau, J., Caplan, R., Barker, S., Connis, R., Cowles, C. et al. (2013) Practice advisory for the prevention and management of operating room fires. *Anesthesiology*, 118, 271–290.

Atlee, J. (2006) *Complications in Anesthesia*, 2nd ed. Philadelphia, PA: Saunders, p. 524.

Dorsch, J. and Dorsch, S. (2011) Hazards of anesthesia machines and breathing systems. In: *A Practical Approach to Anesthesia Equipment.* Philadelphia, PA: Lippincott Williams & Wilkins Health, pp. 218–229, 573–598.

Ellett, A., Shields, J., Ifune, C., Roa, N. and Vannucci, A. (2009) A near miss: a nitrous oxide-carbon dioxide mix-up despite current safety standards. *Anesthesiology*, 110, 1429–1431.

ERCI Institute (2009) New clinical guide to surgical fire prevention. Patients can catch fire – Here's how to keep them safer. *Health Devices*, 38, 314–332.

ERCI Institute (1983) PEEP valves in anesthesia circuits. *Health Devices*, 13, 24.

ERCI Institute (1998) Carbon monoxide exposures during inhalation anesthesia: the interaction between halogenated anesthetic agents and carbon dioxide absorbents. *Health Devices*, 27, 402–404.

Elakkumanan, L., Krishnappa, S., Balachander, H., Vasudevan, A., Pandey, R. and Badhe, A. (2012) Obstruction to scavenging system tubing. *J Anaesthesiol Clin Pharmacol*, 28, 270.

Fang, Z., Eger, E., Laster, M., Chortkoff, B., Kandel, L. and Ionescu, P. (1995) Carbon monoxide production from degradation of desflurane, enflurane, isoflurane, halothane, and sevoflurane by soda lime and baralyme. *Anesth Analg*, 80, 1187–1193.

Federal Drug Administration. Resources and tools for preventing surgical fires. Available from: http://www.fda.gov/Drugs/DrugSafety/SafeUseInitiative/PreventingSurgicalFires/ucm272680.htm [accessed June 23, 2016].

Green, J., Gonzalez, R., Sonbolian, N. and Rehkopf, P. (1992) The resistance to carbon dioxide laser ignition of a new endotracheal tube: Xomed laser-shield II. *J Clin Anesth*, 4, 89–92.

Hart, S.R., Yajnik, A., Ashford, J., Springer, R. and Harvey, S. (2011) Operating room fire safety. *The Ochsner Journal*, 11, 37–42.

Hofstetter, C., Scheller, B., Hoegl, S., Mack, M., Zwissler, B. and Byhahn, C. (2010) Cuff over-inflation and endotracheal tube obstruction: case report and experimental study. *Scand J Trauma Resusc Emerg Med*, 18, 18.

Ioannidis, G., Lazaridis, G., Baka, S., Mpoukovinas, I., Karavasilis, V. et al. (2015) Barotrauma and pneumothorax. *J Thoracic Disease*, 7, S38–S43.

Jawan, B. and Lee, J.H. (1990.) Cardiac arrest caused by an incorrectly filled O_2 cylinder: a case report. *Br J Anaesth*, 64, 749–751.

Jellish, S.W., Nolan, T. and Kleinman, B. (2001) Hypercapnia related to a faulty adult co-axial breathing circuit. *Anesth Analg*, 93, 973–974.

McMillan, M. and Darcy, H. (2015) Adverse event surveillance in small animal anaesthesia: an intervention-based, voluntary reporting audit. *Vet Anaes Analg*, 43, 128–135.

Mitchell, S., McCarthy, R., Rudloff, E. and Pernell, R. (2000) Tracheal rupture associated with intubation in cats: 20 cases (1996–1998). *J Am Vet Med Assoc*, 216, 1592–1595.

Mun, S. and No, M. (2013) Internal leakage of oxygen flush valve. *Korean J Anesthesiol*, 64, 550.

Scott, D.M. (1991) Performance of BOC Ohmeda Tec 3 and Tec 4 vaporisers following tipping. *Anaesth Intensive Care*, 19, 441–443.

Seegobin, R. and van Hasselt, G. (1984) Endotracheal cuff pressure and tracheal mucosal blood flow: endoscopic study of effects of four large volume cuffs. *Br Med J (Clin Res Ed)*, 288, 965–968.

Segal, N., Yannopoulos, D., Truchot, J., Laribi, S., Plaisance, P. and Convertino, V.A. (2013) Improving vital organs perfusion by the respiratory pump: physiology and clinical use. *Ann Fr Anesth Reanim*, 32, 572–579.

Steffey, E., Laster, M., Ionescu, P., Eger, E., Gong, D. and Weiskopf, R. (1997) Dehydration of baralyme increases compound a resulting from sevoflurane degradation in a standard anesthetic circuit used to anesthetize swine. *Anesth Analg*, 85, 1382–1386.

Subrahmanyam, M. and Mohan, S. (2013) Safety features in anaesthesia machine. *Indian J Anaesth*, 57, 472.

Tobias, J. (1998) Administration of sevoflurane using other agent-specific vaporizers. *Am J Ther*, 5, 383–386.

Wissing, H., Kuhn, I., Warnken, U. and Dudziak, R. (2001) Carbon monoxide production from desflurane, enflurane, halothane, isoflurane, and sevoflurane with dry soda lime. *Anesthesiology*, 95, 1205–1212.

10

Components of the Breathing System

Craig Mosley[1] and Amanda Shelby[2]

[1] Specialty Medicine, VCA Canada, Calgary, AB, Canada
[2] Jurox Animal Health, Kansas City, Missouri, USA

10.1 Breathing Systems

Although some parts of the breathing system are built into anesthesia machines (i.e. the circle system carbon dioxide absorbent canister), breathing systems are considered separate from the actual anesthesia machine (i.e. components are upstream of the fresh gas outlet). On any single anesthetic machine, the breathing system may be frequently changed, depending upon the needs of the patient or the circumstances in which anesthetic is delivered (Figure 10.1). The primary purposes of the breathing system are to direct oxygen to the patient, deliver anesthetic gas to the patient, remove carbon dioxide from inhaled breaths (or prevent significant rebreathing of carbon dioxide), and to provide a means of controlling ventilation.

Breathing systems have been classified using numerous schemes, with little uniformity or consensus of nomenclature (i.e. open, semi-open, semi-closed). For this reason, it is suggested that these terms be abandoned and rather a description of the flow rates and breathing system (e.g. circle system, Mapleson D system, etc.) are all that is needed. For clarity, it is easiest to classify the breathing circuits into one of two groups; those designed for rebreathing of exhaled gases (rebreathing or partial rebreathing systems) and those designed to be used under circumstances of minimal to no rebreathing (non-rebreathing systems, i.e. Mapleson systems). This classification may be a bit of a misnomer, since depending upon the specific system used and the fresh gas flow rates, a rebreathing system may have minimal rebreathing occurring (i.e. with excessively high fresh gas flows) or a non-rebreathing system may not completely prevent rebreathing (i.e. with inadequate/low fresh gas flow). To help circumvent this debate, in addition to describing the design of the breathing circuit, the fresh gas flow rate should be provided to fully describe how the system is

being used (Hamilton 1964). The fresh gas flow rate is expressed in mL/kg/min in veterinary medicine, owing to the vast range of patient sizes encountered. Additionally, the degree of rebreathing with breathing circuits can be affected by other factors such as equipment dead-space and the patient's respiratory pattern. In any case, breathing systems have been specifically developed to function as rebreathing or non-rebreathing systems, and should be used in the manner for which they were originally intended.

10.1.1 Rebreathing Systems (Circle and To-and-Fro)

Rebreathing systems are commonly referred to as circle systems; however, they are defined as any system with a means of chemically absorbing carbon dioxide from the breathing circuit. The benefits of this system include conservation of anesthetic, oxygen, patient heat and moisture. The circle system is the most commonly used rebreathing system in veterinary medicine. The circle system is designed to produce a unidirectional flow of gas through the system and has a means of absorbing carbon dioxide from exhaled gases. The components of the circle system include a fresh gas inlet, inspiratory one-way valve, breathing tubes, expiratory one-way valve, adjustable pressure limiting (APL) valve, reservoir bag and carbon dioxide absorber (Figure 10.2).

The fresh gas flows used with a circle system determine the amount of rebreathing. For example, there can be full rebreathing (closed), partial rebreathing (semi-closed or low flow) or minimal rebreathing (high flows). Historically, many terms have been applied to describe the amount of rebreathing, but there is no universally accepted standard or description of these terms. However, the use of the terms "open", "semi-open" and

Veterinary Anesthetic and Monitoring Equipment, First Edition. Edited by Kristen G. Cooley and Rebecca A. Johnson.
© 2018 John Wiley & Sons, Inc. Published 2018 by John Wiley & Sons, Inc.

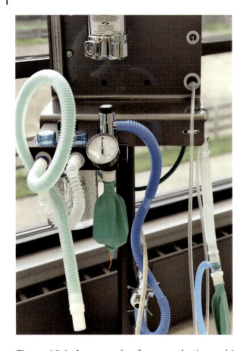

Figure 10.1 An example of an anesthetic machine mounted with both a circle (left) and non-rebreathing (right) circuit connector. Changing gas flow to the circuits is achieved with a switch handle located on the upper right front of the machine. There is no obvious common gas outlet on this machine as it is integrated into the breathing circuit toggle switch (photograph courtesy of Kristen Cooley, University of Wisconsin-Madison, WI).

"semi-closed" are no longer in use to avoid confusion (Dorsch and Dorsch 2008).

The To-and-Fro system is a rebreathing circuit with the carbon dioxide absorbent canister located between the endotracheal tube and reservoir bag and convenient for disassembly and ease of cleaning; however, care should be taken as placement of the carbon dioxide absorbent near the patient's endotracheal tube does allow for potential inhalation of granules. Additionally, gas flow channeling is likely to occur within the CO_2 absorber canister, which contributes to inefficiency (Walker *et al.* 2013). Overall, this type of rebreathing circuit has been replaced by the more convenient, less cumbersome circle system mentioned above.

10.1.1.1 Full (Complete) Rebreathing System

The full (complete) rebreathing system describes a circle system using flow rates equal to, or nearing, the metabolic oxygen consumption of the patient, usually between 3 and 14 mL/kg/min (Haskins 1992). This was described as a closed system, but this term is now obsolete. Noteworthy, is that in a "closed system" the APL is not normally closed, since that could create a potentially dangerous situation should fresh gas flow rates exceed metabolic oxygen requirements.

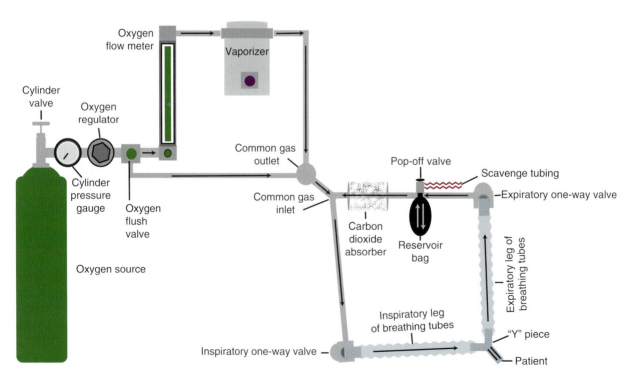

Figure 10.2 Diagram of the basic anesthetic machine and circle breathing system. Exact position of the various components and specific features can vary markedly among manufacturers (illustration courtesy Kristen Cooley, University of Wisconsin-Madison, WI).

10.1.1.2 Partial Rebreathing System

The partial rebreathing system describes a circle system using a flow rate greater than metabolic oxygen consumption (e.g. 20 mL/kg/min), but less than that required to prevent rebreathing. Since this is a very large range, it is often divided arbitrarily into low flow (20–50 mL/kg/min), mid ("so-so") flow (50–100 mL/kg/min) and high flow (100–200 mL/kg/min), although this is not a universally accepted description. With the availability of low volume, low dead-space pediatric and neonatal circle systems coupled with improved patient monitoring (pulse oximetry and end tidal carbon dioxide), it is common to use circle systems with partial rebreathing flow rates (i.e. <1000 mL/min) in small patients (<5 kg).

10.1.1.3 Non-(Minimal) Rebreathing System

The non-(minimal) rebreathing system describes a circle system using flow rates greater than 200 mL/kg/min (flow rates that would normally not be used in most circumstances) (Roth and Howley 1984). This unusually high flow rate may result when circle systems are used for maintenance of anesthesia in very small patients (<5 kg) with flow rates of 1000 mL/min or greater. Frequently, in veterinary medicine it has arbitrarily been suggested that flow rates below 1000 mL/min should not be used. Although this recommendation may be clinically useful for preventing some anesthetic delivery errors, it is wasteful and most modern anesthetic systems (i.e. vaporizers) continue to function optimally down to flow rates of 250–500 mL/min (Andrews 1990).

10.1.1.4 Working with Rebreathing Systems

Working with rebreathing systems is most economical in both terms of oxygen and inhalant anesthetic use, to employ low flow rates when possible. Lower flow rates are also associated with less environmental contamination by halogenated hydrocarbons (all commonly available inhaled anesthetics) and marginally improved maintenance of body temperature. However, lower flow rates are also associated with decreased anesthetic gas delivery (unless higher vaporizer settings are utilized). Additionally, when low carrier gas flows are used (relative to the volume of the circuit), the time required to change anesthetic concentration within the circuit is increased.

Most inhalant anesthetics are delivered initially using relatively high fresh gas flow rates (i.e. 50–100 mL/kg/min) to facilitate rapid inspired concentration increases within the system and to replace large volumes of anesthetic vapor, which are dissolving into patient tissues during the initial uptake period following intravenous anesthetic induction. The flow rates are then decreased (i.e. 20–50 mL/kg/min) after the initial uptake period (e.g. first 10–20 minutes) to economize on gas use and waste. The initial and maintenance recommended flow rates (mL/kg/min) often used clinically tend to be much higher in smaller patients (i.e. cats) relative to larger patients (i.e. horses). This ensures the patient's inspired gas concentration is more reflective of the concentration of anesthetic gas delivered from the vaporizer.

In contrast, when using low fresh gas flows, the inspired patient anesthetic concentration will not necessarily reflect the vaporizer concentration of gas until nearing equilibration. Use of anesthetic agent analyzers to monitor inspired and expired anesthetic partial pressures greatly facilitates decision-making with respect to vaporizer settings and timing changes in gas flows when using lower carrier gas flows. Agent analyzers are also beneficial when using multiple carrier gases (i.e. oxygen and nitrous oxide) to assist in monitoring for hypoxic gas mixtures.

The interaction between the vaporizer output, circuit volume, patient size, and flow rate is often an unfamiliar and difficult concept to grasp. Equating anesthetic delivery to a constant rate infusion of an intravenous drug is perhaps a more familiar comparison for understanding inhalant anesthetic delivery. For example, the loading dose for a constant rate infusion is similar to using a high carrier or fresh gas flow and vaporizer setting to quickly obtain anesthetic doses in the body. This would then be followed by lower infusion rates or lower vaporizer settings during maintenance anesthesia.

10.1.1.5 Components of Circle Rebreathing Systems

The configuration and features of available circle systems vary somewhat, depending upon the manufacturer. In general, a common pattern of gas flow is followed through the fresh gas inlet, the inspiratory one-way valve, the inspiratory and expiratory breathing tubes (into and out of patient, respectively), the expiratory one-way valve, the adjustable pressure limiting valve, the reservoir bag, and the carbon dioxide absorbing canister back to the fresh gas inlet (Figure 10.3). Some circle systems may also have additional incorporated features, such as a switch to automatically engage the mechanical ventilator and oxygen sensor ports (Figure 10.4).

Fresh Gas Inlet The fresh gas inlet is the site of gas delivery to the circle system from the common gas outlet of the anesthetic machine. The fresh gas inlet is normally found after the carbon dioxide absorber and before the inspiratory one-way valve.

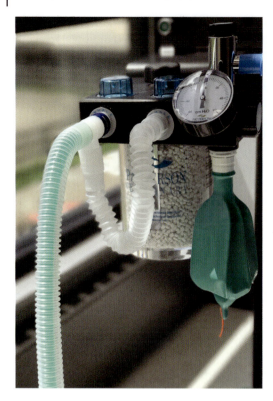

Figure 10.3 An example of a circle rebreathing circuit connected to a small animal machine. The degree of configuration and added details vary markedly among manufacturers, but the essential features and function are similar (photograph courtesy of Kristen Cooley, University of Wisconsin-Madison, WI).

Inspiratory One-Way Valve The function of the one-way valve is to ensure unidirectional gas flow and to prevent rebreathing of exhaled gases. During inspiration, the inspiratory one-way valve opens, allowing gas to move from the fresh gas inlet and reservoir bag to move through the valve into the inspiratory limb of the breathing circuit. These valves normally consist of a clear dome (for direct visualization of valve function), a lightweight valve, and a valve housing (valve seat and valve guides). The valves are normally accessible for cleaning and repair through a removable cover. Alcohol should be avoided on plastic dome valve covers, as it can cause the material to crack and leak.

Condensation can form within the valves and contribute to the disk sticking to the valve housing. If excessive moisture is noted, the valve housing can be opened and allowed to dry. Moisture is more likely to occur in the expiratory valve; however, condensation can form in the inspiratory valve housing as well depending on the machines configuration. Care should be taken not to crack, chip or scratch the disk. During expiration, the inspiratory valve is closed preventing exhaled gas from entering the inspiratory limb of the breathing circuit, forcing it into the expiratory limb of the breathing circuit. At least one system (Matrx circle system, Midmark Animal Health, Versailles, OH) also incorporates a negative pressure relief valve, providing an alternative path of gas flow (room air) to the patient, should the inspiratory valve become stuck in the closed position or when there is insufficient oxygen in the circuit. (Figure 10.5).

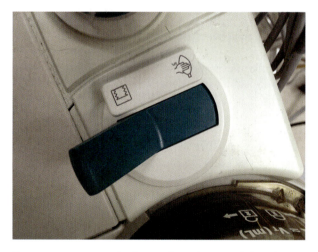

Figure 10.4 An example of a switch used on a circle breathing system and anesthetic machine with a built-in ventilator to engage the ventilator circuit. This can minimize the potential for misconnections, disconnections, or kinked hoses during ventilator set up (photograph courtesy of Kristen Cooley, University of Wisconsin-Madison, WI).

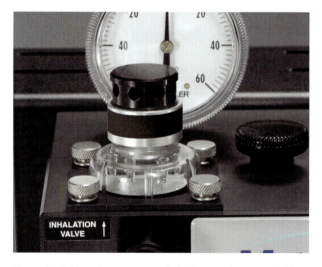

Figure 10.5 Negative pressure relief valves are incorporated into some circle systems and will be activated (allowing the patient to inhale air from the room) should the inspiratory valve become occluded or stuck. This one is located on top of the inspiratory one-way valve.

Typically, there is an O-ring present on the valve housing, which requires replacement as part of routine preventative maintenance.

Breathing Circuit Tubing The most basic breathing circuit is comprised of corrugated plastic or rubber inspiratory and expiratory limbs. The corrugated tubing helps prevent kinking and allows for some expansion if the breathing circuit is subjected to compression or traction. The two breathing limbs are connected via a wye piece (Y-piece), which connects to the endotracheal tube or facemask, typically with a standard 15-mm female connection. There are also various co-axial designs that place the inspiratory limb within the expiratory limb of the breathing circuit (Universal F-circuit; Figure 10.6). Co-axial systems reduce the bulk associated with the breathing system and (at least theoretically) facilitates warming the inspired gases by the expired gases. The Universal F-circuit (a coaxial breathing system) is designed to function with standard circle systems (i.e. 22-mm O.D. connectors of the circle system). Most breathing circuits are adapted for use with all circle systems, as the fitting diameters are standardized. However, a proprietary co-axial circuit is available that utilizes non-standard sized circle system connectors, requiring the use of a proprietary circle system (Moduflex Coaxial breathing circuit, Dispomed, Joliette, QC, Canada).

Several sizes of breathing circuits are available that vary in length, volume and the amount of dead space to meet various anesthetic requirements. Pediatric and neonatal rebreathing circuits are normally low volume and low dead space systems, allowing them to function optimally in small patients (i.e. those with small tidal volumes). Pediatric tubing is 15-mm I.D. and recommended for use in patients of less than 6.8–7 kg (Hartsfield 1987; Bednarski 1993). Standard adult tubing is recommended for patients between 6.8 and 135 kg (Hartsfield 1987). Patients over 135 kg should be placed on large animal equipment with breathing hoses 5 cm in diameter (2 inches), to ensure there is no additional resistance to ventilation resulting from the breathing hoses (Hartsfield 1987; Figure 10.7). Ultimately, when selecting the diameter of hosing for the breathing circuit, it is recommended to utilize hosing larger than the diameter of the patient's endotracheal tube, in an effort to reduce resistance to ventilation.

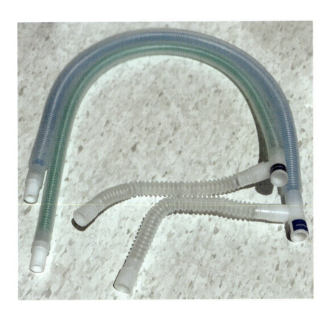

Figure 10.6 An example of an adult Universal F-circuit (22-mm internal diameter, blue) and a pediatric Universal F-circuit (15-mm internal diameter, green). Hoses are designed for one-time use only, but can be cleaned and re-used. Care should be taken to avoid cross-contamination. It is important to remember that the colored inner tube end should attach to the inspiratory port on the anesthesia machine (the sticker may fall off after washing) and the colorless corrugated end attaches to the expiratory port (photograph courtesy of Kristen Cooley, University of Wisconsin-Madison, WI).

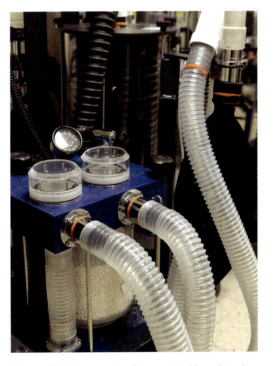

Figure 10.7 An example of large animal breathing hoses with an internal diameter of 5 cm (photograph courtesy of Kristen Cooley, University of Wisconsin-Madison, WI).

Expiratory One-Way Valve The expiratory one-way valve functions together with the inspiratory one-way valve, closing upon inspiration and opening during expiration, to maintain unidirectional gas flow and prevent rebreathing of expired gases. This valve helps direct gas into the expiratory limb of the breathing system, through the expiratory valve and into the reservoir bag. This valve is more likely than the inspiratory valve to collect condensation from moisture in the patient's exhaled breath. This may require opening to allow the valve to dry as moisture can contribute to functional compromise during prolonged procedures. Care should be taken when cleaning this valve and disc. Alcohol should not be used on plastic valve domes, as this will lead to cracks and leaks requiring replacement of the dome cover.

Reservoir Bag The reservoir bag is also referred to as a breathing or rebreathing bag; the latter term should not be used, as the degree of rebreathing depends on the fresh gas flow rate and rarely should significant rebreathing of gas from the bag occur when connected to a non-rebreathing system. Depending on the manufacturer, the location of the reservoir bag in the circuit is downstream (preferable) or upstream of the absorber. Small animal reservoir bags have a 22-mm O.D. port to attach to the anesthesia machine reservoir arm.

The purpose of the reservoir bag is to provide a compliant reservoir of gas, which changes volume with the patient's expiration and inspiration. This compliance becomes particularly important if the APL valve is accidentally closed. Additionally, the reservoir bag serves as a means to manually assist or control ventilation. It is recommended that the reservoir bag be approximately 5–10 times the patient's normal tidal volume (10–20 mL/kg) or roughly equivalent to the patient's minute volume. Ultimately, the reservoir bag should be large enough to provide a reasonably-sized reservoir of gas, but not so large that it becomes difficult to observe movements of the bag associated with breathing.

Subjectively, when properly sized, the reservoir bag can be used by the anesthetist to quantify a patient's respiratory rate and potentially tidal volume, which is helpful when chest excursions are difficult to visualize or when capnography is not in use. In addition, a very large reservoir bag will contribute to the overall functional volume of the rebreathing system (i.e. circle system), contributing to slower rates of change in anesthetic concentration when the vaporizer output is altered. This is not the case when using a non-rebreathing system. Commonly available sizes utilized in small animals include 0.5, 1, 2, 3 and 5 L.

Adjustable Pressure Limiting (APL) Valve The adjustable pressure limiting (APL) valve is also referred to as the overflow, pop-off or pressure relief valve. The APL is a safety valve allowing excess gas to escape from the patient circuit. If the valve is functioning properly and left in the open position, gas should escape if system pressures exceed 1–3 cmH$_2$O. Normally it should be fully open at all times, unless positive pressure ventilation is being used or during routine pre-use positive pressure leak check of the anesthetic machine and breathing circuit. It should be immediately re-opened when positive pressure ventilation ceases or upon completion of the pre-use pressure checking, to prevent excessive pressure from building in the patient circuit resulting in potential patient barotrauma. The APL is partially closed in some instances to prevent collapse of the reservoir bag due the negative pressure/vacuum from the scavenging system. Although this can remedy the situation, it is discouraged, because it can lead to excessive pressure in the patient circuit. If the reservoir bag continually collapses under normal use, simply adjust the central vacuum/scavenge system and/or incorporate a properly functioning scavenging interface to offset this effect.

It is important to recognize that, in most veterinary manufactured machines, the APL valve is *not* a pressure limiting valve. Several manufacturers market products that minimize accidental closure of the APL valve, helping to prevent accidental patient barotrauma. Some of these devices allow temporary closure of outflow to the scavenge system when a button is depressed, while others alarm or automatically allow excessive gases to escape from the system when a preset pressure is exceeded. Some momentary closure systems are built directly into some APL valves or can be added to currently-used APL valves or within the breathing circuit (Figures 10.8 and 10.9). Pressure limiting valves are commercially available and can be placed between the patient circuit and APL valve on both rebreathing and non-rebreathing circuits (Figure 10.10). Pressure alarms (either audible or illuminating), can be placed on existing anesthesia machines. The alarm is triggered when a preset pressure is exceeded. These are valuable additions to the APL valve system and help to prevent excessive pressure that can lead to patient barotrauma or death.

The position of the APL valve does not characterize the circuit (i.e. open, closed, semi-closed) as frequently misleads users. Fresh gas flow rates determine the classification of the circuit as open, closed or semi-closed, as mentioned above and these terms are discouraged from use due to their misleading nature.

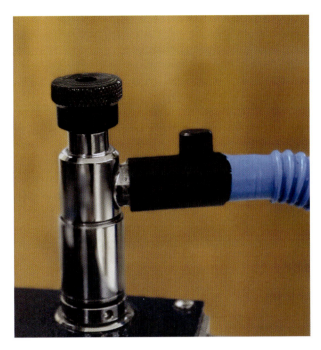

Figure 10.8 An example of a momentary closure valve that can be added to any standard APL valve (photograph courtesy of Kristen Cooley, University of Wisconsin-Madison, WI).

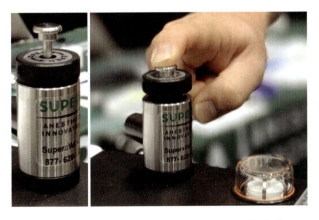

Figure 10.9 An example of a momentary closure valve built into the adjustable pressure-limiting (APL) valve (Supera Anesthesia Innovations, Clackamas, OR). The valve is open in the resting position (left). The valve is only closed when the button is depressed (right) (photograph courtesy of Kristen Cooley, University of Wisconsin-Madison, WI)

Carbon Dioxide Absorber and Canister   The carbon dioxide absorber contains the chemical absorbent for removing carbon dioxide from exhaled gases. There are many types (dual canister, disposable, etc.) and sizes of carbon dioxide absorbers available (Figure 10.11). All contain some type of screen to prevent absorbent granules from entering the breathing circuit and most contain a baffling system to prevent channeling of gases within the absorber canister. Older canisters may have metal screens that

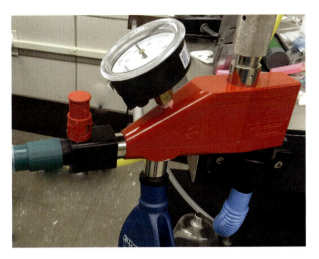

Figure 10.10 Example of a commercially available fixed pressure relief valve placed on a modified Bain circuit (EMC, Alan Cross, Atlanta, GA).

should be inspected regularly, due to the corrosive nature of the absorbent with metal. Newer machines are utilizing plastic screens to avoid this issue. Despite the screens, the absorbent granules and/or dust will occasionally enter the breathing circuit. This is commonly encountered in large animal systems, where relatively high peak flows of gas (associated with inspiration and expiration) are more common. Gas flow patterns within canisters vary considerably, but canister design normally attempts to ensure optimal and efficient absorbent use. Canisters are typically made from plastic and are positioned between the one-way inspiratory and

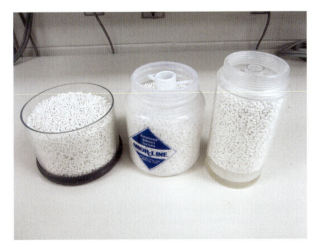

Figure 10.11 Three different absorber canisters. The canister on the far left is a bulk flow-through type canister where the exhaled gas from the patient circuit enters one side (i.e. top) of the canister and exits the other (i.e. bottom) upon inspiration. The two canisters to the right utilize a conducting tube to direct the exhaled or inhaled gases in a predictable pattern through the canister. Gas must enter and exit the canister from the same opening (i.e. the top).

expiratory valves of circle systems. Due to the frequent nature of changing the absorbent, this is a common place for anesthetic leaks to occur.

It has been suggested that the absorber canister must be twice the patient's tidal volume to ensure complete absorption of carbon dioxide, but there is little evidence to support this statement. Most large animal machine canisters rarely have a volume equal to twice the patient's tidal volume and may in fact have a volume less than the patient's tidal volume. Moreover, many carbon dioxide absorbers used in human anesthetic machines have volumes less than the patient's tidal volume. Smaller canisters are often preferred to ensure more frequent changing of the absorbent, lessening the likelihood that toxic products will be produced by desiccated absorbent. However, the relative efficiency of absorption (i.e. the carbon dioxide load absorbed when an absorbent appears exhausted) may improve with larger carbon dioxide absorbers (Davey 2005). Smaller carbon dioxide absorbers will reduce the internal volume of the breathing circuit, leading to vaporizer concentration changes being reflected more rapidly in the inspired gas concentration, but will require more frequent absorbent changes.

10.1.1.6 Carbon Dioxide Absorbents

The general principle of carbon dioxide absorption involves a base (absorbent) neutralizing an acid (CO_2). The products of the reaction are water, formation of a carbonate (e.g. calcium carbonate) and heat production. The principle component of most commonly-used absorbents is calcium hydroxide ($Ca(OH)_2$). There are currently three absorbents available in North America: soda lime, Baralyme (barium lime) and Amsorb (calcium hydroxide lime), with soda lime being the most commonly used. Soda lime is approximately 80% calcium hydroxide, 15% water and 4% sodium hydroxide (NaOH). Baralyme is a mixture of approximately 20% barium hydroxide and 80% calcium hydroxide, and may also contain some potassium hydroxide. Amsorb, marketed as Amsorb⁺ Plus, consists of approximately 80% calcium hydroxide, 1% calcium sulfate hemihydrate, 3% calcium chloride and 15% water. Amsorb is the newest absorbent and is associated with minimal (if any) carbon monoxide production, minimal Compound A production and the least amount of sevoflurane degradation compared to soda lime and Baralyme (Kharasch *et al.* 2002). The absorptive capacities of soda lime and Baralyme are approximately 25 and 27 liters of carbon dioxide per 100 g respectively, with Amsorb absorption being about 50% that of soda lime (Higuchi *et al.* 2001).

The absorption of CO_2 in soda lime occurs through a series of chemical reactions. CO_2 first combines with water to form carbonic acid, which then reacts with the hydroxides to form sodium (or potassium) carbonate,

water and heat. The calcium hydroxide then accepts the carbonate to form calcium carbonate and regenerate sodium (or potassium) hydroxide:

1) $CO_2 + H_2O \leftrightarrow H_2CO_3$

2) $H_2CO_3 + 2NaOH(KOH) \rightarrow Na_2CO_3(K_2CO_3) + 2H_2O + Heat$

3) $Na_2CO_3(K_2CO_3) + Ca(OH)_2 \rightarrow CaCO_3 + 2NaOH(KOH)$

Some CO_2 may react directly with the calcium hydroxide. but the reaction is relatively slow compared to the process utilizing sodium- or potassium hydroxide:

$$H_2CO_3 + Ca(OH)_2 \rightarrow CaCO_3 + 2H_2O + Heat$$

The reaction of Baralyme differs in that more water is liberated by the direct reaction of CO_2 with the barium hydroxide:

1) $Ba(OH)_2 + 8H_2O + CO_2 \rightarrow BaCO_3 + 9H_2O + Heat$

2) $9H_2O + 9CO_2 \rightarrow 9H_2CO_3$, then by direct reactions (below) and by KOH and NaOH (as above)

3) $9H_2CO_3 + 9Ca(OH)_2 \rightarrow 9CaCO_3 + 18H_2O + Heat$

The reaction of Amsorb is simpler with the CO_2 reacting with water to form carbonic acid and the carbonic acid reacting directly with the calcium hydroxide to form calcium carbonate:

1) $CO_2 + H_2O \leftrightarrow H_2CO_3$

2) $H_2CO_3 + Ca(OH)_2 \rightarrow CaCO_3 + 2H_2O + Heat$

When in continuous use, the absorbents may appear exhausted (i.e. indicator color change) before the absorbing capacity of the granules is exceeded. Granules normally turn from white to purple or pink as they become exhausted, depending upon the indicator used (Figure 10.12). Ethyl violet (purple) and phenolphthalein (red) are pH sensitive indicators commonly added to the granules to help identify absorbent exhaustion. The color change should not be used as the only indicator of absorbent exhaustion. It is common for absorbent that has changed color to turn back to white if allowed to stand unused for several hours. Fresh absorbent is normally easily crumbled under pressure, whereas used absorbent becomes hard (calcium carbonate).

Additionally, since the reaction of carbon dioxide absorption produces heat and moisture, activity of the absorbent may be evaluated by looking for evidence of both heat and moisture development within the canister. Also, where available, capnography can be used to detect

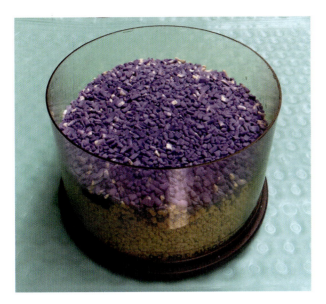

Figure 10.12 Exhausted soda lime particles showing a color change (photograph courtesy of Dr Rebecca Johnson, University of Wisconsin-Madison, WI).

absorbent exhaustion, and inspired carbon dioxide will be shown by an elevated baseline on the capnogram. However, the anesthetist should be aware that exhausted CO_2 absorbent is not the only cause of inspired CO_2 on a capnogram. The rate of absorbent exhaustion will be determined by the size of patient (CO_2 production) and the rate of fresh gas flow (mL/kg/min). Absorbent exhaustion will occur faster in larger patients and when low fresh gas flows are used. The absorbent canister should be filled carefully to avoid overfilling, packing of granules in the canister and spilling granules into the breathing system.

Some degradation of inhalant anesthetics occurs with their exposure to carbon dioxide absorbents. Normally, this degradation is insignificant. However, sevoflurane can decompose to a potentially nephrotoxic compound, Compound A. Factors associated with increasing production of Compound A include a high concentration of sevoflurane, low fresh gas flows, dry absorbent, high temperature and use of barium lime. The significance of Compound A production for human and other animal health effects has been widely debated, but its clinical significance appears to be of little concern in dogs and cats. Carbon monoxide can also be produced when desflurane, enflurane or isoflurane are passed through dry absorbents containing a strong alkali (potassium or sodium hydroxide). Most human cases of carbon monoxide poisoning have been reported to occur during the first general anesthetic administered from a little-used anesthetic machine. In human anesthesia, it is recommended to use only non-desiccated absorbents containing no potassium hydroxide and little or no sodium

hydroxide. Although carbon monoxide poisoning associated with anesthetic use in veterinary medicine seems to be a very rare occurrence (or it is simply not recognized), similar recommendations are probably applicable.

10.1.2 Non-Rebreathing Systems (Mapleson Systems)

Non-rebreathing systems are characterized by the absence of unidirectional valves and a carbon dioxide absorber. Rather than relying on carbon dioxide absorption for removal of CO_2, these systems depend on high fresh gas flow rates to flush CO_2 from the circuit. Non-rebreathing systems are not routinely used for patients exceeding 10 kg, as they become far less economical due to use of high fresh gas flow rates required to prevent rebreathing of CO_2. Recommended flow rates to minimize the rebreathing of expired CO_2 range from 130–300 mL/kg/min, although values as high as 600 mL/kg/min have been recommended (Dorsch and Dorsch 1994). The wide range of recommended flow rates is associated with fact that, in addition to the fresh gas flow rate, the patient's intrinsic respiratory pattern will influence the occurrence of rebreathing.

Non-rebreathing systems have historically been recommended, somewhat arbitrarily, for use in all patients of less than 5 kg, citing lower resistance during breathing, less equipment dead space and less total circuit volume. However, by using newer pediatric, neonatal and small patient specific rebreathing circuits, many of the advantages normally associated with non-rebreathing systems are negated and it is possible to safely maintain patients of less than 5 kg by using rebreathing systems, as long as the patient's tidal volume is adequate to actuate the unidirectional valves. Small patient-specific circuits generally have no more, and in some cases, less dead space and total volume than standard non-rebreathing systems. There is no generally accepted minimum patient size for using a rebreathing system accepted among anesthesiologists. The minimum patient size generally ranges between 3 and 7 kg, although individual anesthetist may choose patient sizes outside this range, depending upon monitoring available (i.e. capnography for evaluation of rebreathing), intended ventilation mode (spontaneous vs. controlled), patient signalment, history and co-existing morbidities (i.e. obesity, pregnancy, etc.).

Although the Mapleson system for classification of anesthetic breathing circuits is still used (Figure 10.13), only a small number of Mapleson systems are used clinically. Although there are often three or more non-rebreathing systems commonly described for use in veterinary medicine in North America, all are nearly

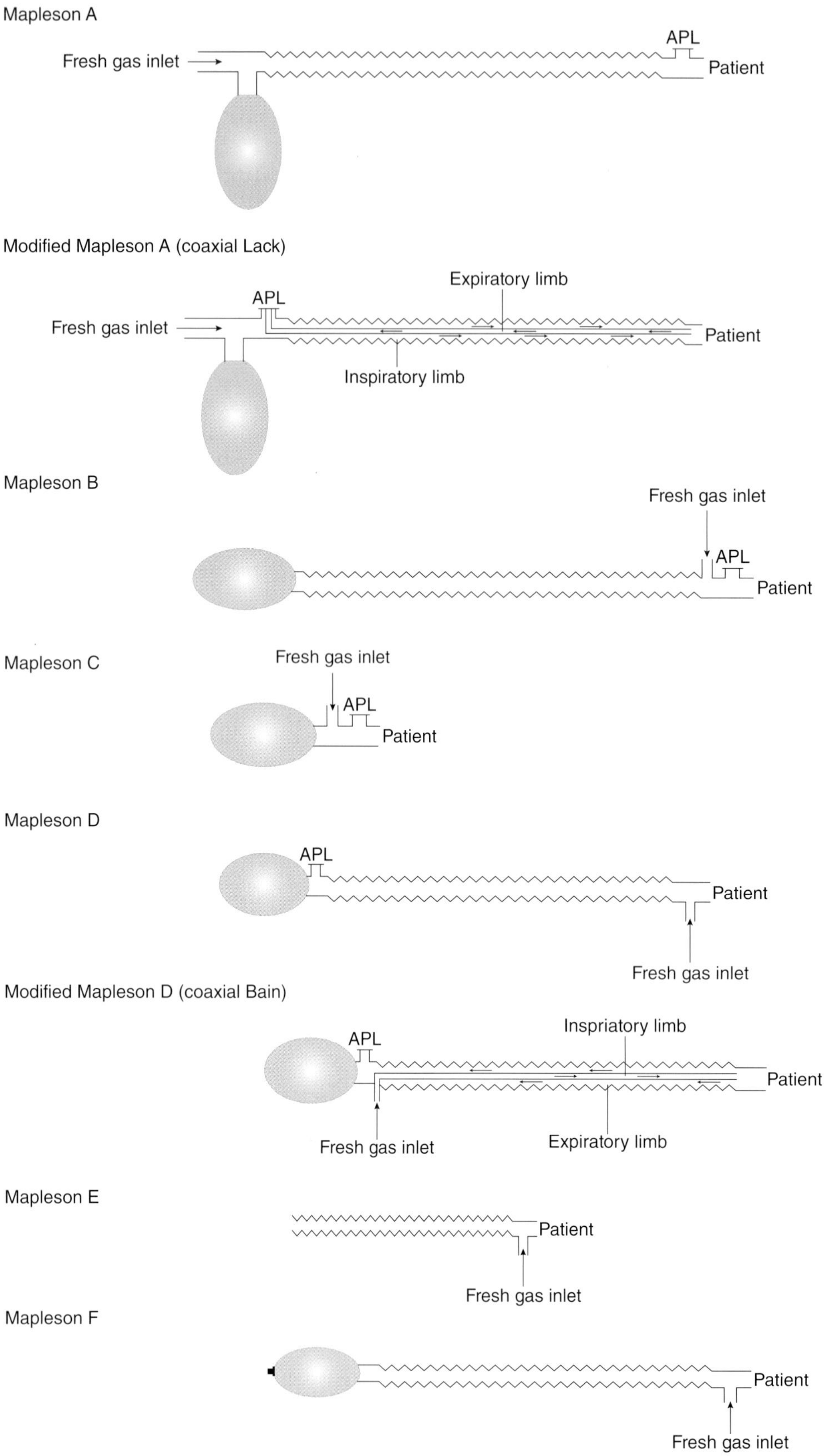

Mapleson A

Modified Mapleson A (coaxial Lack)

Mapleson B

Mapleson C

Mapleson D

Modified Mapleson D (coaxial Bain)

Mapleson E

Mapleson F

Figure 10.13 Diagrams of each of the Mapleson breathing systems (A–F) (illustration courtesy of Kristen Cooley, University of Wisconsin-Madison, WI).

functionally identical and based on two of the six described Mapleson systems: D and F (Figure 10.14).

The non-rebreathing system includes a fresh gas conducting hose, patient connection, exhalation conducting tubing (normally corrugated), excess gas venting system and a reservoir bag. All commonly-used systems have the fresh gas flow entering near the patient connection and rely on the fresh gas inflow to displace the CO_2-containing expired breath down a variable length of conducting tubing toward the reservoir bag and ultimately into the scavenge system. High fresh gas flows are necessary to help minimize the rebreathing of expired gases.

During the expiratory pause, the high fresh gas flow from the fresh gas conducting tube pushes the exhaled gas from the previous expiration down the exhalation conducting tube away from the patient towards the reservoir bag. When the patient inspires, they inspire gas coming from both the fresh gas conducting tube and the

A. Bain with Bain Mount and APL
   (Mapleson D type configuration - coaxial)

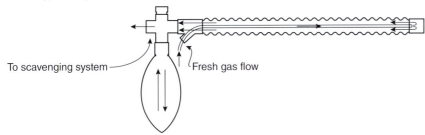

B. Bain with pinch valve distal to bag
   (Mapleson F type configuration - coaxial)

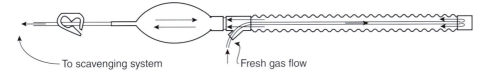

C. Modified Jackson Ree's with relief valve proximal to bag
   (Mapleson D type configuration - non coaxial)

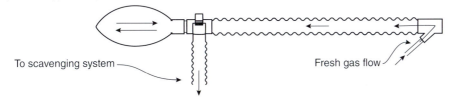

D. Modified Jackson Ree's with pinch valve distal to bag
   (Mapleson F type configuration - non coaxial)

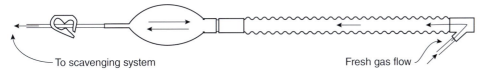

COMMONLY USED NON-REBREATHING SYSTEM CONFIGURATIONS

Figure 10.14 Further diagrams of the Mapleson systems (D and F) used most commonly as the foundation for modern non-rebreathing systems. Most modern non-rebreathing systems are modifications of the Mapleson classification and can no longer be strictly classified as one type or the other. For example, a Bain system is a coaxial system like the Mapleson D system, but can be configured with the exhaust gas exiting prior to the rebreathing bag (Mapleson D – A) or after the rebreathing bag (Mapleson F – B). The Jackson-Rees system, a non-coaxial system, can be configured similarly with the exhaust gas exiting either before (Mapleson D – C) or after the rebreathing bag (Mapleson F – D) (illustration reprinted with permission from John Wiley & Sons).

exhalation conducting tube. In some circumstances (i.e. patients with unusual respiratory patterns), a patient may rebreathe exhaled gases despite seemingly sufficient fresh gas flows. For example, a patient with rapid breathing may not have an expiratory pause of sufficient duration for CO_2 to be washed distally enough from the patient end of the tube to prevent rebreathing, particularly if a sufficiently large breath is taken. End-tidal carbon dioxide monitoring can be useful in determining if adequate fresh gas flows are being used to minimize rebreathing, as increased inspired CO_2 may be present with low fresh gas flows. Alternatively, the high fresh gas flows used with non-rebreathing systems can markedly distort the capnograms produced using a sidestream capnograph.

The Bain system and the Modified Jackson Rees names are commonly applied to most non-rebreathing systems, but they do not adequately describe the systems as they are used in veterinary medicine. Neither system is specifically defined, in that they are not always reliably configured in the same manner. Using the Mapleson descriptions of these circuits, the Bain circuit (based on a Mapleson D system) would have an APL valve proximal to the rebreathing bag, whereas the Modified Jackson Rees (based on a Mapleson F system) would have a pinch or stopcock valve located distal to the rebreathing bag. However, both systems can be adapted for use with a mounting block and various reservoir bag and venting system combinations, making strict classification nearly impossible. Essentially, the main difference between how the two systems function clinically is that one is a coaxial design (Bain) and the other is not (Modified Jackson Rees). Perhaps a less confusing and consistent way to classify the commonly-used non-rebreathing circuits in veterinary medicine would be based on the configuration of the conducting tubing (i.e. coaxial or non-coaxial), location of scavenging system (i.e. proximal or distal to the reservoir bag), and method of scavenging (APL valve, pinch valve or stopcock type valve).

The coaxial design of the Bain system reduces the overall bulk and provides a method for potentially warming the cold inspired gases (although this benefit is disputable when used with high fresh gas flow rates). Mounting blocks are convenient methods for arranging non-rebreathing systems by providing fixed connection points for the breathing circuit, reservoir bag and scavenge tubing (Figure 10.15). Use of a mounting block minimizes the potential for misconnections, disconnections or kinked hoses. The fixed positioning relative to the anesthetic machine also allows the anesthetist to readily assess the integrity of all connections. Non-rebreathing systems used without a mounting block can be placed anywhere in the anesthetic work area and run the risk of being covered by drapes, hanging off surgical tables, or

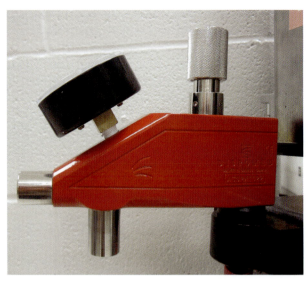

Figure 10.15 A mounting block (sometimes also referred to as a Bain mount, although they are not exclusive for use with Bain circuits only) provides fixed connection points for the non-rebreathing circuit, the reservoir bag and scavenge tubing. Most also incorporate an APL valve and pressure gauge.

being pulled or caught by moving legs or equipment in the operating room, all increasing the possibility for anesthetic complications.

Most mounting blocks also have a pressure manometer built into the system; this is an invaluable addition enabling the user to monitor and assess changes in airway pressure. Most non-rebreathing systems sold to veterinarians are not configured with a pressure manometer as part of the standard system that, along with high fresh gas flows and relatively small circuit volumes, exposes patients to the potential for accidental barotrauma. Disposable pressure manometers designed for use with a resuscitation bag can be used for this purpose (Vetmac, Inc., Rossville, IN). These can be easily placed within all non-rebreathing systems, used repeatedly, and are an inexpensive method of evaluating airway pressures (Figure 10.16). Alternatively, high patient pressure

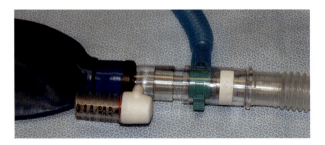

Figure 10.16 An example of a disposable resuscitation bag manometer that can be adapted for use with most non-rebreathing systems. The presence of the manometer will allow the anesthetist to better evaluate airway pressures within the breathing system.

alarms and pressure relief valves are available, which can be inserted into the system between the patient and the valve used to isolate the system from the scavenging.

10.1.2.1 Pre-use Checking of Non-rebreathing System

As with the rebreathing circuits, positive pressure leak testing should be part of the set-up routine. Thorough pressure checking can be difficult to accomplish in non-rebreathing options that lack a patient pressure manometer. Generally, the APL or occlusion valve should be closed or obstructed. While obstructing the patient end of the circuit, the oxygen flow rate should be adjusted to fill the reservoir bag. Once full, the oxygen flow is discontinued and observation of the reservoir bag distention is evaluated. Without a pressure manometer, it is challenging to establish that a slow leak is present or absent. Non-rebreathing circuits with a pressure manometer are positive pressure checked, similar to a rebreathing circuit. An additional pressure check step exists with co-axial Bain circuits; pressure checking the internal or inspiratory hosing. Utilizing the eraser end of a pencil, obstruct the internal hose. Turn on the oxygen flow. The flowmeter float should depress if no leaks exist in the internal hosing.

10.1.3 Servicing Equipment

Manufacturers' recommendations should always be followed regarding servicing. Outside the routine pre-use checks, machines require maintenance. Rubber seals and O-rings require periodic changing. Routinely, machines are inspected or serviced annually. Frequently, the manufacturer or a third-party company may offer service contracts. If servicing in house, it is important to remember only oxygen-appropriate lubricant should be used on equipment.

10.1.4 Cleaning and Maintenance

Currently, no consistent recommendations exist for cleaning of patient breathing circuits. Consideration should be given to extent of use, exposure to transmissible disease, and life expectancy of the material. Equipment made of rubber materials can absorb volatile inhalants and disinfectants. Due to use in the high oxygen environment, certain aspects of the breathing circuit will limit bacterial growth. If chemical disinfectants are used, manufacturer recommendations should be followed for proper dilution, exposure time, rinsing and thorough drying before use on a patient. Co-axial tubing of breathing circuits can be particular time-consuming to dry following liquid chemical disinfection. Drying cabinets are commercially available. Gas sterilization can effectively decontaminate equipment once organic debris is removed and equipment is dry from patient condensation.

10.2 Summary

Having an understanding of the breathing circuits and their purpose is vital to the safe delivery of inhalant anesthetics, fresh oxygen and to appropriate manual or mechanical ventilation of patients. To provide optimal anesthetic care to a veterinary patient, the anesthetist needs a working knowledge of the circuits available for veterinary use, their benefits and intended patient population and how to properly implement their use.

References

Andrews, J. (1990) Inhaled anesthetic delivery systems. In: Miller, R.D. (ed.). *Anesthesia*, 3rd ed. New York: Churchill Livingstone, p. 171.

Bednarski, R. (1993) Anesthetic breathing systems. *Semin Vet Med Surg (Small Anim)*, 8, 82–89.

Davey, A.J. (2005) Breathing systems and their components. In: Davey, A.J. and Diba, A. (eds) *Ward's Anaesthetic Equipment*, 6th ed. Philadelphia, PA: Elsevier Ltd., pp. 107–138.

Dorsch, J. and Dorsch, S. (1994) The Mapleson breathing system. In: *Understanding Anesthesia Equipment*, 3rd ed. Baltimore, MD: Williams & Wilkins, pp. 175.

Dorsch, J.A. and Dorsch, S.E. (2008) The breathing system: general principles, common components, and classifications. In: *Understanding Anesthesia Equipment*, 5th ed. New York: Lippincott Williams & Wilkins, pp 192–205.

Hamilton, W.K. (1964) Nomenclature of inhalation anesthetic systems. *Anesthesiology*, 25, 3–5.

Hartsfield, S.M. (1987) Machines and breathing systems for administration of inhalation anesthetics. In: Short, C.E. (ed.). *Principles and Practice of Veterinary Anesthesia*. Baltimore, MD: Williams & Wilkins, p. 403.

Haskins, S. (1992) Opinions in small animal anesthesia. *Vet Clin North Am Small Anim Pract*, 22, 245–502.

Higuchi, H., Adachi, Y., Arimura, S. and Al, E. (2001) The carbon dioxide absorption capacity of Amsorb is half that of soda lime. *Anesth Analg*, 93, 221–225.

Kharasch, E., Powers, K. and Artru, A. (2002) Comparison of Amsorb, sodaline, and Baralyme degradation of volatile anesthetics and formation of carbon monoxide and compound a in swine *in vivo*. *Anesthesiology*, 96, 173–182.

Roth, P.A. and Howley, J.A. (1984) Anesthesia delivery systems. In: Stoelting, R. and Miller, R. (eds). *Basics of Anesthesia*. New York: Churchill Livingstone, pp. 195–206.

Walker, S.G., Smith, T.C., Sheplock, G., Acquaviva, M.A. and Horn, N. (2013) Breathing circuits. In: Ehrenwerth, J. and Eisenkraft, J. (eds). *Anesthesia Equipment: Principles and Applications*. St Louis, MO: CV Mosby, pp. 95–124.

11

Mapleson Breathing Systems

Tatiana Ferreira

School of Veterinary Medicine, University of Wisconsin, Madison, Wisconsin, USA

11.1 Introduction

The Mapleson breathing systems are characterized by the absence of carbon dioxide (CO_2) absorbents and unidirectional valves. They are also known as non-rebreathing systems; however, this classification is controversial because, depending on the fresh gas flow rate (FGF) used, rebreathing of exhaled gases may still occur.

According to the original description from W.W. Mapleson in 1954 (Mapleson 1954), there are five types of breathing systems (A–E); however, a sixth circuit (F) was added later (Willis *et al.* 1975) (Figure 11.1). The common components within these breathing systems include a patient connection, fresh gas inlet, conducting tubing (usually corrugated), reservoir bag (excluded in the Mapleson E), and excess gas venting system.

The Mapleson systems can be separated into three functionally distinct groups: A, BC and DEF. Within each group, the performance characteristics regarding FGF requirements are similar (Conway 1985; Dorrington and Lehane 1987; Miller 1988). In the Mapleson A (i.e. Magill), the excess venting system is located near the patient end of the system and fresh gas inlet away from the patient. In the B and C systems, the excess venting system and fresh gas inlet are both located near the patient. Lastly, in the D, E and F systems, the fresh gas inlet is near the patient, and the excess venting system is located away from the patient.

11.2 Fresh Gas Flows (FGFs)

Compared to the circle (or rebreathing) systems, the FGFs used with the Mapleson systems are higher in order to avoid rebreathing, thus ensuring fresh inspired gas and elimination of CO_2. All of the Mapleson systems have the fresh gas inlet near the patient, except for the Mapleson A (Figure 11.1), and they depend on the high

FGF to push expired gases through the conducting tubing towards the reservoir bag (if present) and scavenging system. During inspiration, the patient inspires gas from the fresh gas inlet and the conducting tubing, thus it is important that the FGF is high enough to push the expired gases away from the patient during expiration, replacing it with fresh gas, and thereby avoiding rebreathing. Other factors that may influence rebreathing with Mapleson systems include mode of ventilation (spontaneous or controlled), tidal volume and respiratory rate, inspiratory to expiratory ratio, volume of conducting tubing, and especially the duration of the expiratory pause (Mapleson 1954; Sykes 1968; Rose and Froese 1979; Cook 1996a,b).

11.3 Advantages and Disadvantages

The high FGF used in Mapleson systems represents a disadvantage, because it contributes to drying of the respiratory tract, heat loss and increased gas waste (including oxygen and inhaled anesthetics), which increases pollution and anesthesia cost. On the other hand, these systems are associated with several advantages, including their lower equipment cost, simple construction, lightweight design, low resistance to breathing (compared to other breathing systems), small apparatus dead space, and low total circuit volume. Additionally, because of the high FGF and low circuit volume, inspired inhalant concentrations will more rapidly reach vaporizer settings, facilitating anesthetic control and depth changes. CO_2 absorbents are not part of the Mapleson systems, thus there is no risk associated with absorbent dust or inhalant anesthetic breakdown. Lastly, Mapleson systems are disposable, which allows them to be discarded after bacterial contamination.

Veterinary Anesthetic and Monitoring Equipment, First Edition. Edited by Kristen G. Cooley and Rebecca A. Johnson.

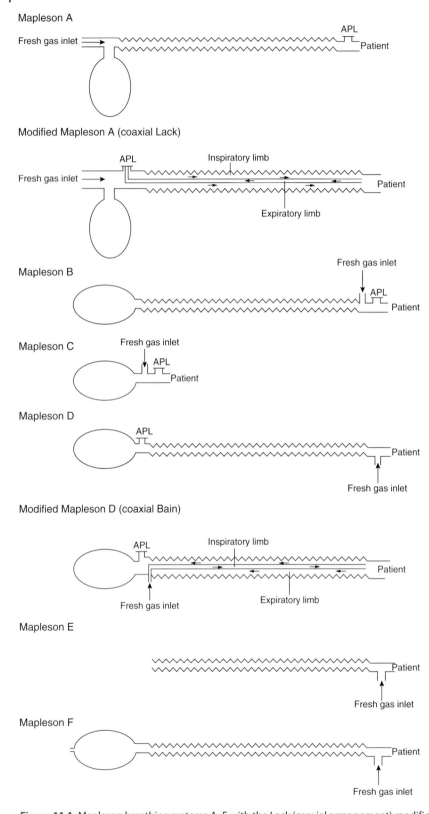

Figure 11.1 Mapleson breathing systems A–F with the Lack (coaxial arrangement) modification of the Mapleson A and Bain (coaxial arrangement) modification of Mapleson D. Image courtesy of Kristen Cooley, University of Wisconsin-Madison, WI.

In general, resistance and work of breathing increases when high FGFs are used with both systems (Mapleson and circle/rebreathing) (Kay *et al.* 1983; Rasch *et al.* 1988). However, the resistance associated with both the Mapleson and circle/rebreathing systems is still lower than breathing through the endotracheal tube alone (Rasch *et al.* 1988). Avoiding the use of conducting tubes with an internal diameter of less than that of the endotracheal tube is necessary to prevent further increase in airway resistance.

The use of Mapleson systems in larger animals (>10 kg) is functionally possible, but is wasteful due to the higher FGFs required to remove CO_2 from the system. This will additionally increase oxygen and inhalant anesthetic waste. The use of Mapleson systems has been historically recommended for animals weighing less than 5–7 kg due to the above-mentioned advantages, including low resistance, small dead space and total circuit volume (Lerche *et al.* 2000; Mosley 2015). However, the advent of lower resistance valves, improved CO_2 absorbent canisters and smaller dead space, has made modern pediatric circle systems a safe and efficient alternative to Mapleson systems for small animals (Rasch *et al.* 1988; Conterato *et al.* 1989). Indeed, resistance from pediatric circle systems might be similar or even lower than some Mapleson systems, especially if excessive FGFs are avoided (Kay *et al.* 1983; Rasch *et al.* 1988; Conterato *et al.* 1989) and circle systems have been used in spontaneously breathing healthy cats weighing as low as 2.5 kg (Hartsfield and Sawyer 1976). Nevertheless, it is imperative that proper functioning of unidirectional valves before and during anesthesia is confirmed and appropriate monitoring for assessment of rebreathing (i.e. capnography) is implemented when circle systems are used for small animals (Rasch *et al.* 1988). Additionally, when using a Mapleson system for assisted/controlled ventilation, partially closing the APL valve can lead to significant increases in resistance, even higher than with the use of a circle system (Rasch *et al.* 1988), which can be an important consideration when trying to decide between Mapleson and circle systems.

11.4 Choice of System

Ultimately, the choice of breathing system is determined by personal preference, availability of equipment, economy, animal size/body composition and health status (i.e. respiratory disease, increased resistance to breathing, etc.) (Hartsfield and Sawyer 1976; Bednarski 1993; Lerche *et al.* 2000). In veterinary medicine, the most commonly used Mapleson systems are A, D, F and some modifications of these systems (Bednarski 1993). There are many variations of the Mapleson systems reported in the veterinary literature (Dickson and Anderson 1988; Holden 2000; Walsh and Taylor 2004; Almubarak *et al.* 2005; Gale *et al.* 2015), but this chapter will focus on the most commonly-used systems and associated modifications described in veterinary anesthesia. Based on the FGF requirements to prevent rebreathing, Mapleson group A is more efficient that DEF during spontaneous breathing and DEF is more efficient than A during controlled ventilation (Mapleson 1954; Waters and Mapleson 1961; Sykes 1968; Miller 1988; Cook 1996a); therefore, the breathing modality may affect the choice of system. There is a wide range of FGFs recommended in the literature for these different individual systems (see below), and capnography is a useful tool to determine optimal flow to prevent rebreathing.

11.5 Specific System Types

11.5.1 Mapleson A

The classic Mapleson A system (i.e. Magill) (Figure 11.1) represents an exception regarding location of the fresh gas inlet, since it is the only Mapleson system where the inlet is positioned away from the patient connection. This circuit has a reservoir bag (also located away from the patient), a corrugated conducting tube and an excess venting system with an adjustable pressure limiting (APL) valve positioned near the patient connection port.

11.5.1.1 Modifications of Mapleson A

The Lack modification (Figure 11.1) has an additional conducting tube carrying the expired gas to an APL valve (Lack 1976). The reservoir bag is positioned on the inspiratory limb of the system and the APL valve on the expiratory limb, both located away from the patient. This arrangement is advantageous as it facilitates gas scavenging, adjustments of the APL valve, and assisted breathing. The Lack system is available with a parallel or coaxial configuration (Lack 1976; Ooi *et al.* 1993a,b). In the coaxial arrangement, the expiratory limb runs concentrically inside the outer inspiratory limb (tube within a tube). However, both configurations can be associated with higher breathing resistance (Ooi *et al.* 1993b). The gas flow dynamics are similar between Lack and classic Magill systems during spontaneous and controlled ventilation.

11.5.1.2 Gas Flow Dynamics

Spontaneous Breathing   The APL valve is kept in the fully open position for spontaneous breathing in the Mapleson A breathing system (Mapleson 1954; Kain and Nunn 1968; Cook 1996b) (Figure 11.2). During inspiration, gas moves from the reservoir bag and conducting tubing

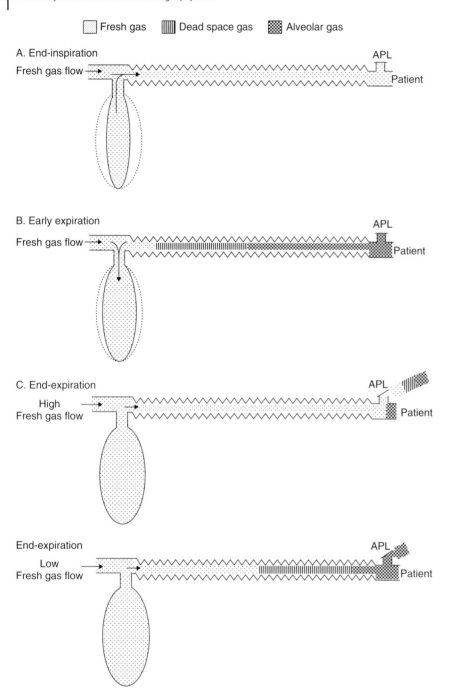

☐ Fresh gas   ▦ Dead space gas   ▨ Alveolar gas

A. End-inspiration

Fresh gas flow →

APL

Patient

B. Early expiration

Fresh gas flow →

APL

Patient

C. End-expiration

High
Fresh gas flow →

APL

Patient

End-expiration

Low
Fresh gas flow →

APL

Patient

Figure 11.2 Gas flow dynamics in the Mapleson A system during spontaneous breathing. Image courtesy of Kristen Cooley, University of Wisconsin-Madison, WI.

toward the patient (Figure 11.2A). During early expiration, expired gas (composed initially of dead space gas followed by alveolar gas) moves through the conducting tubing, displacing the fresh gas towards the bag, while fresh gas is simultaneously flowing into the bag causing it to distend (Figure 11.2B). Pressure inside the circuit increases as the bag fills, leading to opening of the APL valve. Thus, at end-expiration, the continued fresh gas inflow reverses the flow of expired

gases in the conducting tube toward the patient, and alveolar gas moves out the APL valve into the scavenging system (Figure 11.2C). The higher the FGF used, the more expired gas is forced out of the APL, including alveolar and dead space gas, and potentially even fresh gas (Figure 11.2C). If FGF is low, very little alveolar gas is forced out the APL valve (Figure 11.2C). This may cause CO_2 rebreathing during the next inspiration. During the pause after expiration and before inspiration, fresh inflowing gas moves expired gases from the conducting tubing toward the APL valve.

With high FGF, the first gas to be forced out the APL valve in the Mapleson A system is alveolar gas (high in CO_2), followed by dead space gas and finally fresh gas (Figure 11.2C). However, the initial elimination of alveolar gas allows the use of relatively low FGFs with a Mapleson A system, making it an efficient system, as it requires the lowest FGF to prevent rebreathing during spontaneous ventilation when compared to other systems (Mapleson 1954; Cook 1996b). Additionally, changes in respiratory pattern do not significantly affect the rebreathing potential for Mapleson A systems during spontaneous breathing (Cook 1996a,b).

There are some inconsistencies regarding differences in efficiency between the classic Mapleson A and the Lack modification. Some authors claim that the Lack is less efficient than the Magill (Barnes *et al.* 1980) and others show that they are equally efficient (Nott *et al.* 1982; Miller 1988; Chan *et al.* 1989). Clinical reports demonstrate that the Lack seems to be more efficient than the Magill,

requiring lower FGF in anesthetized humans and dogs (Humphrey 1982; Waterman 1986). However, wide ranges of FGF have been used based on the different definitions of rebreathing (Miller 1988; Chan *et al.* 1989; Mapleson 2004), which leads to an overlap in the FGFs recommended for the different Mapleson systems, including the classic configuration (i.e. Magill) and the modification of Mapleson A (i.e. Lack). Studies have shown rebreathing with FGFs of 51–72 mL/kg/min or 0.72–0.78 times patient minute volume (Humphrey 1982; Humphrey *et al.* 1986a; Chan *et al.* 1989; Ooi *et al.* 1993a; Gale *et al.* 2015). Thus, the recommended FGF to prevent rebreathing is 85–130 mL/kg/min or 0.70–1.0 times patient minute volume (Kain and Nunn 1968; Jonsson and Zetterstrom 1986; Waterman 1986; Jonsson *et al.* 1987).

Controlled or Assisted Ventilation Although Mapleson A systems are the most efficient systems during spontaneous breathing, they are the least efficient during controlled ventilation (Sykes 1959, 1968; Waters and Mapleson 1961; Humphrey 1983) (Figure 11.3). The breathing pattern

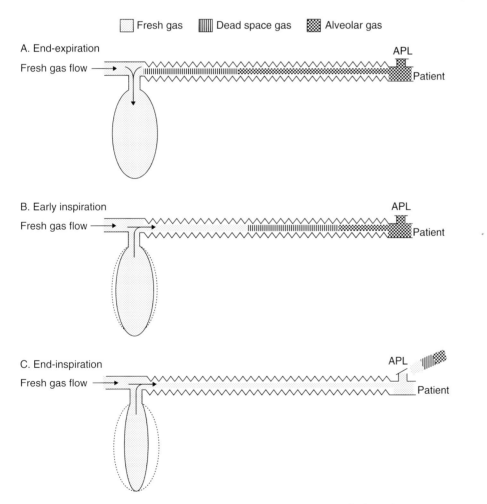

Figure 11.3 Gas flow dynamics in the Mapleson A system during controlled ventilation. Image courtesy of Kristen Cooley, University of Wisconsin-Madison, WI.

affects the efficiency of Mapleson A during controlled ventilation (Sykes 1959; Conway 1985). Very large FGFs are used to prevent rebreathing with Mapleson A, which discourages its use during assisted or controlled ventilation (Sykes 1959; Waters and Mapleson 1961; Humphrey 1983). Additionally, positioning of the APL valve near the patient and away from the reservoir bag makes its use for controlled/assisted ventilation problematic. The Lack modification is advantageous, since the APL valve is away from the patient and close to the reservoir bag; however, high FGFs are still needed during controlled ventilation (Humphrey 1983).

During inspiration using controlled ventilation, the APL valve is kept partially closed while the bag is squeezed, therefore generating sufficient pressure for lung inflation, while some of the gas is also forced out of the APL valve, leaving the reservoir bag partially empty at end-inspiration. During expiration, fresh gas is also continuously flowing into the bag; however, because the bag is almost empty at end-inspiration, the pressure in the system remains low and no gas is forced out the APL valve. Additionally, a large portion of the conducting tubing fills with expired gas (dead space and alveolar gas), which moves towards the bag (Figure 11.3A), potentially even allowing alveolar gas to enter the bag. The APL valve opens during expiration in case the reservoir bag becomes distended, especially if FGF is high. During early inspiration (Figure 11.3B), the expired gas in the conducting tubing moves toward the patient. Since the alveolar gas is closest to the patient, it is inspired first, leading to significant CO_2 rebreathing. As the system pressure builds, the APL valve opens and gas (fresh and expired) flows to the patient and also through the APL valve, leading to waste of fresh gas (Figure 11.3C).

11.5.1.3 Inspection Before Use

System integrity should be inspected before each use. After visual inspection, a leak test can be performed by occluding the patient end, closing the APL valve and pressurizing the system by increasing the FGF or using the oxygen flush valve. The oxygen flow is then stopped and the system should hold pressure, demonstrating no loss of gas (Furst and Laffey 1984). The APL valve is then opened, leading to deflation of the bag and confirming proper functioning of the APL valve.

Additional testing is required in order to assess the inner tube integrity in the Lack modification. One method involves inserting an endotracheal tube into the inner tube at the patient end of the system and blowing through it. The APL valve should remain closed during this test and if a leak is present, the reservoir bag will expand (Furst and Laffey 1984). Another technique requires occluding both the outer and inner tubes at the patient end of the system. The system is then pressurized while leaving the APL valve open until the reservoir bag is inflated. The bag is

squeezed, which will lead to bag collapse if a leak is present (Martin and McKeown 1985).

11.5.2 Mapleson B and C

The Mapleson B and C systems (Figure 11.1) have similar configurations, in that both the fresh gas inlet and APL valve are located near the patient and the reservoir bag is at the opposite end of the system. The difference is that the Mapleson C does not have any conducting tubing. These systems work similarly during spontaneous and controlled ventilation (Sykes 1968; Conway 1985). In the Mapleson B, the corrugated conducting tubing corresponds to an extension of the reservoir bag, which means that the conditions for preventing rebreathing are similar for both systems (Mapleson 1954). However, if rebreathing does occur, the composition of the inspired gas (CO_2 build up) may be different, because the mixing of expired gases with gas in the reservoir bag occurs more efficiently in system C than in system B (Mapleson 1954). These systems are less commonly used in veterinary medicine.

11.5.2.1 Gas Flow Dynamics

Spontaneous Breathing Gas flow within Mapleson B and C systems is similar (Sykes 1968; Cook 1996b). For spontaneous breathing, the APL valve is kept fully opened. During inspiration, gas moves from the reservoir bag and fresh gas inlet toward the patient. During early expiration, expired gas (dead space followed by alveolar gas) moves toward the reservoir bag while fresh gas is continuously flowing, causing the bag to distend. At end-expiration, as the bag is full, the increased circuit pressure leads to APL valve opening and elimination of alveolar gas and fresh gas. All the expired gas beyond the fresh gas inlet and APL valve (that moved toward the reservoir bag) remains in the reservoir bag (and conducting tubing, in the case of Mapleson B) and cannot be eliminated through the APL valve; consequently, it contributes to rebreathing during the next inspiration.

During the expiratory pause before inspiration, only fresh gas moves out of the APL valve. When inspiration starts, the patient inspires fresh and expired gas mixed with fresh gas from the reservoir bag (and conducting tubing for Mapleson B). In the case of Mapleson B, if the tidal volume of the patient is smaller than the volume of the conducting tube, no gas from the reservoir bag would be inspired.

The FGF must be high enough to fill the reservoir bag and allow the APL valve to open early enough in expiration for all the alveolar gas to be eliminated (Cook 1996b). Rebreathing for both systems can be prevented by using FGF of at least 1.5–2 times minute volume (Mapleson 1954; Sykes 1968; Conway 1985; Miller 1988). The main factor affecting their efficiency is the expiratory pause duration as a fraction of the respiratory cycle; the longer the pause, the less efficient (Cook 1996a, b).

Controlled or Assisted Ventilation For controlled or assisted ventilation, the APL valve is kept partially closed during inspiration while the bag is squeezed; the lungs will inflate and some of the gas is also forced out the APL valve. At the beginning of expiration, the bag is partially empty, and the system pressure is low, thus gas flows toward the bag while fresh gas is continuously flowing in the same direction. The alveolar gas will concentrate toward the bag, while fresh gas will accumulate closer to the patient.

At the next inspiration, when the bag is squeezed again, the fresh gas is inspired first and while some of the expired gas might be inspired, it is also eliminated through the APL valve. In system C, because there is no conducting tube, the expired gas and fresh gas will go directly to the bag where they mix. Thus, during inspiration, this mixture and the continuous fresh gas will be inspired. There is less separation of fresh gas than in system B. Therefore, system C might be slightly less efficient than B during controlled ventilation, but both are still more efficient than A (Waters and Mapleson 1961).

Inspired gas composition is significantly influenced by the ventilatory pattern; consequently, performance is inconsistent during controlled ventilation (Conway 1985). For Mapleson B and C, FGF of at least two times minute volume is recommended to reduce rebreathing during controlled ventilation (Sykes 1968; Conway 1985).

11.5.3 Mapleson D, E and F

All of the breathing systems in this group have a common structure with a T-shaped connector (Conway 1985). In this T-piece (Figure 11.4), one port is for the fresh gas inlet, the second one is the patient connection, and the third is for conducting tubing directing expired gases away from the patient (Mapleson 1954; Conway 1985). The conducting tube connections differ between the Mapleson D, E and F systems. Connected to the conduct-

ing tubing (usually corrugated), on the opposite end of the system, the Mapleson D has an APL valve and a reservoir bag; Mapleson E does not have anything but an open length of conducting tube; and the Mapleson F has an open-ended reservoir bag (Mapleson 1954; Willis *et al.* 1975; Conway 1985) (Figure 11.4). A modification of the T-piece, the Norman elbow, has the fresh gas inlet extending inside the T-piece toward the patient connection in order to minimize dead space.

Many modifications of these systems have been used in veterinary medicine (Dickson and Anderson 1988; Walsh and Taylor 2004; Almubarak *et al.* 2005; Gale *et al.* 2015), but only the most common ones used are discussed in this chapter. The Mapleson D, E and F systems work similarly during spontaneous and controlled ventilation (Conway 1985) and similar FGFs are required to prevent rebreathing (Dorrington and Lehane 1987).

11.5.3.1 Mapleson D

The Mapleson D system (Figure 11.1) has the fresh gas inlet near the patient, with corrugated conducting tubing connecting it to the reservoir bag and the excess venting system with an APL valve, both located away from the patient on the opposite end of the system.

Bain Modification The Bain is a modification of the Mapleson D breathing system with a coaxial configuration (Bain and Spoerel 1972). In the Bain breathing system, the fresh gas supply enters the system near the reservoir bag/APL valve and is delivered by the inner tube to exit near the patient; the outer corrugated tube is the expiratory limb (Figure 11.1).

The Bain system may be used with a mounting block, sometimes referred to as a Bain block, which includes a port for the conducting tubing, a port for the reservoir bag, an APL valve with connection for the scavenging system, and a pressure manometer (Figure 11.5). It allows the breathing system to be fixed and more readily accessible to the anesthetist, while avoiding risks of potential disconnections or kinked hoses. Furthermore, the pressure manometer built into the system allows the anesthetist

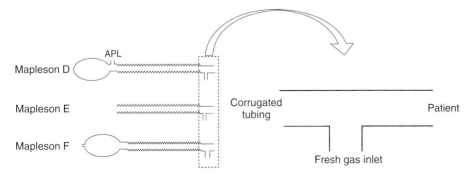

Figure 11.4 T-shaped connector used in Mapleson D, E and F systems. Image courtesy of Kristen Cooley, University of Wisconsin-Madison, WI.

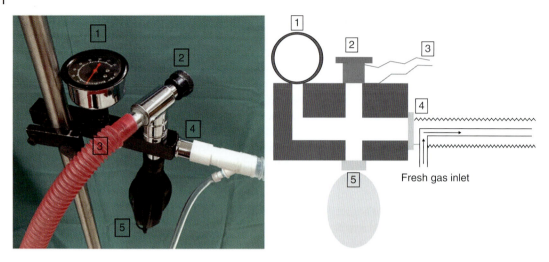

Figure 11.5 Example of a Bain system and mounting block, including: (1) pressure manometer; (2) adjustable pressure limiting valve (APL); (3) connection for the scavenging system; (4) port for the conducting tubing; and (5) port for a reservoir bag. Image courtesy of Kristen Cooley, University of Wisconsin-Madison, WI.

to assess airway pressure. Pressure monitoring is especially important when using Mapleson systems, since the low circuit volume and high FGFs used could potentially lead to significant and very fast increases in airway pressure to levels causing barotrauma and cardiovascular collapse, especially if accidental obstruction or kinks occur.

The commercially available Bain system with added tube length can be used for remote anesthesia, such as during magnetic resonance imaging and radiotherapy. However, they are associated with an increased static compliance and increase in positive end-expiratory pressure (Sweeting *et al.* 2002). Additionally, a decrease in peak inspiratory pressure at the patient end and a decrease in delivered tidal volume with the longest version (9.6 m) are also observed. The decrease in delivered tidal volume was more significant (23% reduction) in the 10-kg lung model when compared to the 20-kg and 70-kg model lungs (Sweeting *et al.* 2002); therefore, ventilator settings should be adjusted as needed, especially for smaller patients. An increase in resistance to spontane-

ous breathing can also be appreciated with the longer Bain system (Sellers and Dykes 2003).

11.5.3.2 Gas Flow Dynamics
Spontaneous Breathing The APL valve is kept fully opened during spontaneous ventilation. During inspiration, gas moves from the reservoir bag/conducting tubing and fresh gas inlet toward the patient. During early expiration, expired gas moves toward the reservoir bag, while fresh gas is continuously flowing causing the bag to distend. Once the reservoir bag is full at late expiration (Figure 11.6), the APL valve opens and this mixture of expired gases and fresh gas that occupies the conducting tubing closer to the bag is partly eliminated. Note that expired dead space/alveolar gas is closer to the bag and APL valve, while fresh gas concentrates closer to the patient.

During the next inspiration, gas in the conducting tubing and fresh gas (added because of the continuous flow from the fresh gas inlet) is inspired by the patient. The gas composition in the conducting tubing at end-expiration and before the next inspiration depends on the FGF; high FGF

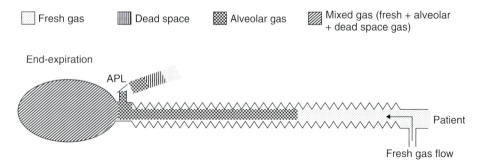

Figure 11.6 Gases at end-expiration in the Mapleson D system during spontaneous breathing. Image courtesy of Kristen Cooley, University of Wisconsin-Madison, WI.

leads to elimination of most of the alveolar gas in the conducting tubing, whereas low FGF will allow more rebreathing of expired gas containing CO_2. Additionally, the respiratory pattern is a major determinant of rebreathing with this group (Dorrington and Lehane 1987; Cook 1996a, b). If an end-expiratory pause is present, fresh gas inflow forms a reservoir at the patient end of the conducting tubing, which becomes the first gas to be inspired by the patient (Figure 11.6). Thus, in contrast to the Mapleson C, the expiratory pause in the Mapleson D system makes it more efficient (Conway 1985; Cook 1996a, b). Additionally, if the patient's tidal volume is higher than the conducting tubing volume, mixed expired and fresh gas from the bag is inspired, leading to further rebreathing (Sykes 1968).

Rebreathing occurs with FGFs of 100–150 mL/kg/min in spontaneously breathing humans (Byrick 1980; Humphrey 1982; Humphrey *et al.* 1986a; Jonsson *et al.* 1987). Due to the different definitions of rebreathing (Miller 1988; Chan *et al.* 1989) and that respiratory patterns have such a dramatic effect on this group of breathing systems (Dorrington and Lehane 1987; Cook 1996a,b), a wide range of FGFs are recommended. For example, an FGF of 100–130 mL/kg/min has been recommended in dogs (Manley and McDonell 1979a,b), 250 mL/kg/min in pigs (Almubarak *et al.* 2005) and 100 200 mL/kg/min in humans (Bain and Spoerel 1972; Jonsson and Zetterstrom 1986). Moreover, 1.52 times minute volume (Dean and Keenan 1982; Meakin and Coates 1983; Conway 1985; Miller 1988; Chan *et al.* 1989) and up to 3 times minute volume, have been recommended in humans (Mapleson 1954; Harrison 1964; Sykes 1968; Conway *et al.* 1977; Rose *et al.* 1978; Lindahl *et al.* 1984; Dorrington and Lehane 1987).

Controlled or Assisted Ventilation For mechanically controlled ventilation, the ventilator hose replaces the reservoir bag and the APL valve is kept fully closed. For manually controlled or assisted ventilation, the APL valve is kept partially closed during inspiration while the bag is squeezed; the lungs will inflate and some gas is also forced out the APL valve.

During controlled ventilation, at the beginning of expiration, the bag is partially empty and the system pressure is low, thus gas flows into the conducting tubing toward the bag, while fresh gas is also continuously flowing in the same direction. The alveolar gas is more concentrated in the conducting tubing toward the bag, while fresh gas accumulates closer to the patient. Similar to Mapleson B and C, at the next inspiration, fresh gas goes directly to the patient and the rest of the tidal volume is made up of gas from the conducting tubing. However, with the Mapleson D, the first gas inspired is rich in fresh gas (closer to the patient) and goes exclusively to the patient instead of being partially eliminated by the APL valve (as occurs in Mapleson B and C). Additionally, with

the Mapleson D, the gas in the bag or closer to the APL valve (richer in alveolar and dead space gas) is partially eliminated through the APL valve during inspiration using manually controlled or assisted ventilation, demonstrating higher efficiency for Mapleson D (Waters and Mapleson 1961; Sykes 1968).

A FGF during controlled ventilation as low as 70–100 mL/kg/min has been recommended for humans and dogs (Bain and Spoerel 1973; Henville and Adams 1976; Manley and McDonell 1979a, b; Rose and Froese 1979; Humphrey *et al.* 1986b) and 2 times minute volume has also been recommended in humans (Rose and Froese 1979).

Inspection Before Use System integrity evaluation is performed first by initial visual inspection (cracked tubes, kinking and disconnection of inner tube, etc.). Then, after closing the APL valve and occluding the patient end, the system is pressurized. The oxygen flow is subsequently discontinued; the system should hold pressure. Afterwards, the APL valve is opened and the bag should deflate easily if the APL valve and scavenging systems are functioning properly.

Additional testing is required to assess the inner tube integrity in the Bain modification. If the inner tube is disconnected, there is a significant increase in apparatus dead space, which will increase rebreathing substantially. The Pethick test involves filling the system using the oxygen flush valve without obstructing the flow at the patient end and with the oxygen flowmeter off (Pethick 1975). The high velocity flow through the inner tube creates a Venturi effect, thus lowering the pressure in the outer tube and reservoir bag, leading to collapse of the bag. If the inner tube is disconnected proximally (opposite end from the patient), the bag can inflate slightly instead of deflate (Pethick 1975). However, this test does not completely assess inner tube integrity (Beauprie *et al.* 1990) or omission (Peterson 1978).

A leak test involving occlusion of the inner tube can be performed by turning on the oxygen flow (2–4 L/min) and occluding only the inner tube with a 3-mL syringe plunger at the patient end for 2–5 seconds (Foëx and Smith 1977; Ghani 1984; Heath and Marks 1991). This produces a rise of pressure within the inner tube and a reduction in the pressure gradient; consequently, the oxygen flowmeter indicator should fall slightly. When the plunger is removed, a "hissing sound" is heard due to the sudden release of accumulated oxygen in the inner tube (Foex and Smith 1977; Ghani 1984; Heath and Marks 1991). The period of occlusion should be as short as possible to avoid damage to the flowmeter (Heath and Marks 1991).

The inner tube occlusion test is effective for many types of defects, except when there are small holes in the inner tube (Heath and Marks 1991). Therefore, along with the effects seen in the previously described occlusion test (inner tube only), the double occlusion test (inner and outer tube) has been recommended to fully assess full inner tube integrity (Heath and Marks 1991). The oxygen flowmeter should be set at 4 L/minute and the APL valve closed. Both inner and outer tubes should be occluded; if the reservoir bag distends, it indicates the presence of a leak between the inner and outer tubes (Heath and Marks 1991).

11.5.2.4 Mapleson E

An example of the Mapleson E system (Figure 11.1) is the Ayre's T-piece, which has a T-piece and conducting tubing. This system was originally described by Ayre in 1937 (Ayre 1937a, b) and later further analyzed (Mapleson 1954; Ayre 1956; Harrison 1964). Many modifications have been described; however, its function depends primarily on the conducting tubing volume (Sykes 1968). For example, this volume may be greater than the patient's tidal volume, which contributes to an increase in dead space and rebreathing (Ayre 1956; Sykes 1968). The tubing volume may also be smaller than the patient's tidal volume, which could potentially lead to inspired gas dilution (Ayre 1937b, 1956). If tubing length is reduced to near zero (Lewis and Spoerel 1961), where rebreathing cannot occur, dilution of fresh gas with room air can only be avoided by using an FGF exceeding peak inspiratory flow (~3 times minute volume) (Sykes 1968).

One difference between Mapleson D and E systems is that during expiration with the Mapleson E, expired gases and fresh gas will move along the conducting tubing and exit into ambient air due to lack of a reservoir bag, which makes scavenging of excess gases difficult. Considering that large-bore tubing is frequently used, resistance of the Mapleson E is very low (Mapleson 1954), because there is no APL valve. The APL valve can lead to a considerable resistance to expiration, particularly when high FGF are used (Kay et al. 1983; Rasch et al. 1988). In order to provide controlled ventilation with a Mapleson E, intermittent occlusion of the conducting tubing can be done, allowing fresh gas flow to inflate the lungs. However, this should be performed with caution, since it can lead to over-inflation and barotrauma due to the absence of a reservoir bag and APL valve.

The conditions necessary to prevent rebreathing are similar to system D (Mapleson 1954; Conway 1985). The FGF recommendation is approximately 1.5–2.5 times minute volume (Mapleson 1954; Ayre 1956; Harrison 1964; Sykes 1968). As with Mapleson D, the breathing pattern also influences rebreathing and FGF requirements (Harrison 1964). Similar considerations apply when ventilation is controlled (Sykes 1968), where 1.5–2 times minute volume has been recommended (Rose and Froese 1979; Hatch et al. 1987), but higher FGF (up to 3 times minute volume) may be required, depending on the expiratory pause, inspiratory and expiratory flow (Harrison 1964).

11.5.2.5 Mapleson F

The Mapleson F system (i.e. Jackson-Rees) (Figure 11.1) is similar to the Mapleson D. However, instead of having an APL valve positioned close to the reservoir bag, the Mapleson F system has an open-ended reservoir bag for venting excess gases, which can make scavenging expired gases difficult, yet reduces breathing resistance. The Jackson–Rees modification of the Ayre's T-piece was initially described by Rees (1950) and then added to the Mapleson breathing systems as system "F" (Willis et al. 1975). Different scavenging systems have been described for the Jackson–Rees system (Chan 1993; Chan and Kong 1993; Prosser 1997; Dhara and Pua 2000).

Controlled or assisted ventilation can be performed by occluding the distal end of the reservoir bag and squeezing the bag. Mechanical ventilation can be performed by replacing the bag with the ventilator hose. Functionally, Mapleson F behaves like the D system, with similar dynamics for gas flow within the system during spontaneous and controlled ventilation, thus similar FGF have been recommended (Conway 1985).

11.6 Combined Systems

There are commercially available options that combine the use of the Mapleson A system and the T-piece (D and/or E) in coaxial or parallel arrangements (Miller 1979; Humphrey 1983; Humphrey et al. 1986a, b; Dickson and Anderson 1988). These systems allow the anesthetist to switch between Mapleson A during spontaneous ventilation and Mapleson D or E during controlled ventilation within a single case, allowing the lowest FGF use with each mode of ventilation. The Humphrey ADE (in A mode) has been evaluated in spontaneously breathing dogs and cats (Alibhai et al. 1999; Gale et al. 2015); an FGF of 100 mL/kg/min prevented rebreathing if less than 15 kg (Gale et al. 2015).

11.7 Respiratory Gas Monitoring

Reliable gas monitoring necessitates an understanding of the limitations and specific requirements of the devices available (Sasse 1985). Factors such as a proper seal around the endotracheal tube and the monitor response speed and gas-sampling rate relative to the respiratory rate and minute ventilation of the patient are vital when considering the accuracy of the expired gas measurements (Sasse 1985). For example, high sampling rates with low tidal volumes from small patients may lead to dilution of the sample with fresh gas, resulting in erroneous low end-tidal CO_2. Causes for end-tidal CO_2 measurement error may also affect anesthetic gas concentration measurements (Schieber *et al.* 1985).

When using Mapleson systems, sampling of expired gases may be associated with dilution by fresh gas due to the high FGF used and the position of the fresh gas inlet in relation to the monitor sampling site. In Mapleson F systems, sampling from the distal end of the endotracheal tube was recommended to obtain accurate end-tidal CO_2 measurements that reliably estimate arterial partial pressure of CO_2 ($PaCO_2$) in small patients (<12 kg) (Badgwell *et al.* 1987). In addition, the ratio between expiratory flow rate and gas sampling rate is important in determining the magnitude of error when gas is sampled from proximal sites (i.e. the elbow connector between endotracheal tube and breathing system).

When using the Bain circuit in animals and humans, site significantly affects gas sampling, especially concerning changing FGF and expiratory flow rates (Gravenstein *et al.* 1985). When gas sampling is near the fresh gas inlet, specifically at the corner of the elbow connector or at the proximal end of elbow (close to the Bain circuit), samples are unreliable, even at low FGFs, due to the mixing of the expired gas with fresh gas. In these situations, arterial blood gas sampling ($PaCO_2$) is recommended to assess ventilation. However, sampling distally (closer to the patient end of the elbow) or at the endotracheal tube adaptor is more accurate (Gravenstein *et al.* 1985), although end-tidal CO_2 can still under-estimate the $PaCO_2$ in some situations (Schieber *et al.* 1985). Additionally, mixing of expired and fresh gas becomes apparent with lower expiratory flow rates (Gravenstein

et al. 1985; Schieber *et al.* 1985) or with the use of uncuffed endotracheal tubes (Schiever *et al.* 1985). Indeed, with Bain circuits, the best sampling site is within the endotracheal tube itself (Miller 1990).

11.8 Potential Hazards

Breathing systems should always be inspected before use, because incorrectly manufactured or assembled systems can lead to potentially severe consequences. For example, if the fresh gas inlet of the Lack is placed adjacent to the APL valve instead of the reservoir bag, significant rebreathing occurs (Jones 1991; Picton and Crosse 1998; Langton *et al.* 2010). Bain systems can also be improperly assembled (Peterson 1978), with manufactured defects (Gooch and Peutrell 2004; Singh *et al.* 2011), defects in the mounting block (Allen 2000), or with inner tubes being disconnected (Hannallah and Rosales 1974; Jackson 1988; Ghai *et al.* 2006; Singh *et al.* 2011), which can lead to a significant increase in apparatus dead space and rebreathing.

Always inspect these systems during use for any potential occlusions, including inadvertently closed APL valves and incompatibility of monitoring equipment (Evans 1998), since the high FGFs and low total volume of the Mapleson circuits can quickly lead to dangerous increases in airway pressure and barotrauma. The use of safety APL valves is recommended, which close the system only when a button is depressed; upon release of the button, the valve automatically opens (Figure 11.7; SafeSigh Nonrebreathing System, Vetamac, Rossville, IN; Safety Pressure Relief Valve, Supera Anesthesia Innovations, Clackamas, OR; Pop Off Occlusion Valve, Smiths Medical, Dublin, OH). High pressures can also occur if the oxygen flush valve is used when the Mapleson system is connected to the patient; therefore this practice should be avoided.

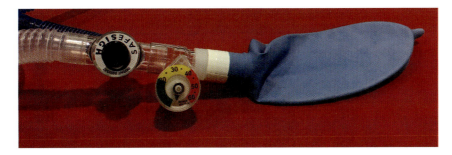

Figure 11.7 Example of a safety APL valve (SafeSigh) that remains open until the button is depressed to administer a breath. Once released, the valve is automatically opened. In this situation, it is placed between the rebreathing bag and non-rebreathing circuit. However, they may also be used in rebreathing systems. A plastic (single-use) manometer is also shown in this photograph (Vetamac, Rossville, IN).

References

Alibhai, H.I.K., Lilja, A.S. and Clarke, K.W. (1999) Evaluation of the Humphrey ADE circuit during spontaneous ventilation in dogs. *Vet Anaesth Analg*, 26, 38.

Allen, P. (2000) Bain circuit adapter fault. *Anaesth Intensive Care*, 28, 333.

Almubarak, A., Clarke, K. and Jackson, T.L. (2005) Comparison of the Bain system and Uniflow universal anaesthetic breathing systems in spontaneously breathing young pigs. *Vet Anaesth Analg*, 32, 314–321.

Ayre, P. (1937a) Anesthesia for intracranial operation – a new technique. *The Lancet*, 1, 561–563.

Ayre, P. (1937b) Endotracheal anesthesia for babies: with special reference to Hare-Lip and Cleft Palate operations. *Anesth Analg*, 16, 330–333.

Ayre, P. (1956) The T-piece technique. *Br J Anaesth*, 28, 520–523.

Badgwell, J.M., McLeod, M.E., Lerman, J. and Creighton, R.E. (1987) End-tidal PCO_2 measurements sampled at the distal and proximal ends of the endotracheal tube in infants and children. *Anesth Analg*, 66, 959–964.

Bain, J.A. and Spoerel, W.E. (1972) A streamlined anaesthetic system. *Can Anaesth Soc J*, 19, 426–435.

Bain, J.A. and Spoerel, W.E. (1973) Flow requirements for a modified Mapleson D system during controlled ventilation. *Can Anaesth Soc J*, 20, 629–636.

Barnes, P.K., Conway, C.M. and Purcell, G.R. (1980) The Lack anaesthetic system. *Anaesthesia*, 35, 393–394.

Beauprie, I.G., Clark, A.G., Keith, I.C. and Spence, D. (1990) Pre-use testing of coaxial circuits: the perils of Pethick. *Can J Anaesth*, 37, S103.

Bednarski, R.M. (1993) Anesthetic breathing systems. *Semin Vet Med Surg (Small Anim)*, 8, 82–89.

Byrick, R.J. (1980) Respiratory compensation during spontaneous ventilation with the Bain circuit. *Can Anaesth Soc J*, 27, 96–105.

Chan, A.S., Bruce, W.E. and Soni, N. (1989) A comparison of anaesthetic breathing systems during spontaneous ventilation. An *in-vitro* study using a lung model. *Anaesthesia*, 44, 194–199.

Chan, M.S. (1993) A new T-piece scavenging system. *Anaesth Intensive Care*, 21, 899.

Chan, M.S. and Kong, A.S. (1993) T-piece scavenging – the double-bag system. *Anaesthesia*, 48, 647.

Conterato, J.P., Lindahl, S.G., Meyer, D.M. and Bires, J.A. (1989) Assessment of spontaneous ventilation in anesthetized children with use of a pediatric circle or a Jackson-Rees system. *Anesth Analg*, 69, 484–490.

Conway, C.M. (1985) Anaesthetic breathing systems. *Br J Anaesth*, 57, 649–657.

Conway, C.M., Seeley, H.F. and Barnes, P.K. (1977) Spontaneous ventilation with the Bain anaesthetic system. *Br J Anaesth*, 49, 1245–1249.

Cook, L.B. (1996a) The importance of the expiratory pause. Comparison of the Mapleson A, C and D breathing systems using a lung model. *Anaesthesia*, 51, 453–460.

Cook, L.B. (1996b) Respiratory pattern and rebreathing in the Mapleson A, C and D breathing systems with spontaneous ventilation. *A theory. Anaesthesia*, 51, 371–385.

Dean, S.E. and Keenan, R.L. (1982) Spontaneous breathing with a T-piece circuit: minimum fresh gas/minute volume ratio which prevents rebreathing. *Anesthesiology*, 56, 449–452.

Dhara, S.S. and Pua, H.L. (2000) A non-occluding bag and closed scavenging system for the Jackson Rees modified T-piece breathing system. *Anaesthesia*, 55, 450–454.

Dickson, L. and Anderson, I.L. (1988) Evaluation of a non-rebreathing circuit for small animal anaesthesia. *NZ Vet J*, 36, 194–197.

Dorrington, K.L. and Lehane, J.R. (1987) Minimum fresh gas flow requirements of anaesthetic breathing systems during spontaneous ventilation: a graphical approach. *Anaesthesia*, 42, 732–737.

Evans, A.T. (1998) Anesthesia case of the month. Pneumothorax, pneumomediastinum and subcutaneous emphysema in a cat due to barotrauma after equipment failure during anesthesia. *J Am Vet Med Assoc*, 212, 30–32.

Foëx, P. and Smith, A.C. (1977) A test for co-axial circuits. *Anaesthesia*, 32, 365–367.

Furst, B. and Laffey, D.A. (1984) An alternative test for the lack system. *Anaesthesia*, 39, 834.

Gale, E., Ticehurst, K.E. and Zaki, S. (2015) An evaluation of fresh gas flow rates for spontaneously breathing cats and small dogs on the Humphrey ADE semi-closed breathing system. *Vet Anaesth Analg*, 42, 292–298.

Ghai, B., Makkar, J.K. and Bhatia, A. (2006) Hypercarbia and arrhythmias resulting from faulty Bain circuit: a report of two cases. *Anesth Analg*, 102, 1903–1904.

Ghani, G.A. (1984) Safety check for the Bain circuit. *Can Anaesth Soc J*, 31, 487–488.

Gooch, C. and Peutrell, J. (2004) A faulty Bain circuit. *Anaesthesia*, 59, 618.

Gravenstein, N., Lampotang, S. and Beneken, J.E. (1985) Factors influencing capnography in the Bain circuit. *J Clin Monit*, 1, 6–10.

Hannallah, R. and Rosales, J.K. (1974) A hazard connected with re-use of the Bain's circuit: a case report. *Can Anaesth Soc J*, 21, 511–513.

Harrison, G.A. (1964) The effect of the respiratory flow pattern on rebreathing in a T-piece system. *Br J Anaesth*, 36, 206–211.

Hartsfield, S.M. and Sawyer, D.C. (1976) Cardiopulmonary effects of rebreathing and non-rebreathing systems during halothane anesthesia in cats. *Am J Vet Res*, 37, 1461–1466.

Hatch, D.J., Yates, A.P. and Lindahl, S.G. (1987) Flow requirements and rebreathing during mechanically controlled ventilation in a T-piece (Mapleson E) system. *Br J Anaesth*, 59, 1533–1540.

Heath, P.J. and Marks, L.F. (1991) Modified occlusion tests for the Bain breathing system. *Anaesthesia*, 46, 213–216.

Henville, J.D. and Adams, A.P. (1976) The Bain anaesthetic system. An assessment during controlled ventilation. *Anaesthesia*, 31, 247–256.

Holden, D.J. (2000) Clinical evaluation of a valveless non-absorber breathing system in spontaneously breathing canine patients. *J Small Anim Pract*, 41, 198–201.

Humphrey, D. (1982) The Lack, Magill and Bain anaesthetic breathing systems: a direct comparison in spontaneously-breathing anaesthetized adults. *J R Soc Med*, 75, 513–524.

Humphrey, D. (1983) A new anaesthetic breathing system combining Mapleson A, D and E principles. A simple apparatus for low flow universal use without carbon dioxide absorption. *Anaesthesia*, 38, 361–372.

Humphrey, D., Brock-Utne, J.G. and Downing, J.W. (1986a) Single lever Humphrey A.D.E. low flow universal anaesthetic breathing system. Part I: Comparison with dual lever A.D.E., Magill and Bain systems in anaesthetized spontaneously breathing adults. *Can Anaesth Soc J*, 33, 698–709.

Humphrey, D., Brock-Utne, J.G. and Downing, J.W. (1986b) Single lever Humphrey A.D.E. low flow universal anaesthetic breathing system. Part II: Comparison with Bain system in anaesthesized adults during controlled ventilation. *Can Anaesth Soc J*, 33, 710–718.

Jackson, F.J. (1988) Tests for co-axial systems. *Anaesthesia*, 43, 1060–1061.

Jones, P.L. 1991. Hazard – single-use parallel lack breathing system. *Anaesthesia*, 46, 316–317.

Jonsson, L.O., Johansson, S.L. and Zetterstrom, H. (1987) Rebreathing and ventilatory response to different fresh gas flows in the Bain and Lack systems. A clinical study. *Acta Anaesthesiol Scand*, 31, 179–186.

Jonsson, L.O. and Zetterstrom, H. (1986) Fresh gas flow in coaxial Mapleson A and D circuits during spontaneous breathing. *Acta Anaesthesiol Scand*, 30, 588–593.

Kain, M.L. and Nunn, J.F. (1968) Fresh gas economics of the Magill circuit. *Anesthesiology*, 29, 964–974.

Kay, B., Beatty, P.C., Healy, T.E., Accoush, M.E. and Calpin, M. (1983) Change in the work of breathing imposed by five anaesthetic breathing systems. *Br J Anaesth*, 55, 1239–1247.

Lack, J.A. (1976) Theatre pollution control. *Anaesthesia*, 31, 259–262.

Langton, S., Flaherty, D., Pawson, P. and Auckburally, A. (2010) A serious breathing system fault identified by capnography. *Vet Anaesth Analg*, 37, 581–582.

Lerche, P., Muir, W.W. 3rd and Bednarski, R.M. (2000) Non-rebreathing anesthetic systems in small animal practice. *J Am Vet Med Assoc*, 217, 493–497.

Lewis, A. and Spoerel, W.E. (1961) A modification of Ayre's technique. *Can Anaesth Soc J*, 8, 501–511.

Lindahl, S.G., Charlton, A.J. and Hatch, D.J. (1984) Accuracy of prediction of fresh gas flow requirements during spontaneous breathing with the T-piece. *Eur J Anaesthesiol*, 1, 269–274.

Manley, S.V. and McDonell, W.N. (1979a) Clinical evaluation of the bain breathing circuit in small animal anesthesia. *J Am Anim Hosp Assoc*, 15, 67–72.

Manley, S.V. and McDonell, W.N. (1979b) A new circuit for small animal anesthesia: the Bain coaxial circuit. *J Am Anim Hosp Assoc*, 15, 61–65.

Mapleson, W.W. (1954) The elimination of rebreathing in various semi-closed anaesthetic systems. *Br J Anaesth*, 26, 323–332.

Mapleson, W.W. (2004) Editorial I: Fifty years after – Reflections on "The elimination of rebreathing in various semi-closed anaesthetic systems". *Br J Anaesth*, 93, 319–321.

Martin, L.V.H. and McKeown, D.W. (1985) An alternative test for the Lack system. *Anaesthesia*, 40, 80–81.

Meakin, G. and Coates, A.L. (1983) An evaluation of rebreathing with the Bain system during anaesthesia with spontaneous ventilation. *Br J Anaesth*, 55, 487–496.

Miller, D.M. (1979) A new universal anaesthetic circuit using a preferential-flow T-piece. *S Afr Med J*, 55, 721–725.

Miller, D.M. (1988) Breathing systems for use in anaesthesia. Evaluation using a physical lung model and classification. *Br J Anaesth*, 60, 555–564.

Miller, D.M. (1990) Early detection of "rebreathing" in afferent and efferent reservoir breathing systems using capnography. *Br J Anaesth*, 64, 251–255.

Moseley, C.A. (2015) Anaesthesia equipment. In: Grimm, K.A., Lamont, L.A., Tranquilli, W.J., Greene, S.A. and Robertson, S.A. (eds). *Veterinary Anaesthesia and Analgesia, The Fifth Edition of Lumb and Jones.* Ames, IA: John Wiley & Sons Inc., pp. 23–85.

Nott, M.R., Walters, F.J. and Norman, J. (1982) The Lack and Bain systems in spontaneous respiration. *Anaesth Intensive Care*, 10, 333–339.

Ooi, R., Lack, J.A., Soni, N., Whittle, J. and Pattison, J. (1993a) The parallel Lack anaesthetic breathing system. *Anaesthesia*, 48, 409–414.

Ooi, R., Pattison, J. and Soni, N. (1993b) The additional work of breathing imposed by Mapleson A systems. *Anaesthesia*, 48, 599–603.

Peterson, W.C. (1978) Letter to the editor – Bain Circuit. *Can Anaesth Soc J*, 25, 532.

Pethick, S.L. (1975) Letters to the editor. *Can Anaesth Soc J*, 22, 115.

Picton, P. and Crosse, M.M. (1998) A serious breathing system fault. *Anaesthesia*, 53, 1229–1231.

Prosser, D.P. (1997) The "hourglass" reservoir bag. A closed scavenging system for the Jackson Rees modification of Ayre's "T"-piece. *Paediatr Anaesth*, 7, 177.

Rasch, D.K., Bunegin, L.L., Ledbetter, J. and Kaminskas, D. (1988) Comparison of circle absorber and Jackson-Rees systems for paediatric anaesthesia. *Can J Anaesth*, 35, 25–30.

Rees, G.J. (1950) Anaesthesia in the newborn. *Br Med J*, 2, 1419–1422.

Rose, D.K., Byrick, R.J. and Froese, A.B. (1978) Carbon dioxide elimination during spontaneous ventilation with a modified Mapleson D system: studies in a lung model. *Can Anaesth Soc J*, 25, 353–365.

Rose, D.K. and Froese, A.B. (1979) The regulation of $PaCO_2$ during controlled ventilation of children with a T-piece. *Can Anaesth Soc J*, 26, 104–113.

Sasse, F.J. (1985) Can we trust end-tidal carbon dioxide measurements in infants? *J Clin Monit*, 1, 147–148.

Schieber, R.A., Namnoum, A., Sugden, A., Saville, A.L. and Orr, R.A. (1985) Accuracy of expiratory carbon dioxide measurements using the coaxial and circle breathing circuits in small subjects. *J Clin Monit*, 1, 149–155.

Sellers, W.F. and Dykes, S. (2003) Don't pre-oxygenate with a 3-metre Bain circuit. *Anaesthesia*, 58, 916.

Singh, I., Gupta, M. and Singh, T.K. (2011) Hypercapnia resulting from a faulty co-axial (Bain) circuit. *Indian J Anaesth*, 55, 402–404.

Sweeting, C.J., Thomas, P.W. and Sanders, D.J. (2002) The long Bain breathing system: an investigation into the implications of remote ventilation. *Anaesthesia*, 57, 1183–1186.

Sykes, M.K. (1959) Rebreathing during controlled respiration with the Magill attachment. *Br J Anaesth*, 31, 247–257.

Sykes, M.K. (1968) Rebreathing circuits. *Br J Anaesth*, 40, 666–674.

Walsh, C.M. and Taylor, P.M. (2004) A clinical evaluation of the "mini parallel Lack" breathing system in cats and comparison with a modified Ayre's T-piece. *Vet Anaesth Analg*, 31, 207–212.

Waterman, A.E. (1986) Clinical evaluation of the Lack coaxial breathing circuit in small animal anesthesia. *J Sm Anim Pract*, 27, 591–598.

Waters, D.J. and Mapleson, W.W. (1961) Rebreathing during controlled respiration with various semi-closed anesthetic systems. *Br J Anaesth*, 33, 374–381.

Willis, B.A., Pender, J.W. and Mapleson, W.W. (1975) Rebreathing in a T-piece: volunteer and theoretical studies of the Jackson-Rees modification of Ayre's T-piece during spontaneous respiration. *Br J Anaesth*, 47, 1239–1246.

12

The Circle System

Geoffrey Truchetti[1] and Trish Anne Farry[2]

[1] *Centre Vétérinaire Rive Sud, Brossard, QC, Canada and Centre Vétérinaire Laval, Laval, QC, Canada*
[2] *The University of Queensland, Gatton, Queensland, Australia*

12.1 Introduction

Classification of breathing systems is complex and multiple classifications have been devised over time. However, none is truly faultless. The circle system is the most commonly used rebreathing system. Descriptions of other rebreathing systems, such as the Waters to-and-fro, can be found in other veterinary textbooks (Hartsfield 2007) and chapters within this book. Gas flow through a circle system is unidirectional and follows a circular pathway, hence the name of the system. As with any breathing system, a circle system can direct oxygen to the patient, allow inhalant anesthetic agent delivery, facilitate removal of CO_2 from exhaled gases, and can be used as a means to control ventilation.

12.2 Components

Although the components vary slightly between machines, most fundamental pieces can be found in every circle system. Some of these components have previously been discussed in Chapter 10; however, they will be expanded upon in this chapter.

12.2.1 Carbon Dioxide (CO_2) Absorber

The carbon dioxide (CO_2) absorber may be attached or can be separate from the anesthetic machine. The components that make up the absorber assembly are ports for connection to the breathing system and reservoir bag, a fresh gas inlet, inspiratory and expiratory valves and an adjustable pressure limiting (APL) valve.

12.2.1.1 Canister

The CO_2 absorbent is contained in a single or double canister system. The canister sides are usually clear so that color changes of the absorbent can be monitored.

Canisters vary in size or capacity. Larger canisters may require fewer changes in absorbent, but this will also increase the internal volume of the breathing system, which will increase the time necessary for changes in gas concentration (see time-constant below). Conversely, a smaller canister may need to be changed more frequently, but the decreased internal volume will allow more rapid changes in the concentration delivered.

12.2.1.2 Housing

The canister housing adds space for incoming gases to disperse before passing through the absorbent, and outgoing gases to collect before passing through the system. In addition, this space in the housing also allows dust from the absorbent and moisture to accumulate.

12.2.1.3 Baffles

Baffles are rings that direct the gas flow preferentially through the middle of the absorber canister to compensate for increased resistance to flow. This allows for a more homogenous flow through the canister.

12.2.1.4 Side or Center Tube

From the canister, gas flows back to the patient through a side or a center tube (Figure 12.1). When on the side, the reservoir bag can be connected to that tube.

12.2.1.5 Bypass

Canister housing may incorporate a switch that will bypass the canister to facilitate changing of the absorbent canister when the machine is in use (Figure 12.2).

12.2.1.6 Absorbents

The absorbent is contained in the absorber canister. The general principle of CO_2 absorption is a base neutralizing an acid. The products of the chemical reactions are carbonate, water and heat. Absorbents are available in pellets

Veterinary Anesthetic and Monitoring Equipment, First Edition. Edited by Kristen G. Cooley and Rebecca A. Johnson.
© 2018 John Wiley & Sons, Inc. Published 2018 by John Wiley & Sons, Inc.

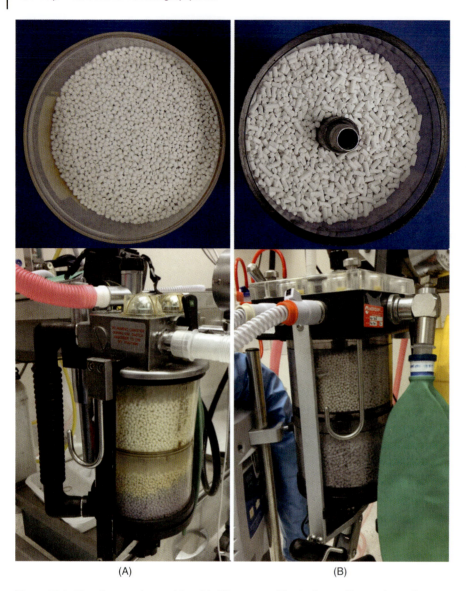

(A)   (B)

Figure 12.1 Absorbent canisters with a side (A) or center (B) tube for gas flow to the patient.

or granules. The most common size of granules is 4–8 mesh (0.125–0.25 inch diameter). Smaller granules will provide a greater surface area but will also increase the resistance to flow through the absorber. In addition to the composition of each of the absorbents, most granules also contain small amounts of silica and other agents for hardening and reduction of dust. One of the most common absorbents used is soda lime (Parthasarathy 2013). Two other types are Baralyme and Amsorb (see Chapter 10). Different compositions of absorbents will have varying absorptive capacity. The absorption rate will depend on the chemical composition of the granules, the size of the patient (the larger the patient the greater the CO_2 production), and the fresh gas flow rate. Chemical reactions occurring during neutralization of CO_2 are discussed in Chapter 10 and are illustrated in Table 12.1.

Exhausted or desiccated absorbent must be changed. Absorbents are supplied in re-sealable containers or single-use, pre-filled, canisters. Once a container is opened, it should be resealed as promptly as possible to prevent moisture loss, indicator deactivation, and reactions to CO_2 in the atmosphere. Each absorbent should be stored as per manufacturer's recommendations. When refilling a multi-use absorbent canister, personnel should be aware that absorbent dust can be irritating to the eyes and respiratory tract, and that absorbents may be caustic to the skin. Appropriate personal protective equipment should be worn. Tap gently on the side of the canister while filling it, to ensure homogenous packing of the granules to avoid a channeling effect (see below). The absorbent canister should be filled leaving a small space at the top to promote even gas flow through the canister.

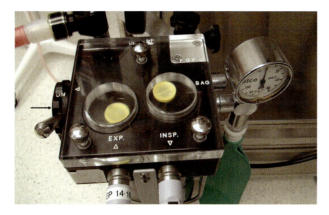

Figure 12.2 Absorbent canister with a bypass switch (arrow) to facilitate changing of absorbent when the system is in use.

If a pre-filled disposable canister is being used, the outer wrapping must be removed to ensure that gas can flow once fitted to the absorbent housing. The absorber canister should be roughly twice the tidal volume of the patient, even though there is scant evidence to support this statement (Mosley 2015).

12.2.1.7   Reactions Between Absorbents and Anesthetic Agents

Absorbent can also react with inhalant agents. Sevoflurane can be degraded into Compound A, which has the potential to be nephrotoxic (Gonsowski *et al.* 1994). Factors influencing Compound A generation include low fresh gas flow, use of Baralyme instead of soda lime, high concentrations of sevoflurane, high absorbent temperature and dry absorbent (Lerche *et al.* 2000). Evidence of Compound A toxicity in veterinary medicine is lacking. For example, the concentration of Compound A obtained in the system during low-flow anesthesia in dogs was below the nephrotoxic dose (Muir

and Gadawski 1998). Therefore, the significance of Compound A seems to be of little concern in veterinary medicine (Mosley 2015).

Carbon monoxide (CO) can also be generated when inhalant agents pass through the absorbent. Potentially harmful concentrations can be obtained, even though clinical reports of CO intoxication are lacking in veterinary medicine. Factors influencing CO production include dry absorbent, barium hydroxide lime (Baralyme), high temperature, high anesthetic concentration, and increased anesthesia duration (Lerche *et al.* 2000). Magnitude of CO production is influenced by the inhalant used. For example, inhalants likely to produce CO are desflurane > enflurane > isoflurane > halothane = sevoflurane (Coppens *et al.* 2006). Therefore, as dryness of the absorbent is a factor for both Compound A and CO production, guidelines should be followed to prevent incidents (Coppens *et al.* 2006). Gas flow should be turned off after each anesthesia, especially at the end of the day. Absorbent should be changed routinely, even more if the machine is not used frequently. The absorbent should be changed if a fresh gas flow is maintained over a prolonged period, independent of whether a patient is connected to the breathing system and of the absorber exhaustion state. Interestingly, during low-flow anesthesia, CO may accumulate, but moisture will be kept within the system, which should decrease the incidence of CO production.

12.2.1.8   Absorbent Exhaustion Measurement

Measuring Inspired CO₂   Measuring inspired CO_2 with a capnometer or capnograph is the most reliable method to detect absorbent exhaustion. During inspiration, the patient rebreathes CO_2 and the curve does not return to zero during inspiration. The shape of the tracing is normal, and the end-tidal CO_2 value may be increased if the patient cannot compensate for the inspired CO_2 (Figure 12.3).

Table 12.1 Composition, absorptive reactions and capacity of different absorbent (Mosley 2015).

Absorbent	Composition	Absorptive reactions	Absorptive capacity/100 g
Soda lime	80% calcium hydroxide 15% water 4% sodium hydroxide	$CO_2+H_2O \leftrightarrow H_2CO_3$ $H_2CO_3 +2\,NaOH(KOH) \rightarrow NaCO_3(K_2CO_3)$ $+2\,H_2O+heat$ $NaCO_3(K_2CO_3)+Ca(OH)_2 \rightarrow CaCO_3+2\,NaOH(KOH)$	25 L CO_2
Baralyme (barium lime)	80% calcium hydroxide 20% barium hydroxide	$Ba(OH)_2+8\,H_2O+CO_2 \rightarrow BaCO_3+9\,H_2O+heat$ $9\,H_2O+9\,CO_2 \leftrightarrow 9\,H_2CO_3$ $9\,H_2CO_3+9\,Ca(OH)_2 \rightarrow 9\,CaCO_3 + 18\,H_2O + heat$	27 L CO_2
Amsorb (calcium hydroxide lime)	80% calcium hydroxide 15% water 1% calcium sulphate 3% calcium chloride	$CO_2+H_2O \leftrightarrow H_2CO_3$ $H_2CO_3+Ca(OH)_2 \rightarrow CaCO_3 + 2\,H_2 0 + heat$	~15 L CO_2

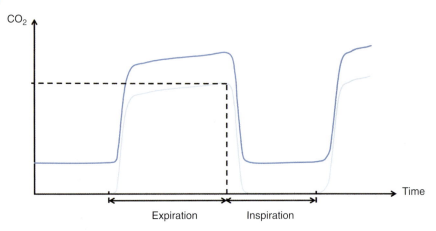

CO_2

Expiration   Inspiration   Time

Figure 12.3 Typical capnogram obtained when soda lime is exhausted (blue trace), compared to a normal waveform (grey trace). During inspiration, the curve does not return to 0 mmHg, and the shape of the waveform is normal. End-tidal CO_2 value is increased in this example.

Indicator Color Change When CO_2 reacts with the absorbent, heat and water are formed and pH changes. The latter causes the indicator contained in the absorbent to change color, indicating that the absorbent is near the point of exhaustion. Two common indicators are phenolphthalein and ethyl violet, which change the absorbent color to pink and purple, respectively.

Absorbent should be replaced when two-thirds of the canister has changed color (Mosley 2015). The color may revert to its pre-exhaustion color when not in use. Upon subsequent use, the indicator color will rapidly return to its exhausted state. Therefore, a rested canister can give a false sense of security. For this reason, inspection of the absorbent color should be made during, or just after, anesthesia.

Additionally, if the absorbent is not packed properly in the canister, channeling can occur; the gas flow passes through a channel in the absorbent, exposing only a small part of the absorbent to CO_2. As absorbent along

the channel becomes exhausted quickly, the patient rebreathes CO_2. The rest of the absorbent remains white, delaying the identification of a potentially harmful event if only relying on absorbent color changes (Figure 12.4). Therefore, indicator color change is useful, but is not always reliable.

Alternative Signs As stated above, during CO_2 absorption, heat and water are formed. Therefore, during anesthesia, the canister should be slightly warm to the touch and water droplets should be visible on its wall. The amount of heat and water vapor is proportional to the amount of absorbed CO_2. If a high oxygen flow is used (100–200 mL/kg/min), CO_2 is not completely eliminated from the system by the absorbent; in this situation, the canister could remain cold. However, if the canister remains cold with an appropriate oxygen flow (~20 mL/kg/min), it is imperative to check for other signs of absorbent exhaustion.

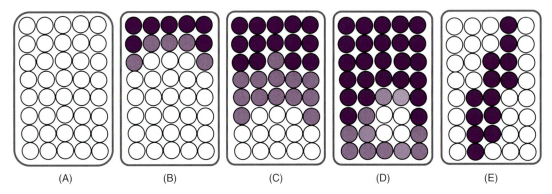

(A)   (B)   (C)   (D)   (E)

Figure 12.4 Pattern of CO_2 absorption in the canister. Purple circles represent exhausted soda lime; white circles represent fresh soda lime. (A) Unused canister, or appearance of the canister after some time unused; all granules are white. (B) After limited use; absorption of CO_2 has occurred primarily at the inlet and to a lesser extent along the sides. (C) After extensive use; the canister appears nearly completely purple as granules on the side are exhausted. (D) Exhausted soda lime; CO_2 is filtering through the canister and the only granules that are still capable of absorbing CO_2 are in the distal third. (E) A channeling effect as gas passes through the soda lime preferentially through a channel; absorbent in this channel is quickly exhausted, and the patient breathes CO_2, even though the canister remains white if the channel is not along the wall.

When a patient inspires CO_2, clinical signs may include increased respiratory rate, increased amplitude of respiratory movement, increased sympathetic tone (increased heart rate and blood pressure), vasodilation and red mucous membranes. A blood gas analysis may reveal a respiratory acidosis. Without a capnometer, if those clinical signs are present, it is important to consider absorbent exhaustion in the list of differential diagnoses.

Physical properties of the granules can also be used as an indicator. Granules should fragment easily. If not, this suggests that the absorbent may be exhausted. This is easily assessed when changing absorbent; if the hardness of the absorbent is different than usual, it may suggest it is already exhausted.

Without a capnometer, even if the color of the absorbent does not change, it is recommended to change the absorbent after a given amount of time. For a standard anesthesia machine, some manufacturers recommend changing the absorbent after 14 hours of use. However, the absorbent may be exhausted more rapidly than in 14 hours. In addition, if dust is in the canister, or if the canister is cracked or not completely filled, the absorbent should be changed. Finally, it is best to change the absorbent before the patient actually inspires CO_2. Changing the absorbent during anesthesia requires changing the canister or the system, potentially exposing personnel to waste anesthetic gases, delaying the procedures and exposing the patient to anesthesia for a longer time.

12.2.2 Unidirectional Valves

The unidirectional valves may also be referred to as flutter, non-return, one-way, dome, or inspiratory and expiratory valves. These valves are integral in a circle system to ensure that one arm of the circle conducts gas to the patient (inspiratory), and the other takes expired gas away from the patient (expiratory). The identification of each valve is usually marked with the word "inspiration" or "expiration" or by a directional arrow (Figure 12.5). The aim is to prevent the mixing of inspired and expired gases, preventing rebreathing. These valves may be contained as part of the absorbent canister or located as part of the structure of the breathing system. The valves are mounted under transparent domes so they can be observed during use. Most commonly, they are positioned horizontally, but may also be seated vertically (Figure 12.5). The valves are commonly flat discs that have a cage or retainer above to prevent the discs from becoming displaced. Valves may also be constructed of deformable rubber (Figure 12.5). The pressure generated by the patient's ventilation causes the valve to rise and allows gas to pass in one direction only.

Malfunction of the unidirectional valves may result in hypercapnia due to rebreathing of expired gases, ventilation failure or barotrauma. The result of valve failure will depend on the source of the valve failure (inspiratory or expiratory). For example, failure in the closed position

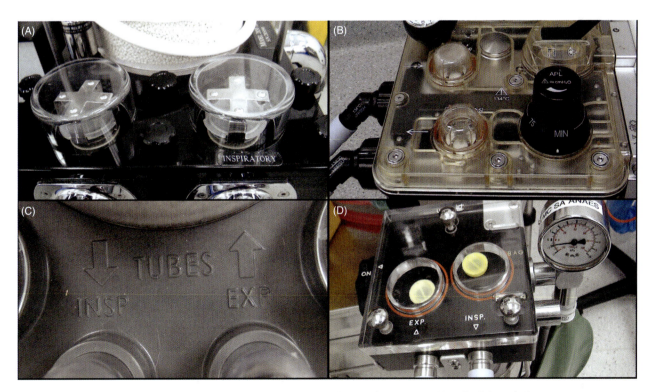

Figure 12.5 Identification of inspiratory and expiratory valves with either words (A), arrows (B), or both (C and D).

will not allow the patient to exhale or inhale. Failure in the open position will result in rebreathing of CO_2. If the inspiratory valve stays open, exhaled CO_2 will enter the CO_2-free inspiratory limb of the breathing system which, in turn, will be rebreathed by the patient during inspiration (Lee *et al.* 2013). If the expiratory valve stays in the open position, exhaled CO_2 in the expiratory limb of the breathing system will be rebreathed during inspiration.

12.2.3 Inspiratory and Expiratory Ports

Inspiratory and expiratory ports are part of the absorber assembly. The breathing system is connected to these ports to provide gas flow to the patient. The inspiratory port is located in close proximity to the inspiratory unidirectional valve and the expiratory port close to the expiratory unidirectional valve. These ports usually have 22-mm male connecters.

12.2.4 Y-Piece

The Y-piece (sometimes referred to as the wye-piece) is the three-way adapter that connects the breathing tubes to the patient. The patient connection end is a 15-mm female connector allowing attachment of an endotracheal tube or supraglottic airway device, and a 22-mm outer diameter connector to allow attachment of some facemasks. Some Y-pieces swivel, which may be beneficial in patient positioning.

12.2.5 Fresh Gas Inlet

The fresh gas inlet is connected to the common gas outlet on the anesthetic machine. This connection may be via flexible tubing, which is visible to the operator, or on newer equipment it may be a direct connection that is not visible to the operator.

12.2.6 Adjustable Pressure-Limiting Valve (APL)

The Adjustable Pressure-Limiting (APL) valve may also be designated as a pop-off valve, spill valve, exhaust valve, scavenging valve, expiratory valve, pressure relief valve, venting port, relief valve, overspill valve, overflow valve, dump valve, blow-off valve, safety relief valve, excess valve, Heindebrink valve, adjustable pressure limiter, excess venting valve, excess gas valve, pressure release valve, or release valve. The function of the valve is to limit the maximum pressure in the breathing system and to release waste gases. It does not allow room air to enter the breathing system. The APL valve has an adjustment dial or knob that when turned will increase or decrease the outlet size to allow pressure control in the breathing system.

12.2.7 Pressure Gauge

Many anesthetic machines have an analog pressure gauge or manometer attached to the absorber assembly. It displays pressure changes in the breathing system. It is usually attached to the exhalation pathway and is commonly of the diaphragm type. Two diaphragms contained in the manometer respond to changes in pressure by moving outward or inward. This pressure is transmitted to a pointer on a calibrated display. The scale on the manometer scale is in units of cmH_2O and/or kPa. Newer anesthetic machines may have the capability to electronically monitor and digitally display breathing system pressures.

12.2.8 Breathing Tubing

Breathing tubing or limbs convey gases to and from the patient. Each limb connects to either the inspiratory or the expiratory port at one end and connects to the patient at the other end. They are constructed of rubber or plastic and are corrugated to allow for expansion and flexibility. Newer breathing tubing has a smooth internal bore as this creates less turbulence and resistance during respiration. Breathing tubing comes in various diameters and lengths to allow for different patient sizes and flexibility. Due to the unidirectional gas flow, the length of the tubing does not increase dead space or rebreathing. However, increasing length and diameter will increase the total volume and resistance of the system, as explained below.

An adaptation of the circle system with a tube within a tube is a coaxial breathing tube. Some circle systems have specific inspiratory and expiratory ports, and use specific breathing tubes (Figures 12.6B and C). A universal F circuit can be used on a standard circle system (Figure 12.6A). In a coaxial breathing tube, the inner tubing is usually the inspiratory limb and the outer tubing is the expiratory limb. Benefits of the coaxial tube include thermal efficiency (Mizrak *et al.* 2011) as the exhaled gases warm the inspired gases and it is less bulky than the standard circle system breathing tubes.

12.2.9 Reservoir Bag

The reservoir bag is usually made of rubber, plastic or latex and is an integral component of the circle system. The reservoir bag increases compliance of the system by acting as a reserve for inspiration and accommodates the gas flow during expiration. By doing so, it protects the patient from excessive pressure in the breathing system. The bag can also be used as a means to administer manual ventilation, a visual monitor for respiratory rate, and a very basic indication of tidal volume. An experienced

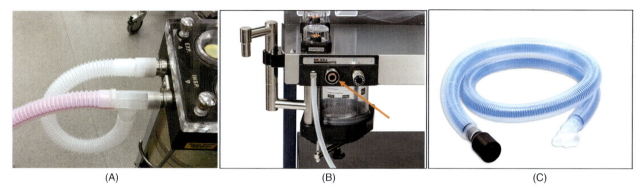

Figure 12.6 (A) Universal F-circuit. (B) Specific inspiratory and expiratory ports (arrow). (C) Coaxial tubing used for rebreathing system (photographs B and C courtesy of Dispomed, QC, Canada).

operator can also assess changes of pulmonary compliance during ventilation.

Reservoir bags are available in various sizes and the size of the bag chosen will be dependent on the breathing system and patient size. Recommendations in veterinary anesthesia are commonly 5–10 times the patient's tidal volume (10–20 mL/kg) or a volume similar to the patient's minute volume (Mosley 2015). Practically, using a bag size of 1 L per 10 kg is appropriate. A reservoir bag that is too small will not provide sufficient reserve for the patient to take an adequate breath, and may result in development of negative pressure during inspiration. An overly-large reservoir bag will impede adequate monitoring of movements of the bag. Additionally, the volume of the bag needs to be taken into account when calculating the time constant (see below) and may delay reaching equilibrium of anesthetic agent concentration in the system.

12.2.10 Bag/Ventilator Switch

Some circle systems may have a reservoir bag/ventilator selection switch (Figure 12.7). This allows the operator to switch between manual/spontaneous ventilation and automatic ventilation, without the need to remove the bag or attach the ventilator hose to the reservoir bag connector. In those circle systems, when the ventilator switch is in the "ventilator" position, the APL valve is isolated, which eliminates the need to close it when doing IPPV.

12.2.11 Optional Equipment

12.2.11.1 Positive End Expiratory Pressure (PEEP) Valves and Humidifiers

Positive end expiratory pressure (PEEP) valves, humidifiers and heat and moisture exchangers (HMEs) can be used in a circle system (Chapter 7). PEEP valves are usually connected between the expiratory limb and the expiratory unidirectional valve.

HME filters are usually placed between the endotracheal tube and the breathing system. They help conserve heat and moisture of inhaled gas during anesthesia and may also be the most efficient way to conserve both heat and moisture during pediatric anesthesia (Mizrak *et al.* 2011; Bicalho *et al.* 2014). For example, in human medicine, circle systems can be used with a low-flow technique to reach a humidity level of 20 mg H_2O/L (Henriksson *et al.* 1997; Yamashita *et al.* 2007; de Castro *et al.* 2011,). However, when using those systems for pediatric anesthesia, an HME was needed to reach appropriate humidity

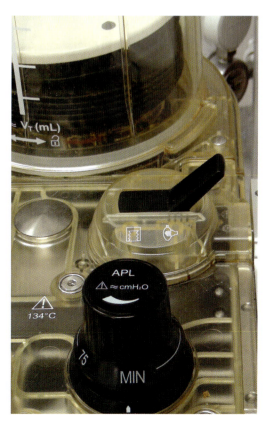

Figure 12.7 Reservoir bag/ventilator selection switch.

levels (Bicalho *et al.* 2014). In veterinary medicine, one study (Hofmeister *et al.* 2011) did not show HMEs to be useful in medium- to large-sized dogs undergoing orthopedic surgery. More studies are needed to assess the use of HME filters in veterinary patients.

12.2.12 Filters

Filters can be added to a breathing system to protect both the equipment and patients from cross contamination. Correct location of filters is detailed in Table 12.2.

12.3 Component Arrangement

There are many variations on the arrangement or sequence of components in the circle system. The fol-

lowing concerns should be kept in mind when determining the best arrangement of components in the circle system.

12.3.1 Desiccation of Absorbent

Absorbent desiccation has been identified as a source of carbon monoxide and by-product of inhalant degradation. Therefore, desiccation of absorbent should be minimized by limiting the amount of fresh gas going through the absorber. Desiccation can be limited by placing the fresh gas inlet tube downstream of the absorber.

12.3.2 Venting Only Expired Gas

Although gas flows through the breathing system in a circle, fresh gas flow may be vented through the APL valve

Table 12.2 Typical location and possible arrangement of the different components typically found in a circle system.

	Common location	Other locations
Fresh gas inlet	Upstream of inspiratory unidirectional valve and downstream of absorber.	1) Upstream of the absorber. 2) Downstream of the inspiratory unidirectional valve. 3) Upstream of the expiratory unidirectional valve. 4) Upstream of the reservoir bag and the APL valve.
Reservoir bag	Between the expiratory unidirectional valve and the absorber.	1) Between the patient and either inspiratory or expiratory unidirectional valves. 2) Upstream of the absorber.
Unidirectional valves	Attached to the absorber.	
APL	Downstream of the expiratory unidirectional valve (near the reservoir bag) and upstream of the absorber.	1) Between the fresh gas inlet and the patient. 2) Upstream of the expiratory unidirectional valve.
Filters	Between the Y-piece and the patient.	1) Between the inspiratory limb and the Y-piece. 2) Between the y-piece and the expiratory limb. 3) Between the inspiratory limb and the inspiratory unidirectional valve. 4) Between the expiratory limb and the expiratory unidirectional valve.
PEEP valves	Between the expiratory limb and the expiratory unidirectional valve (disposable).	1) Downstream of the expiratory unidirectional valve and upstream of the absorber (built in). 2) Between the ventilator and breathing system (bidirectional PEEP valve).
Pressure gauge	Same side of the unidirectional valves as the PEEP valves.	
Respirometer	In the expiratory limb on either side of the expiratory unidirectional valve.	1) Between the patient and the Y-piece.
Airway pressure sensor	Between the patient and the breathing system.	1) On the expiratory limb downstream from the APL valve and the expiratory unidirectional valve. 2) On the expiratory limb upstream from the APL valve.
Ventilator	Upstream of the absorber.	1) Upstream of the inspiratory unidirectional valve.

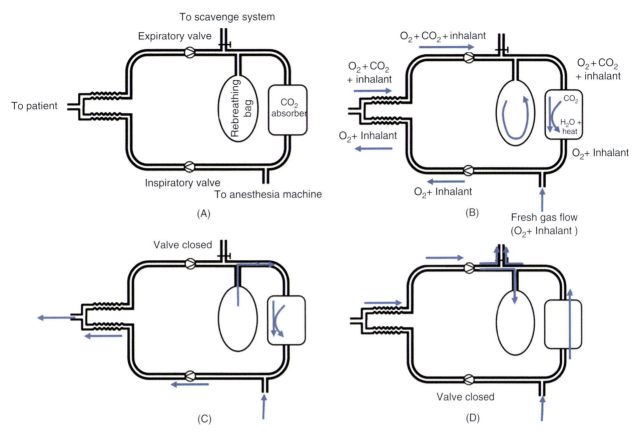

Figure 12.8 Diagram of circle system. (A) Arrangement of typical circle system. (B) Overall gas flow through the system (arrows). (C) Gas flow during inspiration. (D) Gas flow during expiration.

(Figure 12.8). Keeping the fresh gas flow within the circle while venting mainly expired gas will improve the rate at which the partial pressure of gas changes in the breathing system. This is more important at low flow rates.

12.3.3 Decreasing Absorbent Consumption

The APL valve position within the circle influences absorbent consumption. Preferably, any vented gas should not pass through the absorbent first. Additionally, to decrease absorbent consumption, much of the alveolar gas (late exhalation) should be vented through the APL valve, reducing dilution of the exhaled gas with fresh gas entering the circle. At low flows, as all exhaled gas passes through the absorbent, absorbent consumption cannot be decreased.

12.3.4 Maintaining Heat and Moisture

As exhaled gas goes through the absorbent, heat and moisture are produced during the chemical reaction.

Ensuring that the warmed humidified air is not subsequently vented is preferable. The position of the APL valve relative to the absorbent canister is important for this.

12.3.5 Reducing Mechanical Dead Space

Dead space and resistance can interfere with patient ventilation. Therefore, minimizing dead space with appropriately-sized connectors between the patient and the breathing system and decreasing resistance to flow during ventilation cycle are critical.

12.3.6 Ease of Use

Ease of use should always be considered. The size of the breathing system should be optimized for each patient, especially in situations where the breathing system needs to be moved from one location to another. Having the breathing system fixed to the same structure as the anesthetic machine simplifies their use. Finally, when in use, making sure that the breathing system does not pull on the endotracheal tube will prevent accidental disconnection or extubation.

The most common arrangement of components is classified as the classic circle system. Table 12.2 illustrates the common location and some variations of the arrangement of components in the circle system. In clinical situations, the arrangement of components may be altered on a case-by-case basis. For example, minimization of dead space for pediatric patients may be achieved by variations in the common location of components such as filters.

Systems have been developed for their ease of use in multiple species and to maximize efficiency. For example, the Humphrey ADE–Circle (Anaequip-Vet UK, Worthen, Shrewsbury) has been developed for use in human and veterinary patients. It is a compact system that is used in multiple species (reportedly 30 g–100 kg), with or without an absorber. A lever switches between spontaneous, manual and ventilator respiration modes. The reservoir bag on the inspiratory limb (rather the more common placement within the expiratory side), and a 4-phase exhaust valve, which stays closed at the beginning of expiration to automatically preserve the dead space gas or gas for recycling while eliminating only alveolar gas, enhances efficiency and saves fresh gas (rather than expired gas).

Even though not usually part of the breathing system, certain types of vaporizers can be used in-circuit. This technique is still in use in certain countries (Nicholson and Watson, 2001). Those vaporizers are detailed elsewhere in this book (see Chapter 5). Using a vaporizer-in-circuit necessitates the operator to have a thorough understanding of the underlying factors influencing vapor output.

12.4   Gas Flow

12.4.1   Gas Flow Direction

Gas flow through the most common configurations of the circle system is illustrated in Figure 12.8. During inspiration, the fresh gas flows from the fresh gas flow inlet, toward the inspiratory valve, and is mixed with gas from the reservoir bag. The relative amount of fresh gas and rebreathed gas determines the rate of change of inspired gas concentration in the system. The inspiratory valve opens and the expiratory valve is closed. The CO_2 is absorbed when the gas flows through the absorbent, in exchange for heat and water, as explained above.

During the inspiratory or expiratory pause, and whenever the fresh gas flow rate is higher than the inspired flow rate, the excess fresh gas flow passes through the inspiratory valve, to the expiratory valve via the Y-piece, then to the scavenging system and the reservoir bag. The excess fresh gas can also flow backward through the absorbent to the scavenging system and the reservoir bag.

During expiration, the expired gas flows through the expiratory valve to the scavenging system and the reservoir bag. The inspiratory valve closes and prevents backward flow from the patient to the inspiratory limb. The fresh gas cannot flow toward the patient, as the expiration increases pressure and resistance. Instead, the fresh gas flows backward through the absorbent, to the scavenging system or the reservoir bag.

12.4.2   Fresh Gas Flow Rate

As CO_2 is removed from the circle system by the absorbent, rebreathing of gas is possible in a circle system. Therefore, fresh gas flow is typically lower than in non-rebreathing systems, in which high flows are required to rid the system of CO_2. The role of the fresh gas flow in a circle system is to deliver enough O_2 to the system to compensate for the O_2 consumption of the patient, supply enough inhalant anesthetic agent to keep an adequate plane of anesthesia, and compensate for any loss caused by an overly active scavenging system.

Oxygen consumption is approximately 3–10 mL/kg/min (Lerche *et al.* 2000). This is dependent on the patient's metabolic rate, which is based on the body surface area, the species and the activity (Brody 1945). At such low flow rates, the volume of fresh gas is small compared to the volume of the system. The mixing of fresh gas and rebreathed gas will result in the dilution of components in each gas. At low fresh gas flow rates, heat and moisture will be preserved. However, any changes of inhalant concentration will be slow.

The time constant of the system is calculated as the total volume divided by the flow rate (Figure 12.9). It represents the time required for the concentration to change to 63% of the new concentration (Lerche *et al.* 2000; Davis and Kenny 2003b). To reach 98% of the new concentration, it requires approximately 4–5 time constants. A 20-kg dog may only need a 5 mL/kg/min oxygen flow rate to provide for its metabolic needs (total of 0.1 L/min). With a 1 L reservoir bag, the total volume of all of the system components approaches approximately 5 L. Therefore, in this example, the time constant is 5 L × 1 min/0.1 L = 50 minutes. It would take 50 minutes to reach 63% of the new concentration, and approximately 200 minutes (4 × 50 min) to reach 98% of the new concentration. These calculations do not take into account the uptake of inhalant by the patient, which may increase the time to reach the new concentration. Therefore, using low flow rates may be unsuitable, especially when a change of anesthesia planes is urgently required.

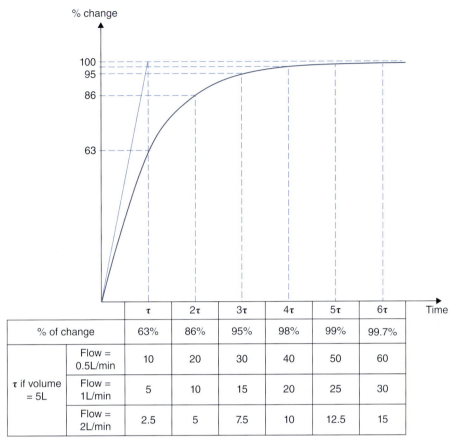

Figure 12.9 Illustration of time constants (time at which the process would have been completed had the initial rate of change continued). A time constant is often designated as tau. The straight line (A) represents how the concentration would have changed had the initial rate of change continued. The curve (B) is how concentrations change in the circuit. The table illustrates tau and multiples of tau for a 5-L circuit at different fresh gas flow rate.

To overcome difficulties encountered when using low flow rates, flow rates above the metabolic oxygen consumption are commonly used, typically between 20 and 100 mL/kg/min (Lerche *et al.* 2000; Mosley 2015). Flow rates above O_2 requirements can be provided as an inert gas. For example, medical grade air is often used, and the total O_2 flow is calculated to match at least the O_2 requirement, making sure to avoid hypoxemia. The higher the flow rate, the lower the amount of rebreathing. The rebreathing system classification is usually based on flow rates and/or degree of rebreathing (Table 12.3). Higher flow rates are appropriate during periods of anesthesia when rapid depth change is required, such as induction, recovery or complications. After the induction, or when changing anesthesia systems, it is necessary to use higher flow rates to remove the nitrogen (N_2) present in the breathing system and to reach an appropriately elevated inspired fraction of O_2 (F_iO_2). Once anesthesia depth is stable and removal of N_2 from the system is completed, fresh gas flow rates can be lowered.

12.4.3 Relationship Between Inspired and Delivered Concentrations

At the beginning of anesthesia, anesthetic agent concentration needs to rapidly increase to reach effective concentrations before the injectable induction agent is redistributed out of the brain. Additionally, N_2 is present in the breathing system and the lungs, and needs be removed until an appropriate F_iO_2 is reached (denitrogenation process). Calculating the time-constant helps determine how long it will take to reach equilibrium. Other factors will affect the anesthetic agent concentration, such as uptake by the patient and the breathing system components, uptake and elimination of other gases by the patient, and degradation by the absorbent.

At the end of anesthesia, once the vaporizer is turned off, inhalant agents are eliminated in the exhaled gas, and none is provided in the fresh gas flow. The patient becomes the source of inhalant for the breathing system. If the oxygen flow rate is high enough, inhalant will be removed from the system more rapidly. Therefore,

Table 12.3 Classification of flow rates used in circle system. Definition of low/intermediate/high flow not universally accepted (Mosley 2015).

	Fresh gas flow rates	% of rebreathing	Pop-off valve	Advantages/Disadvantages
Low-flow	3–10 mL/kg/min (O_2 requirement)	Full	Can be closed	+ Economical, heat and moisture preserved, reduce atmospheric pollution - Technically more challenging, slow changes of inhalant concentration
Intermediate-flow	20–50 mL/kg/min	Partial	Open	+ Intermediate easy to perform, preserve some heat and moisture, quite economical - Rate of change still slow if rapid changes needed
High-flow	100–200 mL/kg/min	Minimal	Open	+ Easier to perform, rapid changes of depth - Economical, no preservation of heat and moisture

when changes of depth of anesthesia are needed, increasing fresh gas flow will help reach equilibrium faster.

12.5 Resistance and Work of Breathing in the Circle System

Resistance to flow of a gas in the breathing system can be described using the Poiseuille-Hagen law: $R = 8\eta l/\pi r^4$ (Tamul and Ault 2013), where resistance (R) is proportional to the viscosity (η) and length (l), and inversely proportional to the radius (r) to the power of 4. Therefore, the resistance in a circle system will be higher when using longer tubing, and in any part where the diameter is small.

This equation is only valid when the flow is laminar, which is not always the case in a breathing system. Changes in direction of the flow (valves, elbows, kinks in tubing, etc.) or flow through an absorber, will result in turbulent flow, which will increase resistance. Higher flow rates, such as during inspiration and expiration, can also cause turbulent flow (Davis and Kenny 2003a). Resistance to flow is generally not an issue when using systems as per manufacturer's recommendations. Very small patients (cats weighting between 2.5 and 4.3 kg) have been anaesthetized using rebreathing systems without apparent issues (Hartsfield and Sawyer 1976). However, small resistances can be enough to interfere with patient respiratory mechanics (Davis and Kenny 2003a).

Pediatric and adult systems differ by the diameter of the tubing. Pediatric tubing has a smaller diameter and should therefore have a higher resistance. However, when used on a patient of an appropriate size (usually <7 kg – Dunlop 1992), resistance to flow is not an issue, even during peak flow, and the smaller volume is preferable. Some pediatric tubing also has less dead space. Work of breathing is the work required to overcome resistance to flow. Even if typical breathing systems have

low resistance, the work of breathing increases by around 27% when using a typical breathing system (Davis and Kenny 2003a).

Generally, non-rebreathing systems are considered as having lower resistance, but this may not be true as previously reported (Rasch *et al.* 1988; Conterato *et al.* 1989). Resistance in the breathing system is likely to change from one manufacturer to another. It is therefore advisable to use breathing systems as per manufacturer's recommendations, and to closely monitor the patient for signs of respiratory fatigue or pulmonary edema.

12.6 Dead Space

Definition of apparatus dead space (or mechanical dead space) differs among authors. It is either defined as:

1) the volume of breathing system occupied by gases that is rebreathed without any change in their composition (Hughes 2016); or
2) the volume that extends from the patient port to the partition between the inspiratory and exhalation tubing (Dorsch and Dorsch 2008).

A Y-piece with a septum decreases dead space in definition (2). Both definitions have limitations. In a rebreathing system, even if the absorbent does not neutralize CO_2, there are changes in composition due to dilution by fresh gas flow, which can be significant at high fresh gas flow rates. Such an event is not taken into consideration in definition (1). Additionally, a malfunction of the system, such as dysfunctional unidirectional valves, may cause rebreathing and increased dead space (Dorsch and Dorsch 2008). Such an event is not taken into consideration in definition (2).

Therefore, apparatus dead space associated with the breathing system should likely be defined as the volume of gas that is rebreathed without changes in composition.

Dilution by fresh gas flow can then be considered as adding a volume of fresh gas to a volume of rebreathed gas. That volume of rebreathed gas is dead space if no changes of composition occur. Additionally, backlash is defined as a backwards flow of gas in the tubing until the unidirectional valves close. The increased dead space is insignificant if the unidirectional valves are competent (Dorsch and Dorsch 2008).

12.7 Heat and Moisture

The optimal airway humidity level is approximately 20–30 g H_2O/L (Wilkes 2011), which may be difficult to achieve during inhalant anesthesia. Administration of dry, cold, fresh gas can be deleterious to the patient. Dysfunction caused by dehydration of airways is important (Wilkes 2011), and includes thickening of mucus, slowing of mucociliary transport, cellular damage, decreased compliance and functional residual capacity, and can cause the formation of atelectasis.

Breathing cold, dry gas may also contribute to the development of hypothermia peri-operatively (Johansson *et al.* 2003). As mentioned, in dogs, the use of an HME filter did not decrease heat loss (Hofmeister *et al.* 2011), and in cats, the choice of the breathing system had no impact on the development of hypothermia during anesthesia (Kelly *et al.* 2012). Heat and moisture are produced during the neutralization of CO_2 by the absorbent. The patient also exhales moist and warmed gas. However, the fresh gas delivered by the anesthetic machine is cold and dry. Therefore, the humidity in the system will be influenced by the relative amount of cold, dry, fresh gas flow and the rebreathed, warm, moist gas. In addition, arrangement of the breathing system components will interfere with the capacity of the breathing system to retain heat and moisture. Co-axial tubing may maintain heat and moisture better than normal tubing (Mizrak *et al.* 2011).

12.8 Maintenance

12.8.1 Routine Maintenance

All personnel using the equipment have the responsibility to ensure that it is in working order each time a patient is connected to a breathing system. Maintenance of the circle absorber is of the highest importance for patient safety. As described previously in this chapter, the circle absorber is made up of many components. Each of these components has the ability to compromise patient safety due to malfunction or damage. Testing the system, as described below and in Chapter 27, will alert personnel to faulty equipment prior to the use on a patient, therefore improving the quality and outcome of the anesthesia. Cleaning of the breathing system should be done according to the manufacturer's recommendations.

12.8.2 Leaks

There are numerous methods of checking a circle system for leaks. Checking the anesthetic machine is necessary as well (see Chapter 27). Machines and breathing systems should be checked every time they are used. Below is a brief example of the steps needed to check a breathing system:

1) Assemble the breathing system:
   a) Attach a hose from the common gas outlet to the absorber.
   b) Attach the scavenging system.
   c) Assemble components of breathing system: reservoir bag, expiratory and inspiratory tubing, manometer and any other additional equipment (PEEP valve, filters, etc.).
2) Integrity check:
   a) all components present;
   b) no holes, no obstructions, no foreign bodies;
   c) inner tube of the coaxial system attached at both ends; and
   d) adequate quantity of absorbent (check exhaustion).
3) Check for leaks:
   a) Occlude the patient connector.
   b) Close the APL valve.
   c) Using the oxygen emergency flush, fill the breathing system up to ~30 cmH_2O. If there is no manometer, fill the breathing system until the wrinkles in the reservoir bag disappear.
   d) Wait 10–20 seconds. Pressure should hold if no leaks are present. If leaks are present, quantify the leak by turning the oxygen flowmeter on; slowly increase the flow from 0 L/min until the pressure stops dropping.
   e) If the leak is <200 mL/min, or if there is no leak, open the APL valve to release pressure and check its function.
4) Check function of unidirectional valves:
   a) Partly fill the reservoir bag.
   b) Attach a small reservoir bag to the patient connector to act as the patient's lungs.
   c) Squeezing the reservoir bag at the patient connector will test the function of the expiratory valve.
   d) Squeezing the reservoir bag from the breathing system will test the function of the inspiratory valve.
5) Always leave the APL valve open at the end of the check.

Table 12.4 Advantages and disadvantages of circle system.

Advantages	Disadvantages
Economical	Inability to alter rapidly inspired agent concentration
Decreased work environment pollution	Accumulation of undesired gas in the system
Decreased environmental pollution	Potential for malfunction higher (multiple interconnected parts)
Heat and moisture conservation	Higher compliance
Less danger of barotrauma if low fresh gas flow	Possible higher resistance

12.9   Advantages/Disadvantages

Using a circle system has both advantages and disadvantages (Table 12.4). Overall, circle systems are economical and decrease pollution of the work environment and the atmosphere (Gadani and Vyas 2011; Sherman *et al.* 2012). However, they require more attention, and changes in anesthesia depth can be slow. Finally, as explained above, this system has the potential of having higher resistance.

References

Bicalho, G.P., Braz, L.G., De Jesus, L.S., Pedigone, C.M., De Carvalho, L.R. *et al.* (2014) The humidity in a Drager Primus anesthesia workstation using low or high fresh gas flow and with or without a heat and moisture exchanger in pediatric patients. *Anesth Analg*, 119, 926–931.

Brody, S. (1945) Basal energy and protein metabolism in relation to body weight. In: Brody, S. (ed.). *Bioenergetics and Growth, with Special Reference to the Efficiency Complex in Domestic Animals*. New York: Reinhold, pp. 352–403.

Conterato, J.P., Lindahl, S.G., Meyer, D.M. and Bires, J.A. (1989) Assessment of spontaneous ventilation in anesthetized children with use of a pediatric circle or a Jackson-Rees system. *Anesth Analg*, 69, 484–90.

Coppens, M.J., Versichelen, L.F., Rolly, G., Mortier, E.P. and Struys, M.M. (2006) The mechanisms of carbon monoxide production by inhalational agents. *Anaesthesia*, 61, 462–468.

Davis, P.D. and Kenny, G.N.C. (2003a) Breathing and scavenging systems. In: *Basic Physics and Measurement in Anaesthesia*, 5th ed. Boston, MA: Butterworth-Heinemann, pp. 237–252.

Davis, P.D. and Kenny, G.N.C. (2003b) Natural exponential functions. In: *Basic Physics and Measurement in Anaesthesia*, 5th ed. Boston, MA: Butterworth-Heinemann, pp. 51–63.

De Castro, J. Jr., Bolfi, F., De Carvalho, L.R. and Braz, J.R. (2011) The temperature and humidity in a low-flow anesthesia workstation with and without a heat and moisture exchanger. *Anesth Analg*, 113, 534–538.

Dorsch, J.A. and Dorsch, S.E. (2008) The breathing system – general principles, common components, and classification. In: *Understanding Anesthesia Equipment*, 5th ed. Philadelphia, PA: Wolters Kluwer Health/ Lippincott Williams & Wilkins, pp. 191–278.

Dunlop, C.I. (1992) The case for rebreathing circuits for very small animals. *Vet Clin North Am Small Anim Pract*, 22, 400–403.

Gadani, H. and Vyas, A. (2011) Anesthetic gases and global warming: Potentials, prevention and future of anesthesia. *Anesth Essays Res*, 5, 5–10.

Gonsowski, C.T., Laster, M.J., Eger, E.I., Ferrell, L.D. and Kerschmann, R.L. (1994) Toxicity of compound A in rats. Effect of a 3-hour administration. *Anesthesiology*, 80, 556–565.

Hartsfield, S.M. (2007) Anesthetic machines and breathing systems. In: Tranquilli, W.J., Thurmon, J.C. and Grimm, K.A. (eds) *Veterinary Anesthesia and Analgesia*, 4th ed. Ames, IA: Wiley-Blackwell, pp. 453–493.

Hartsfield, S.M. and Sawyer, D.C. (1976) Cardiopulmonary effects of rebreathing and non-rebreathing systems during halothane anesthesia in the cat. *Am J Vet Res*, 37, 1461–1466.

Henriksson, B.A., Sundling, J. and Hellman, A. (1997) The effect of a heat and moisture exchanger on humidity in a low-flow anaesthesia system. *Anaesthesia*, 52, 144–149.

Hofmeister, E.H., Brainard, B.M., Braun, C. and Figueiredo, J.P. (2011) Effect of a heat and moisture exchanger on heat loss in isoflurane-anesthetized dogs undergoing single-limb orthopedic procedures. *J Am Vet Med Assoc*, 239, 1561–1565.

Hughes, L. (2016) Breathing systems and ancillary equipment. In: Duke-Novakovski, T., De Vries, M. and Seymour, C. (eds). *British Small Animal Veterinary Association Manual of Canine and Feline Anaesthesia and Analgesia*, 3rd ed. Quedgeley, Gloucester: British Small Animal Veterinary Association, pp. 45–64.

Johansson, A., Lundberg, D. and Luttropp, H.H. (2003) The effect of heat and moisture exchanger on humidity and body temperature in a low-flow anaesthesia system. *Acta Anaesthesiol Scand*, 47, 564–568.

Kelly, C.K., Hodgson, D.S. and McMurphy, R.M. (2012) Effect of anesthetic breathing circuit type on thermal loss in cats during inhalation anesthesia for ovariohysterectomy. *J Am Vet Med Assoc*, 240, 1296–1299.

Lee, C., Lee, K.C., Kim, H.Y., Kim, M.N., Choi, E.K. *et al.* (2013) Unidirectional valve malfunction by the breakage or malposition of disc – two cases report. *Korean J Anesthesiol*, 65, 337–340.

Lerche, P., Muir, W.W. and Bednarski, R.M. (2000) Rebreathing anesthetic systems in small animal practice. *J Am Vet Med Assoc*, 217, 485–492.

Mizrak, A., Bilgi, M., Koruk, S., Ganidagli, S., Karatas, E. *et al.* (2011) Comparison of the coaxial circle circuit with the conventional circle circuit. *Eurasian J Med*, 43, 92–98.

Mosley, C.A. (2015) Anesthesia equipment. In: Grimm, K.A., Lamont, L.A., Tranquilli, W.J., Greene, S.A. and Robertson, S.A. (eds). *Veterinary Anesthesia and Analgesia. The Fifth Edition of Lumb and Jones*. Ames, IA: Wiley Blackwell, pp. 23–85.

Muir, W.W. and Gadawski, J. (1998) Cardiorespiratory effects of low-flow and closed circuit inhalation anesthesia, using sevoflurane delivered with an in-circuit vaporizer and concentrations of compound a. *Am J Vet Res*, 59, 603–608.

Nicholson, A. and Watson, A. (2001) Survey on small animal anaesthesia. *Aust Vet J*, 79, 613–619.

Parthasarathy, S. (2013) The closed circuit and the low flow systems. *Indian J Anaesth*, 57, 516–524.

Rasch, D.K., Bunegin, L., Ledbetter, J. and Kaminskas, D. (1988) Comparison of circle absorber and Jackson-Rees systems for paediatric anaesthesia. *Can J Anaesth*, 35, 25–30.

Sherman, J., Le, C., Lamers, V. and Eckelman, M. (2012) Life cycle greenhouse gas emissions of anesthetic drugs. *Anesth Analg*, 114, 1086–1090.

Tamul, P.C. and Ault, M.L. (2013) Respiratory function in anaesthesia. In: Barash, P.G., Cullen, B.F., Stoelting, R.K., Cahalan, M.K., Stock, M.C. and Ortega, R (eds). *Clinical Anesthesia*, 7th ed. Philadelphia, PA: Wolters Kluwer/ Lippincott Williams & Wilkins, pp. 263–286.

Wilkes, A.R. (2011) Heat and moisture exchangers and breathing system filters: Their use in anaesthesia and intensive care. Part 1: History, principles and efficiency. *Anaesthesia*, 66, 31–39.

Yamashita, K., Yokoyama, T., Abe, H., Nishiyama, T. and Manabe, M. (2007) Efficacy of a heat and moisture exchanger in inhalation anesthesia at two different flow rates. *J Anesth*, 21, 55–58.

13

Laryngoscopes

Erin Wendt-Hornickle

College of Veterinary Medicine, University of Minnesota, St Paul, Minnesota, USA

13.1   History

This history of laryngoscope use is fairly convoluted. Several different men are credited with the invention and evolution of the laryngoscope: Leverete in 1743, Bozzini in 1807, Babington in 1829, and Baume and Liston in 1838–1840. Interestingly, Babington was the first to use a light source (the Sun) to indirectly visualize the upper portions of the larynx (Bailey 1996). However, it was Manuel Garcia, a voice teacher whose greatest ambition was to visualize the glottis, who became known as the "father of the laryngoscope". A clear description of his instrument, presented to the Royal Society in 1855, is lacking, although it seemed to involve a mirror to visualize the glottis and epiglottis (Garcia 1855). In any case, Garcia was the first man to indirectly visualize the vocal cords clearly and repeatedly (Bailey 1996).

Two men are credited for advancing Garcia's work in clinical applications, Ludwig Turck and Johan Czermak (Bailey 1996). Nevertheless, the first man recognized for direct visualization of the glottis was Alfred Kirstein in 1895. He used a modified esophagoscope, which he called an autoscope (Hirsch *et al.* 1986). In 1913, Chevalier Jackson was the first to report the use of the laryngoscope as an aid in successful tracheal intubations of humans. Jackson introduced a laryngoscope that moved the light source from the proximal portion to the distal tip of the instrument (Zeitels 1998). During the same year, Henry Harrington Janeway, an American anesthesiologist, made several modifications to the instrument. These included the inclusion of batteries within the handle, a central notch in the blade for maintaining the tracheal tube in the midline of the oropharynx during intubation, and the addition of a curve to the distal tip of the blade to help guide the tube through the glottis (Janeway 1913). Over the next century, many advances to this relatively simple instrument were made. Most of our present-day laryngo-

scopes are slight modifications of instruments used by these men in the early 1900s.

13.2   Laryngoscope Use

The most common use for laryngoscopes is to provide visualization for tracheal intubation during anesthesia (Figure 13.1) or cardiopulmonary resuscitation. Laryngoscopes are also used for evaluating oral, pharyngeal and laryngeal structure and function. They aid in the detection of neoplastic conditions, laryngeal paralysis and collapse, and the etiology of partial or complete airway obstructions. Laryngoscopes are also utilized during placement of esophagostomy tubes and transesophageal echocardiogram probes.

13.3   Description

13.3.1   Rigid Laryngoscopes

Rigid laryngoscopes are most commonly used in veterinary medicine. They are available as a single piece or as detachable handle and blade pieces.

13.3.1.1   Handle

The handle piece (Figure 13.2) is the part held in the operator's hand while using the device. It provides the connection point for the blade and a hinge pin, as well as a power source for the light or an LED light, and frequently batteries. The point of connection between the blade and handle is made of metal, completing an electrical circuit between the lamp bulb and batteries while in the correct operating position. There are two methods of light illumination, a lamp-in-blade system or a fiber optic system using a halogen or argon light bulb. Handles are

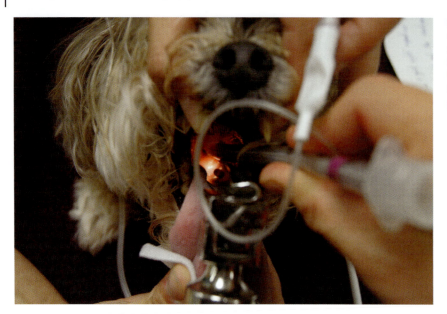

Figure 13.1 Direct laryngoscopic visualization for intubation. The anesthetist is using a Miller blade with a flange present. Note the position of the flange potentially interfering with visualization and endotracheal tube placement.

found in varying sizes from a thin, penlight handle to an extra-large-diameter handle, although it is most common to use a handle in between these two extremes.

13.3.1.2 Blade

The blade (Figure 13.3) is the part of the laryngoscope that is inserted into the patient's mouth. It has several important parts: the base, heel, tongue, flange, web, tip, lock and light source (Figures 13.4 and 13.5). Bulb-in blades also have electrical contact within the blade base, while fiber optic blades have an encased fiber optic bundle that transmits light from the source found in the han-

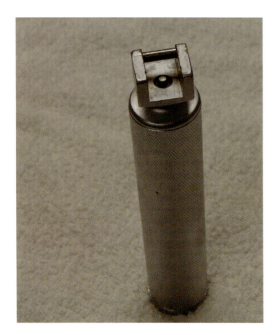

Figure 13.2 Laryngoscope handle, showing the hinge pin.

dle or blade (e.g. DarvallVet/Advanced Anesthesia Specialists, Payson, AZ). There are more than 40 types of laryngoscope blades designed for intubation in humans. The most common type of blades encountered in veterinary medicine are the straight Miller blade, the curved MacIntosh blade and a Miller-style long blade (~300 mm).

Miller blades were originally designed in 1941 by an American anesthesiologist, Dr Robert Miller (Miller 1972). They have a straight tongue with a slight curve toward the tip. The flange (if present) is positioned over the tongue creating a "C" shape in cross-section (Figures 13.4 and 13.6) and can interfere with visualization (Figure 13.1). Miller blades come in many sizes (Table 13.1). The smallest size (000), though rarely used, was originally designed for premature infant intubation. More commonly, size 00 is used in very small dogs and cats. The largest size (5) can be used for giant breed dogs, though a size 4 is generally sufficient.

The extra-long Miller-style blade (Figure 13.3) is similar in structure to the typical Miller blades, though much longer. It is used primarily in the intubation of swine, camelids and small ruminants.

An English anesthesiologist, Sir Robert MacIntosh (Scott and Baker 2009), designed MacIntosh blades. This type of blade is commonly used for human patients and is described as "the most numerously and widely made durable item in the history of anesthesia" (Scott and Baker 2009). It has a curved tongue and the flange (if present) is positioned away from the tongue creating a "Z" in cross-section (Figure 13.7). The blade also comes in a left-handed version, in which the flange is located on the opposite side. Since many veterinary patients are intubated in sternal recumbency, this configuration may improve visualization while intubating. MacIntosh blades come in several sizes (Table 13.1).

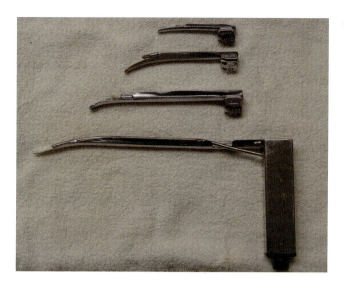

Figure 13.3 Detachable straight Miller blades (top three) and single piece extra-long Miller-style blade (bottom).

13.3.2 Other Laryngoscopes

Other types of laryngoscopes have been described. In 2006, Robert Molthen described in elaborate detail how to construct an inexpensive, effective laryngoscope for rat intubation. The three variations he describes vary in length from 85–100 mm end to end and can be used with a light source to successfully intubate rats from 200–450 g (Molthen 2006). In addition, otoscope cones have been fashioned to connect to an otoscope handle (Figure 13.8). When lit by the base, they can be effectively used to visually intubate rodents and other small patients.

Modifications of many laryngoscope blades have been used in veterinary medicine, due to the unique consid-erations when intubating such diverse species. For exam-ple, straight Wisconsin laryngoscope blades with added length and the flange/light source extending to the distal end (~41 cm) have been made to intubate difficult spe-cies such as swine and small ruminants, to increase the visual field (Figure 13.9).

Cost-effective, disposable laryngoscopes are also com-mercially available for use in veterinary medicine (Timesco™ Callisto Green Fitting Disposable Laryngoscope Systems, Smiths Medical, Dublin, OH). These laryngo-scopes have a permanent LED light source, require no bat-teries, reduce cross contamination, and minimize equipment and processing costs. They come with both Miller and MacIntosh blade types.

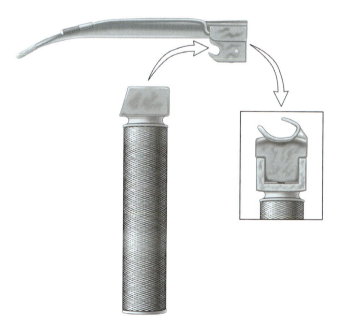

Figure 13.4 Example of laryngoscope blade and handle assembly. The left arrow depicts where the handle fits into the blade. The right arrow points to an image of the handle and blade from the vantage point of the anesthetist when positioned correctly for intubation.

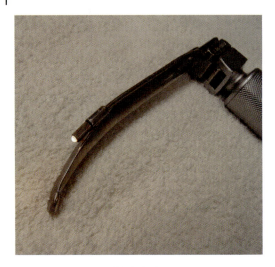

Figure 13.5 Lamp-in-blade light source.

13.4 Fiber Optic Endoscopes

Flexible fiber optic endoscopes can be used to assist the anesthetist with intubation of a difficult airway in companion animals, as well as in small mammals and other exotic species (Johnson 2010) (Figures 13.10 and 13.11). They can be used to aid in the placement of double-lumen tracheal tubes and bronchial blockers. These instruments are also utilized in horses for performing airway examinations and diagnosing causes of respiratory difficulty that occur during exercise, such as laryngeal hemiplegia. The endoscope consists of a handle, light source and insertion piece. Cameras can be attached directly or wirelessly for remote viewing. If using the endoscope for assistance with intubation, the insertion piece can be placed into an endotracheal tube with an internal diameter that is minimally 1 mm larger than the external diameter of the inser-

Table 13.1 Approximate lengths for Miller and MacIntosh laryngoscope blades.

Type	Size	Approximate Length (mm)
Miller	00	65
	0	78
	1	102
	2	154
	3	195
	4	205
MacIntosh	00	68
	0	80
	1	92
	2	100
	3	130
	4	155
	5	175

tion piece (Dorsch and Dorsch 2008). These endoscopes are versatile and are used to intubate small rodents (BioLite Intubation System, Braintree Scientific, Inc. Braintree, MA; Figure 13.9) as well as larger species such as canids, swine, etc. (Figure 13.10).

Rigid fiber optic endoscopes can also be used to facilitate intubation or visualization of laryngeal structures, especially in small mammals (Jekl and Knotek 2007). The major limitation is the inability to move the distal end of the scope independently of rest of the unit.

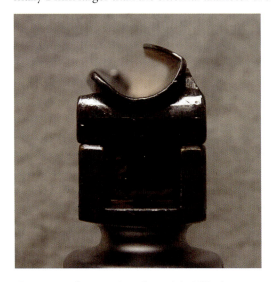

Figure 13.6 Cross-section of a straight Miller laryngoscope blade. Note the "C" shape of the blade.

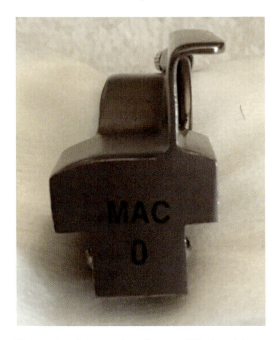

Figure 13.7 Cross-section of a curved MacIntosh laryngoscope blade. Note the "Z" shape of the blade.

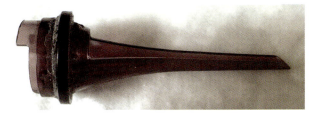

Figure 13.8 An otoscope cone modified dorsally. It fits on the handle of a conventional otoscope and is used to intubate rodents and other small patients.

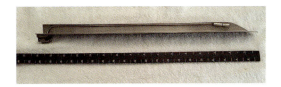

Figure 13.9 A modified Wisconsin laryngoscope blade with straight flange used in difficult airways, such as those encountered in swine and small ruminants.

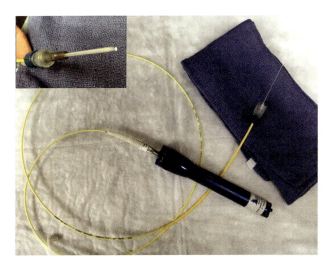

Figure 13.10 A commercially available fiber optic scope used for tracheal intubation in rodents. The tracheal tube (an intravenous catheter) is slipped over the small fiber optic light (upper left), which is used to directly visualize the larynx.

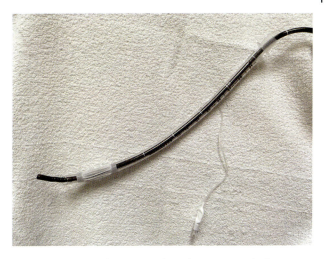

Figure 13.11 An endoscope used as a laryngoscope/stylet to visualize the larynx in larger species such as dogs, pigs, camelids, small ruminants, etc. The tracheal tube is placed over the endoscope and is slid off to intubate the trachea once visualized.

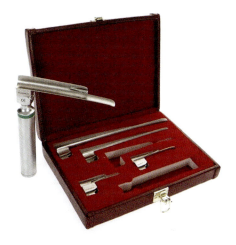

Figure 13.12 Example of a commercially available veterinary laryngoscope kit directed specifically to the veterinary patient. Blades can be purchased individually or as a set and come in left- and right-handed versions (pictured here) with the LED source in the base (image courtesy of DarvallVet/Advanced Anesthesia Specialists (Payson, AZ)).

13.5 Veterinary-Specific Laryngoscopes

Recently, laryngoscopes manufactured specifically for veterinary use have been commercially developed, since the laryngoscope is held in an opposite position to intubate many veterinary species compared with human intubation techniques (DarvallVet/Advanced Anesthesia Specialists, Phoenix, AZ; Figure 13.12). These laryngoscopes have the light on the opposite side, can be made for right- or left-handed intubation, and have the LED source located within the waterproof handle. They are made in a variety of sizes but frequently have straight blades from 3 inches to 12–14 inches in length for small animals as well as sheep, goats, pigs, marine and zoo animals.

13.6 Summary

In summary, laryngoscopes are an essential piece of equipment for all anesthesia personnel. The numerous types and blade choices allow the anesthetist to choose which best suits the unique needs of the situation and patient.

References

Bailey, B. (1996) Laryngoscopy and laryngoscopes – who's first? the forefathers/four fathers of laryngology. *Laryngoscope*, 106, 939–943.

Dorsch, J.A. and Dorsch, S.E. (2008) Medical gas cylinders and containers. In: *Understanding Anaesthesia Equipment*, 5th ed. Philadelphia, PA: Lippincott Williams & Wilkins, pp. 520–560.

Garcia, M. (1855) Observations on the human voice. *Proceedings of the Royal Society of London*, 7, 399–410.

Hirsch, N.P., Smith, G. and Hirsch, P.O. (1986) Alfred Kirstein. Pioneer of direct laryngoscopy. *Anaesthesia*, 41, 42–45.

Janeway, H.H. (1913) Intra-tracheal anesthesia from the standpoint of the nose, throat and oral surgeon with a description of a new instrument for catheterizing the trachea. *The Laryngoscope*, 23, 1082–1090.

Jekl, V. and Knotek, Z. (2007) Evaluation of a laryngoscope and a rigid endoscope for the examination of the oral cavity of small mammals. *Vet Rec*, 160, 9–13.

Johnson, D.H. (2010) Endoscopic intubation of exotic companion mammals. *Vet Clin North Am Exot Anim Pract*, 13, 273–289.

Miller, R.A. (1972) The development of the laryngoscope. *Anaesthetist*, 21, 145–147.

Molthen, R.C. (2006) A simple, inexpensive, and effective light-carrying laryngoscopic blade for orotracheal intubation of rats. *J Am Assoc Lab Anim Sci*, 45, 88–93.

Scott, J. and Baker, P.A. (2009) How did the MacIntosh laryngoscope become so popular? *Paediatr Anaesth*, 19, 24–29.

Zeitels, S.M. (1998) Chevalier Jackson's contributions to direct laryngoscopy. *J Voice*, 12, 1–6.

14

Supraglottic Airway Devices and Tracheal Tubes and Stylets

Jennifer Sager

College of Veterinary Medicine, University of Florida, Gainesville, Florida, USA

14.1 Introduction

Maintenance of general anesthesia in veterinary medicine can be achieved through a variety of methods, including inhalant, total intravenous and partial intravenous anesthesia. Early methodology of controlling inhalant anesthesia involved the use of ether dripped over a mask secured to a patient's face. Evolution in the study of anesthesia has shown us that this method is less than desirable. Inability to adequately control anesthetic depth, the airway patency, and proper waste gas scavenging, along with the possible sequelae of complications including esophageal regurgitation and aspiration, could result in an increase in morbidity and mortality. Adapted from human medicine, supraglottic devices such as laryngeal mask airways (LMAs), veterinary-gel (v-gel®) airway devices, and endotracheal tubes assist the anesthetist in maintaining an adequate airway for ventilation in both small and large animal patients.

14.2 Laryngeal Mask Airway (LMA)

Developed by a British anesthesiologist, Dr Archie Brain in 1988, the LMA was an alternative for endotracheal intubation in human medicine (Mosley 2015). LMAs sit outside the trachea, but still provide a gas-tight airway (Dorsch and Dorsch 2011a). Applications in veterinary medicine have become more popular in recent years, especially in cats, rodents, rabbits and pigs (Goldmann *et al.* 2005). The applicable use in dogs is more difficult due to breed and anatomical variances, but is still a non-invasive alternative to the standard endotracheal tube (Reed and Iff 2012).

14.2.1 Description

The laryngeal mask airway (LMA) is a silicone rubber tube that opens into a small elliptical mask with an inflatable outer rim (Figure 14.1). Sizes range from 1–6, depending on the body weight of the patient, with 1 being the smallest, accepting an endotracheal tube of 3.5 mm if needed through the device. These supraglottic airway devices are designed to be placed over the glottis and larynx without insertion into the trachea, still providing an airway seal (Reed and Iff 2012).

14.2.1.1 LMA-Classic™

The LMA-Classic™ (LMA, LMA-C, cLMA) is a silicone-curved tube, with an elliptical 30-degree angle spoon-shaped mask. Eight sizes are available, ranging from 1, 1.5, 2, 2.5 through size 6. The inflatable outer rim is connected to a pilot balloon, which is attached to the proximal or patient end of the device. This LMA is equipped with a standard 15-m breathing circuit connector. Two rigid lines connect the shaft to the mask, preventing obstruction from the epiglottis.

These LMAs can be sterilized after use with ethylene oxide. Standard endotracheal tubes, cuffed or uncuffed, can be passed through the classic device up to size 7.0 mm I.D. This type is most commonly used in veterinary patients due to ease of use (Dorsch and Dorsch 2011a).

14.2.1.2 LMA-Unique™

The LMA Unique™ is an inexpensive single-use disposable item (DLMA) made of polyvinyl chloride (PVC). Compared to the LMA-Classic™, these tubes are stiff, with less compliant cuffs, but similar in design (Dorsch and Dorsch 2011a). Due to the stiffness of the tube, it is helpful to warm them prior to use.

Veterinary Anesthetic and Monitoring Equipment, First Edition. Edited by Kristen G. Cooley and Rebecca A. Johnson.
© 2018 John Wiley & Sons, Inc. Published 2018 by John Wiley & Sons, Inc.

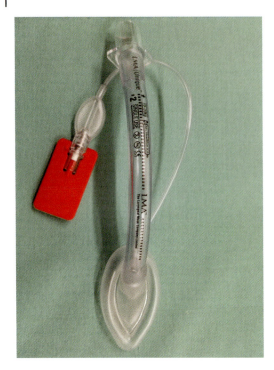

Figure 14.1 Laryngeal Mask Airway device (LMA; LMA-Unique™, size 2).

14.2.1.3 LMA-Fastrach™

Similar in design to the LMA-Classic™, the LMA-Fastrach™ accommodates all standard size endotracheal tubes up to 9.0-mm I.D. It is a latex-free stainless steel curved tube with metal handle and epiglottic elevating tool (Dorsch and Dorsch 2011a).

14.2.1.4 LMA-ProSeal™

The LMA-ProSeal™ is a silicone, latex-free LMA with the standard cuff, inflation line, and tube of an LMA-Classic™. It has an additional drain or gastric recess tube. Unlike the cLMA, this device is shorter with a smaller diameter, but is wire reinforced allowing for more flexibility in the tube. The drain is parallel to the airway, and when placed correctly, the tip will cover the opening of the esophagus (Boldizar *et al.* 2007).

14.2.1.5 LMA-Supreme™

Similar in specification to the LMA-ProSeal™, the LMA-Supreme™ has a built-in bite block (Dorsch and Dorsch 2011a).

14.2.2 Placement Techniques

The LMA is designed for quick insertion without the necessitation of a laryngoscope or even direct visualization of the larynx (Weiderstein *et al.* 2006). Before place-

ment, the LMA should be inflated with air only, no liquid, to ensure proper cuff enlargement. Once a viable cuff has been confirmed, the air should be removed to completely deflate the rim. After appropriate induction agents are administered, one person should open the mouth, grasping the top jaw behind the canines, and extrude the tongue. With the tip of a rigid laryngoscope, press on the base of the tongue to move the epiglottis ventral opening the airway. Hold the LMA between your thumb and forefinger, close to the base of the tube and mask, and advance the LMA into the oral cavity. The tip of the cuff should be pointed toward the esophagus and the lateral aspect of the cuff should slide over the arytenoids (Weiderstein *et al.* 2008). Inflate according to manufacture pressure limits (up to 60 cmH$_2$0) to create a further seal, and confirm placement via capnography. The black marker line on the LMA should be midline between the incisors.

14.2.3 Complications

Inappropriate sizing of the LMA can result in environmental exposure of inhalant gases during ventilation if too small, aspiration of stomach contents (noted in pigs), a sore throat (noted in humans), discomfort upon tracheal palpation post-extubation in dogs, or pressure on lingual nerves if too large (Goldmann *et al.* 2005).

14.3 Veterinary-gel (v-gel®) Airway Device

Originally developed for the human market as an i-gel device in 1990 (second-generation LMA), the v-gel® supraglottic airway product was created specifically for veterinary patients by Docsinnovent Ltd (www.docsinnovent. com) (Figure 14.2). The v-gel® for cats and the v-gel® for rabbits are designed as an alternative to endotracheal tubes in these species. They cause less tissue damage to the larynx or trachea, but still maintain a patent airway for inhalant and gas exchange. Future devices are being developed for canine and equine patients.

14.3.1 Description

The v-gel® device creates an airtight seal using a soft, non-inflatable cuff that contours to the anatomical features of the patient pharyngeal and laryngeal structures (Oostrom *et al.* 2013). The airtight seal creates not only a patent airway for maintenance of general anesthesia, but also minimal pollution of anesthetic gases, and it works with mechanical ventilators. This device also contains an esophageal seal to prevent the possible aspiration of gastroesophageal reflux, and does not cause laryngeal spasm.

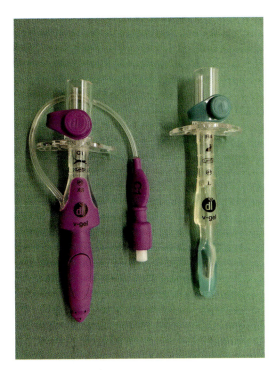

Figure 14.2 V-gel® devices designed specifically for veterinary patients. Two types of v-gel® devices are available, the v-gel® for cats (left) and the v-gel® for rabbits (right).

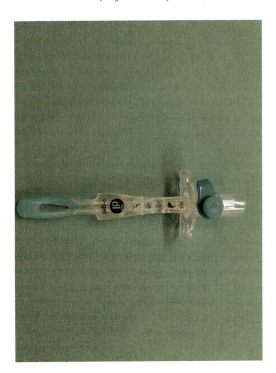

Figure 14.3 V-gel® device for rabbits (size 4). Note the lack of inflatable dorsal pressure adjuster.

There are up to six sizes available for each of the feline and rabbit type of v-gel® device, depending on the weight and breed of the animal. V-gels® can be reused up to 40 times, provided autoclave sterilization is carried out in between each use at 121°F (49.4°C) cycle (Mosby 2015).

14.3.1.1 V-gel® for Cats

The v-gel® for cats product specifications include an airway channel, a cuff tip, a monitoring port and a bite-block. The airway channel is a large channel that minimizes airway resistance. The cuff tip is a soft gel-like material that contours to the anatomy of the pharyngeal area. The monitoring port can attach to a luer lock sampling line for gas analysis and the bite-block protects the device and airway from collapsing if a patient bites down. On the dorsal side, an inflatable valve and inflation line allows for the adjustment of the initial seal pressure when needed. A rotation resistant shoulder provides a safety stop while inserting the device into the airway. Two winged sections on the proximal end of the bite-block exist to secure the device to the patient, preventing maladjustment of position. Also on the dorsal surface is an information block or quick guide for size reference, species type and maximum use indication.

14.3.1.2 V-gel® for Rabbits

The v-gel® for rabbits has the same specifications as the v-gel® for cats (Figure 14.3), except for the absence of the inflatable dorsal pressure adjuster. Placement can be challenging due to the anatomical features of the rabbit larynx, but it is a good alternative to a standard endotracheal tube (Uzun *et al.* 2015).

14.3.2 Placement Techniques

Extend the head of the patient and extrude the rostral end of the tongue. Place the device into the pharyngeal area exerting minimal pressure until resistance is felt. Confirm placement via capnography and secure the device to the patient with a tie (gauze, tape, etc.) around the head via attachment through the winged sections of the bite-block (Figure 14.4).

14.3.3 Complications

Endotracheal intubation is associated with complications in cats, such as laryngeal spasm, tracheal damage, and rupture. In rabbits, changes in heart rate and blood pressure are associated with standard endotracheal intubation (Toman *et al.* 2015). The v-gel® airway device has not been linked to any major post-operative complications and has less reported changes in hemodynamic status (Barletta *et al.* 2015).

14.4 Endotracheal Tubes

Most endotracheal tubes are developed for humans, but can be used in small animal patients and are commonly

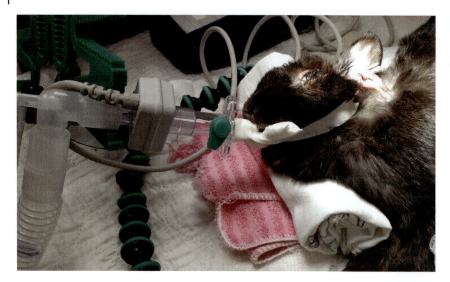

Figure 14.4 V-gel® secured to a rabbit patient using tape. The tubes are secured with a holder (green and black, d-grip, Jorgensen Laboratories, Loveland, CO) designed to reduce torque on the airway devices.

used to maintain airways via oral or nasal intubation over the newer supraglottic airway devices (Dorsch and Dorsch 2011b).

14.4.1 Description

Endotracheal tubes (ETT) are comprised of some universal features and some unique features, depending on the type of tube in question. The two most common types of endotracheal tubes are classified as a Murphy or Magill type, and can further be classified as cuffed or non-cuffed.

The endotracheal tube is cylindrical in shape, with a beveled edge at the patient end. The size of the endotracheal tube is labeled according to both the internal (I.D.) and external or outer diameter (O.D.). Sizes are referenced from the endotracheal tube's internal diameter, which can range from size 2.0–30.0 mm. Selection of the appropriately-sized endotracheal tube is determined by the outer diameter of the tube, whereas the I.D. determines the resistance to airflow. The O.D. can be influenced by the material used to manufacture the tube (rubber, silicone or polyvinyl chloride), and depending on the thickness, can reduce the internal airway diameter. A thin-walled tube will offer less resistance than a thicker tube.

Due to the cross-over from human medicine, endotracheal tubes must be labeled with I.D. and O.D. measurements, tube characteristics or intended use (oral nasal, oral/nasal), as well as the scale for the depth of insertion (Figure 14.5) (Mosley 2015).

All small animal endotracheal tubes will have a 15-mm I.D. connector that will universally fit all breathing circuits. These can be removed from regular endotracheal tubes and replaced with specially designed port sampling adapters or those designed for small patients in order to reduce mechanical dead space (Figure 14.6).

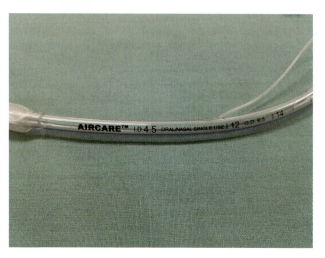

Figure 14.5 Endotracheal markings with I.D., O.D., type, and cm measurements.

Tubes with cuffs will have an inflation valve that can be connected to a syringe and used to inflate the cuff. Cuffs should not be inflated in excess of the maximum pressure limit, as designated by the manufacturer.

14.4.2 Materials

Endotracheal tubes can be manufactured from rubber, silicone and polyvinyl chloride (PVC). Red rubber endotracheal tubes are opaque and can be reused after sterilization via ethylene oxide. They also make good tubes for those patients undergoing Computed Tomography (CT) scanning, because there are no external markings to interfere with image quality. Red rubber endotracheal tubes have a tendency to kink when flexed, compromising adequate airflow and patency of the patient airway. Over time, red rubber tubes will degrade, hardening and becoming sticky with prolonged use (Mosley 2015).

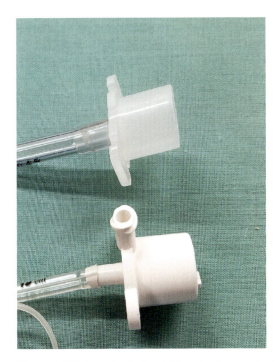

Figure 14.6 Endotracheal tube with low dead space adapters for use in small patients. The one on the bottom is adapted for gas sampling.

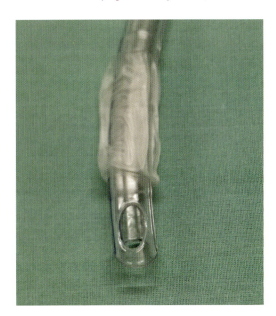

Figure 14.7 Endotracheal tube with Murphy's eye, providing an alternative gas pathway in the event of obstruction.

Silicone endotracheal tubes are less opaque and have a slightly thicker wall than red rubber or PVC tubes, resulting in a smaller I.D. for patients. They can be sterilized in ethylene oxide or steam autoclaved, affording multiple uses. However, they are more expensive than the others. Silicone tubes can often be floppy, therefore the use of a stylet or intubation assisted device is necessary to ensure proper placement.

Polyvinyl chloride (PVC) tubes are widely used and inexpensive. They are clear and reusable (after sanitation), are less likely to kink compared to red rubber tubes and are stiff at room temperature, so a stylet is not necessary. They are manufactured with a radio-opaque line that confirms placement via radiography. PVC tubes will soften at body temperature, allowing the tube to conform to the anatomy of the upper airway (Hass *et al.* 2014).

14.4.2.1 Murphy-type

The hole at the distal or patient end of the endotracheal tube opposite the side of the bevel is called the Murphy's eye (Figure 14.7). Tubes that have this hole are referred to as Murphy tubes. In the event of occlusion, this eye provides an alternative pathway for gas exchange. Less mucosal damage is noted during nasal intubation with a Murphy-type tube.

14.4.2.2 Magill-type

Endotracheal tubes without the distal hole are referred to as Magill-type tubes (Figure 14.8). The one advantage

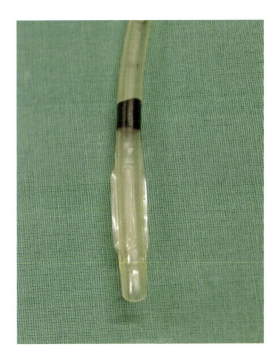

Figure 14.8 Magill style endotracheal tube with the cuff located close to the tube end.

of this style of tube is that the absence of a hole allows the cuff to be placed close to the end of the tube, reducing the incidence of endobronchial intubation.

14.4.3 Cuffed Endotracheal Tubes

Cuffed tubes have a latex or soft plastic inflatable sleeve at the distal end of the endotracheal tube which, when inflated, helps to provide a seal between the tube and the tracheal wall. This is beneficial in ensuring less environmental pollution of anesthetic gas and helps in the prevention of aspiration of gastro-esophageal reflux during regurgitation.

14.4.3.1 High-Volume, Low-Pressure Cuff

Two different types of endotracheal tube cuffs exist (Figure 14.9). A high-volume, low-pressure cuff is a cuff made out of thin compliant material that enables a seal with the tracheal wall with minimal stretching of the tracheal mucosa. These cuffs have a large resting volume and diameter and are associated with reduced frequency of cuff-induced damage following prolonged use. However, the larger surface area of the cuff may obscure direct visualization during intubation, and studies have shown that these types of tubes are less effective against aspiration of fluid. Inflation of these cuffs should follow posted manufacture guidelines for maximum cuff pressure, with adjustments made during changes in muscle tone.

14.4.3.2 Low-Volume, High-Pressure Cuff

The second type of cuff has a small diameter at rest and low residual volume, requiring a high pressure to create an adequate seal with the tracheal wall. Although the contact area of the trachea is small, and offers a greater seal against potential aspiration of fluid, prolonged use can cause ischemic damage to the tracheal mucosa. As such, inflation of these cuffs should be performed with the minimum amount of air needed to create a seal. Low-volume, high-pressure cuffs with their smaller area of contact, will distort the trachea to a circular shape to create a seal. However, the aforementioned high-volume, low-pressure cuffs conform to normal tracheal lumen contour (Dorsch and Dorsch 2011b).

14.4.4 Non-Cuffed Endotracheal Tubes

Cole-style endotracheal tubes are cuffless tubes used for oral intubation only. The distal end of the tube is of a smaller diameter than the proximal end (Figure 14.10). The idea is that the smaller end will slide into the trachea and the larger end will sit atop the larynx to form a seal. The Cole-style tube is not recommended for long-term use.

14.4.5 Alternative Cuffed Endotracheal Tubes

The K9 Safe-Seal™ Endo Tube (Jorgensen Labs, Loveland, CO) is a medical-grade silicone tube that utilizes a series of baffles that form a seal within the trachea instead of an inflatable cuff (Figure 14.11). This design eliminates the risk of cuff over- or under-inflation, because the soft, flexible silicone baffles create a seal without pressure

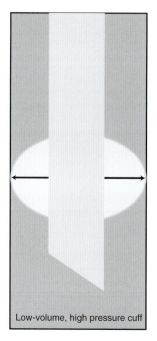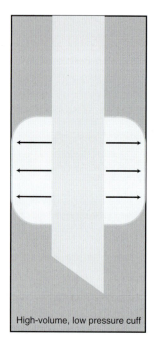

Low-volume, high pressure cuff   High-volume, low pressure cuff

Figure 14.9 Schematic representing a low-volume, high-pressure endotracheal tube cuff compared to the high-volume, low-pressure endotracheal tube cuff. Notice how all the pressure of the low-volume, high-pressure cuff is concentrated into one small area of the trachea, whereas the high-volume, low-pressure cuff is more evenly distributed (illustration courtesy of Kristen Cooley, University of Wisconsin-Madison, WI).

points. The tube is very flexible and a stylet is recommended to facilitate placement. The one-piece construction of medical-grade silicone is safe to sterilize in the autoclave between uses. The tube comes in only 4 sizes and is said to fit dogs weighing from 10–200 pounds; it is not marketed for cats.

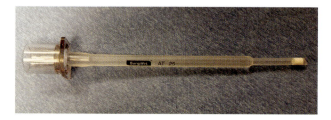

Figure 14.10 Cole-type endotracheal tube with a smaller distal end that is inserted into the trachea.

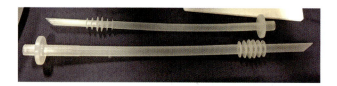

Figure 14.11 Endotracheal tube for use in dogs with baffles in the place of the cuff to create a seal.

14.4.6 Placement Techniques

Selection of an appropriately-sized endotracheal tube is often done by palpation of the trachea, or assessment of the width of the nares, which is less reliable (Shelby and McKune 2014). Direct tracheal palpation tends to overestimate tube size, whereas choosing a tube based on which size fits between the nares tends to underestimate tube size. A more reliable method is to base endotracheal tube size on the patient's lean body weight and breed. Note that brachycephalic breeds, both canine and feline, will have smaller tracheas than similarly-sized animals of another species.

Length should be predetermined prior to induction. This is achieved by placing the endotracheal tube alongside the patient with the distal or patient end falling between the larynx and the thoracic inlet. Note where the tube exits the mouth, as this will be your advancement guide. Endotracheal tubes are often longer than necessary, mainly because there is such a size variation between species and breeds. PVC tubes can be cut down in length to minimize mechanical dead space and the rebreathing of expired carbon dioxide.

Patients can be in either sternal or lateral recumbency, depending on the presenting complaint; sternal recumbency affords the easiest view of the laryngeal folds. A rigid laryngoscope can be used to visualize and illuminate the larynx. With gentle pressure placed on the base of the tongue by the tip of the laryngoscope, the epiglottis will fold ventrally, allowing direct visualization of the larynx. The use of a stylet, bougie or intubation-assisted device can facilitate the placement of the bevel tip at the laryngeal fold into the trachea (see below). The endotracheal tube should be advanced to the predetermined measurement and secured to the patient.

14.4.7 Securing the Tube

Different options exist concerning securing the endotracheal tube to the patient. The goal is to use something that can be cinched down securely onto the tube (without compromising the lumen). The material should be either disposable or of a material that can be easily sanitized between patients. It should be able to withstand moisture and not slip when manipulated or wet.

The most commonly used materials include roll gauze, IV tubing and Trinity Trach-Tube Ties (www.trachtubeties.com). Other materials used include glue, rubber bands, shoelaces, tape, umbilical tape, towel clamping to the lip, or suturing the tube to the lip. These materials have some potential drawbacks, including unnecessary hair removal/pulling (glue, rubber band, tape), decreased security (shoelace, umbilical tape) and tissue damage (towel clamp, suture), but find their way into veterinary practices nonetheless. Trinity Trach-Tube Ties are superior as they are designed for this purpose, they have good security, and are able to be sanitized and reused.

Most frequently, tubes are placed oro- or naso-tracheally. However, for oral or head procedures, pharyngotomy or transmylohyoid placement of the tracheal tubes with a finger trap suture or butterfly tape and suture is recommended. These methods allow for optimal oral cavity visibility during maxillofacial surgery (Soukup and Snyder 2015).

The method by which the material is tied onto the tube is also of importance. A half-hitch knot (Figure 14.12A) provides better security compared to forming a loop by passing the tie ends through the loop (Figure 14.12B). A standard "bow tie" or quick release knot is best when securing the tube, either atop the muzzle or behind the ears. The tube should be snug to avoid movement and potential extubation, but care should be taken to not make it too tight, causing edema of the muzzle.

14.4.8 Complications

One of the most common complications is inadvertent esophageal intubation. Proper placement can be confirmed through use of capnography as well as the presence of condensation on the inside of the endotracheal tube. Signs of esophageal intubation include a light plane of anesthesia, abdominal distention, regurgitation and absence of expired CO_2 on the capnograph.

Endobronchial intubation can also occur during initial intubation or through movement of the patient. Ensure proper length of the tube before induction by measuring from the midway between the larynx and thoracic inlet to the nares.

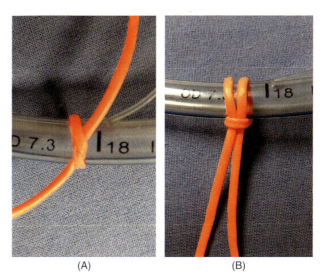

(A)   (B)

Figure 14.12 (A) Half hitch knot cinched down tightly to the endotracheal tube. (B) Less secure loop-through method of securing the tube (photographs courtesy of Kristen Cooley, University of Wisconsin-Madison, WI).

Tracheal rupture can occur, more commonly in cats, when the patient is manipulated into another position without disconnecting the breathing system. Always disconnect the patient from the breathing system before a change in recumbency. Accidental extubation can occur during patient transport or surgical manipulation. To avoid this, a stress anchor is recommended.

Changes in hemodynamic status, such as a catecholamine release, and possible changes in heart rate, blood pressure and intraocular pressure have been reported in both canine and feline patients (Ismail *et al.* 2011). A rapid sequence induction and intubation is recommended to reduce patient stress.

14.5 Large Animal Endotracheal Tubes

14.5.1 Description

The large animal Murphy-type tube consists of silicone or reinforced PVC tubing with a segmented polyurethane coated latex cuff (Kissinger and Hughes 1984). All PVC endotracheal tubes come with a plastic or rubber universal adapter (Figure 14.13), which fits over the Y-piece (50 mm). The inner diameter of the plastic bulb is the same size as the internal diameter of the tube, creating an airtight seal. The rubber adapter can also be removed and fitted with standard metal or plastic adapters (Figure 14.14). Sizes available for equine oral endotracheal tubes range from 24–30 mm ID, although smaller tubes from 16–22 mm are available for foals and large ruminants.

Nasal intubation can be performed when an obstructive airway precludes routine intubation or post-operatively for oxygen insufflation. These tubes are usually longer and

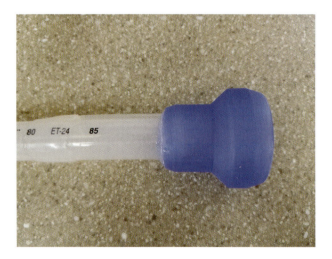

Figure 14.13 Large animal endotracheal tube adapter that fits on the end of the Y-piece.

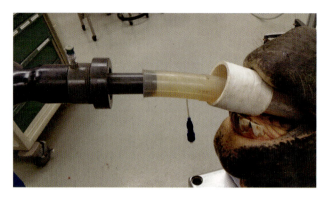

Figure 14.14 Large animal endotracheal tube with rubber adapter removed and fitted with an alternative plastic adapter.

silicone-based, with a standard 15-mm ETT adapter, ranging in internal diameter from 8.0–12 mm.

Typically, large animal tubes are multi-use products, with sterilization according to the autoclave cycle (121°F/49.4°C) between each use, to reduce potential transmission of infectious agents between patients.

14.5.2 Placement Techniques

Oral intubation of an equine patient is generally performed in lateral recumbency. Although for the sick colic horses with large amounts of gastroesophageal reflux preoperative, intubation can be performed in sternal recumbency to lessen the incidence of aspiration pneumonia. Once induced, a mouth gag (usually made of a piece of PVC tube with the rough edges wrapped with Elasticon or other similar material), is placed between the incisors. The head is extended cranially using caution with the down eye to avoid dragging it across the induction floor. Extend the tongue to allow for more space in the pharynx and feed the preselected endotracheal tube through the mouth gag. This is a blind intubation technique; there are no laryngoscopes available for visualization of the equine airway. In rare instances where intubation is extremely difficult, a fiber optic assisted scope can be used to help facilitate intubation if necessary. Once the endotracheal tube reaches the retropharyngeal area, apply slight pressure to advance. If the tube will not advance, remove the tube slightly, turn it 180 degrees and try to advance again. Confirmation of correct placement can be achieved via capnography, and the presence of air being expressed when the chest is compressed.

14.5.3 Complications

Similar complications with the use of small animal endotracheal tubes can arise with large endotracheal tubes, including esophageal intubation and damage to the laryngeal and tracheal mucosa. The latex cuff is thin and can be damaged when sliding over the teeth of the patients, causing an inappropriate seal within the trachea.

14.6 Reinforced Tubes

Commonly referred to as guarded, armored or wire tubes, reinforced endotracheal tubes are used in small animal anesthesia patients that are undergoing procedures where extreme flexion of the neck or head will occur (i.e. ophthalmic and neurologic procedures such as CSF collection). Unlike standard endotracheal tubes, these guarded tubes will not kink when flexed, thus ensuring adequate airflow (Figure 14.15) (Campoy *et al.* 2003). Smiths-Medical Bivona® Small Diameter Aire-Cuf®, Small Diameter TTS Air-Cuff® and Intersurgical's InTube™ are the most popular brands on the market at this time.

14.6.1 Description

Reinforced endotracheal tubes are a Murphy or Magill-type and they are made of silicone, rubber, latex or PVC, with a spiral-wound wire incorporated into the walls of the tube. The coil is kink resistant, but not bite resistant. The tubes are manufactured similarly to regular endotracheal tubes, with the inner and outer diameter labeled on the surface, universal 15-mm O.D. breathing circuit adapter, left-facing bevel tip and pilot balloon. Reinforced tubes have high-volume, low-pressure barrel-shaped cuffs, or they can be uncuffed. Uncuffed tubes are generally limited to sizes of less than 5.0-mm I.D.

Unlike standard endotracheal tubes, wire reinforced tubes do not contain a radio-opaque line, because the wire itself will show up on radiographs. The endotracheal tube adapter is also non-detachable. The walls of the silicone endotracheal tubes, to accommodate the wire shaft, are slightly thicker, making the outer diameter greater than that of a standard tube of the same internal

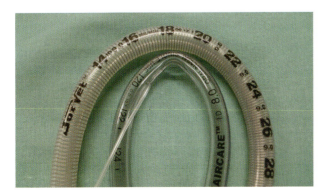

Figure 14.15 Comparison of the flexion capabilities of wire reinforced (top) compared with PVC (bottom) endotracheal tubes.

diameter. The sizes that are available range from 4–12 mm I.D. Reinforced endotracheal tubes are designed for single-use application, but can be resterilized using ethylene oxide (Aircare 2012).

14.6.2 Placement Techniques

Use of reinforced endotracheal tubes is similar to the procedure for the non-complicated endotracheal intubation method.

14.6.3 Complications

Due to the spiral wire, these tubes cannot be cut to a custom length, therefore appropriate measurements must be taken to avoid endobronchial intubation. A stylet should be used to help facilitate the placement of the endotracheal tube past the laryngeal folds into the trachea, as the tubes are fairly flaccid. Reinforced endotracheal tubes are generally considered MRI-conditional and generally safe to use in the MRI unit, meaning the wire will not heat up in the presence of the magnet. However, the metal within the tube causing scatter and poor-quality imaging (Dorsch and Dorsch 2011b) will directly affect picture quality.

14.7 Laser Safe Tubes

Laser safe endotracheal tubes are specially designed for use during surgical laser procedures of the head, neck and thoracic region, to avoid accidental rapid combustion of oxygen. These tubes are labeled as laser resistant and certain tubes can only be used with certain lasers (CO_2, YAG or Potassium-Titanyl-Phosphate [KTP]).

14.7.1 Description

Laser safe tubes can be made of metal or manufactured wrapped in a protective aluminum and/or Teflon coating. You can also wrap a normal endotracheal tube with reflective tape; however, caution should be taken with rough edges and the amount of tape, to avoid causing tracheal mucosal damage (Figure 14.16) (Mosley 2015).

14.7.1.1 Sheridan Laser Tracheal® Tube

The Laser Tracheal® tube by Sheridan is a red-rubber tube wrapped with an initial layer of copper foil tape, overlaid by a water absorbent fabric that must be saturated before use. These tubes are compatible with CO_2 and KTP lasers but have a thicker wall, and therefore reduced I.D. with reduced airflow. They have a high-pressure, low-volume cuff and a standard 15-mm connector (Dorsch and Dorsch 2011b).

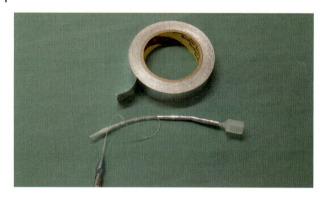

Figure 14.16 Endotracheal tube adapted for laser with aluminum wrap.

14.7.1.2   Laser-Shield II Tube
The Laser-Shield II tube is a silicone endotracheal tube with an outside Teflon coating and inner aluminum wrap, compatible with CO_2 and KTP lasers. The cuffs on these tubes are not laser resistant and a small portion of the proximal and distal end is also exposed. The Laser-Flex™ endotracheal tube will eventually replace these tubes.

14.7.1.3   Mallinckrodt™ Laser-Flex Endotracheal Tube
The Mallinckrodt™ Laser-Flex Endotracheal tube is a flexible, stainless steel Murphy-type, dual-cuffed, or Magill-type uncuffed endotracheal tube. Each has a standard 15-mm connector and incorporates a reinforced tube to prevent obstruction of the airway during extreme flexion. The surface reflects the beam of the laser and is compatible with the CO_2 and KTP lasers. The sizes available range from 3.0–4.0 mm I.D. for the Magill type, and 4.5–6.0 mm I.D. for the Murphy type, and they can be used for oral or nasal intubation. These tubes utilize a dual cuff technology with separate pilot lines to maintain and ensure proper endotracheal tube seal if the laser damages one cuff (Dorsch and Dorsch 2011b).

14.7.2   Placement Techniques

Intubation with these types of tubes is similar to standard intubation with oral or nasal endotracheal tubes. It is best practice to place these tubes using a rigid laryngoscope to visualize anatomical landmarks and a stylet to facilitate intubation.

14.7.3   Complications

Failure of the tube during the laser procedure could be catastrophic to the patient. Areas of the endotracheal tube that are not laser resistant, extreme proximal and distal ends, as well as the cuffs, can become exposed to the laser. Care should be taken to properly measure all endotracheal tubes prior to intubation. If reflective aluminum tape is used over manufactured laser endotracheal tubes, rough edges could potentially damage laryngeal and tracheal mucosa.

14.8   Single Lung Intubation

Certain thoracic surgeries require the isolation of one lung with the use of a double-lumen endotracheal or bronchial blocking tube. Bronchial blocking devices, unlike DLTs, are thin tubes than can be passed through a standard single lumen endotracheal tube into the main stem bronchus (Bussieres *et al.* 2016). DLTs are designed for human use and adapted for veterinary patients.

14.8.1   Description

14.8.1.1   Double Lumen Tubes (DLTs)
Double Lumen Tubes (DLTs) are two single lumen PVC tubes of different lengths combined in one apparatus. The longer tube is placed 1–2 cm into the bronchus and the shorter is used for tracheal intubation. Each tube has a separate channel, pilot balloon and endotracheal tube adapter. These are available as a left or right blocker, designating which lung they will fit best. The three most commonly used DLTs are the Robertshaw, Carlens and White (Mosley 2015). Each tube has two cuffs, one occludes the trachea and the other occludes the bronchus. These cuffs are often color coded, with corresponding pilot balloons, to differentiate between the two; the bronchial blocking cuff is blue and the tracheal cuff is white. The tube has an angled tip to help facilitate placement into the respective bronchus. The internal diameter of the tracheal portion is oval-shaped, with sizes ranging from 26–41 Fr, limiting the use of these tubes to patients between 5 and 20 kg (Mosley 2015).

Right-sided DLTs are used to help ventilate the right cranial lung lobe in humans, and are often less effective in the canine patient due to anatomical differences in the proximal end of the lung lobe. Left-sided DLTs are more effective in veterinary medicine and can be positioned to block either left- or right-sided thoracic cavities.

14.8.1.2   Endobronchial Blockers
Not as anatomically specific as DLTs, endobronchial blockers are adaptable for a wide range of patient sizes. These devices are long catheters made of silicone with an inflatable round or elliptical cuff, usually colored blue to differentiate between normal endotracheal tube cuffs (Figure 14.17). The most common types of endobronchial blockers are Arndt, Cohen and EZ-blocker. The EZ-blocker is unique in that it has a Y-shaped tip that can be placed at the bifurcation of the trachea into the separate bronchi (Niwal *et al.* 2011).

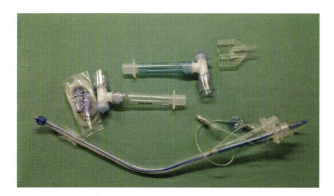

Figure 14.17 Endobronchial blocking tube for use in single lung ventilation techniques.

Swivel adapters are available to connect to the endotracheal tube to allow the anesthetist to pass the bronchial blocker coaxial with the endotracheal tube, or the blocker can be inserted into the trachea and advanced into either bronchus. There is typically an extra port on the adapter for a bronchoscope to assist in placement of these blockers.

As an alternative, if a bronchial blocker is not available, a Foley catheter can be used as a bronchial blocker, but they do not have the same color differentiation as the endotracheal tube. Bronchial blockers offer an advantage over DLTs in that they can be used to isolate separate lung lobes within the existing endotracheal tube (Mosley 2015).

14.8.2 Placement Techniques

Placement of endobronchial blockers is less complicated than DLTs, in that they can be placed through a pre-existing endotracheal tube into the bronchus of choice. Inflate the cuff prior to intubation to verify validity of the balloon. Disconnect the endotracheal tube from the breathing circuit and pass the tube inside the ET tube. A bronchoscope can then be passed to verify correct placement; insufflate the balloon, collapsing the lung lobe, and resume ventilation via the original endotracheal tube.

DLT cuffs should also be checked prior to placement. Then:

1) Place the stylet inside the tracheal tube channel.
2) Pass the DLT into the trachea, rotating toward the right or left side, depending on which lung field you want to ventilate.
3) Insufflate the tracheal cuff to ensure bilateral lung sounds.
4) Clamp the tracheal lumen temporarily; insufflate the bronchial balloon until there is no air leak.
5) Unclamp the tracheal lumen, verifying correct placement and that there is no obstruction of the opposite bronchi.
6) Clamp the bronchial lumen, and verify unilateral chest movement.

14.8.3 Complications

Less control of ventilation, inadvertent bronchial collapse, and inability to control anesthetic depth can be common complications from use of these devices (Dorsch and Dorsch 2011b). Bronchial blockers must be removed and placed in the contralateral bronchus in order to facilitate independent lung ventilation (Mosley 2015), and do not adapt to suction devices as effectively as DLTs (Niwal *et al.* 2011).

14.9 Stylets

The use of a stylet can help facilitate intubation of the patient. In smaller patients, visualization of the airway can be obscured by the use of a laryngoscope, and in larger patients, such as ruminants, the laryngoscope is often too small and ineffective in visualizing the larynx (Figure 14.18).

14.9.1 Description

The most common type of stylet is a plastic coated metal with a smooth distal end. These stylets are of small enough diameter to fit inside the endotracheal tube, and can be malleable to changes in shape (Quandt 2002). The proximal end of the stylet can come with an adjustable stopper or be bent to ensure the stylet does not protrude past the distal end of the endotracheal tube causing trauma to the trachea.

A bougie is a thin resin-coated, polyester-based stylet, airway exchange catheter or introducing guide. The classic bougie is usually a hollow tube with an angled or straight tip. The bougie can be shaped to help facilitate intubation by placing a wire into the shaft of the endotracheal tube (Figure 14.19).

A lighted intubation stylet or use of a flexible fiber optic scope can also be used to assist in more difficult intubation scenarios. The lighted intubation stylet has a handle with a malleable stylet covered in plastic with a light on the distal end. This technique is common in human medicine to illuminate the larynx and tissues during a "blind" intubation technique (Dorsch and Dorsch 2011b). A flexible fiber optic scope is more expensive and is preferred when patients are unable to be intubated using a rigid laryngoscope. The scope can be threaded inside the endotracheal tube and guide the insertion of the endotracheal tube past the larynx (Sanuki *et al.* 2011).

14.9.2 Placement Techniques

The use of a stylet can be accomplished by two different methods. The first technique can be accomplished by

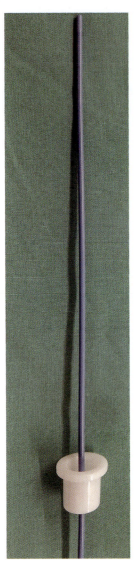

Figure 14.18 One example of a commonly used stylet in small animal intubation. The stylet is placed within the tracheal tube and the length is determined by adjusting the large adapter (bottom) to ensure the stylet tip is not distal to the tube opening.

sliding the plastic or metal stylet inside the endotracheal tube, careful not to extend past the end of the tube (Muir *et al.* 2000). This allows the anesthetist to change the shape of the endotracheal tube, aiding in intubation.

The use of a small wire, with a blunted end, plastic stylet or even smaller diameter endotracheal tube can be beneficial when conditions such as trauma or tissue enlargement obscure direct visualization of the larynx. The wire can be placed through the laryngeal folds, and an endotracheal tube is then passed over the wire. A small amount of pressure may need to be applied to slide past any enlarged tissue. The endotracheal tube is then secured and the wire or other facilitative device removed (Dorsch and Dorsch 2011b).

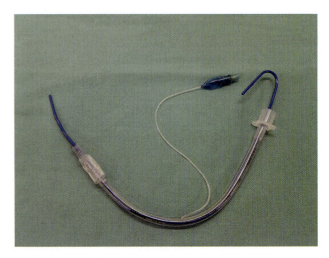

Figure 14.19 Example of a thin polyester coated bougie.

In large animal patients, such as ruminants and camelids, the use of a propylene plastic catheter can be used as described above, as a guide for an "over the wire" technique. More often, the anesthetist will have to use their hand to guide the catheter or endotracheal tube into place, as direct visualization of the larynx is almost impossible without use of a flexible lighted endoscope.

14.9.3 Complications

Caution must be taken when using a stylet as a primary guide for endotracheal intubation. Trauma to the laryngeal folds and esophagus, as well as tracheal rupture and endobronchial foreign body, can all result from inappropriate techniques. Accidental extubation can occur when removing the stylet from the endotracheal tube.

14.10 Cuff Pressure Manometers

The endotracheal tube cuff is the dynamic portion of the tube that is inflated to a pressure range, in order to form a seal with the walls of the trachea. LMAs and endobronchial tubes, as well as other types of airways, all use a cuff system. Under-inflated cuffs may lead to aspiration of stomach contents or allow for waste anesthetic gas leakage. Damage to the delicate tracheal walls can occur when the endotracheal tube cuff is over-inflated, leading to a high mucosal contact pressure and subsequent local ischemia (Bunegin *et al.* 1993). Optimal cuff pressures should be maintained in the range of 20–30 cmH_2O (Sengupta *et al.* 2004).

Of the typical techniques used to inflate the endotracheal tube cuff, none have proven to be accurate (Briganti *et al.* 2012; White *et al.* 2017). These traditional methods include direct palpation of the pilot balloon, minimal occlusive pressure of 20 cmH$_2$O and incremental deflation until an audible leak is heard. Direct measurement of cuff pressure with a manometer is recommended (Briganti *et al.* 2012).

Different products exist to help guide the anesthetist to properly inflate the airway tube cuff. Aneroid manometer cuff pressure inflators such as The Posey Cufflator™ Tracheal Cuff Inflator and Monitor (Posey® Company, Arcadia, CA) (Figure 14.20), the Rusch Endotest (Teleflex, Morrisville, NC) and the Ambu® Cuff Pressure Gauge (Ambu Inc, Columbia, MD) are designed to inflate and monitor the pressure in high-volume low-pressure endotracheal tube cuffs. These products can also be used with LMAs and endobronchial tubes. They all possess an easy-to-read gauge calibrated in cmH$_2$O, along with a one-handed operation design. The T.L.F Cuff (ICST Corporation, Saitama, Japan; Figure 14.21) is similar to the aneroid manometer-style pressure gauge, but with an LCD display and three inflation modes (T-mode [endotracheal tube], L-mode [LMA] and F-mode [no restrictions]). The screen is backlit for better visibility in low light and the display changes color with

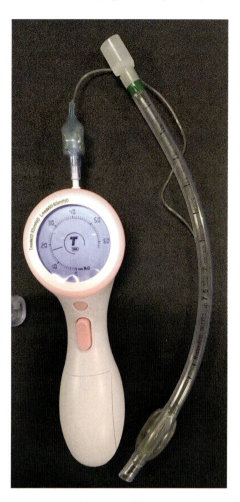

Figure 14.21 The T.L.F. Cuff has a digital display of the cuff pressure and three modes to ensure safe pressures are not exceeded in specific airway devices. This device is in T-mode and reads a pressure of 17 cmH$_2$O m (photograph courtesy of Dr Rebecca Johnson, University of Wisconsin-Madison, WI).

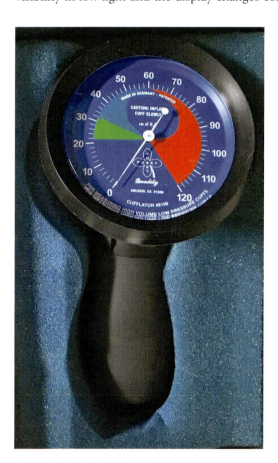

Figure 14.20 The Posey Cufflator used to measure pressure of the cuff in high-volume low-pressure endotracheal tubes (photograph courtesy of Dr Rebecca Johnson, University of Wisconsin-Madison, WI).

pressure changes. As an additional safety feature, the different modes do not allow additional pressure to be applied once the pre-set maximum is met (T-mode max is 32 cmH$_2$O; L- and F-mode maximum is 60 cmH$_2$O).

Other products include the Tru-Cuff (AES, Black Diamond, WA; Figure 14.22), a tracheal tube inflation syringe with cuff pressure indicator built in. It is available for both LMAs (cuff pressure of 40–60 cmH$_2$O) and small animal endotracheal tubes (20–30 cmH$_2$O). This product is less expensive but also less durable compared to the hand-held inflation manometers. The AG Cuffill is a similar device with a digital display for an accurate reading (Hospitech Respiration Ltd., Mercury Medical, Clearwater, FL). The PressureEasy Cuff-Pressure Controller (Smiths Medical, St Paul, MN; Figure 14.23) is a disposable single-patient use product that is used to rapidly inflate and maintain cuff pressures between 18

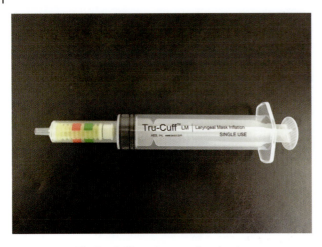

Figure 14.22 The Tru Cuff is an inexpensive, simple way to measure cuff pressure in LMAs (shown here) and tracheal tubes (photograph courtesy of Dr Rebecca Johnson, University of Wisconsin-Madison, WI).

and 27 cmH$_2$O. It has an optional adapter that can adjust the cuff pressure as intrathoracic pressures change, such as with mechanical ventilation.

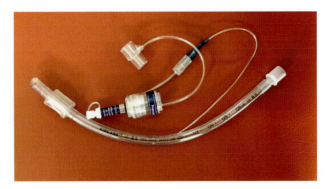

Figure 14.23 The PressureEasy Cuff-Pressure Controller is a disposable single-patient use monitor for cuff pressures. The cuff is inflated to a set pressure through a small tube attached to the pilot (blue). An optional adaptor (unattached in this picture) can be used on the tracheal tube to allow adjustments in cuff pressure with simultaneous changes in intrathoracic pressure (photograph courtesy of Dr Rebecca Johnson, University of Wisconsin-Madison, WI).

14.11   Summary

There are many options available to the practitioner to establish a patent airway. Each has its own advantages and disadvantages. However, most are easily placed and help in anesthetized patient management.

References

Aircare (2012) *Aircare® Endotracheal Tubes Instructions Manual.* Smiths Medical ASD, Inc.

V-gel (2014) *V-gel®® Advanced Veterinary Airway Management System Tech Sheet.* JorVet, Inc.

Barletta, M., Kleine, S.A. and Quandt, J.E. (2015) Assessment of v-gel® supraglottic airway device placement in cats performed by inexperienced veterinary students. *Vet Rec,* 10, 1136.

Boldizar, M., Pelikan, K., Repel, D., Vidrickova, P. and Sevcik, A. (2007) LMA ProSealTM in the veterinary anaesthesia – the animal is patient as well: 19AP2-3. *Eur J Anesth,* 24, 194.

Briganti, A., Portela, D.A., Barsotti, G., Romano, M. and Breghi, G. (2012) Evaluation of the endotracheal tube cuff pressure resulting from four different method of inflation in dogs. *Vet Anaesth Analg.* 39, 488–494.

Bunegin, L., Albin, M.S. and Smith, R.B. (1993) Canine tracheal blood flow after endotracheal tube cuff inflation during normtension and hypotension. *Anesth Analg,* 76(5), 1083–1090.

Bussieres, J., Somma, J., Del Castillo, J.L., Lemieux, J., Conti, M. *et al.* (2016) Bronchial blocker versus left double lumen endotracheal tube in video-assisted thoracoscopic surgery: a randomized-controlled trial examining time and quality of lung deflation. *Can J Anaesth,* 63, 818–827.

Campoy, L., Hughes, J.M., McAllister, H. and Bellenger, C.R. (2003) Kinking of endotracheal tubes during maximal flexion of the atlanto-occipital joint in dogs. *J Sm Anim Prac,* 44, 3–7.

Dorsch, J.A. and Dorsch, S.E. (2011a) Supraglottic airway devices. In: *A Practical Approach to Anesthesia Equipment.* Philadelphia, PA, Lippincott Williams & Wilkins, pp. 266–310.

Dorsch, J.A. and Dorsch, S.E. (2011b) Tracheal tubes and associated equipment. In: *A Practical Approach to Anesthesia Equipment.* Philadelphia, PA, Lippincott Williams & Wilkins, pp. 336–412.

Goldmann, K., Kalinowski, M. and Kraft, S. (2005) Airway management under general anaesthesia in pigs using LMA-ProSeal™: a pilot study. *Vet Anaesth and Analg,* 32, 308–313.

Hass, C.F., Eakin, R.M., Kinkle, M.A. and Blank, R. (2014) Endotracheal tubes: old and new. *Respir Care,* 59, 933–952.

Ismail, S., Bisher, N.A., Kandil, H.W., Mowafi, H.A. and Atawia, H.A. (2011) Intraocular pressure and hemodynamic responses to insertion of the i-gel, laryngeal mask airway or endotracheal tube. *Eur J Anaesth,* 28, 443–448.

Kissinger, J.T. and Hughes, H.C. (1984) Fabrication method for endotracheal tubes for sheep, goats, and calves. *Lab Anim Sci,* 34, 97–97.

Mosley, C.A. (2015) Anesthesia equipment. In: Grimm, K.A., Tranquilli, W.J., Greene, S.A. and Roberson, S.A. (eds). *Veterinary Anesthesia and Analgesia: The Fifth Edition of Lumb and Jones.* Ames, IA: John Wiley & Sons, Inc., pp. 23–84.

Muir, W., Hubbell, J.A., Skarda, R.T. and Bednarski, R.M. (2000) Anesthetic procedures and techniques in dogs and cats. In: *Handbook of Veterinary Anesthesia*, 3rd ed. St Louis, MO: Mosby, Inc., pp. 14–330.

Niwal, N., Ranganathan, P. and Divatia, J. (2011) Bronchial blocker for one-lung ventilation: an unanticipated complication. *Indian J Anaseth*, 55, 636–637.

Oostrom, H., Krauss, M. and Sap, R. (2013) A comparison between the v-gel® supraglottic airway device and the cuffed endotracheal tube for airway management in spontaneously breathing cats during isoflurane anaesthesia. *Vet Anaesth Analg*, 40, 265–271.

Quandt, J.E. (2002) Airway maintenance. In: Greene, S.A. (ed.). *Veterinary Anesthesia and Pain Management Secrets*. Philadelphia, PA: Hanley & Belfus, Inc., pp. 1–13.

Reed, F. and Iff, I. 2012. Use of a laryngeal mask airway in a brachycephalic dog with masticatory myositis and trismus. *Can Vet J*, 53, 287–290.

Sanuki, T., Son, H., Sugioka, A., Komi, N., Hirokane, M. et al. (2011) Comparison of metal stylet, small tracheal tube and combined introducer-aided insertions of flexible reinforced laryngeal mask airway with conventional method: a Manikin study. *J Anesth Clinic Res*, 2, 147.

Sengupta, P., Sessler, D.I., Maglinger, P., Wells, S., Vogt, A. et al. (2004) Endotracheal tube cuff pressure in three hospitals, and the volume required to produce an appropriate cuff pressure. *BMC Anesthesiol*, 4, 8.

Shelby, A.M. and McKune, C.M. (2014) Anesthesia in patients with concurrent disease. In: *Small Animal Anesthesia Techniques*. Ames, IA: John Wiley & Sons, Inc., pp. 172–173.

Soukup, J.W. and Snyder, C.J. (2015) Transmylohyoid orotracheal intubation in surgical management of canine maxillofacial fracture: an alternative to pharyngotomy endotracheal intubation. *Vet Surg*, 44, 432–436.

Toman, H., Erbas, M., Sahin, H., Kiraz, H.A., Uzun, M. and Ovali, M.A. (2015) Comparison of the effects of various airway devices on hemodynamic response and QTc interval in rabbits under general anesthesia. *J Clin Monit Comput*, 29, 727–732.

Uzun, M., Kiraz, H.A., Ovali, M.A., Sahin, H., Erbas, M. and Toman, H. (2015) The investigation of airway management capacity of v-gel® and cobra-PLA in anaesthetised rabbits. *Acta Cir Bras*, 30, 80–86.

Weiderstein, I.., Auer, U. and Moens, Y. (2006) Laryngeal mask airway insertion requires less propofol then endotracheal intubation in dogs. *Vet Anaesth Analg*, 33, 201–206.

Weiderstein, I. and Moens, Y. (2008) Guidelines and criteria for the placement of laryngeal mask airways in dogs. *Vet Anaesth Analg*, 35, 374–382.

White, D.M., Redondo, J.I., Mair, A.R. and Martinez-Taboada, F. (2017) The effect of user experience and inflation technique on endotracheal tube cuff pressure using a feline airway simulator. *Vet Anesth Analg*, 44, 1076–1084

15

Oxygen Delivery Systems

Jonathan Bach

School of Veterinary Medicine, University of Wisconsin, Madison, Wisconsin, USA

15.1 Introduction

Oxygen supplementation is an important aspect of veterinary care and typically occurs during one of three settings:

1) treatment of shock and resuscitation in emergencies;
2) supportive care of hospitalized critical care patients with hypoxemia; and
3) the management of anesthetic patients, including supplementing oxygen peri-anesthetically.

Nearly 40% of recovering anesthetic patients without pulmonary disease have transient hypoxemia (Jackson and Murison 2010).

Hypoxemia is a common indication to provide supplemental oxygen. While it is valuable to objectify the level of hypoxemia, measurement of an arterial blood gas or applying a pulse oximeter should not supersede providing supplemental oxygen to a patient in respiratory distress. Clinical signs of respiratory distress often include tachypnea, increased respiratory effort, orthopnea (head/neck extended and elbows abducted), and possibly cyanosis. However, cyanosis is an insensitive marker of hypoxemia.

Hypoxemia is defined as the partial pressure of arterial oxygen (PaO_2) of less than 80 mmHg; severe hypoxemia is defined as a PaO_2 of less than 60 mmHg. An arterial blood gas and measurement of PaO_2 is the gold standard determinant of hypoxemia. Since there may be limited access to blood gas analyzers and obtaining an arterial blood gas may be technically challenging, particularly in a patient suffering from respiratory distress, a pulse oximeter can be used to assess hypoxemia and a patient's response to supplemental oxygen (see Chapter 18).

The hemoglobin-oxygen dissociation curve depicts a relationship between PaO_2 and the percent of hemoglobin saturated with oxygen (SpO_2). The curve is dynamic and can be affected by temperature, pH, carbon dioxide in blood, and red blood cell 2–3 diphosphoglycerate

(2–3 DPG) levels. Regardless, SpO_2 can be used to estimate the PaO_2. In most species, an SpO_2 of approximately 94% correlates with a PaO_2 of approximately 80 mmHg (below which is hypoxemia), and an SpO_2 of approximately 90% correlates with a PaO_2 of approximately 60 mmHg (below which is *severe* hypoxemia). Caution should be exercised when interpreting values obtained on a pulse oximeter, which can obtain erroneous values from numerous causes, including motion artifact, weak pulse signal, pigmented tissues, and other causes. The heart rate obtained by the pulse oximeter should be similar to the patient's heart rate. In addition, the pulse quality measured by the pulse oximeter, either indicated by a series of LED lights or graphically on a plethysmograph, should indicate a strong signal.

15.2 Oxygen Supplementation Techniques

15.2.1 Flow-by Delivery

Flow-by oxygen is a simple and easy method (Figure 15.1) to achieve an increased fraction of inspired oxygen (F_IO_2). For example, in dogs, flow rates of 0.25 L/min–10 L/min held within 2 cm of the nose, achieve an average F_IO_2 of 37.2% (range: 29.5–48%). Flow rates of 0.5 L/min–10 L/min held 4 cm from the nose achieve an average F_IO_2 of 32.9% (range: 24.0–42.5%) (Loukopoulos and Reynolds 1997). Although technically easy and comprising some effectiveness, certain challenges with this technique should be recognized. High flow rates toward the patient's nose or face often lead to patient agitation, which can exacerbate respiratory distress as they attempt to avoid the high flow rates; most patients do not comply with continuously delivered flow-by oxygen within 2–4 cm of their nose. Flow-by oxygen requires an attentive staff member to hold the tubing near the patient's nose or mouth; higher oxygen flow rates are recommended for larger patients

Veterinary Anesthetic and Monitoring Equipment, First Edition. Edited by Kristen G. Cooley and Rebecca A. Johnson.
© 2018 John Wiley & Sons, Inc. Published 2018 by John Wiley & Sons, Inc.

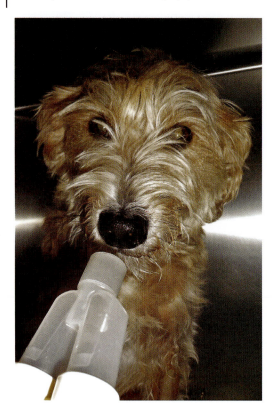

Figure 15.1 The technique of flow-by oxygen delivery to a dog. In this case, an anesthetic Y-piece and hoses are used for delivery.

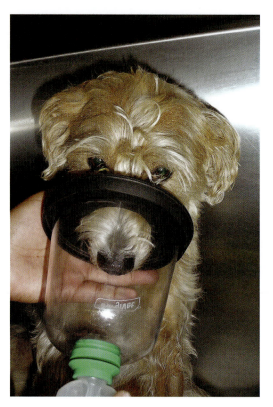

Figure 15.2 Administration of oxygen using a tight fitting mask in a dog. Note that, similar to flow-by oxygen, personnel must be present to ensure delivery.

(i.e. 5–10 L/min when >15 kg). In lieu of these challenges, it remains a commonly used approach for a patient presenting in respiratory distress, and pre- and post-anesthesia, and offers patient benefit, especially in short-term situations.

15.2.2 Mask Delivery

Supplemental oxygen delivered by a tight fitting mask with minimal leak (Figure 15.2), can achieve average F_IO_2 concentrations of 46.5% (range: 30.0–70.6%) in dogs (Loukopoulos and Reynolds 1997). However, many veterinary patients will actively move away from oxygen administered by mask. In addition, approximately one-third of people report feelings of suffocation when a non-rebreathing mask is utilized (Booth 2003). Similar to flow-by oxygen, an attentive staff member is often needed, and higher oxygen flow rates are recommended for larger patients. However, patients may not be able to move away from an oxygen mask (e.g. severely ill or injured, or moderately sedated patients). In such instances, an oxygen mask can be easily held in place by implementing a loose fitting muzzle around the device to keep it attached to the animal. An overly tight fitting mask may lead to hyperthermia and/or carbon dioxide

rebreathing, particularly when inspiratory gas flow rates are lower (<10 L/min) (Loukopoulos and Reynolds 1997).

In larger species, mask delivery of oxygen can be challenging, with varying efficacy. In respiratory depressed calves (induced by heavy sedation), mask administration of 5 L/min oxygen was well tolerated and increased PaO_2 moderately; however, addition of continuous positive airway pressure did not greatly affect PaO_2 (Donnelly *et al.* 2016). In contrast, non-sedated horses usually must be trained to the mask, and even at 10 L/min, this technique is not exceedingly successful in raising PaO_2 (Mason *et al.* 1987). Increasing the oxygen flow rates in horses with heaves increased the F_IO_2 to 60–80%, and PaO_2 increased from 66 mmHg to 108 mmHg (Dixon 1978); however, alternative techniques may be more tolerable and efficacious in large animals.

15.2.3 Nasal Administration

15.2.3.1 Traditional Nasal Delivery Techniques

Providing supplemental oxygen via one or two nasal catheters is a simple and practical technique for patients needing supplemental oxygen for extended periods (i.e. hours to days). An appropriately sized feeding tube (e.g. 3, 5, 8 or 10 French, possibly larger in larger species) is passed into the ventral meatus of the nasal cavity following application of topical anesthetic solution. The catheter is premeasured and advanced to the level of the medial canthus of the eye (Figure 15.3); water-soluble lubricant is applied to the catheter prior to placement, taking care not to plug the holes. After advancing the catheter to the desired level, it is secured at the mucocutaneous junction lateral to the alar fold. Utilizing a butterfly tape tab works well, as does the Chinese finger trap suture pattern. Few patients require systemic sedation for the procedure; however, when required, intravenous sedatives such as butorphanol (0.1–0.4 mg/kg) or dexmedetomidine (1–3 μg/kg) may be used for this procedure in small animals, depending on the individual patient's condition and co-morbidities. In addition, nasal prongs, which are manufactured for human use and only advance approximately 1 cm into the nasal passages, can be used as well (Figure 15.4). The cinch can be tightened behind the patient's ears. Nasal oxygen catheters can preemptively be placed in patients under general anesthesia, who are likely to need ongoing supplemental oxygen upon recovery.

Following placement of a nasal catheter, an Elizabethan collar is required in most patients to prevent tube dislodgement. Dry cold air can result in turbinate desiccation and jet lesions to the mucosa. Thus, nasal oxygen is routinely humidified with a bubbler (Figure 15.5). The bubblers are cleaned or sterilized between patients. Unfortunately, bubble humidifiers do not routinely provide adequate relative humidity and mucosal injuries may still occur, especially at high flow rates (Darin *et al.* 1982). When dogs breath quietly, the F_IO_2 delivered via nasal catheter(s) is reliably increased (Table 15.1) (Fitzpatrick and Crowe 1986; Dunphy *et al.* 2002). It is unknown how effective nasal oxygen delivery is when dogs pant or breathe through the mouth. In such cases, it is likely preferable to advance nasal catheters into the nasopharynx; the base of the ear is used as the external measurement landmark (Figure 15.6).

In larger species, nasal oxygen delivery (catheter measured to the medial canthus of the eye as previously described) increases F_IO_2 in normal and premature foals (Rose *et al.* 1983; Stewart *et al.* 1984). In normal adult horses, nasal oxygen delivery in a single catheter at rates of up to 15 L/min increased F_IO_2 and PaO_2 from a baseline of approximately 21% and 102 mmHg to approximately

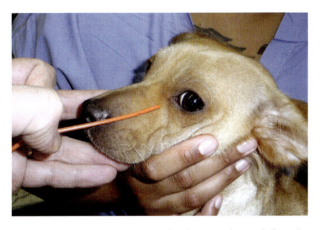

Figure 15.3 Pre-measuring a nasal catheter to the medial canthus of the eye in a dog.

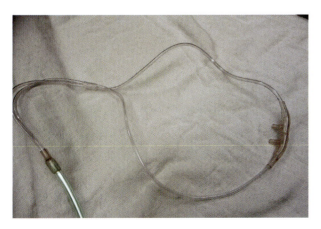

Figure 15.4 Example of commercially available nasal prongs that are placed in both nostrils and wrapped behind the ears to secure.

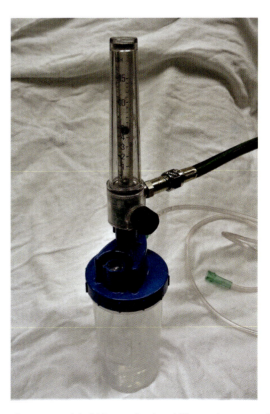

Figure 15.5 A bubbler used to humidify nasal oxygen prior to administration.

Table 15.1 F_IO_2 concentrations (mean ± standard deviation) in dogs administered supplemental oxygen via nasal catheter(s) at varying flow rates (modified from Dunphy *et al.* 2002).

Oxygen Flow Rate	Unilateral Nasal Catheter	Bilateral Nasal Catheters
50 mL/kg/min	29.8 ± 5.6	36.4 ± 5.9
100 mL/kg/min	37.3 ± 5.7	56.0 ± 11.9
200 mL/kg/min	57.9 ± 12.7	77.3 ± 13.5

49.5% and 249 mmHg, respectively (Wilson *et al.* 2006). When bilateral nasal catheters were placed and 15 L/min delivered into both nostrils (total of 30 L/min), F_IO_2 and PaO_2 increased to approximately 71.2% and 319 mmHg, respectively (Wilson *et al.* 2006). Interestingly, in horses with recurrent airway obstruction, PaO_2 also increased with unilateral or bilateral nasal oxygen delivery; however, values were always lower than in their normal counterparts (Wilson *et al.* 2006). Flow rates of 20 L/min were well tolerated, but 30 L/min was associated with some coughing and gagging (Wilson *et al.* 2006).

15.2.3.2 Newer Nasal Delivery Techniques

A novel technique for administering oxygen in small animals, called high flow oxygen therapy (HFOT), has become available. The technology utilizes an integrated heated, medical grade vapor humidification system, which provides warmed, fully humidified oxygen. Supplemental oxygen can be delivered without causing desiccation of the nasal mucosa, and higher flow rates may be delivered. Traditional nasal oxygen flow rates are not able to exceed 8–10 L/min; HFOT devices can achieve 40–70 L/min (Dysart *et al.* 2009). A case series of six dogs described successful increases in PaO_2 after changing from traditional nasal oxygen to HFOT deliv-

ered at flow rates of 0.5–1.7 L/kg/min (Keir *et al.* 2016). HFOT requires specialized equipment, and its use is currently limited. However, it may become more widely utilized and affordable.

15.2.4 Oxygen Hood or Elizabethan Collar

Supplemental oxygen may be provided via commercially available oxygen hoods (Figure 15.7). An oxygen line is passed into the hood along the patient's neck, and adhered to the side of the hood. The amount the cover is open can be modified by opening or closing the zipper. It should remain approximately 25% open to allow CO_2 and heat to escape. Alternatively, the front of an Elizabethan collar can be covered with saran wrap; an open vent at the top is made to allow CO_2 and heat to escape. An oxygen hood or Elizabethan collar has the advantages of being affordable, not requiring advanced equipment, and the patient is highly accessible. Delivered oxygen concentrations will vary; concentrations are affected by oxygen flow rates, how snug the collar is on the patient's neck, size of the vent hole, and respiratory rate. In small animals, F_IO_2 concentrations of 34.8–48.6% can be achieved when oxygen is delivered at 0.75 L/min (Loukopoulos and Reynolds 1996). Alternatively, F_IO_2 concentrations of 95% could be achieved with flow rates of 300 mL/kg/min (Crowe 1995).

15.2.5 Oxygen Cage

An oxygen cage provides a sealed environment in which supplemental oxygen can be delivered; F_IO_2 concentrations can be set to a desired level, typically to a maximum of 60% (Figure 15.8). The oxygen cage can also regulate temperature, humidity, and eliminate accumulated CO_2. Custom-built oxygen cages that utilize a Plexiglas front to replace

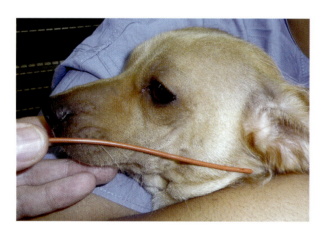

Figure 15.6 Pre-measuring a nasal catheter to the ear base to approximate the nasopharynx in dogs that may be panting or open-mouth breathing.

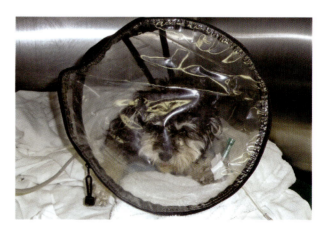

Figure 15.7 An oxygen hood used to deliver increased inspired oxygen levels to a dog. The tubing is placed inside the hood near the patient's neck. The green tubing end taped to the front of the clear hood delivers the oxygen.

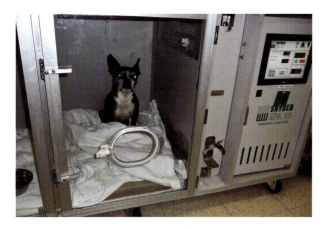

Figure 15.8 A dog in the oxygen cage with an inside temperature of 74°F, humidity of 71% and an inspired concentration of 37% O_2.

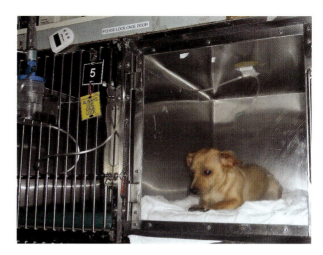

Figure 15.9 The use of a Plexiglas cage door in a conventional dog cage. Although this helps to increase the inspired oxygen levels (using the tubing seen here), it does not allow control of environmental conditions or CO_2 removal.

cage bars are not able to control environmental settings, and risk CO_2 accumulation (Figure 15.9). Oxygen cages are a non-invasive method to deliver supplemental oxygen. However, they are costly pieces of equipment, and consume large amounts of oxygen. Patients in an oxygen cage are effectively semi-isolated from clinicians and nursing staff, limiting access. Additionally, when the door is opened, the elevated interior F_1O_2 concentrations rapidly equilibrate with room air; during this period, patients may deteriorate. Supplemental oxygen administration via another route (e.g. face mask, flow by) is advised for patients that are highly oxygen dependent when cage doors are opened.

15.2.6 Transtracheal Oxygen

Transtracheal oxygen administration is rarely utilized in small animal practice, although the technique is highly effective in increasing F_1O_2 and subsequently PaO_2 levels; it has also been used in foals (Hoffman and Viel 1992). In small animals, lower oxygen flow rates are recommended (10 mL/kg/min), which may achieve up to 97% hemoglobin saturation in dogs; flow rates may need to be gradually increased for patients with severe parenchymal disease (Mann *et al.* 1992). Recommended oxygen flow rates in foals are 5–10 L/min (Hoffman and Viel 1992). Placement of a transtracheal catheter involves sterilely preparing the skin on the neck over the trachea, instillation of local anesthetic, and placement of a large catheter (e.g. 12–16 gauge) between two tracheal rings

relatively close to the larynx. The catheter is advanced down the trachea toward the tracheal bifurcation, the needle is removed, and the catheter secured with suture and a light bandage. Transtracheal catheter placement should be avoided in coagulopathic patients, those with tracheal collapse, and patients with pyoderma affecting the ventral neck at the insertion site.

15.3 Hyperbaric Oxygen

Hyperbaric oxygen therapy has limited applications, and is rarely utilized in the treatment of primary pulmonary diseases. Severe carbon monoxide (CO) poisoning is a valid application of this treatment. Patients with CO poisoning have carboxyhemoglobin, which is unable to deliver oxygen to tissues; by increasing the amount of oxygen dissolved in plasma through the use of higher pressure (thus, hyperbaric), adequate oxygen delivery can be achieved. Additionally, high oxygen concentrations shorten the half-life of CO and hasten recovery (Jasani 2015). Treatment sessions are administered within a specialized contained chamber that is pressurized to 1 or 2 atmospheres while 100% oxygen is administered. Patients are inaccessible during treatments, and costly equipment is required.

References

Booth, J.L. (2003) Nose breathing mask for a medical patient; and method. US 20050051171 A1. United States patent application US 10/369,743. Available from: http://www.google.sr/patents/US20050051171 [Accessed September 10, 2003].

Crowe, D.T. (1995) Use of an oxygen collar. *Vet Pract*, 7, 27–28.

Darin, J., Broadwell, J. and MacDonell, R. (1982) An evaluation of water-vapor output from four brands of unheated, prefilled bubble humidifiers. *Respir Care*, 27, 41–50.

Dixon, P.M. (1978) Pulmonary artery pressures in normal horses and in horses affected with chronic obstructive pulmonary disease. *Equine Vet J*, 10, 195–198.

Donnelly, C.G., Quinn, C.T., Nielsen, S.G. and Raidal, S.L. (2016) Respiratory support for pharmacologically induced hypoxia in neonatal calves. *Vet Med Int*, EPub ahead of print.

Dunphy, E.D., Mann, F.A., Dodam, J.R., Branson, K.R., Wagner-Mann, C.C. *et al.* (2002) Comparison of unilateral versus bilateral nasal catheters for oxygen administration in dogs. *J Vet Emerg Crit Care*, 12, 245–251.

Dysart, K., Miller, T.L., Wolfson, M.R. and Shaffer, T.H. (2009) Research in high flow therapy: mechanisms of action. *Respir Med*, 103, 1400–1405.

Fitzpatrick, R.K. and Crowe, D.T. (1986) Nasal oxygen administration in dogs and cats: experimental and clinical investigations. *J Am Anim Hosp Assoc*, 22, 293–300.

Hoffman, A.M. and Viel, L. (1992) A percutaneous transtracheal catheter system for improved oxygenation in foals with respiratory distress. *Equine Vet J*, 24, 239–241.

Jackson, Z.E. and Murison, P.J. (2010) Influence of oxygen supplementation on hypoxaemia during recovery from anaesthesia in dogs. *Vet Rec*, 166, 142.

Jasani, S. (2015) Smoke inhalation. In: Silverstein, D. and Hopper, K. (eds). *Small Animal Critical Care Medicine*, 2nd ed. St Louis, MO: Elsevier, pp. 785–788.

Keir, I., Daly, J., Haggerty, J. and Guenther, C. (2016) Retrospective evaluation of the effect of high flow oxygen therapy delivered by nasal cannula on PaO$_2$ in dogs with moderate-to-severe hypoxemia. *J Vet Emerg Crit Care*, 26, 598–602.

Loukopoulos, P. and Reynolds, W. (1996) Comparative evaluation of oxygen therapy techniques in anaesthetised dogs: Intranasal catheter and Elizabethan collar canopy. *Austral Vet Pract*, 26, 199.

Loukopoulos, P. and Reynolds, W. (1997) Comparative evaluation of oxygen therapy techniques in anaesthetised dogs: face mask and flow-by technique. *Austral Vet Pract*, 27, 34–39.

Mann, F.A., Wagner-Mann, C., Allert, J.A. and Smith, J. (1992) Comparison of intranasal and intratracheal oxygen administration in healthy awake dogs. *Am J Vet Res*, 53, 856–860.

Mason, D.E., Muir, W.W. and Wade, A. (1987) Arterial blood gas tensions in the horse during recovery from anesthesia. *J Am Vet Med Ass*, 190, 989–994.

Rose, R.J., Hodgson, D.R., Leadon, D.P. and Rossdale, P.D. (1983) Effect of intranasal oxygen administration on arterial blood gas and acid base parameters in spontaneously delivered, term induced and induced premature foals. *Res Vet Sci*, 34, 159–162.

Stewart, J.H., Rose, R.J. and Barko, A.M. (1984) Response to oxygen administration in foals: effect of age, duration and method of administration on arterial blood gas values. *Equine Vet J*, 16, 329–331.

Wilson, D.V., Schott, H.C. Robinson, N.E., Berney, C.E. and Eberhart, S.W. (2006) Response to nasopharyngeal oxygen administration in horses with lung disease. *Equine Vet J*, 38, 219–223.

16

Gas Monitoring

Louise O'Dwyer

Clinical Support Manager, VetsNow, Dunfermline, UK

16.1   Introduction

Respiratory gas monitoring is an essential part of anesthesia in which oxygen, nitrous oxide, carbon dioxide and inhalant levels are measured. Inspired and expired gas monitoring ensures that gas going to (and from) the patient contains sufficient amounts of oxygen and volatile agents, which helps to prevent hypoxemia and aids in maintaining a stable anesthetic plane. Gas monitoring via capnography will also ensure adequacy of ventilation and provides information concerning circulation. Gas monitoring, although once believed to be expensive and a "luxury", is now becoming commonplace in veterinary practice.

16.2   Capnometry/Capnography

16.2.1   Physiology

Carbon dioxide (CO_2) is transported in the body in three forms:

1) as bicarbonate ions (60–70%);
2) bound to protein (20–30%); and
3) dissolved in plasma (5–10%; Marshall 2004).

Only the dissolved form is measured during arterial blood gas analysis as the partial pressure of carbon dioxide ($PaCO_2$). End-tidal carbon dioxide ($ETCO_2$) measures expired CO_2 from the alveoli by a sensor or adaptor placed at the end of the tracheal tube or a catheter fed down the trachea (uncommon). Under normal circumstances, $ETCO_2$ typically underestimates the $PaCO_2$ by a clinically insignificant 2–5 mmHg (Marshall 2004). Therefore, because of the extremely close proximity of gas exchange between the alveoli and pulmonary capillaries, in the normal animal, $ETCO_2 \sim PaCO_2 \sim$ alveolar

CO_2 ($PACO_2$) (Reuss-Lamsky 2010). These relationships hold true, assuming that:

1) Capillary blood and alveolar gas CO_2 are in equilibrium.
2) End-tidal CO_2 approximates the time weighted average of the ventilation weighted $PaCO_2$.
3) Significant ventilation/perfusion (V/Q) mismatch does not exist.
4) Tidal volumes are large enough to displace dead space.
5) Fresh gas flow is low enough to prevent dilution, and sample aspiration is low enough not to entrain gas or interfere with patient ventilation.

Fundamentally, the basis of CO_2 measurement is simple: cells produce CO_2, which is carried to the lungs and expelled from the body when expiration occurs. All cells within the body undergo respiration; that is, they take in oxygen, use sugars and release energy and CO_2 as a byproduct. The rate of CO_2 production is usually directly related to metabolic rate. For example, if an animal is running, the metabolic rate will be greater than if that animal was sleeping. Most anesthetized patients will have a steady, low metabolic rate with little variation in exertion or effort and hence metabolic rate remains fairly constant.

CO_2 produced in cells is brought to the right side of the heart via venous blood, which is rich in CO_2 (~50 mmHg $PvCO_2$). It travels through the pulmonary artery to the lungs and rapidly diffuses into the alveoli until the levels in the alveoli and pulmonary circulation are equal. The blood leaving the lungs is now rich in newly acquired oxygen and has CO_2 levels of approximately 40 mmHg. Blood travelling from the lungs has not lost all of its CO_2 (e.g. 50 mmHg arrives to the lungs, 40 mmHg leaves the lungs); the amount left in the blood that returns to the left side of the heart is at the same level as in the alveoli (Simpson 2014a,b).

Veterinary Anesthetic and Monitoring Equipment, First Edition. Edited by Kristen G. Cooley and Rebecca A. Johnson.
© 2018 John Wiley & Sons, Inc. Published 2018 by John Wiley & Sons, Inc.

CO_2 levels are closely related to the blood pH. Changes in CO_2 levels result in changes in blood pH, which has dramatic effects on ventilation, organ perfusion and oxygen carriage (Reuss-Lamky 2010; Simpson 2014a). If homeostasis is disrupted (e.g. with anesthetic or analgesic agents), physiologic changes occur, depending on severity and duration of CO_2 alteration. For example, elevated CO_2 levels may result in cerebral vasodilation and increased cranial pressure, peripheral vasodilation through direct effects, secondary tachycardia, and eventual peripheral vasoconstriction via the sympathetic nervous system. In addition, CNS and myocardial depression are common with severe cases. Variations in CO_2 levels quickly change respiratory drive and alter the oxygen loading/unloading due to shifts in the oxygen-hemoglobin dissociation curve.

16.2.2 Measurement Technique

Since 1943, when Luft introduced the first CO_2-measuring and recording device based on the principle that carbon dioxide absorbs infrared light, capnography has become an essential part of monitoring anesthetized and critical care patients (Krauss and Hess 2007). Since that time, other methods of measuring end-tidal CO_2 ($ETCO_2$) have been documented (e.g. laser-based molecular correlation spectrography, Raman spectrography, magnetic-based mass spectrography, and photoacoustic spectrography), but infrared technology (see below), as well as colorimetric methods, remain the most compact, least expensive, and most popular method of $ETCO_2$ measurement.

Capnography produces a graphical representation of CO_2 levels over time, usually in addition to displaying numerical measurements as those seen in capnometry. However, the two terms have been (incorrectly) used interchangeably in some instances. Colorimetric methods are currently used as qualitative monitors of $ETCO_2$, but do not display precise numbers (e.g. Colorimetric CO_2 Detector, Covidien Ltd., Dublin, Ireland). These methods change color due to changes in the pH, as carbonic acid is formed as a product of the reaction between CO_2 and water (Long *et al.* 2017). For quantitative information, capnometry is required.

The use of capnography reduces the need to obtain repeated arterial blood gas samples, therefore providing a useful non-invasive monitoring and diagnostic tool (Marshall 2004). Another alternative to arterial blood gas analysis (see below) is the use of transcutaneous PCO_2 sensors that use Severinghaus temperature-stabilized, tissue CO_2 electrodes (e.g. SenTec Digital Monitoring System, SenTec Inc., Fenton, MO) (Huttmann *et al.* 2014). However, the use of these monitors is not widespread in veterinary medicine.

$ETCO_2$ is a product of three major determinants:

1) the rate of CO_2 production by the tissues (metabolism);
2) the rate of exchange of CO_2 from the blood to the alveoli (cardiac output); and
3) the rate of CO_2 removal by alveolar ventilation [(tidal volume − dead space) × frequency].

Thus, $ETCO_2$ provides information regarding metabolism, circulation and ventilation. For example, it is useful during anesthesia, when effects of injectable drugs and inhalants are likely to cause respiratory depression, or during long-term ventilatory assistance with the use of a mechanical ventilator. Normal $ETCO_2$ values in most non-anesthetized patients are approximately 35–45 mmHg (Marshall 2004), but vary somewhat by species. Readers are referred to other physiology books for further details. During anesthesia, end-tidal CO_2 values greater than 45 mmHg may indicate that either there is an excess production of CO_2 (infrequent) or there is a degree of hypoventilation. A strong indication for mechanical (or manual) ventilation is severe, prolonged hypoventilation, with a $PaCO_2$ (or $ETCO_2$) approaching 60 mmHg or greater (Hopper 2012).

In addition, capnography is also superior over pulse oximetry for the prompt identification of apnea and circulatory issues. Changes in the percentage of hemoglobin saturated with oxygen as read by pulse oximetry (SpO_2) will be delayed as compared to the instantaneous changes that occur with $ETCO_2$ when the next breath fails detection. For example, an abrupt decrease in $ETCO_2$ can be an early and reliable indication of an impending cardiovascular collapse or cardiac arrest when the patient is inspiring 100% O_2. In addition, since delivery of CO_2 from the lungs requires blood flow, cellular metabolism and alveolar ventilation, the presence of $ETCO_2$ can also be used to assess the effectiveness of cardio-pulmonary cerebral resuscitation (CPCR) efforts (Jandrey 2006).

As previously mentioned, most capnographs used in clinical monitoring use infrared absorption spectroscopy to determine the concentration of carbon dioxide in the expired gas. Infrared light, at wavelengths absorbed by CO_2, is passed through the expired gas sample and the concentration is determined according to the Lambert-Beer law, which says that the amount of infrared light absorbed is proportional to the amount of absorbing substance. Capnography is a more straightforward technology than pulse oximetry, in that the sample is removed from the patient and is not subject to corrections for patient's background interference (Jandrey 2006).

16.2.3 Units of CO_2 Measurement

CO_2 is quantified in mmHg, percent or kPa. Most capnographs have the option to switch between units. The average atmospheric pressure at sea level is approximately

760 mmHg. If the reported CO_2 value is 40 mmHg, that represents $40/760 \times 100\% = 5.3\%$. In locations with lower atmospheric pressure (e.g. ~625 mmHg), the same partial pressure of 40 mmHg would represent a percentage value of $40/625 \times 100\% = 6.4\%$. As a rough guide, conversion from mmHg to percent is a division by 8 (the actual value should be division by 7.6, but 8 will approximate values near enough for making clinical decisions (e.g. 45 mmHg = 45/8 or ~5.5%). Some countries use kPa as the unit of measure for capnography. Because atmospheric pressure in kPa is around 100 kPa (actually value is 101.3 kPa), it means that the partial pressure in kPa is practically the same as the number in percent (i.e. 5.1 kPa = $5.1/101.3 \times 100\% = 5.03\%$). This small error of less than 0.1% is likely to not be clinically relevant; thus, as sea level, kPa can be approximated by the percent and vice versa.

16.2.4 Infrared Light Absorption Technology

Although capnometers may use infrared technology, colorimetric detectors, Raman scattering or mass spectroscopy for measurement of CO_2, the most commonly used is the previously mentioned infrared light absorption. Mass spectroscopy is also used and separates gases and vapors of differing molecular weights; this is discussed in detail later. Mass spectroscopy units are more expensive and bulkier than infrared units, and are generally considered impractical for the majority of veterinary clinics, but may be seen in referral centers.

Infrared light is invisible to the human eye and has a lower frequency wavelength than red light (hence infrared). Infrared light absorption uses the principle that polyatomic gases (non-elemental gases, i.e. nitrous oxide and CO_2 with two or more dissimilar elements) and water vapor selectively absorb infrared light (Davis and Kenny 2007b). For example, CO_2 maximally absorbs light with a wavelength of 4.3 μm. The infrared light is emitted by a hot wire and the frequency needed is obtained as the radiation is passed through a filter. Infrared technology uses either solid-state or non-solid-state detectors. Solid-state detectors are durable and use a beam splitter to measure the light at two wavelengths, one that is absorbed by CO_2 and a reference sample.

Non-solid-state detectors use a chopper wheel that can measure the sample, a sealed reference gas and no gas to determine the absorbance of CO_2. Although the sample is easier to amplify and has less drift, these detectors are fragile. The amount of light absorbed by CO_2 (measured with capnometry) is directly proportional to the concentration of absorbing molecules (Davis and Kenny 2007b). Infrared CO_2 monitoring does have limitations. For example, water vapor condensation interferes with $ETCO_2$ values (Marshall 2004). In addition, collision broadening (discussed below) occurs when two gases have similar absorbance wavelengths, collide with each other and the energy at which they absorb infrared radiation is altered slightly (e.g. nitrous oxide, which absorbs wavelengths of 4.5 μm and CO_2 at 4.3 μm; Davis and Kenny 2007b).

16.2.5 Mainstream Monitors

Mainstream or sidestream capnometry describes the location of the measurement chamber or airway sampling site. Mainstream capnometers place the measurement chamber within the airways, at the head of the ET tube, so all exhaled gas passes through the chamber itself. The absorbance is quantified with a detector on the opposite side of the chamber and thus, must be made of material that allows infrared light to pass through, such as sapphire. Mainstream technology allows for an almost instantaneous measurement of CO_2 (fast response time). However, the sensors are easily damaged, increase mechanical dead space, and water condensation (infrequent due to sensor heating) or secretions on the sensor interfere with readings (Figure 16.1). Recently, more lightweight, battery powered mainstream devices have shown excellent promise in veterinary medicine (Figure 16.2; EMMA Mainstream Capnometer, Masimo, Irvine, CA). They have minimal warm-up time, are somewhat durable and display a numerical bar graph with the measurements; capnography is also available on some monitors.

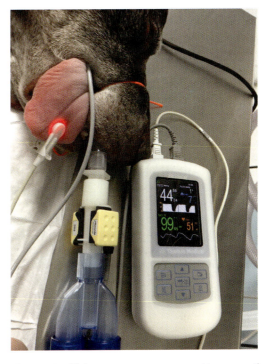

Figure 16.1 Mainstream capnometer used in an anesthetized dog. The sensor is usually made from sapphire for optimal infrared light transmittance. The response time is fast; however, the sensor is heavy for small patients and can accumulate secretions.

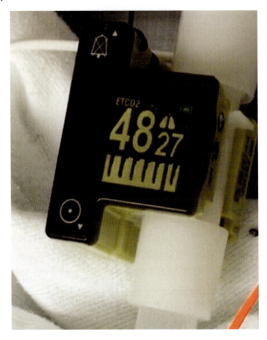

Figure 16.2 Example of a portable, battery operated mainstream capnograph (EMMA, Masimo, Irvine, CA).

16.2.6 Sidestream Monitors

Sidestream capnometers continually aspirate gas from the airway through fine bore tubing and transport it to a distant analyzing sensor outside the device (Figure 16.3). An advantage is that the units often measure other gases as well (i.e. O_2, inhalants) and the adapters are light-weight. However, slight delays in measurement (longer response time) may occur due to long tubing, and this technique becomes inaccurate in small patients with small tidal volumes. For example, the sampling rate is the rate at which the unit draws gas, and is frequently between 50 and 200 mL/minute. This volume can become significant, as removing even 50 mL/min in a patient with only a 30 mL tidal volume (e.g. a small kitten) would draw all of the expired breath as well as additional fresh gas. This will artificially lower the $ETCO_2$ and be reflected in poor, small waveforms. High respiratory rates can also result in an under-estimation of the $ETCO_2$ value, due to inadequate alveolar emptying. In this situation, the response time of the analyzer may be reprogrammed to less than the respiratory cycle time of the patient. In addition, secretions from the airway may easily obstruct the tubing.

Many manufacturers of sidestream capnometers exist for veterinary patients including, but not limited to, LifeSense® and RespSense™ (Nonin Medical Incorporated, Plymouth, MN), Nellcor™ N-85 Monitor and Microstream™ Capnography (Medtronic, Covidien, Minneapolis, MN), V9004 Series Capnograph (Surgivet, Smiths Medical,

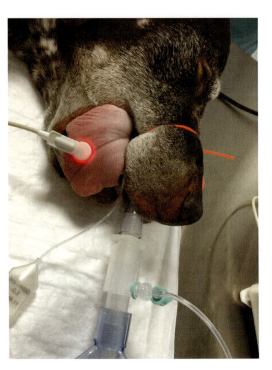

Figure 16.3 Sidestream capnometry used in an anesthetized dog. The adaptor draws the sample away from the patient to a distant site for analysis. The port should be vertically placed to reduce the amount of water condensation transported to the unit. These devices incorporate filters and water traps to reduce this problem.

Dublin, OH), Capnocheck II® (Smiths Medical, Dublin, OH), Novametrix Tidal Wave (DRE Veterinary, Avante Health Solutions, Louisville, KY), and (ISA™ CO_2 Module, Masimo, Irvine, CA) among others. All have unique features and many can incorporate pulse oximetry or inhalant analyses (ISA™) as well. For example, some monitors draw very low volumes of gas, making them useful in small patients (Nellcor™ Microstream™). In addition, some are available with both mainstream and sidestream technology (Tidal Wave). Readers are referred to the specific manufacturer's website for more detailed information.

16.2.6.1 Sampling Issues

The analyzer response time is comprised of two factors:

1) the delay or transit time, which is the time it takes for the sample to travel from the patient's airway to the analyzer itself; and
2) the rise time, which is the time required for an analyzer to respond to within 90–95% of a change in gas concentration.

The rise time depends on the sample chamber and the gas flow (Davis and Kenny 2007b). Sidestream monitors typically have longer response times than mainstream monitors; however, use of short, narrow lines helps to reduce response times. In addition, scavenging of the sample must occur when expired gases containing volatile agents are sampled; frequently the excess sample is returned to the breathing system or is scavenged with a passive scavenger.

Atmospheric pressure does not affect $ETCO_2$ readings, as most capnometers have internal calibration devices that adjust for atmospheric changes. In addition, halogenated anesthetic agents absorb infrared light at different wavelengths, and their concentrations are generally very low in the gaseous mixture, thus their presence does not significantly affect levels. However, as described above, dilution of the sample by other gases may result in falsely low $ETCO_2$ values and affect the waveform shape. This is more frequently seen with sidestream units rather than mainstream analysis, and this issue can be compensated for by reducing the fresh gas flow rate to 10–30 mL/kg/min, which is generally considered a moderate flow rate for anesthesia maintenance (Marshall 2004).

16.2.6.2 Positioning

When using sidestream capnographs, the sampling line is connected to the common gas flow portion of the circuit (i.e. where both inspired and expired gas is flowing). Usually this is at the end of the endotracheal tube, before it connects to the Y-piece connector. The adaptors range from low dead space adaptors for very small patients (Figure 16.4) to in-line adaptors where the sampling line connects for larger patients (Figure 16.3). Care should be taken that the sampling line does not fill with fluid; this is usually accomplished with inclusion of complicated filters or water traps in the system. The sidestream sampling take-off point should be pointed upward, so that it is always at the highest vertical point, reducing the amount of condensation accumulating in the sampling line, prolonging the filter life and protecting the sensor from damage.

16.2.7 Capnogram Interpretation

The normal capnogram (www.capnometry.com) (Figure 16.5) compares the CO_2 level on the *y*-axis with time on the *x*-axis. In most normal mammals, $ETCO_2$ is

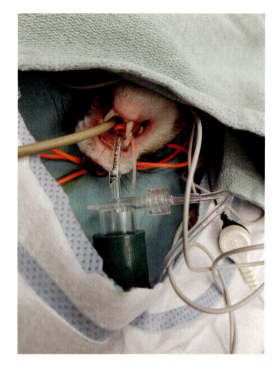

Figure 16.4 Example of a low dead space adapter used for sidestream capnometry in an anesthetized ferret. This adapter helps to reduce response time and increases accuracy due to low volumes.

approximately 35–45 mmHg, or 4.5–5.0%. The inspired $ETCO_2$ should closely approach zero. Newer, standardized terminology divides the capnogram into four main phrases:

Phase I: Phase I starts at the end of inspiration as the direction of gas flow reverses with expiration. During early expiration, the exhaled gas comes from anatomic dead space; this gas has not undergone any gas exchange, and as a result the gas from this area is identical to inspired gas (i.e. contains no CO_2).

Phase II: Phase II is where the upstroke of the waveform corresponds to the part of exhalation where CO_2-containing alveolar gas starts to be exhaled in a mixture with gas from the anatomical dead space. As expiration continues, the expired gas is composed of rapidly

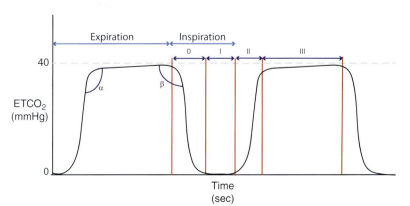

Figure 16.5 The normal capnogram is divided into 4 main phases. Phase 0: rapid downstroke of inspiration; Phase I: end inspiration; Phase II: expiratory upstroke; and Phase III: end-expiratory plateau. The alpha angle should measure 100–110 degrees between Phases II and III; the beta angle should be ~90 degrees between Phase III and 0.

increasing proportions of alveolar gas, and the CO_2 levels quickly begin to rise.

Phase III and Phase IV: The plateau of the capnogram is the point where $ETCO_2$ is normally almost constant as alveolar gas is exhaled and is termed Phase III. $ETCO_2$ is measured as the maximal value at the end of Phase III, just prior to inspiration. Expiration ends partway through this phase and is usually followed by a pause. During this pause, $ETCO_2$ does not greatly change on the capnogram, despite there being no gas flowing in or out of the patient. This is because there is expired alveolar gas remaining stationary within the region of the breathing circuit from which the gas is being sampled. This part of the plateau may be shortened by small tidal volumes, high fresh gas flow rates, and/or high gas sampling rates. The angle between phases II and III of the capnogram is known as the alpha (α) angle and is normally around 100–110 degrees. If there is a terminal upswing at the end of Phase III, it is termed Phase IV. Phase IV is seen most frequently in pregnant or obese patients, and is determined by the expiratory characteristics of fast and slow alveoli. It can be responsible for higher $ETCO_2$ compared with $PaCO_2$ in some patients (Shankar *et al.* 1986).

Phase 0: The rapid downstroke on the capnogram corresponds to inspiration. During this phase, fresh inspired gas (which should be free of CO_2) passes the sampling port as it is inspired into the lungs. The angle between phases III and 0 is known as the beta (β) angle and is normally around 90 degrees. The level should reach zero at its minimum, unless inspired CO_2 is detected.

If all alveoli emptied simultaneously and evenly, the capnogram would be square, with Phase II being an upward straight line. However, this does not occur, and it takes time for the CO_2 to mix with the fresh gas in the dead space area, creating a steep, yet gradual slope in Phase II.

To interpret the capnogram (Barter 2012), all four phases of the waveform should be clearly identified. There should be:

1) A distinct plateau in Phase III. If a plateau is present, the sampling rate and subsequent $ETCO_2$ measurement should be working appropriately. Occasionally, Phase III is short; assess the overall waveform to ensure values are appropriate or compare with an arterial blood gas analysis of $PaCO_2$;
2) A steady rise in Phase II; and
3) A noticeable "knee" where Phase II changes to Phase III. Phase II should rise steadily. Observing Phase II is useful in patients with rapid respiratory rates, as there is often very little time for Phase III (the plateau), resulting in "spiked" waveforms compared to more squared-off waves. This may result in inaccurate sampling, frequently

from sample dilution. $ETCO_2$ values displayed can be much lower than the $PaCO_2$ values and should be verified with arterial blood gas analyses.

If these are not present, the capnogram cannot be appropriately analyzed. In some instances, the waveform will be completely absent. For example, if there is a disconnect in the system, the waveform may abruptly transition from a normal shape to zero. In addition, capnography is the gold standard to assure tracheal intubation. For example, if after induction and intubation, the waveform is absent or the $ETCO_2$ begins low and goes quickly to zero, the tube is most likely not in the trachea and is probably within the esophagus. Examples of the most common alterations in the normal capnogram are described below. For more detailed information, readers are referred to other physiology textbooks.

16.2.7.1 Rebreathing of CO_2

Phase I of the capnogram is altered when values do not return to baseline during inspiration, especially when the response time is adequate for the patient and the waveform has a normal shape (Figure 16.6). This suggests a degree of inspired CO_2 in the system, resulting from insufficient expiratory time, inadequate fresh gas flow rates when using non-rebreathing systems, exhausted CO_2 absorbent within a rebreathing system, excessive mechanical dead space, or a malfunctioning or missing one-way (commonly expiratory) valve in a circle system. If the patient cannot compensate for the increased inspired CO_2, the $ETCO_2$ is frequently elevated as well.

16.2.7.2 Abnormal Phase II

Phase II is affected when slow sampling rates of sidestream capnographs decrease the slope of Phase II, shorten the alveolar plateau, and decrease the slope of Phase 0. This delay in response time will commonly cause an increase in the alpha and beta angle of the capnogram. If the slope of Phase II is decreased in the absence of delayed equipment response time, it suggests a slow expiration time. Causes of slow expiration include partially obstructed (e.g. mucus plug) or kinked endotracheal tubes or physical conditions that cause a narrowing of the airway such as severe broncho-constriction. This waveform is known as the "shark fin" (Figure 16.7).

16.2.7.3 Hypercapnia

Phase III or peak $ETCO_2$ values in healthy, conscious patients are only slightly lower than $PaCO_2$ levels. A normal-shaped capnograph with an elevated alveolar plateau indicates hypercapnia (Figure 16.8). In anesthetized or sedated patients, this is frequently associated with hypoventilation, but can also be associated with

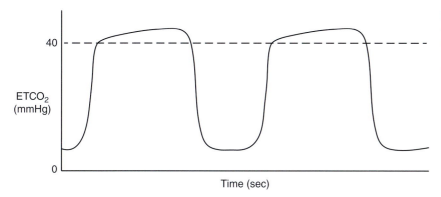

Figure 16.6 CO_2 rebreathing results in an elevated baseline on the capnogram following inspiration (Phase 0 to Phase I). The ETCO$_2$ is frequently, but not necessarily, elevated.

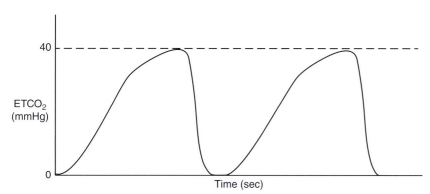

Figure 16.7 Phase II of the capnogram changes with slow response times or, more commonly, obstruction to exhalation. Obstructions can occur within the tracheal tube lumen or within the patient, such as that seen with severe bronchoconstriction. These result in the classic "shark fin" waveform.

increased production of CO_2 (e.g. malignant hyperthermia, pyrexia, etc.), although this reason is less likely.

16.2.7.4 Hypocapnia

An appropriately-shaped capnogram with a lower than normal Phase III plateau demonstrates hypocapnia (Figure 16.9). Similar to hypercapnia (Figure 16.8), the capnogram has a sharp rise to Phase II, a clear "knee" transition to Phase III, and a clear plateau in Phase III. Common causes of hypocapnia during anesthesia are spontaneous patient hyperventilation (i.e. too light or painful), overzealous mechanical ventilation, hypothermia, or decreased delivery of CO_2 to the lungs (low cardiac output). Leaks in the sampling line can also cause low ETCO$_2$ values; however, usually the plateau has a

"bump" at the end of Phase III, corresponding to the next inspiration when non-diluted end-tidal gas is sampled (Figure 16.10).

Although ETCO$_2$ levels may be in the normal range, they may be significantly lower than PaCO$_2$ levels. For example, significant alveolar dead space (ventilated but under-perfused alveoli) may occur secondary to diseases such as pulmonary thrombo-embolism. This creates a situation in which peak ETCO$_2$ levels are substantially lower than PaCO$_2$ measurements. Under-perfused alveoli will not have participated in gas exchange and so contain gas identical in composition to inspired gas, which is normally CO_2 free. During expiration, this gas mixes with the gas from perfused alveoli, thereby diluting the ETCO$_2$ in the sample. Blood-gas analysis is required to diagnose this situation.

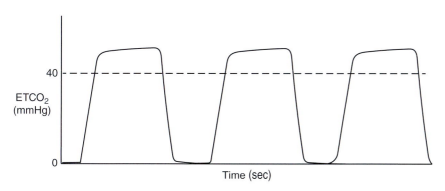

Figure 16.8 Example of a capnogram showing hypercapnia. The waveform, although normally shaped, has a higher than normal ETCO$_2$ value at the end of Phase III.

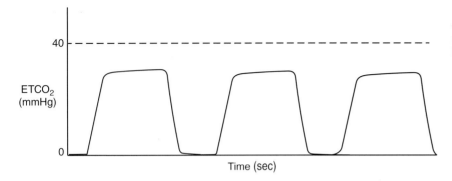

Figure 16.9 Example of a capnogram displaying hypocapnia. The waveform is normally shaped but the ETCO$_2$ value is lower than normal.

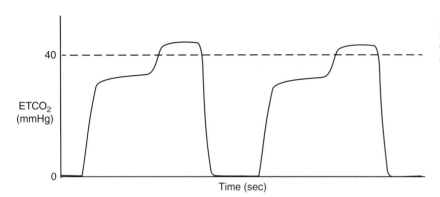

Figure 16.10 If the sampling tube of a sidestream monitor is not patent, the capnogram, although initially normal, will contain a "bump" at the end.

16.2.7.5 Irregular Phase III Plateau

The normal alveolar plateau is roughly horizontal and smooth (Figure 16.5). Irregularities in the Phase III plateau may result from pressure on the thorax of an anesthetized patient, resulting in gas moving in and out of the lungs. In addition, if a patient is mechanically ventilated, spontaneous ventilatory efforts may be interspersed amongst mechanical breaths, resulting in dips or clefts in the alveolar plateau. These are sometimes referred to as "curare clefts", as they are seen as the neuromuscular blockade wearing off, especially in human patients. Causes of these respiratory efforts should be investigated and may include insufficient anesthetic depth, inadequate mechanical ventilation, hypoxemia, inadequate analgesia and hyperthermia (Figure 16.11).

16.2.7.6 Cardiogenic Oscillations

Cardiogenic or cardiac oscillations are undulations in the capnogram from end expiration through Phase 0, which are synchronous with cardiac contractions. They are commonly seen on the capnogram, but particularly in deep-chested breeds (e.g. greyhounds). These movements of the capnogram are seen as contraction of the right ventricle, and filling of the pulmonary vasculature results in the expulsion of a small volume of gas from the lungs with each beat; posture also affects cardiogenic oscillations (Figure 16.12).

16.2.7.7 Abnormal Phase III to Phase 0 Transition

During Phase 0, the capnogram should quickly return to baseline as fresh gas is inspired and replaces CO$_2$-containing

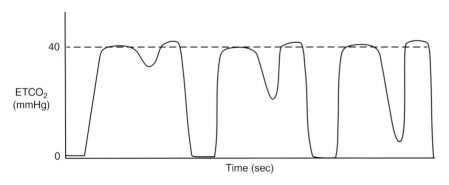

Figure 16.11 Irregularities in the plateau of Phase III are common. These can result from personnel pushing on the patient's chest or spontaneous attempts made at breathing over a mechanical ventilator.

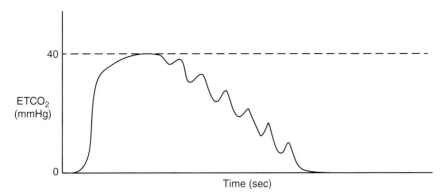

Figure 16.12 Cardiogenic oscillations seen to correlate to each heartbeat, especially in deep chested dogs with slow respiratory rates.

gas at the sampling site; the resulting beta angle is approximately 90 degrees. If the slope of Phase 0 blends in with the plateau of Phase III, the slope of Phase 0 is reduced (i.e. increased beta angle) and the plateau is rounded. This frequently indicates there is a leak within the breathing system or at the patient. There also may be CO_2 in the inspired gas (frequently the baseline would not return to zero in this situation) (Figure 16.13).

16.2.7.8 Exponential Decreases in ETCO$_2$
An exponential drop in ETCO$_2$ indicates a serious problem (Figure 16.14). When the shape of consecutive waveforms look normal, but the ETCO$_2$ is progressively decreasing, it usually indicates severe pulmonary thrombo-embolism has occurred or CO_2 delivery to the lung is greatly reduced, usually from impaired reduced cardiac output. This is seen

with impending cardiovascular collapse or cardiac arrest. Frequently, the ETCO$_2$ drops lower and lower with subsequent breaths until complete cessation of perfusion occurs. In contrast, if the ETCO$_2$ drops abruptly (within one breath), assess the system for disconnections.

16.3   Oxygen Measurement

The measurement of oxygen concentrations within the breathing system ensures that delivery of a hypoxic gas mixture does not occur, especially important when mixtures are delivered (oxygen, medical air and nitrous oxide). In healthy patients undergoing anesthesia, the minimum concentration of inspired oxygen delivered to the patient should be 30–35% (McDonell and Kerr 2015).

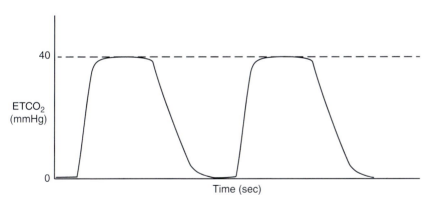

Figure 16.13 Leaks within the breathing system or in the patient frequently result in an abnormal Phase III to 0 transition.

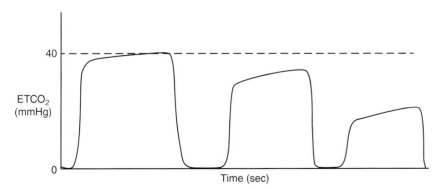

Figure 16.14 Gradual decreases in ETCO$_2$ indicate that cardiac output is impaired and not returning CO_2 back to the lungs appropriately. Diligent patient assessment should occur as this exponential decrease frequently implies impending cardiovascular collapse. If an acute drop occurs, the system should be checked for disconnections within the system.

There are several ways of measuring the oxygen concentration in inspired and expired gases, but the simplest technique is with the use of an oxygen sensor that uses a fuel cell (Davis and Kenny 2007c).

16.3.1 Fuel Cells

The inspired oxygen concentration (FiO_2) is commonly measured using electrochemical (galvanic, polarographic) or paramagnetic methods (Al-Shaikh and Stacey 2007). The galvanic and polarographic analyzers have a slow response time of around 20–30 seconds, since they rely on membrane diffusion; thus, they mainly measure mean oxygen levels. For example, the galvanic fuel cell (Hersh cell) contains two electrodes in a potassium hydroxide solution. Oxygen enters a Teflon-coated membrane where it picks up electrons from a negatively charged gold mesh cathode, combines with water, and diffuses to the positively charged anode (usually lead). The flow of electrons is proportional to the partial pressure of oxygen. The polarographic analyzer (Clark electrode) is similar to the galvanic cell, but it requires a battery and has a shorter response time. The oxygen enters through the Teflon membrane and picks up electrons from the negative platinum cathode. It then combines with water and travels to the positive silver anode. Again, the flow of electrons is proportional to the partial pressure (Davis and Kenny 2007c).

16.3.1.1 Paramagnetic Analyzers

Paramagnetic techniques rely on the fact that oxygen is paramagnetic due to an unpaired electron, and is attracted to a magnetic field. Most other gases are weakly diamagnetic and are repelled by a magnetic field (Davis and Kenny 2007c). In this analyzer, a gas-tight cell containing two glass spheres (filled with nitrogen) in a dumb-bell arrangement, is suspended in a magnetic field. When a sample containing oxygen is passed through a magnetic field, the glass spheres containing nitrogen will be displaced. The deflection of the dumb-bell is measured by attaching it to a mirror, which reflects a light beam and provides an indication on a scale (Davis and Kenny 2007c). In addition, an alternated paramagnetic analyzer contains a pressure transducer. The movement of oxygen into the magnetic field reduces the pressure of a volume of gas situated between the field and a flow restriction upstream of the field. This causes a deflection in the pressure gauge. When the magnetic field is turned off, the differential pressure is gone and the transducer diaphragm returns to its resting position. The magnitude of the alternating pressure differences is proportional to the partial pressure of oxygen (Davis and Kenny 2007c). Paramagnetic analyzers have a short response time, are commonly used, and can accurately measure inspired and expired oxygen levels as a percentage.

16.3.1.2 Transcutaneous Oxygen Analyzers

Transcutaneous oxygen electrodes are available, although they are not routinely used in veterinary practice due to inaccuracies in various species (e.g. SenTec Digital Monitoring System, SenTec Inc., Fenton, MO). However, they use a platinum or gold cathode surrounded by a silver anode, both within a thin layer of electrolytes in a membrane permeable to oxygen, creating a polarographic electrode (Davis and Kenny 2007c). They require a heat source that can cause burns if malfunction occurs. Although less accurate than blood gas analysis, they do provide continuous readings.

16.4 Nitrous Oxide and Inhalation Agent Analyzers

Modern monitors are capable of measuring the concentrations of all the current inhalation agents available, including nitrous oxide, halothane, isoflurane, enflurane, sevoflurane and desflurane, on a breath-by-breath basis. Historically, this was done using gas chromatography. Currently, this is most commonly performed with infrared or piezoelectric analyzers, but often concentrations are still confirmed with gas chromatography if required. Mass spectrometry, Raman spectroscopy and ultraviolet absorption (in the case of halothane) can also be used.

16.4.1 Infrared Analyzers

Similar to $ETCO_2$ measurements, infrared absorption analyzers are used with the sampled gas entering a chamber where it is exposed to infrared light (Davis and Kenny 2007b). A photodetector measures the light reaching it across the correct infrared wavelength band. Absorption of the infrared light is proportional to the vapor concentration. The electrical signal is then analyzed and processed to give a measurement of the agent concentration.

Optical fibers are used to select the desired wavelength. Nitrous oxide absorbs light at 4.6 μm, whereas newer machines that measure inhalational agents use higher wavelengths, usually between 8 and 9 μm. This avoids interference from methane and alcohol, which absorb at the lower 3.3 μm band, as inhalants can as well (Al-Shaikh and Stacey 2007; Hendrickx *et al.* 2008). Modern sensors can automatically identify and measure concentrations of up to three agents present in a mixture and produce a warning message to the user if multiple agents are detected.

In multi-agent sensors, up to five sensors are used to produce a spectral signal of the agent(s) present in the sample. This signal is then compared with the spectral shapes stored in the memory of the sensor and used to identify the agent. The amplitude of the spectral shape represents the amount of vapor present in the mixture and is inversely proportional to the amount of agent present. The infrared source is kept constant with a continuous supply of current. Optical fibers (mentioned above) are used to filter the desirable wavelengths. Due to the auto-detection, individual calibration for each agent is unnecessary (Al-Shaikh and Stacey 2007). Advantages of this system include the sample gas returning to the breathing system, no individual calibration necessary, and water vapor has minimal effect on the performance and accuracy of the analyzer.

16.4.1.1 Collision Broadening

Collision broadening describes the effects of nitrous oxide on CO_2 measurements, since they absorb infrared light at similar wavelengths (Davis and Kenny 2007b). As previously mentioned, nitrous oxide absorbs infrared light at 4.5 μm, whereas CO_2 absorbs at 4.3 μm; the presence of nitrous oxide can give falsely high CO_2 readings. Using an infrared filter that only transmits at 4.3 μm minimizes this effect. In addition, because their absorption peaks are so close, collision of CO_2 and nitrous oxide causes the CO_2 spectral peak itself to broaden when nitrous oxide is present, called collision broadening. Suggested correction factors for CO_2 when nitrous oxide is present are approximately 0.90 when 70% nitrous oxide is used (corrected PCO_2 = observed PCO_2 × 0.90) to approximately 0.94 when 50% nitrous oxide is used. Although some monitors compensate for this effect, calibration of the monitor with a gas containing both nitrous oxide and CO_2 will eliminate the errors.

16.4.2 Piezoelectric Quartz Crystal Oscillation Analyzers

Piezoelectric quartz crystal oscillations can be used to measure the concentration of volatile agents. A lipophilic-coated piezoelectric quartz crystal undergoes changes in its natural resonant frequency when exposed to the lipid-soluble inhalation agents. The change in frequency is directly proportional to the partial pressure of the agent (Al-Shaikh and Stacey 2007). However, this technique does not permit measurement of agent specificity and it is sensitive to water vapor.

16.4.3 Gas Chromatography

A gas chromatograph can detect inhalational anesthetics in clinical patients, as well as trace waste anesthetic gases in the environment (Davis and Kenny 2007a). It can also analyze barbiturates, phenothiazines, benzodiazepines, steroids and catecholamines, after techniques have been used to change them into volatile compounds (Davis and Kenny 2007a). Briefly, a gas chromatograph contains a stationary and a mobile phase in a thermostatically-controlled environment. The stationary phase contains the chromatographic column and is usually packed with very small silica-alumina particles that are coated with polyethylene glycol or silicone oil. A carrier gas (nitrogen, argon, helium) passes through this column and forms the mobile phase. The gas sample is injected into this mobile phase, which travels through the column at a speed depending on their solubility between the two phases. The column is usually a long coiled glass tube; the longer the column, the better the sample separation. At the outlet, a recorder monitors the appearance of the sample components. Three types of detectors exist; the flame ionization detector, the thermal conductivity detector (katharometer; used mainly for inorganic gases, i.e. nitrous oxide and oxygen) and the electron capture detector (used for halogenated anesthetics) (Davis and Kenny 2007a).

16.4.4 Mass Spectrometry

Mass spectrometry can be used to identify and measure, on a breath-to-breath basis, the concentration of oxygen, CO_2 and halogenated anesthetics. The sample is drawn into the machine and is bombarded with electrons to charge the particles of the sample. They are accelerated and forced through a magnetic field, are deflected, and are separated into a spectrum according to their specific mass:charge ratios (David and Kenny 2007a).

The creation and manipulation of the ions is done in a high vacuum (10^{-5} mmHg) to avoid interference by outside gas and to minimize random collisions among the ions and the residual gas. The relative abundance of ions at specific mass:charge ratios is determined and is related to the fractional composition of the original gas mixture. Because of the high expense, multiplexed mass spectrometer systems are used with several patient sampling locations on a time-shared basis.

16.4.5 Raman Spectrography

When radiation is exposed to a sample, it may be completely absorbed (such as in infrared technology discussed above) or may have some transfer of energy between the radiation and the molecules (Davis and Kenny 2007a). This is termed the Raman Effect, where the energy transfer affects the vibration of bonds between atoms in the molecule, and absorption of radiation is associated with a certain type of bond. The energy of radiation is proportional to the frequency of radiation and the transfer of energy from the radiation to the molecule changes the wavelength of the radiation, usually by decreasing it. This decrease in wavelength length is unique to each molecule; thus, many agents can be measured using Raman technology. For more detailed information regarding this technique, please refer to other physics textbooks (Davis and Kenny 2007a).

16.5 Blood Gas Analysis: Partial Pressures of Oxygen and CO$_2$

16.5.1 Oxygen

When measuring oxygen tensions in a blood gas, oxygen is measured using a Clark electrode or a polarographic electrode, similar to techniques described above (Davis and Kenny 2007c). A platinum cathode and silver/silver chloride anode are placed within a solution containing potassium chloride. A voltage of 0.6 V is applied and the current measured. Electrons are supplied by the anode from the reaction of silver and chloride. At the cathode, oxygen combines with electrons and water such that:

$$O_2 + 4e^- + 2H_2O \rightarrow 4OH^-. \quad (16.1)$$

The more oxygen measured, the more electrons taken up and the greater the current flow (Davis and Kenny 2007c).

16.5.2 Carbon Dioxide (CO$_2$)

The measurement of CO$_2$ in a blood sample relies on the equation:

$$CO_2 + H_2O \leftrightarrow H_2CO_3^- \leftrightarrow H^+ + HCO_3^- \quad (16.2)$$

In a Severinghaus electrode (see Section 16.2.2 above), a hydrogen ion sensitive glass is surrounded by electrodes and a film of sodium bicarbonate. A nylon mesh is fixed over the tip by an O-ring. The sample is separated from the electrode by a plastic membrane that is only permeable to CO$_2$. CO$_2$ diffuses through the membrane into the mesh and combines with water according to the above equation. The change in hydrogen ions is measured and the partial pressure of CO$_2$ displayed.

16.6 Conclusion

Gas monitoring, and particularly capnography, provides anesthetists with valuable tools in the assessment and monitoring of patients under anesthesia. Capnography is considered useful as it gives us information not only about a patient's ventilation, but also because CO$_2$ production, metabolism and excretion is closely linked to cardiopulmonary function, circulation and metabolism. The capnogram waveform also provides information about intubation, equipment function, airway obstruction, hypoventilation and hypotension. Gas monitoring as part of multiparameter monitors is becoming more commonly used within veterinary practice. It is essential that staff participating in the anesthesia of patients have a good working knowledge and understanding on the interpretation of values, trends and waveforms, and how to deal with issues when they are detected.

References

Al-Shaikh, B. and Stacey, S. (2007) Non-invasive monitoring. In: *Essentials of Anaesthetic Equipment*, 3rd ed. London, UK: Elsevier, pp. 145–175.

Barter, L.S. (2012) Capnography. In: Burkitt Creedon, J.M. and Davis, H. (eds). *Advanced Monitoring and Procedures for Small Animal Emergency and Critical Care*. Chichester, UK: Wiley & Sons, pp. 340–348.

Davis, P.D. and Kenny, G.N.C. (2007a) Further techniques of gas and vapour analysis. In: *Basic Physics and Measurement in Anaesthesia*, 5th ed. Philadelphia, PA: Butterworth Heinemann, Elsevier Ltd, pp. 199–210.

Davis, P.D. and Kenny, G.N.C. (2007b) Hydrogen ion and carbon dioxide measurement. In: *Basic Physics and Measurement in Anaesthesia*, 5th ed. Philadelphia, PA: Butterworth Heinemann, Elsevier Ltd, pp. 211–218.

Davis, P.D. and Kenny, G.N.C. (2007c) Oxygen measurement. In: *Basic Physics and Measurement in*

Anaesthesia, 5th ed. Philadelphia, PA: Butterworth Heinemann, Elsevier Ltd, pp. 199–210.

Hendrickx, J.F.A., Lemmens, H.J.M., Carette, R., De Wolf, A.M. and Saidman, L.J. (2008) Can modern infrared analyzers replace gas chromatography to measure anesthetic vapor concentrations? *BMC Anesthesiology*, 8, 2.

Hopper, K. (2012) Mechanical ventilation. In: Burkitt Creedon, J.M. and Davis, H. (eds). *Advanced Monitoring and Procedures for Small Animal Emergency and Critical Care*. Chichester, UK: Wiley & Sons, pp. 349–356.

Huttmann, S.E., Windisch, W. and Storre, J.H. (2014) Techniques for the measurement and monitoring of carbon dioxide in the blood. *Annals ATS*, 11, 645–652.

Jandrey, K.E. (2006) Capnography: What is the evidence? *12th International Veterinary Emergency and Critical Care Symposium* (conference proceedings), San Antonio, TX.

Krauss, B. and Hess, D.R. (2007) Capnography for procedural sedation and analgesia in the emergency department. *Annals Emerg Med*, 50, 172–180.

Marshall, M. (2004) Capnography in dogs. *Compendium*, October, 761–778.

Long, B., Koyfman, A. and Vivirito, M.A. (2017) Capnography in the emergency department: a review of uses, waveforms, and limitations. *J Emerg Med*, Epub ahead of print.

McDonell, W.N. and Kerr, C.L. (2015) Physiology, pathophysiology, and anesthetic management of patients with respiratory disease. In: Grimm, K.A., Lamont, L.A., Tranquilli, W.J., Greene, S.A. and Robertson, S.A. (eds). *Veterinary Anesthesia and Analgesia: The Fifth Edition of Lumb and Jones*. Ames, IA: Wiley Blackwell, pp. 513–557.

Reuss-Lamky, H. (2010) Understanding capnography – It's breathtaking! *23rd Conference Proceedings of the International Veterinary Emergency and Critical Care Symposium*. Nashville, TN.

Shankar, K.B., Moseley, H., Kumar, Y. and Vemula, V. (1986) The arterial to end-tidal carbon dioxide tension difference during Caesarean section anaesthesia. *Anaesthesia*, 41, 698–702.

Simpson, K. (2014a) Capnography for veterinary nurses. Part 1: The basics. *Vet Nurs J*, 29, 358–361.

Simpson, K. (2014b) Capnography for veterinary nurses. Part 2: Capnograms and the respiratory cycle. *Vet Nurs J*, 29, 396–397.

17

Airway Volumes, Flows and Pressures
Andrew Claude[1] and Alanna Johnson[2]

[1] *College of Veterinary Medicine, Michigan State University, East Lansing, Michigan, USA*
[2] *College of Veterinary Medicine, University of Florida, Gainesville, Florida, USA*

17.1   Introduction

Patients undergoing general anesthesia require multiparameter monitoring that is generally comprised of cardiovascular, respiratory, thermoregulatory, anesthetic depth and analgesic parameters. Respiratory parameter monitoring frequently includes ventilation (PCO_2), oxygenation (PO_2) and pulmonary dynamics. In human medicine, airway volumes, flows and pressures are routinely recorded over time, to help evaluate pulmonary performance during spontaneous ventilation (SV) or intermittent positive pressure ventilation (IPPV). In veterinary medicine, monitoring of pulmonary dynamics is customarily applied in ICU settings; however, these parameters have recently been more broadly applied in general anesthetic settings. In order to utilize monitoring of pulmonary dynamics, including airway volumes, flows and pressures, a thorough understanding of pulmonary physiology, respiratory cycles and terminology must be mastered.

17.2   Definitions (Dorsch and Dorsch 2008)

- *Compliance:* The ratio of a change in volume versus a change in pressure. Compliance is a measure of dispensability, typically expressed in milliliters per centimeter of water (mL/cmH_2O). For the anesthetized patient, compliance usually refers to the chest wall and lungs; however, compliance may also be applied to specific components of breathing systems. For example, breathing tubes and reservoir bags have compliance.
- *Expiratory Flow Rate:* The rate at which gas is exhaled by the patient. It is expressed as volume per unit of time (mL/min or L/min).
- *Expiratory Flow Time:* The time between the beginning and end of expiratory flow.
- *Expiratory Pause Time:* The time between the end of expiratory flow and start of inspiratory flow.
- *Expiratory Phase Time:* The time between the start of expiratory flow and start of inspiratory flow. It is the sum of expiratory flow time and expiratory pause time.
- *Inspiratory Flow Time:* The time between the beginning and end of inspiratory flow.
- *Inspiratory Pause Time:* The time during inspiration, during which the lungs are held inflated at a fixed pressure or volume (zero flow rate). It is also referred to as the inspiratory hold or inspiratory plateau.
- *Inspiratory Phase Time:* The time between the start of inspiration and start of expiration. It is the sum of the inspiratory flow and inspiratory pause times. It can be used in a ratio between inspiratory pause time and phase time ($T_{IP}:T_I$).
- *Inspiratory:Expiratory Phase Time Ratio (I:E ratio):* The ratio of inspiratory phase time to expiratory phase time. Typically, the inspiratory phase time is shorter compared to expiratory phase time, unless the ratio is inverted (inverted I:E ratio). The I:E ratio is a function of the minute ventilation cycle (60-second cycle). For example, consider an I:E ratio of 1:2 at 10 breaths per minute (BPM). Ten BPM = 6 second I:E cycle (60 seconds/10 BPM = 6 seconds per breathing cycle). An I:E ratio of 1:2 means there will be 2 seconds for the inspiratory phase and 4 seconds for the expiratory phase. On a mechanical ventilator, I:E ratios can be manually changed or will change according to adjustments in breaths per minute, inspiratory flow or tidal volume delivered to the patient, depending upon available ventilator settings.
- *Inspiratory Flow Rate:* The gas flow rate into the patient during inspiration. It is typically expressed in volume over time (mL/min or L/min).

Veterinary Anesthetic and Monitoring Equipment, First Edition. Edited by Kristen G. Cooley and Rebecca A. Johnson.
© 2018 John Wiley & Sons, Inc. Published 2018 by John Wiley & Sons, Inc.

- *Minute Ventilation or Volume (V_E):* The volume a patient breathes in 1 minute. It is calculated by multiplying the patient's tidal volume by the respiratory frequency ($V_E = V_T \times f$) and is expressed as volume per time (L/min).
- *Peak Inspiratory Pressure (PIP):* The maximum airway pressure during the inspiratory phase time. It is usually expressed in cmH$_2$O.
- *Plateau Pressure:* The resting airway pressure during the inspiratory pause. Usually during the inspiratory pause, airway pressure decreases slightly below PIP. This lower pressure is called the plateau pressure.
- *Positive End Expiratory Pressure (PEEP):* The positive pressure within the breathing circuit (and airway) at the end of expiration. Typically, the pressure within the breathing circuit drops to zero cmH$_2$O at the end of expiration. PEEP occurs when airway pressure remains above zero cmH$_2$O at the end of expiration. PEEP may be either extrinsic, from an external force such as a PEEP valve or ventilator, or intrinsic, due to an incomplete exhalation.
- *Resistance:* The ratio of the change in driving pressure to the change in flow rate. It is expressed in centimeters of water per liter per second (cmH$_2$O/L/sec).
- *Spirometry:* The measurement of gas flow and volumes during breathing. A spirometer is a device used to measure the patient's volume of gas during breathing.
- *Tidal volume:* The volume of gas a patient breathes during the inspiratory or expiratory phase time.
- *Respiratory (Ventilatory) Rate or Frequency (f):* The number of breaths per unit time, usually per minute (breaths per minute, BPM).
- *Work of Breathing:* The energy expended by the patient and/or ventilator during inspiratory and expiratory phases. It is the ratio of work to volume of gas moved, typically expressed as joules per liter. It includes the energy required to overcome the elastic properties of the chest wall and lungs and the flow-resistant forces (gas turbulence and densities) of both the respiratory system and ventilatory equipment.

17.3   Volume and Flow Measurement Devices

Several devices are currently available for the measurement of gas volumes and flows in clinical patients. In general, devices measuring gas flows or volumes should have low resistance, minimal dead space, accuracy across a wide range of clinically-relevant values, rapid response to allow breath-by-breath analyses, and measurements that are unaffected by any alterations in gas composition or temperature. Many of these devices are not routinely used in veterinary medicine. However, the American Society of Anesthesiologists (ASA) has strongly recom-

mended the measurement and monitoring of the volume of expired gases, and modern anesthetic workstations in human medicine incorporate this capability (ASA 2015).

17.3.1   Respirometers/Volumeters

Respirometers and volumeters are devices that measure a volume of gas passing through a flow pathway over a given time period. Historically, respirometers were strictly mechanical devices, but modern respirometers incorporate electronic signal conversions and displays. Respirometers may help detect patient circuit disconnections, occlusions, apnea, leaks and ventilator failure. They are usually placed either on the expiratory limb of the breathing circuit or in between the patient and the breathing circuit. These devices are not extremely common, but are easy to use and provide useful information about the patient's respiratory volume.

17.3.1.1   Wright's Respirometer

The Wright's respirometer is a mechanical device that functions via tangential slots in a cylinder, which allow gas to flow into the central compartment, thereby rotating a vane in the respirometer (Medical Support Products, Lancaster, PA; Figure 17.1). The vane is connected to the gauge needle via a gear system which, when rotated, causes the needle on the dial to move an amount corresponding to the volume of gas passing through the system. These devices may have multiple vanes and gauges, allowing for measurement of varied volume scales. For example, the original Wright's respirometer is the Mark 8; the small inner dial records volumes from 0–1 L and the larger outer dial records 0–100 L. In contrast, the small dial on the Mark 12 reads up to 10 L per revolution and the large dial reads up to 1 L per revolution. The Mark 20 has concentric dials and measures up to 100 L per revolution.

Wright's respirometers are typically placed in the expiratory limb of the anesthetic circuit and may be used to measure patient tidal and/or minute volume. However, no timer is built into this device, so calculation of minute volume requires the observer to measure time separately. The Wright's respirometer is easy to use and dead space is minimal, with neonatal attachments available to further decrease the dead space volume. They have push buttons for on/off and reset controls, and can be sterilized using low-temperature gas systems. However, these units are known to read falsely low at lower flows and falsely high at higher flows (Dorsch and Dorsch 2008).

17.3.1.2   Dräger Volumeter

The Dräger volumeter appears and operates in a similar way to the Wright's respirometer, except it has two lightweight, dumbbell-shaped interlocking rotors. This device

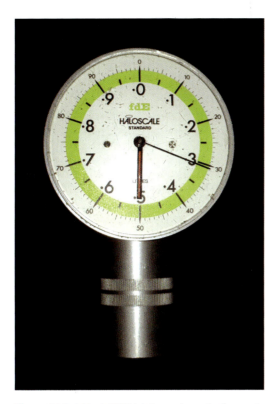

Figure 17.1 A Mark 20 Wright's respirometer for use in veterinary medicine. The concentric dials measure up to 1 L (inner) and 100 L (outer). It can be placed in the breathing system to measure tidal volume, but must be used with the breathing frequency to obtain minute ventilation (photograph courtesy of Dr Rebecca Johnson, University of Wisconsin-Madison, WI).

may measure volumes more accurately than Wright's respirometer (Wernerus *et al.* 1978; Mandal 2008). However, these devices are not widely available and are seldom used.

17.3.1.3 Digital Respirometers

Digital respirometers are similar to the Wright's respirometer, except they have photosensors and a light source behind the vanes; the photosensor counts the rotation of the vanes across this light source. These frequently have electronic LCD displays, minimizing difficulties associated with reading a dial and numbers (Anesthesia Associates, San Marcos, CA; Figure 17.2). Many of these devices read up to 200 L (Dorsch and Dorsch 2008).

17.3.1.4 Ventilator-associated Volumes

One of the simplest and frequently used ways to estimate respiratory volumes is to use the scales provided on the wall of the bellows housing (Hallowell EMC, Pittsfield, MA; Figure 17.3). These scales may be used to estimate the volume delivered into the breathing circuit, but not the patient's tidal volume, as wasted ventilation due to gas compression and circuit distension will not be

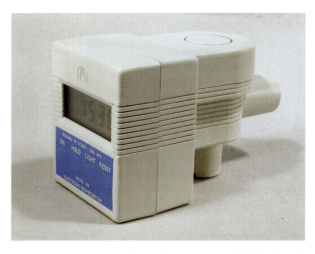

Figure 17.2 An example of a digital respirometer, which displays the breathing volume (this example has measured 15.3 L) (photograph courtesy of Anesthesia Associates Inc., San Marcos, CA).

quantified (Dorsch and Dorsch 2008). Many practices have ventilators with these scales, and this is a common method to estimate delivered volumes.

17.3.2 Flow Detectors

17.3.2.1 Hot-Wire Anemometer

The hot-wire anemometer is not often used clinically, unless it is incorporated into a full anesthesia workstation, as are used in human clinical practice. This anemometer measures flow via the principle of thermal dissipation. Gas flows can be measured in several ways, such as constant current, constant voltage and constant temperature techniques. Using Ohm's law, which states that the current flowing through the circuit is equal to the voltage difference across the circuit divided by the circuit resistance, the output produces results from a circuit within the device, maintaining stability of the specific variable (current, voltage or temperature) (Jewitt and Thomas 2012).

Commonly, in clinically used anemometers, gas flows around a thin, heated platinum (or tungsten) wire. This heating level is usually very low, and the outside of the sensor will not be hot to the touch. However, as the gas flows by, heat is dissipated; cooling occurs in the wire, and thus resistance drops. The higher the volume of gas flow, the more heat dissipation will occur; the resultant changes in resistance are quantified via a Wheatstone bridge circuit, allowing flow to be measured. On the other hand, in some systems, the temperature of the wire is kept constant and the current used to do so is directly proportional to the air velocity (Mandal 2008).

This device is more accurate at low flow rates, and it cannot indicate direction of flow without using two monitors. If the sensor is impacted by air flow in two

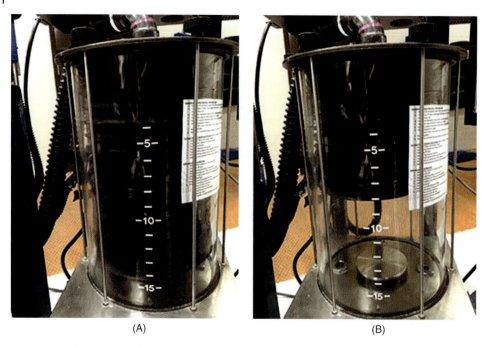

(A)   (B)

Figure 17.3 The use of ventilator bellows markings to estimate delivered volume. In this instance, the descending large animal bellows at end-expiration are near the 15-L mark (A). During inspiration, they approach the 8-L line (B), delivering 7 L to the breathing circuit (photograph courtesy of Dr Rebecca Johnson, University of Wisconsin-Madison, WI).

directions, it could measure higher than actual flows (Dorsch and Dorsch 2008).

17.3.2.2   Peak Flowmeters

A peak flowmeter is an inexpensive, portable, handheld device (Medline, Northfield, IL; Figure 17.4). This variable-orifice flowmeter is composed of a three-compartment metallic cylinder. Expiration of gas causes enlargement of the flow orifice, which in turn moves a vane inside the monitor. The final position of the vane corresponds to the peak flow rate. A ratchet holds this vane in place after expiration, and must be released prior to the next measurement (Mandal 2008). These are commonly used for asthmatic patients (Cross and Nelson 1991).

17.3.2.3   Ultrasonic Flowmeters

Ultrasonic flow sensors measure gas flow via the use of measuring the transmission times between two crystals. The flow of gas affects the signal of two transducers transmitting in opposite directions. When the gas flows in the same direction as the ultrasound waves, an increase in velocity occurs, and when gas flows in the opposite direction, a decrease in velocity occurs. When there is no flow, the velocity of the signals is equal, but during flow, a difference in transmission times occurs, allowing the flow rate to be determined. These monitors are incorporated into some advanced anesthesia workstations.

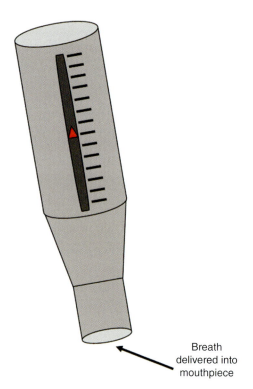

Breath delivered into mouthpiece

Figure 17.4 Illustration demonstrating an example of a peak flowmeter. Patients must breathe into an orifice and the indicator rises to the level of the breath volume. It is locked in place until released before the next breath (illustration courtesy of Dr Rebecca Johnson, University of Wisconsin-Madison, WI).

17.3.2.4 Venturi Tube Flowmeter

A Venturi tube uses the Bernoulli principle to determine flow. This principle states that gas flow across a constriction will experience a drop in pressure in order to maintain flow rate (Figure 17.5). In the Venturi tube, there are at least two ports that measure the pressure – one prior to and one following the constriction in the gas flow pathway. The change in pressure across this constriction is used to calculate the flow rate. Venturi meters are incorporated into some multiparameter monitoring systems or workstations.

17.3.2.5 Pitot Tube Flowmeter

The Pitot tube has two tubes placed in the flow pathway (Figure 17.6). One of these tubes faces the fluid flow and measures the pressure of impact, and the other tube faces away from the flow and measures the static flow pressure. These two tubes are connected to a differential pressure transducer, which allows the flow to be calculated based on the difference in the two values (Mandal 2008).

17.3.2.6 Rotameter

The rotameter is a fixed pressure, variable orifice flowmeter that consists of a calibrated vertical tube of varying diameter (Thorpe tube; Figure 17.7). A bobbin is suspended by the gas flow and indicates the flow rate of gas around it. Flow is laminar near the bottom of the flowmeter, but is turbulent at the top (Mandal 2008). If the bobbin is a sphere, the flow should be read at its widest point. If the bobbin body is cylindrical in shape, the flow should be read at the top of the bobbin. These meters are frequently gas-specific (Dorsch and Dorsch 2008). Rotameters are one of the most commonly seen methods of measuring a continuous flow volume of gas in the anesthesia machine.

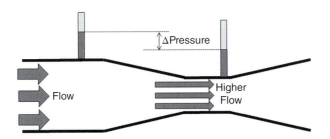

Figure 17.5 Illustration demonstrating the underlying principles of a Venturi tube flowmeter. As the flow is compressed through a smaller diameter, there is a change in pressure, which is used to calculate the actual flow rate (illustration courtesy of Dr Rebecca Johnson, University of Wisconsin-Madison, WI).

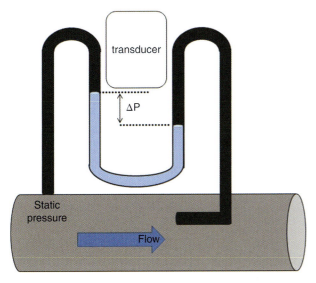

Figure 17.6 Illustration of a Pitot tube. One end faces the flow and the other measures static conditions. The pressure change between the two is used to measure the actual flow rate (illustration courtesy of Dr Rebecca Johnson, University of Wisconsin-Madison, WI).

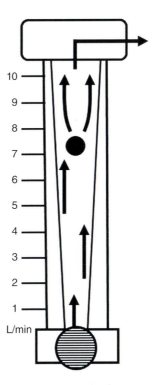

Figure 17.7 Example of a rotameter in which the gas flows through the bottom of a tube when a knob is opened and pushes an indicator upwards, indicating the flow. There are multiple manufacturers and sizes. This example measures 0–10 L (illustration courtesy of Dr Rebecca Johnson, University of Wisconsin-Madison, WI).

17.3.2.7 Pneumotachograph

The pneumotachograph measures both flow and volume using the Hagen–Poiseuille equation. It is a variable pressure, fixed orifice device, in which a resistance is placed in the path of gas flow (Rudolph Linear Pneumotachograph, Hans Rudolph, Inc., Shawnee, KS; Figure 17.8). A differential pressure transducer measures the pressure drop across the resistance, and in laminar flow, this means that the flow rate is proportional to the pressure drop. The tidal volume is then determined by integrating the flow signal over the period of inspiration and expiration (Jewitt and Thomas 2012).

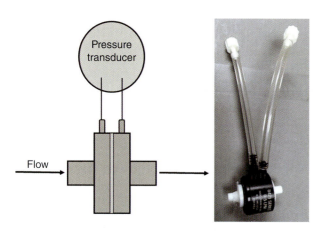

Figure 17.8 Illustration (left) and photograph (right) of a pneumotachograph. A membrane is located within the device that provides resistance to flow. The pressures measured on each side of this resistance are sent to a transducer to calculate actual flows (courtesy of Dr Rebecca Johnson, University of Wisconsin-Madison, WI).

17.4 The Ventilatory (Respiratory) Cycle

17.4.1 Components

During controlled inspiration, there is an initial rise in airway pressure, with the rate of rise being dependent on airflow (Figure 17.9). Peak pressure during inspiration will increase with high inspiratory flow rates, elevated airway resistance and decreased compliance. A decrease in peak pressure can be due to a leak in the system, spontaneous inspiration (bucking the ventilator), a decrease in resistance, and an increased compliance. A pause at the end of inspiration causes a plateau pressure at the end of inspiration (Figure 17.9). Plateau pressure is a function of tidal volume and the total compliance, but is independent of resistance. Inspiration is followed by an expiratory period and frequently an expiratory pause, where airway pressures return to zero in the normal animal, unless positive pressure is purposely applied (Dorsch and Dorsch 2008).

17.4.2 Compliance and Resistance

17.4.2.1 Compliance

Compliance is defined as the change in volume (V) over the change in pressure (P), and its measurement may be classified as dynamic or static. Total compliance represents the elastic properties of the lungs, thorax, abdomen and breathing system. For example, muscle relaxants increase chest wall compliance, but will not affect lung compliance; therefore, changes in compliance are due to alterations in the lungs in patients with neuromuscular blockade.

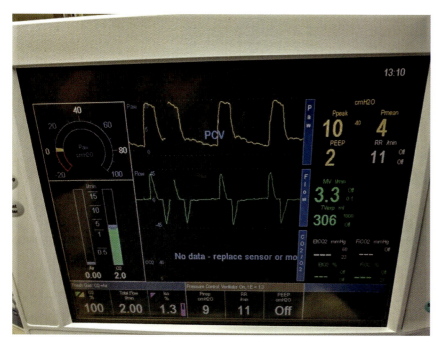

Figure 17.9 Airway pressure graph during mechanical ventilation using pressure-control mode. Airway pressure (paw, yellow waveform) increases as flow (green waveform) increases until a plateau is reached (slightly below the PIP). This is followed by expiration and an expiratory pause prior to the next breath (photograph courtesy of Dr Rebecca Johnson, University of Wisconsin-Madison, WI).

Dynamic Compliance Dynamic compliance is the change in volume over the change in pressure ($\Delta V/\Delta P$) at two points during the respiratory cycle; it is frequently calculated using the following formula: $V_T/(PIP - PEEP)$, where V_T = tidal volume, PIP = peak inspiratory pressure and PEEP = positive end-expiratory pressure (see definitions above). Due to the continued gas flow during its measurement, dynamic compliance is variable and is affected by changes in airway resistance (Khorasani *et al.* 1999).

Static Compliance Static compliance is calculated using the end-inspiratory occlusion pressure. An inspiratory hold, or occlusion of the expiratory port, will allow airway pressure to reach a constant value, resulting in no gas flow. Alternatively, gas flow can be transiently discontinued during the breath hold for this measurement. The pressure at the point of inspiratory hold is called the plateau pressure and represents the elastic recoil of the entire respiratory system, while eliminating any effects of altered airway resistance. Static compliance is calculated by ($V_T/$ [Plateau pressure – PEEP]); see Dynamic compliance above (Tobin 1992; Bardoczky and Engelman 1996).

17.4.2.2 Resistance

Resistance (R) to airflow through a tube is represented by the airway pressure difference between two points (ΔP) divided by the flow (Q), as described by the hydraulic analogy of Ohm's Law: $R = \Delta P/Q$ (the pressure differential is used as the electrical voltage drop, flow is in place of electric current, and vascular resistance is similar to electrical resistance). For example, during mechanical ventilation, increased inspiratory airway resistance will require higher driving pressures in order to maintain flow and/or a lower flow in order to maintain optimum airway pressures.

Total airway resistance may differ between inspiration and expiration and is the sum of the resistance of the patient's airway, endotracheal tube and the breathing system. Accordingly, issues such as broncho-constriction, secretions, edema, tumors or a foreign body can cause increased patient airway resistance. Endotracheal tube resistance depends primarily on the internal tube diameter. For example, tube kinking and airway secretions can cause partial or complete tube obstruction, resulting in increased resistance. Breathing system resistance is also largely affected by the internal diameter and length of the tubes; resistance is increased with sharp bends and restrictions, as these may cause less efficient (turbulent) flow.

Total airway resistance can be estimated by subtracting plateau pressures from peak inspiratory pressures. In humans, normal total resistance is approximately 2–5 cmH_2O; however, normal total resistance in veterinary patients is largely unknown and is likely species dependent.

As described above, increased total airway resistance will require higher peak pressures to maintain flow. However, plateau pressure largely depends on compliance and will not be affected by resistance (Dorsch and Dorsch 2008).

17.5 Airway Pressure Monitoring

Airway pressure monitoring is used to detect high- or low-pressure conditions within the patient or the breathing circuit. These monitors may be stand-alone units, or they may be associated with a ventilator or anesthesia machine. Some conditions that may trigger an alarm from an airway pressure monitor are low peak inspiratory pressure, sustained elevated pressure, high peak inspiratory pressure, and sub-ambient pressure. Portable veterinary anesthesia machines do not traditionally have this feature built into them; however, anesthesia workstations may have these integrated into the system. If used, the monitoring port is ideally placed as near to the patient's airway as is feasible (Figure 17.10B) (Dorsch and Dorsch 2008).

17.5.1 Pressure Monitoring Devices

Airway pressures are commonly measured with manometers and transducers, similar to those used for cardiovascular pressure monitoring. For detailed explanations of these devices, see Chapter 19. In fully incorporated multiparameter monitors in the modern anesthesia workstation (GE Healthcare, Wauwatosa, WI), transducers are used with digital displays for continuous airway pressure monitoring. The transducers are usually calibrated at the manufacturing stage, but should be zeroed to atmospheric conditions. The waveforms are smaller than arterial pressure waves and the scale is usually set from 0–30 cmH_2O on the display.

Single-use, disposable, commercially available manometers are a convenient way for veterinary professionals to monitor airway pressures, especially when expensive multiparameter monitors are unavailable or non-rebreathing systems not connected to a machine are used (Vetamac Inc., Rossville, IN; Figure 17.11). Although traditional manometers may be heavy, especially when placed near the airway of a small patient, these newer plastic pressure manometers can be easily used in the breathing system.

17.6 Spirometry Loops

Spirometry loops are plotted to represent the relationship between two variables such as pressure and volume, or flow and volume. Spirometers are available on anesthetic multiparameter monitors, or they may be incorporated into anesthesia machines and critical care ventilators

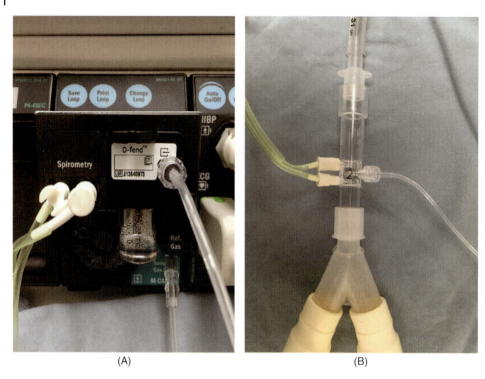

(A)   (B)

Figure 17.10 (A) Spirometry module as part of an integrated small animal anesthesia work system containing a multiparameter monitor and mechanical ventilator. (B) The airway pressure monitoring port and spirometry tubing is positioned between the patient's tracheal tube and breathing circuit (photograph courtesy of Dr Rebecca Johnson, University of Wisconsin-Madison, WI).

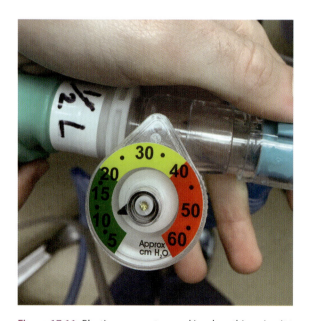

Figure 17.11 Plastic manometer used in a breathing circuit to measure airway pressures, especially during positive pressure ventilation techniques (sighs, assisted ventilation or controlled mechanical ventilation). The "safe" airway pressures are indicated in the green area and extremely high pressures are in the red zone. In this instance, the manometer is placed between the non-rebreathing hoses (with occlusion valve [light blue]) and the green rebreathing bag. A peak inspiratory pressure near 10 cmH$_2$O is measured (photograph courtesy of Dr Rebecca Johnson, University of Wisconsin-Madison, WI).

(Figure 17.10A). The use of spirometry loops is not performed in many routine veterinary anesthesia cases, but are a useful tool in patients with suspected alterations in respiratory drive or breathing mechanics (Aisys CS^2; GE Healthcare, Madison, WI); they are described in more detail elsewhere (Bark *et al.* 2007; Bradbrook *et al.* 2013; Moens 2013). In addition, these measurements are frequently used in the veterinary ICU setting for patients that must be placed on a ventilator (Corona and Aumann 2011; Mellema 2013).

17.6.1   Pressure-Volume Loops

Pressure-volume loops are used to illustrate compliance, as compliance is the ratio of change in volume to change in pressure. This graph typically depicts the *x*-axis as pressure and the *y*-axis as volume (Figure 17.12A). The tidal volume is the highest point reached on the *y*-axis, and the peak pressure is the highest value reached on the *x*-axis. If a line is drawn from the zero point on the graph to the endpoint of inspiration, that line represents the compliance. Normally, this line will be at an angle of approximately 45 degrees or less (in relation to the *y*-axis). A decrease in compliance will be reflected by shifting this line toward the horizontal. In animals and people, a decrease in compliance may be due to such things as pulmonary edema, pneumonia, pulmonary fibrosis and severe pulmonary

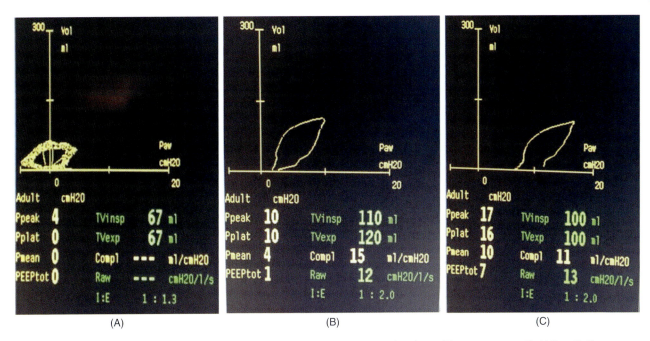

Figure 17.12 Pressure-volume loops in a 5-kg anesthetized dog during spontaneous ventilation (A), pressure controlled (10 cmH$_2$O), mechanical ventilation with 1-cmH$_2$O PEEP (B), and pressure controlled (10 cmH$_2$O), mechanical ventilation with 7 cmH$_2$O PEEP (C). In (A), many loops are superimposed to compare waveform structure over time. During spontaneous ventilation, the inspiratory and expiratory volumes are lower (67 mL) compared with pressure-controlled, mechanically ventilated volumes (˜100–120 mL). In addition, airway pressures are low during spontaneous ventilation and center around 0 cmH$_2$O. Addition of PEEP during mechanical ventilation shifts the loop to the right and increases the peak, plateau and mean airway pressures to 6–7 cmH$_2$O accordingly. Compliance slightly decreased from 15 mL/cmH$_2$O to 11 mL/cmH$_2$O, possibly due to the high levels of PEEP used in this demonstration; however, lower PEEP levels will predictably increase compliance (Suter *et al.* 1978) (photograph courtesy of Dr Rebecca Johnson, University of Wisconsin-Madison, WI).

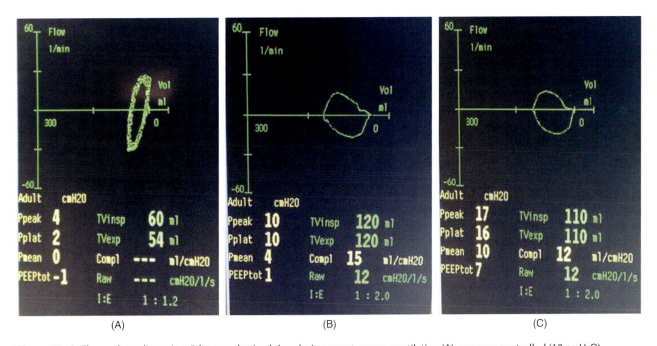

Figure 17.13 Flow-volume loops in a 5-kg anesthetized dog during spontaneous ventilation (A), pressure controlled (10 cmH$_2$O), mechanical ventilation with 1-cmH$_2$O PEEP (B), and pressure controlled (10 cmH$_2$O), mechanical ventilation with 7-cmH$_2$O PEEP (C). In (A), many loops are superimposed to compare waveform structure. During spontaneous ventilation, the inspiratory and expiratory volumes are lower (˜50–60 mL) compared with pressure-controlled, mechanically ventilated volumes (˜110–120 mL). Addition of PEEP during mechanical ventilation increases the peak, plateau and mean airway pressures to 6–7 cmH$_2$O accordingly (photograph courtesy of Dr Rebecca Johnson, University of Wisconsin-Madison, WI).

contusions (Rozanski and Hoffman 1999). The area inside the loop represents the work of breathing, and the direction of flow of the loop depends upon whether the patient is undergoing spontaneous or positive-pressure ventilation (Figure 17.12B). Also, if a patient has PEEP, it will shift the curve to the right (Figure 17.12C).

17.6.2 Flow-Volume Loops

Flow-volume loops (Figure 17.13) are used to illustrate resistance and have volume on the x-axis and flow on the y-axis. Classically, the zero point is shifted to the right on the horizontal axis, which corresponds to the functional residual capacity. Flow rate increases during inspiration (negative deflection), but goes back to zero as inspiration ends. The tidal volume is the point where the loop crosses the x-axis and flow returns to zero. This part of the loop will have a variable shape, depending upon the nature of the patient's ventilation, such as volume-controlled, pressure-controlled or spontaneous ventilation (Figure 17.13). Exhalation occurs in the part of the loop that is above the x-axis. In this part of the curve, the shape is dependent upon the rate of lung deflation (determined by the elastic recoil of the lungs and the chest wall) and the resistance of the conducting airways and equipment.

References

American Society of Anesthesiologists (2015) Standards for basic anesthesia monitoring. Practice Guidance Resources. Available from: http://www.asahq.org/quality-and-practice-management/practice-guidance-resource-documents/standards-for-basic-anesthetic-monitoring [accessed October 2017].

Bardoczky, G. and Engelman, E. (1996) Comparison of airway pressures from different measuring sites. *Anesth Analg*, 83, 887.

Bark, H., Epstein, A., Bar-Yishay, E., Putilov, A. and Godfrey, S. (2007) Non-invasive forced expiratory flow-volume curves to measure lung function in cats. *Respir Physiol Neurobiol*, 155, 49–54.

Bradbrook, A., Clark, L., Dugdale, A., Burford, J. and Mosing, M. (2013) Measurement of respiratory system compliance and respiratory system resistance in healthy dogs undergoing general anaesthesia for elective orthopaedic procedures. *Vet Anaesth Analg*, 40, 382–389.

Corona, T. and Aumannm M. (2011) Ventilator waveform interpretation in mechanically ventilated small animals. *J Vet Emerg Crit Care*, 21, 496–514.

Cross, D. and Nelson, H. (1991) The role of the peak flowmeter in the diagnosis and management of asthma. *J Allergy Clin Immunol*, 87, 120–128.

Dorsch, J. and Dorsch, S. (2008) Airway volumes, flows and pressures. In: *Understanding Anesthesia Equipment*, 5th ed. Philadelphia, PA: Lippincott Williams & Wilkins, 728–772.

Jewitt, H. and Thomas, G. (2012) Measurement of flow and volume of gases. *Anesth Intensive Care Med*, 13, 106–110.

Khorasani. A., Candido, K., Saatee, S. and Khorasani, A. (1999) The relationship between dynamic compliance and inspiratory flow. *Anesth Analg*, 88, 465.

Mandal, N. (2008) Measurement of volume and flow in gases. *Anesth Intensive Care Med*, 10, 52–56.

Mellema, M. (2013) Ventilator waveforms. *Top Companion Anim Med*, 28, 112–123.

Moens, Y. (2013) Mechanical ventilation and respiratory mechanics during equine anesthesia. *Vet Clin North Am Equine Pract*, 29, 51–67.

Rozanski, E. and Hoffman, A. (1999) Pulmonary function testing in small animals. *Clin Tech Small Anim Pract*, 14, 237–241.

Suter, P., Fairley H. and Isenberg M. (1978) Effect of tidal volume and positive end-expiratory pressure on compliance during mechanical ventilation. *Chest*, 73, 158–162.

Tobin. M. (1992) Monitoring of pressure, flow and volume during mechanical ventilation. *Resp Care*, 37, 1081–1096.

Wernerus, H., Silva, G. and Wanner, A. (1978) Accuracy of Dräger and Wright ventilation meters. *Respir Care*, 23, 856–859.

18

Pulse Oximetry

Odette O

Canada West Veterinary Specialists, Vancouver, BC, Canada

18.1   Introduction

Pulse oximetry, as part of the monitoring protocol for anesthetized patients, has become the standard of care for veterinary medicine in recent years. The American Animal Hospital Association's Anesthesia Monitoring Guidelines for Dogs and Cats recommends the use of a pulse oximeter during the peri-anesthetic period, in order to help ascertain information about the patient's physiological parameters while under the influence of anesthetic agents (Bednarski *et al.* 2011). In addition, the American College of Veterinary Anesthesia and Analgesia released updated Anesthetic Monitoring Guidelines in 2009. This document emphasizes the importance of vigilant monitoring of physiological parameters during the peri-anesthetic period by trained personnel, with the goal of improving anesthetic outcomes by early detection of possible complications. Pulse oximetry provides important information about both patient circulation and ventilation via oxygenation. Its use is recommended from induction through the recovery period in anesthetized patients, as well as along with oxygen supplementation in sedated animals (acvaa.org 2016).

18.2   History

The pursuit of increasing anesthetic safety through advancements in monitoring has been examined in human medicine. Despite its invention in the 1940s and first publications for its use in anesthetized humans in the 1950s, routine use of pulse oximetry did not become popular until the 1980s (Lee *et al.* 1991; Tremper and Barker 1989). Since then, the contribution of pulse oximetry to anesthetic safety has been recognized as so important in this field, that it has been amongst the most published topics since the 1980s (Kissin and Valassakov

2015). Its contribution to anesthetic safety is undisputable and pulse oximetry has been referred to as the fifth vital sign (Mower *et al.* 1997, 1998).

The pulse oximeter has been in regular use in veterinary medicine since the 1990s (Butinar *et al.* 1991). Nonetheless, a questionnaire-based study performed more than a decade later found that a large number of veterinary students and general practice veterinarians still had poor overall knowledge of this device. Knowledge was lacking in how pulse oximeters function and how to apply the obtained information for optimal patient benefit (Hofmeister *et al.* 2005).

Vast strides have been made over the past decade, with incorporation of knowledge and use of the pulse oximeter at veterinary teaching institutions in combination with continuing education forums. Currently, pulse oximeters are very accessible and are an expected part of patient monitoring for both anesthetized and heavily sedated veterinary patients. In addition to increasing patient safety, the clinical practicality of pulse oximetry contributes to its popularity. It provides real-time pulse rate and non-invasive measurement of hemoglobin saturation (SpO_2), either as a small, affordable, portable unit or as part of a multiparameter monitor.

18.3   Importance of Pulse Oximetry

Pulse oximetry assesses both the cardiovascular and pulmonary systems of the patient, since both adequate peripheral blood flow and alveolar gas exchange are required for normal pulse oximetry readings. Use of a pulse oximeter immediately after induction can potentially detect signs of anesthetic-related issues such as esophageal or endobronchial intubation, oxygen supply problems, and significant hypoventilation, earlier than relying on clinical signs such as tachycardia or cyanosis. As such, the pulse oximeter should be placed on the

Veterinary Anesthetic and Monitoring Equipment, First Edition. Edited by Kristen G. Cooley and Rebecca A. Johnson.
© 2018 John Wiley & Sons, Inc. Published 2018 by John Wiley & Sons, Inc.

patient immediately after induction and remain in use until after extubation whenever possible.

18.4   Function

Hemoglobin is a complex molecule responsible for carrying oxygen in the erythrocytes. Various forms of hemoglobin exist and absorb light differently (deoxyhemoglobin, oxyhemoglobin, methemoglobin and carboxyhemoglobin); these can be differentiated using a co-oximeter. However, conventional pulse oximeters specifically function on the premise that oxygenated hemoglobin (oxyhemoglobin) absorbs a greater amount of light in the near infrared spectrum (940 nm) and reduced hemoglobin (deoxyhemoglobin) absorbs more light in the visible red spectrum (660 nm).

The principle on which the pulse oximeter works is based on the Beer–Lambert law which states:

$$A = a(\lambda) \times b \times c \qquad (18.1)$$

where A is the measured absorbance, $a(\lambda)$ is the wavelength dependent absorptivity coefficient, b is the path length, and c is the analyte concentration (Grosenbaugh *et al.* 1997). Since there is a linear relationship between the absorbance and concentration of a substance, the concentration of a known substance can be determined if the absorbance, path length of light traveled, and wavelength-dependent absorptivity coefficient is known. The absorbance spectra of the hemoglobin of various domestic species, including human, dog, cat, horse, cow and pig, has been examined. They have been determined as similar enough not to be a limiting factor in pulse oximeters that use human algorithms to be used in these veterinary species (Grosenbaugh *et al.* 1997; Sendak *et al.* 1988).

Taylor and Whitwam (1988) compared five different pulse oximeter models in a clinical setting and found the pulse oximeter useful in monitoring trends and changes in arterial hemoglobin oxygen saturation, especially with sudden drops in oxygen saturation, since an audible alarm is triggered. The pulse oximeter models examined had the tendency to underestimate true saturation, which increases safety since intervention would occur sooner, and that most models are accurate within an SpO_2 range of 80–100% (Taylor and Whitwam 1988). Nonetheless, more recent evidence suggests that over 30% of the monitors tested did not meet manufacturer specifications, even though they claimed accuracy within ±2–3% when the SpO_2 is within the range of 70–100% (Milner and Mathews 2012). Hence, this emphasizes the importance of understanding how the pulse oximeter functions and its use for monitoring trends along with other clinical tools.

18.5   Pulse Oximeter Probes

Pulse oximeter probes are designed to either reflect light onto a tissue bed from a light-emitting diode (LED) to a photosensor located on the same side (reflectance probe), or transmit light from the LED through a tissue bed then onto a photodiode located on the opposite side (transmittance probe) (Figure 18.1). Site selection is important when placing probes, as adequate tissue perfusion and the ability of light to travel through tissue are important to reading accuracy. The red and infrared bands of light created by the LEDs in the probe flash hundreds of times per second, thereby determining the trough (capillary and venous blood) and peak (capillary, venous and arterial blood) of each pulse wave. This light-based data is collected by the photodetector in the probe

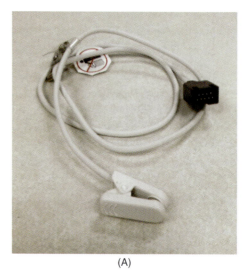

(A)

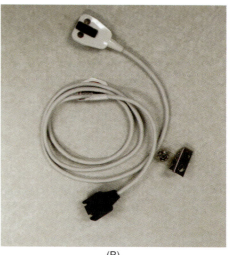

(B)

Figure 18.1 Examples of the numerous commercially available pulse oximetry probes. (A) Transmittance probe. (B) Reflectance probe.

and translated into electrical signals. An empirical algorithm is used to relate the ratio of these wavelengths to the oxygen saturation of arterial blood, thus providing the percentage of oxyhemoglobin compared to total hemoglobin (SpO_2). During this process, both pulse rate and SpO_2 are determined (Tremper and Barker 1989).

18.6   Uses

Under normal circumstances, SpO_2 provides us with an approximation of SaO_2 (oxyhemoglobin compared to all other hemoglobin as determined by a co-oximeter), both of which are directly related to the partial pressure of arterial oxygen dissolved in the blood (PaO_2). PaO_2 is important because it reveals the ability of the patient to transport oxygen from the environment into the bloodstream. PaO_2 is related to SpO_2 by the oxyhemoglobin dissociation curve (Figure 18.2).

The sigmoid shape of this curve reveals no difference in SpO_2 when the PaO_2 is 100 mmHg versus 500 mmHg; the SpO_2 is 100% regardless. It should be noted that this can be a challenge for early detection of oxygen desaturation when monitoring an anesthetized patient who is inspiring an enriched oxygen mixture. Under these circumstances, the SpO_2 reads 100% until oxygenation of the patient decreases from 500 mmHg to below 100 mmHg. At this point, there is only a small further drop until the minimum physiologically normal level of PaO_2 (80 mmHg), which correlates with an SpO_2 of more than 95%, is reached. At an SpO_2 below 90% (PaO_2 ˜60 mmHg) the patient is hypoxemic; the curve suddenly becomes steep and a patient can quickly desaturate further. Although a wide range exists in the literature, capillary reduced hemo-globin cyanosis occurs with an SpO_2 of between 73 and 78%, with a corresponding PaO_2 of approximately 40 mmHg (Martin and Khalil 1990).

18.7   Oxyhemoglobin Dissociation Curves in Different Species

Pulse oximeters were designed using the human oxyhemoglobin dissociation curve. However, the oxyhemoglobin curve is not identical across various species. As such, it is important to consider the magnitude of impact that this may have on its accuracy when used in various veterinary species, if any.

P_{50} is defined as the PO_2 at which 50% of hemoglobin is saturated with oxygen. The P_{50} value varies not only between species, but has also been found to be different within breeds of dogs and can be shifted to the left or right for various physiological reasons (e.g. increased temperature, 2,3-DPG or decreased pH will shift it to the right and vice versa). For human hemoglobin, the P_{50} value is 26.6 mmHg, canine hemoglobin is 28.8 (25.9–35.8) mmHg, equine hemoglobin is 23.8 mmHg, bovine hemoglobin is 25.0 mmHg (Clerbaux *et al.* 1993), and feline hemoglobin is 35.6 mmHg (Herrmann and Haskins 2005). Potentially, this could mean that if using a pulse oximeter calibrated using human data, for any given SpO_2, the corresponding PaO_2 could potentially be more largely underestimated in feline patients, as well as an underestimate in canine and an overestimate in bovine and equine patients. However, clinically-based species–specific studies may be the best way to determine if, in fact, this is true and to what extent it may influence patient management.

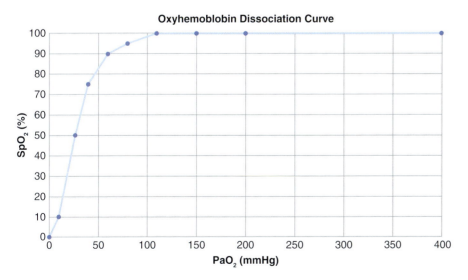

Figure 18.2 A human oxyhemoglobin dissociation curve where the P_{50} is ˜27 mmHg.

The use of pulse oximeters in the anesthetic monitoring of special species remains controversial. In subjects more similar to humans, pulse oximetry seems to be a reliable monitoring tool. In anesthetized cynomolgus monkeys (*Macaca fascicularis*), pulse oximetry was useful for clinical assessment of hypoxemia (Young *et al.* 2002). Pulse oximetry underestimated oxygenation determined by co-oximetry by a small margin in anesthetized late gestation pregnant sheep, but was overall accurate and reliable in these subjects (Quinn *et al.* 2012). However, the P_{50} values of many species remains unknown, and even if known, use of human hemoglobin calibrated pulse oximeters continue to be market standard and may possibly affect accuracy.

The use of human-validated pulse oximeters may result in several potential errors. For example, in avian patients, specifically parrots and pigeons, human pulse oximeters underestimated actual saturation in birds, even though one of the pulse oximeters had been specifically modified to accommodate high avian pulse rates. As a result, the pulse rate obtained was similar to actual heart rate and trends in oxygenation may have been detected; however, motion artifact once the surgical procedure commenced resulted in significant interference and overall the monitor was unsatisfactory in consistently detecting critical events (Schmitt 1998).

Alternatively, reptiles often present with extremely low heart rates, which may also present a challenge when using pulse oximetry. In addition, the variety that exist in this taxa, with their unique cardiopulmonary anatomy and physiology, make validation of this monitor challenging and extrapolation of any validated data from one species to another potentially without merit. Reptiles may demonstrate increased levels of methemoglobinemia that may also negatively affect pulse oximeter readings (Perry 1998). Nonetheless, pulse oximetry in green iguanas (*Iguana iguana*) may be useful for assessing oxygen saturation trends, as no statistically significant differences were found between SaO_2 and SpO_2 (Diethelm 2001). Pulse oximetry in white rhinoceros (*Ceratotherium simum*) with human hemoglobin calibrated pulse oximeters was unreliable, with both a large variation in recorded SpO_2 values as well as values greatly lower than actual oxygen saturation (Haymerle *et al.* 2016).

18.8   Patient Factors

Patient factors can contribute to the reliability of pulse oximetry – appropriate probe size and placement adds to readings that are more accurate from this monitor (Figure 18.3). Transmittance probes may be placed on multiple locations in veterinary patients, including mucous membranes such as the tongue, prepuce/vulva, ear and interdigital skin. Reflectance probes may be placed on hairless,

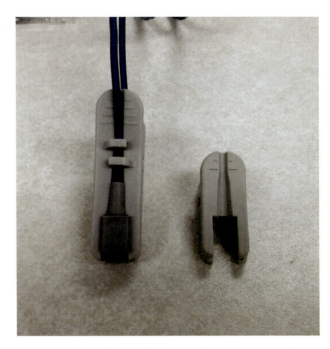

Figure 18.3 Examples of various sizes of transmittance probes.

flat surfaces, including ventral tail base, medial aspect of distal limbs, and even in the oral or rectal cavities and esophagus (Figure 18.4). Poor placement of the probe should be avoided, as it may result in optical shunting, where the LED light reaches the photodetector before passing through a tissue bed and increases error.

Many additional patient causes can interfere with proper LED light signal detection, including dense hair coat, dark pigment and motion/shivering. The pulse oximeter needs to detect peak and trough pulsations, making adequate peripheral blood flow to the tissue bed of paramount importance to accuracy. Vasoactive drugs resulting in intense vasoconstriction and poor perfusion of the tissue, hypotension, hypothermia, abnormally low saturation levels, and even compression of tissues from the probe itself are common causes of absent or inaccu-

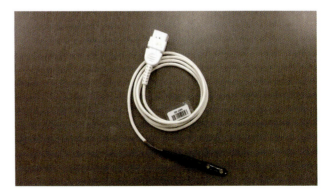

Figure 18.4 A reflectance probe used for rectal or esophageal placement.

rate readings from the pulse oximeter. Indeed, compression of the blood supply is a clinical concern as ischemic damage can occur, especially is very small patients or patients with hypotension (Figure 18.5).

18.9 Abnormal Hemoglobin

Large amounts of abnormal hemoglobin can also alter pulse oximeter reliability (Ralston *et al*. 1991). Carboxyhemoglobin is formed because of exposure to carbon monoxide and absorbs light in a similar spectrum to oxyhemoglobin. Patients with carbon monoxide poisoning will demonstrate an SpO_2 with an artefactual elevation by the percent of carboxyhemoglobin present. In an anesthetic setting, this can be especially dangerous when desiccated soda lime is used with modern volatile anesthetics in a rebreathing anesthetic system, where carbon monoxide will be produced in significant amounts (Keijzer *et al*. 2005).

Methemoglobin is the portion of hemoglobin that exists where iron is in its ferric (Fe^{3+}) instead of the regular ferrous (Fe^{2+}) state. Normal amounts of this type of hemoglobin exist in blood; however, excessive amounts adversely affect oxygen transport, since this form is unable to carry oxygen. Abnormal amounts of methemoglobin may be caused by the administration of certain drugs, such as some local anesthetics (benzocaine), antibiotics (sulfonamides), nitroprusside and acetaminophen toxicity in cats. In addition, it can be a genetically inherited disor-

der reported in certain species including dogs (Harvey 1974). Methemoglobin absorbs both infrared and red light proportionately, so increasing amounts of methemoglobin will cause the pulse oximeter to read towards a saturation of 85%, thereby overestimating true values below 85% and underestimating saturations in patients with a true value greater than 85% (Figure 18.6).

Severe anemia can also negatively affect pulse oximeter accuracy, leading to an overestimate of SpO_2, which may be more important at low saturations. However, the level of anemia must truly be severe for this to happen (Lee *et al.* 1991). Conversely, extreme polycythemia may result in the underestimation of SpO_2 due to the increased presence of hemoglobin binding sites in a patient with normal oxygen content.

18.10 Sources of Error

Equipment issues contributing to pulse oximeter inaccuracy include using a probe inappropriate to the monitor; manufacturers state that the use of a probe not made for their monitor may result in poor function. In addition, optical interference from light sources with frequencies similar to that of the pulse oximeter LED may result in spurious readings (Webster 1997). Sources of light that may cause optical interference include excessive ambient light from sunlight, fluorescent lighting, operating room lights, heating lamps, flash photography, etc. Covering the probe with gauze, white tape or a drape may help to alleviate this malfunction (Figure 18.7). Electrical interference from simultaneous use of an electrosurgical unit can also occur, possibly resulting in erroneously low saturations and/or additional pulse

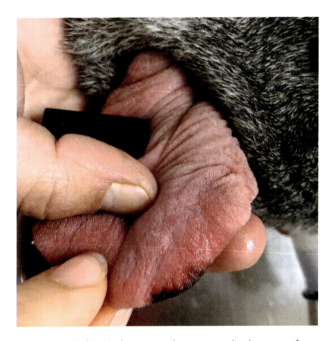

Figure 18.5 Ischemic damage to the tongue edge because of a large, tight pulse oximeter probe (not present in this picture) placed during anesthesia.

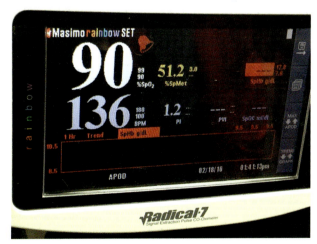

Figure 18.6 Use of a co-oximeter (Masimo Corporation, Irvine, CA) to diagnose congenital methemoglobinemia in a dog. The pulse oximeter is reading an SpO_2 of 90% and a methemoglobin saturation (SpMet) of 51.2%.

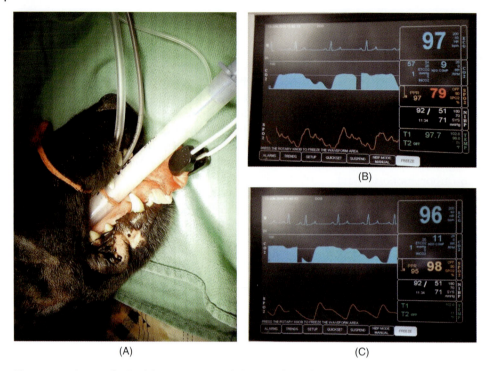

Figure 18.7 An anesthetized dog experiencing light optical interference. (A) The patient probe is exposed to surgical light interference. (B) The pulse oximeter is reading erroneously low (79%, orange trace) and the waveform is abnormal. (C) After the probe is covered from light, SpO$_2$ is now reading 98% with a normally shaped waveform.

counts. This artifact may potentially be minimized by placing the pulse oximeter probe as far away as possible from the surgical site (Ralson *et al.* 1991). Many modern pulse oximeters have tools to assist the user in determining accuracy. A pulse oximeter that displays a pulse waveform (plethysmograph) is always preferable, as the user is able to ensure a normal pulse tracing in order to help determine accuracy; that is, readings are accurate with an appropriate accompanying pulse wave tracing. Other monitors may have a display that alerts the user to pulse quality, a necessary parameter for accurate pulse oximeter readings.

18.11 Perfusion Index (PI) and Plethysmograph Variability Index (PVI)

In today's medical monitoring equipment market, countless models of pulse oximetry are available. While it is beyond the scope of this chapter to review every available pulse oximeter currently obtainable, there are some commonly-used models in veterinary medicine that are manufactured both by human and veterinary equipment providers. Since they measure changes in peripheral blood volume beat by beat, pulse oximeters that display a waveform are known as (photo)plethys-

mographs. The typical arterial waveform with a dicrotic notch (aortic valve closure) may be seen with minimal distortion in the pulse oximetry wave as well, depending on a variety of factors including probe location, monitor type and filters used, etc. These waveforms and related waveform analysis have utility in assisting assessment of patient perfusion and volume status, arrhythmias resulting in the absence of a peripheral pulse, signal integrity, and more.

Human studies have correlated pulse oximeter plethysmograph waveform amplitude variation to blood volume status and have attempted to predict fluid responsiveness in mechanically-ventilated patients (Cannesson *et al.* 2011; see Chapters 19 and 23). The premise of using the pulse oximeter tracing to assess patient volume status during mechanical ventilation is that there will be a greater difference in waveform variation (maximum to minimum peaks of tracing) during the positive pressure portion of the respiratory cycle in the face of hypovolemia (Shamir *et al.* 1999) (Figure 18.8). However, it is important to note that a reliable waveform in a well-perfused tissue bed is important to the accuracy of this technique. Studies on the utility of plethysmographic indices to predict fluid responsiveness in ventilated patients are favorable (Sandroni *et al.* 2012), but may not be completely reliable (Antonsen and Kirkebøen 2012). Application of these techniques in veterinary medicine requires further investigation, but is also encouraging.

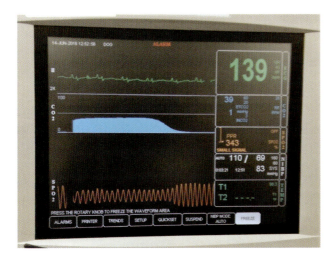

Figure 18.8 Pulse plethysmograph waveform variation (lower screen, compressed trace), likely due to hypovolemia seen in mechanically ventilated patient.

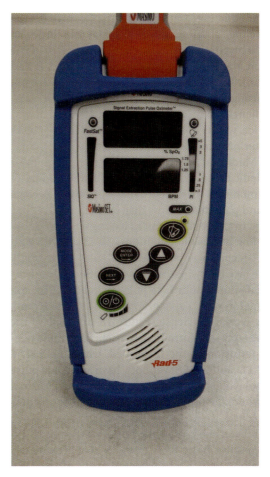

Figure 18.9 Massimo Rad 5 pulse oximeter with PI quantified on the right-hand side of the numerical display.

Masimo Corporation (Irvine, CA) has a wide range of small, portable pulse oximeters that employ patented Signal Extraction Technology (SET), which permits improved accuracy over a wide range of challenges affecting accuracy, including patient motion, poor tissue perfusion, excessive ambient light, and interference from electrosurgical units (Goldman *et al.* 2000). Some of these monitors directly and non-invasively measure perfusion index (PI; Figure 18.9) and calculate their patented plethysmograph variability index (PVI). PI reflects the amplitude of the pulse oximeter waveform itself, indicating peripheral perfusion status; whereas the PVI measures the dynamic changes in PI over time with the respiratory cycle. PI is location- and patient-specific, but trends may be helpful in assessing peripheral perfusion status and patient circulatory status.

At a minimum, PI can be used to determine when a probe is not accurate due to poor perfusion in the tissue bed where it is placed, so that the anesthesia care provider may move it to a potentially better-perfused area. Interestingly, PI has also been used to assess locoregional anesthetic success in both human and canine patients. Since the administration of local anesthetics induces vasodilation in the affected area, it is expected that PI will increase. An increased PI in dogs 10–15 minutes after a sciatic nerve block was administered (as assessed by placement of a pulse co-oximeter probe between the 3rd and 4th digits of these patients) correlated to block success, whereas lack of an increased PI potentially indicated partial or complete failure of the anesthetic block (Gatson *et al.* 2016).

PVI technology makes the use of plethysmography waveform monitoring as a tool to assess fluid responsiveness clinically convenient and a number of references

supporting this methodology is available on their website (www.Masimo.com). In light of recent human medicine publications, both in support and challenging this methodology, further studies in veterinary medicine are warranted to ensure applicability of this tool for fluid resuscitation under various circumstances in our veterinary patients. The Masimo Corporation also markets a number of other patient monitoring products, including a popular, affordable combined pulse oximeter and carbon monoxide (co-oximeter).

18.12 Other Pulse Oximeter Models

Medtronic (Covidien, Minneapolis, MN) manufactures the Nellcor pulse oximeter with OxiMax technology, where a digital memory chip with calibration and operating systems is located in the sensor, permitting the monitoring of a diverse range of patients. The use of this pulse oximeter technology, along with their respiration

References

American College of Veterinary Anesthesia and Analgesia Small Animal Monitoring Guidelines. Available from: http://acvaa.org [Accessed May 15, 2016].

Antonsen, L. and Kirkebøen, K. (2012) Evaluation of fluid responsiveness: Is photoplethysmography a noninvasive alternative. *Anesthesiol Res Pract*, 1–10.

Bednarski, R., Grimm, K., Harvey, R., Lukasik, V., Penn, W. *et al.* (2011) AAHA anesthesia guidelines for dogs and cats. *J Am Anim Hosp Assoc*, 47, 377–385.

Butinar, J., Petrun-Ulaga, M., Cestnik, V., Pavlica, Z. and Frantar, B. (1991) Pulse oximetry and capnometry-methods of monitoring in veterinary anaesthesia. *Vet Anaesth Analg*, 18, 87–88.

Cannesson, M., Le Manach, Y., Hofer, C., Goarin, J., Lehot, J. *et al.* (2011) Assessing the diagnostic accuracy of pulse pressure variations for the prediction of fluid responsiveness. *Anesthesiology*, 115, 231–241.

Clerbaux, T., Gustin, P., Detry, B., Cao, M. and Fran, A. (1993) Comparative study of the oxyhaemoglobin dissociation curve of four mammals: man, dog, horse and cattle. Part A: Comparative biochemistry and physiology. *Physiology*, 106, 687–694.

Diethelm, G. (2001) The effect of oxygen content of inspiratory air (FiO$_2$) on recovery times in the Green Iguana (*Iguana iguana*). PhD Dissertation, University of Zurich, Zurich, Switzerland.

Gatson, B., Garcia-Pereira, F., James, M., Carrera-Justiz, S. and Lewis, D. (2016) Use of a perfusion index to confirm the presence of sciatic nerve blockade in dogs. *Vet Anaes Analg*, 43, 662–669.

Goldman, J., Petterson, M., Kopotic, R. and Barker, S. (2000) Masimo signal extraction pulse oximetry. *J Clin Monit Comput*, 16, 475–483.

Grosenbaugh, D., Alben, J. and Muir, W. (1997) Absorbance spectra of inter-species hemoglobins in the visible and near infrared regions. *J Veter Emer Crit*, 7, 36–42.

Harvey, J., Ling, G. and Kaneko, J. (1974) Methemoglobin reductase deficiency in a dog. *J Am Vet Med Assoc*, 164, 1030–1033.

Haymerle, A., Knauer, F. and Walzer, C. (2016) Two methods to adapt the human haemoglobin-oxygen dissociation algorithm to the blood of white rhinoceros (*Ceratotherium simum*) and to determine the accuracy of pulse oximetry. *Vet Anaes Analg*, 43, 566–570.

Herrmann, K. and Haskins, S. (2005) Determination of P50 for feline hemoglobin. *J Veter Emer Crit*, 15, 26–31.

Hofmeister, E., Read, M. and Brainard, B. (2005) Evaluation of veterinarian and veterinary student knowledge and clinical use of pulse oximetry. *Vet Anaesth Analg*, 32, 2–3.

Keijzer, C., Perez, R. and De Lange, J. (2005) Carbon monoxide production from five volatile anesthetics in dry sodalime in a patient model: halothane and sevoflurane do produce carbon monoxide; temperature is a poor predictor of carbon monoxide production. *BMC Anesthesiol*, 5, 6.

Kissin, I. and Vlassakov, K. (2015) A quest to increase safety of anesthetics by advancements in anesthesia monitoring: scientometric analysis. *Drug Design Devel Therapy*, 11, 2599–2608.

Lee, S., Tremper, K. and Barker, S. (1991) Effects of anemia on pulse oximetry and continuous mixed venous hemoglobin saturation monitoring in dogs. *Anesthesiology*, 75, 118–122.

Martin, L. and Khalil, H. (1990) How much reduced hemoglobin is necessary to generate central cyanosis? *Chest*, 97, 182–185.

Masimo Corporation (2016) Available from: http://masimo.com/index.htm [Accessed May 22, 2016].

Milner, Q. and Mathews, G. (2012) An assessment of the accuracy of pulse oximeters. *Anaesthesia*, 67, 396–401.

Mower, W., Sachs, C., Nicklin, E. and Baraff, L. (1997) Pulse Oximetry as a fifth pediatric vital sign. *Pediatrics*, 99(5), pp. 681–686.

Mower, W., Myers, G., Nicklin, E., Kearin, K., Baraff, L. and Sachs, C. (1998) Pulse oximetry as a fifth vital sign in emergency geriatric assessment. *Acad Emerg Med*, 5, 858–865.

Nonin (2016) Available from: http://www.nonin.com/veterinary [Accessed May 22, 2016].

Perry, S.F. (1998) Lungs: comparative anatomy, functional morphology, and evolution. In: Gans, C. and Gaunt, A.S. (eds). *Biology of the Reptilia*, vol. 19: *Morphology of Visceral Organs*. St Louis, MO: Society for the Study of Amphibians and Reptiles, pp. 1–92.

Pulse Oximetry (2016) Available from: http://www.medtronic.com/covidien/products/pulse-oximetry [Accessed August 7, 2016].

Quinn, C., Raisis, A. and Musk, G. (2012) Evaluation of Masimo signal extraction technology pulse oximetry in anaesthetized pregnant sheep. *Vet Anaesth Analg*, 40, 149–156.

Ralston, A., Webb, R. and Runciman, W. (1991) Potential errors in pulse oximetry. Part III: Effects of interference, dyes, dyshaemoglobins and other pigments. *Anaesthesia*, 46, 291–295.

Sandroni, C., Cavallaro, F., Marano, C., Falcone, C., De Santis, P. and Antonelli, M. (2012) Accuracy of plethysmographic indices as predictors of fluid responsiveness in mechanically ventilated adults: a systematic review and meta-analysis. *Intensive Care Med*, 38, 1429–1437.

Schmitt, P., Göbel, T. and Trautvetter, E. (1998) Evaluation of pulse oximetry as a monitoring method in avian anesthesia. *J Avian Med Surg*, 12, 91–99.

Sendak, M., Harris, A. and Donham, R. (1988) Accuracy of pulse oximetry during arterial oxyhemoglobin desaturation in dogs. *Anesthesiology*, 68, 111–114.

Shamir, M., Eidelman, L., Floman, Y., Kaplan, L. and Pizov, R. (1999) Pulse oximetry plethysmographic waveform during changes in blood volume. *Brit J Anaesth*, 82, 178–181.

SurgiVet ® (2016) Veterinary anesthesia and monitoring equipment. *Smiths Medical*. Available from: http://surgivet.com/ [Accessed May 15, 2016].

Taylor, M. and Whitwan, J. (1988) The accuracy of pulse oximeters. *Anaesthesia*, 43, 229–232.

Tremper, K. and Barker, S. (1989) Pulse oximetry. *Anesthesiology*, 70, 98–108.

Veterinary equipment and supply store. Available from: http://www.dreveterinary.com/ [Accessed May 15, 2016].

Websters J. (1997) *Design of Pulse Oximeters*. New York: Taylor & Francis Group.

Young, S., Skeans, S., Lamca, J. and Chapman, R. (2002) Agreement of SpO_2, SaO_2 and ScO_2 in anesthetized cynomolgus monkeys (*Macaca fascicularis*). *Vet Anaesth Analg*, 29, 150–155.

19

Cardiovascular Monitoring

Anderson Favaro da Cunha[1] *and Rebecca A. Johnson*[2]

[1] *School of Veterinary Medicine, Louisiana State University, Baton Rouge, Louisiana, USA*
[2] *School of Veterinary Medicine, University of Wisconsin, Madison, Wisconsin, USA*

19.1 Introduction

Blood pressure (BP) relies on complex physiological interactions between the heart and vascular systems. It ultimately results from the product of cardiac output and systemic vascular resistance. BP is the most important determinant of afterload, and influences myocardial contractility and cardiac output (Haskins 2015). Clinically, the monitoring of BP helps the veterinary healthcare provider to assess the patient's cardiovascular status and to have an acceptable understanding of tissue perfusion quality, especially since exact tissue perfusion cannot be easily quantified.

19.2 Definitions

Normal BP values vary among species. For example, in healthy, conscious dogs, systolic arterial pressure (SAP) is 150 mmHg, mean arterial pressure (MAP) is 100 mmHg and the diastolic arterial pressure (DAP) is approximately 85 mmHg (Bodey and Michell 1996; Redondo *et al.* 2007). In cats, SAP is approximately 130 mmHg, the MAP is 105 mmHg and the DAP is 90 mmHg (Brown *et al.* 2007). A useful summary of many publications regarding normal BPs for dogs and cats is available in the *Guidelines for the Identification, Evaluation and Management of Systemic Hypertension in Dogs and Cats*, published by the American College of Veterinary Internal Medicine (Brown *et al.* 2007).

In normal, healthy horses, BP is affected by breed and is variable. For example, in one study of 296 horses, SAP was 86–159 mmHg and DAP was 45–97 mmHg. If MAP is estimated as the DAP + ⅓(SAP-DAP), then the calculated MAP for those values (not specifically reported) would be 58–117 mmHg (Parry *et al.* 1984). For birds, the arterial pressures again greatly depend on the species;

anesthetics further alter BP values. For example, SAP was 88 mmHg for anesthetized pigeons (Touzot-Jourde *et al.* 2005) and 232 mmHg for conscious great horned owls (Hawkins *et al.* 2003). For additional normal values, refer to Schnellbacher *et al.* (2014).

Hypotension is a common complication of general anesthesia and is usually defined as MAP of less than 60 mmHg for small animals and less than 70 mmHg for larger species (Brodbelt 2009). Hypertension, although not as common during general anesthesia, is often defined as a MAP of more than 160 mmHg for dogs and cats (Brown *et al.* 2007). Both hypotension and hypertension should be prevented to avoid the negative impact of abnormal tissue perfusion. For example, renal, cerebral and myocardial ischemia are often associated with hypotension (Wagner and Brodbelt 1997) and retinal damage, and kidney, heart and brain injuries are associated with hypertension (Littman 1994, Bartges *et al.* 1996). Even though the clinical significance of hypo- or hypertension depends on the severity and duration of the underlying cause and the level of the hypo- or hypertensive episode (Cooper 2015; Hopper and Brown 2015), the early recognition of pressure abnormalities is key when choosing the optimal treatment for cardiovascular support (Haskins 2015). For blood pressure evaluation, there are many techniques available that can be divided in two major categories: invasive arterial catheterization and indirect, non-invasive means.

19.3 Measurement Techniques

19.3.1 Invasive Blood Pressure (IBP)

The invasive blood pressure (IBP) method is the gold standard of BP measurement and provides accurate, reliable, beat-to-beat monitoring of SAP, DAP and MAP. MAP is calculated as the area under the pressure curve

Veterinary Anesthetic and Monitoring Equipment, First Edition. Edited by Kristen G. Cooley and Rebecca A. Johnson.
© 2018 John Wiley & Sons, Inc. Published 2018 by John Wiley & Sons, Inc.

divided by the beat period and averaged over consecutive heartbeats (Schroeder *et al.* 2015). MAP is frequently estimated as one-third of the pulse pressure added to the diastolic pressure. However, this relationship is the most accurate at slower pulse rates, since tachycardia reduces the proportion of time in diastole (Stouffer 2008; Schroeder *et al.* 2015).

In adult human patients, arterial catheterization for invasive BP monitoring has a low complication rate (<1%), but rare complications such as distal ischemia, hemorrhage, hematoma, embolization, infection, etc. are reported (Scheer *et al.* 2002; Schroeder *et al.* 2015). Similarly, no serious complications were associated with arterial catheters used for intra-operative BP monitoring in dogs (Trim *et al.* 2017). However, some consider the technique technically challenging, uncomfortable for the patient and unsuitable for many clinical situations (Binns *et al.* 1995; Branson *et al.* 1997; Brown and Henik 1998). In any case, the advantages related to understanding the patient's cardiovascular status, the ability to make timely informed patient decisions based on pressure waveform alterations and pressure measurements, and the ability to perform arterial blood gas analysis frequently outweigh disadvantages associated with the technique.

This method is often called the "direct method" for BP measurement; however, this term should be used cautiously since the invasive technique usually requires a transducer to convert the mechanical pulsations from the artery into an electrical signal that can be displayed on a monitor and, therefore, this is an indirect method. However, if the arterial catheter is connected directly to an aneroid manometer without a transducer (infrequently performed), this would be considered a direct technique in that scenario.

Commonly, IBP requires an intra-arterial catheter connected to a microprocessor and display screen (i.e. multifunction monitor) via a fluid filled, disposable, non-compliable extension set (Figure 19.1) connected to a BP transducer (Figure 19.2). The non-compressible fluid column formed by blood and saline is connected to the pressure transducer, creating a "hydraulic coupling" that pressurizes a diaphragm plate located inside the transducer. In newer transducers, this diaphragm is directly connected to four strain gauges that are incorporated into a sensitive Wheatstone bridge (Figure 19.3). The mechanical pressure variations associated with arterial pulsations will lead to pressure applied to the diaphragm and compression of two strain gauges with simultaneous stretching of the other two. The variation in length and diameter of the strain gauges, associated with their compression or stretch, leads to a variation in resistance. The bridge becomes unbalanced and the potential difference generated is proportional to the pressure applied. The resistance variance is then converted into an electrical

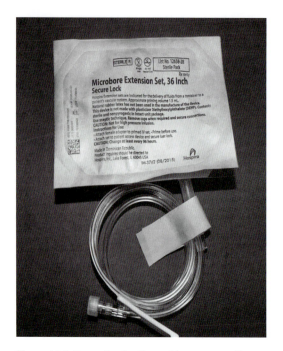

Figure 19.1 Example of a disposable, non-compliant extension set that connects to an IBP pressure transducer (many manufacturers, e.g. Microbore Extension Set, Hospira, Lake Forest, IL).

signal, which is processed, amplified and then displayed graphically and numerically by the BP monitor (Davis *et al.* 1995; Dorsch and Dorsch 2008; Schroeder *et al.* 2015). This type of Wheatstone bridge is four times more sensitive than a single strain gauge and compensates for temperature changes as all gauges are affected equally.

For research situations, special BP transducers can be connected to digital recording systems that allow high definition IBP data collection (e.g. Power Lab, ADInstruments, New South Wales, Australia; BIOPAC®, BIOPAC® Systems, Inc., Goleta, CA). These systems provide higher

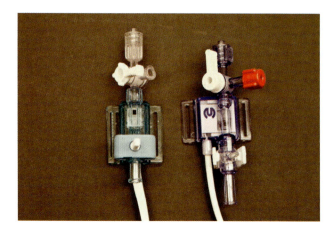

Figure 19.2 Examples of IBP transducers for use in clinical veterinary medicine (many manufacturers, e.g. Argon Medical Devices, Wheeling, IL).

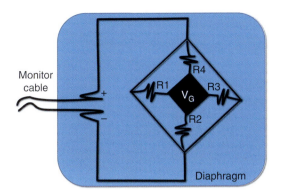

Figure 19.3 The Wheatstone bridge circuit connected to a diaphragm and four resistors (R1-4). The galvanometer (V_G) measures the potential difference, which is proportional to the pressure.

precision data collection when compared with clinical transducers. For example, a special pressure transducer system (ADInstruments, New South Wales, Australia) uses a transducer that generates an output impedance of $1000 \, \Omega$ and input impedance of $700 \, \Omega$, with a sensitivity of $5 \, \mu V/V/mmHg$. This system can collect hundreds of datasets per second, increasing the definition of the data collected. Also, an intra-arterial pressure transducer is available for research (Mikro-tip® pressure catheter, Millar Inc., Houston, TX) that can collect BP data without the need of a fluid filled extension set, reducing the possibility of common equipment errors associated with over- or under-damping of the pressure signal (see below).

19.3.1.1   Calibration Check

To check the calibration, a pressurizing bulb is connected to one air-filled non-compliant extension set and this air-filled set in further connected to a fluid-filled non-compliant extension via a three-way stopcock (Figure 19.4). The air-filled extension set is attached to a mercury manometer and the fluid-filled extension set to

a pressure transducer. The pressure transducer is placed at the same level as the "zero" of the mercury manometer and the pressure transducer of the IBP monitor is zeroed in accordance to the manufacturer's instructions. The air-filled system should be pressurized to 50 mmHg and the stopcock closed to the bulb to connect both extensions; the pressure is held constant for 3–5 seconds. Then the process is repeated at a higher pressure (e.g. 150 mmHg) and observed for another 3–5 seconds. The IBP monitor should display the same pressures as the mercury manometer. Remember, this is just a quality assurance technique for the clinical transducer to *check* the calibration. It is *not* a technique to calibrate the transducer.

19.3.1.2   Patency

While in use, the transducers may be connected to a pressurized (300 mmHg) bag of heparinized (1 U/mL) 0.9% saline to allow continuous flush and to prevent clot formation at the tip of the catheter. Most transducers, when connected to a pressurized saline bag, will allow the delivery of a continuous rate infusion of flush at a rate of 1–3 mL/h (although caution is recommended not to volume overload very small patients) (Schroeder *et al.* 2015). When continuous flush is not an option, hourly, heparinized saline flushes are recommended. Again, be cautious not to over-heparinize the patient with this technique.

19.3.1.3   Zeroing

The modern clinical transducer requires zeroing but not calibration. The zeroing process allows the microprocessor to recognize the atmospheric pressure and then compare it with the arterial pressures being measured. This process does not necessarily need to be performed at the level of the heart. However, it should be performed several times per day to eliminate any baseline drift according to the manufacturer's instructions. Frequently it

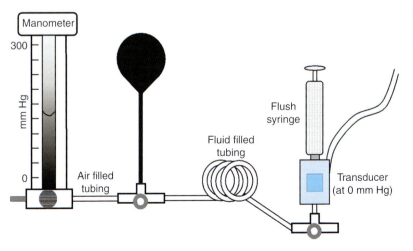

Figure 19.4 The system used to test the calibration of an IBP monitor using a mercury manometer.

entails opening the stopcock attached to the transducer to atmospheric air and pressing the "zero" button on the monitor. A faulty transducer can be sometimes be detected by opening the stopcock to air multiple times during the anesthetic procedure; the transducer should always read zero with no shifts in the baseline.

19.3.1.4 Transducer Positioning

To improve accuracy of the BP readings, the IBP transducer should be placed at the same level as the base of the right atrium (aortic root pressure) during monitoring. Gravity and hydrostatic pressures associated with the fluid-filled extensions do interfere with the pressure transducers accuracy. The BP reading will be inaccurately elevated if the transducer is placed below the heart level, and similarly, BP will be lowered if the pressure transducer is placed above the heart level. Each 1 cm change in height will alter the pressure reading by 0.75 mmHg (Ortega *et al.* 2017).

19.3.1.5 Transducer Physics and Fast Flush Test

Wave Analysis Pressure systems rely on three properties: elasticity, mass and friction, which determine the system's operating features. Many factors influence the shape of the waveform, including the fundamental wave (the pulse rate) and harmonic waves, which are smaller waves with frequencies that are multiples of the fundamental frequency. For example, if the fundamental frequency is 2 Hz, the harmonic waves would have frequencies of 4 Hz, 6 Hz, 8 Hz, etc. The arterial blood pressure waveform is created by Fourier analysis, which sums many sine waves of differing amplitudes and frequencies into a complex waveform. In the IBP system, this complex waveform is broken down by the microprocessor into individual sine waves, and then reformed from the fundamental and harmonic waves to give a more accurate representation of the waveform (Schroeder *et al.* 2015).

Natural Frequency and Resonance System operation also depends on the natural frequency and resonance (Schroeder *et al.* 2015). The natural frequency of an IBP system is the frequency at which it freely oscillates. If the natural frequency is close to the frequency of any of the sine waves incorporated into an arterial waveform, the IBP system with resonate, causing excessive amplification of the waveform with falsely wide and tall peaks. Thus, the system should have the highest natural frequency as possible (Schroeder *et al.* 2015). A normal arterial waveform with a steep systolic upstroke and peak, dicrotic notch (closure of the aortic valve) and diastolic run off (Figure 19.5), can be formed by as little as two sine waves, the fundamental frequency and another harmonic. However, 6–10 harmonics (preferably 8) are

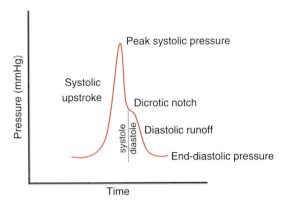

Figure 19.5 Schematic of a normal arterial waveform. The MAP corresponds to the area under the curve (waveform) divided by the duration of the pulse wave and averaged over several waveforms. The pulse pressure results from the difference between the SAP and DAP. The dicrotic notch represents the closure of the aortic valve.

needed to result in a distortion-free arterial pressure waveform (Geddes 1991; Schroder *et al.* 2015). For example, a cat with a pulse rate of 180 bpm (3 cycles/sec or 3 Hz) will require a system with a dynamic response of 18–30 Hz. Patients with faster heart rates and steeper systolic upstrokes will require systems with greater dynamic responses to produce accurate waveforms (Schroder *et al.* 2015). The system's natural frequency is increased by reducing the length of the catheter and tubing, using non-compliant tubing, using low-density fluid to fill the system, and increasing the catheter and tubing diameter.

Damping Systems may experience under- or over-damping of the signals. All systems have some signal damping, mainly from friction by the fluid; the normal damping co-efficient will be approximately 0.7, which stems from the optimal speed of response and best accuracy. Some transducer-based systems are under-damped (damping coefficient <0.7), where the system's natural frequency is too low, resulting in resonation and exaggerated waveforms (Figure 19.6). The systolic pressures overshoot and small oscillatory waves may be present. This system is quick to respond and over-reads systolic and under-reads diastolic pressures. In contrast, over-damped waveforms (damping coefficient >1) have a delayed upstroke, no dicrotic notch and a narrowed pulse pressure. The systolic pressures under-read and the diastolic pressures over-read, although MAP may remain close to normal. Extra stopcocks, bubbles and clots, vasospasm, narrow, long or compliant tubing, and kinks can also cause system over-damping.

To rule out errors associated with the system's dynamic responses, the fast flush test has been recommended

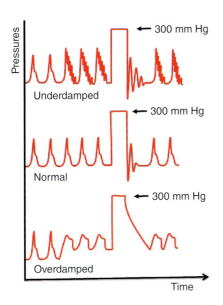

Figure 19.6 Damped signals and the fast flush test. Underdamped signals (top tracing) are over-responsive with erroneously elevated SAP and diminished DAP. Overdamped signals loose definition and have reduced pulse pressures (bottom tracing).

(Figure 19.6), especially for times where accurate SAP and DAP are important. If MAP is the only measurement required, then the dynamic responses are of little significance (Gardner 1981). This test is also known as the "square wave test", which is performed by pressing the flushing mechanism of the pressure transducer, holding it for one or two seconds to allow pressure equilibration with the pressurized flushing bag and then releasing it abruptly. The sudden pressure change after the flush causes oscillations that are used to calculate the harmonic frequency of the system. Well-regulated systems only allow one or two oscillations before the waveform returns to baseline. A system is considered inadequate when it is under-damped or over-damped (Gardner 1981).

As previously mentioned, when the system is under-damped, systolic pressure is overshot and additional small resonant pressure waves will affect the waveform. For example, three or more oscillations will occur before the waveform returns to baseline (system is too responsive), leading to an over-estimation of SAP. On the other hand, the over-damped pressure waveform has a decreased pulse pressure compared to normal. When the system is over-damped, no oscillations will be observed (system response is too slow), leading to an under-estimation of SAP. The DAP is also affected by inadequate systems; however, it is more tolerant of dynamic response inadequacies than SAP (Gardner 1981). Readers are referred to Gardner (1981) for further detailed explanations regarding the calculation of the natural frequency of a system and its damping coefficient.

19.3.1.6 Arterial Pressure Waveform Morphology

As previously mentioned, the normal central arterial (aortic root) waveform has a steep systolic upstroke ending in the SAP, followed by a downstroke containing the incisura (dicrotic notch), which ends at the end-diastolic pressure (Figure 19.5). As the waveform travels to the peripheral arteries, the systolic upstroke becomes steeper, the dicrotic notch is delayed and the diastolic wave becomes more prevalent with a lower end-diastolic pressure (Schroeder *et al.* 2015). This effect is termed "distal pulse amplification". MAPs change very little from the aorta to the peripheral arteries, since there is little resistance to flow; it is not until blood reaches the arterioles where resistance increases dramatically and blood pressure significantly decreases.

New techniques using the changes in the arterial waveform morphology are being used as a starting point for hemodynamic therapeutic interventions. For example, systolic pressure variation (SPV) and pulse pressure variation (PPV) are currently being used to monitor volume responsiveness in veterinary patients. Further information on this topic can be found in Chapter 23.

19.3.1.7 Other Possible Errors

Since the catheter size and type, extension tubing, stopcocks and transducer can affect the pressure signal, the IBP monitoring system should be visually inspected for air bubbles, kinks, fluid leaks, obstructions and clots that can lead to damping of the system response. When the catheter is removed, pressure should be applied to the insertion site for 2–5 minutes to prevent hematoma formation. Even though complications are uncommon, skin infection and complete obstruction of the blood flow have been reported.

19.3.1.8 Anatomical Locations for Arterial Catheterization

The preferred location for arterial catheterization depends on the species and clinical experience of personnel. The most common peripheral arteries that can be catheterized in dogs are the dorsal pedal and median sacral (Figure 19.7), even though the superficial palmar, lingual and median auricular arteries can also be catheterized. However, BP variability between sites has been reported in dogs (Acierno *et al.* 2015; Mooney *et al.* 2017). For example, SAP measured at the dorsal pedal artery was as much as 43 mmHg higher or 11 mmHg lower than simultaneous SAP measured at the superficial palmar arch, when anesthetized dogs were either in dorsal or lateral recumbency (Acierno *et al.* 2015). Similarly, in anesthetized dogs, MAP measured from the dorsal pedal, auricular and coccygeal arteries is underestimated, compared with aortic pressures; however, these changes are relatively small and unlikely to change

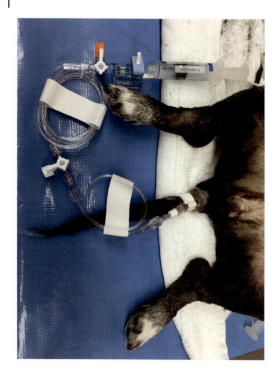

Figure 19.7 Example of a 22-gauge arterial catheter and extension set placed in the median sacral artery in a dog. Following sterile preparation and catheter placement, a non-porous dressing (Tegaderm, 3M Medical, St Paul, MN) is placed to reduce contamination and secure the catheter. It is attached to a transducer for IBP monitoring.

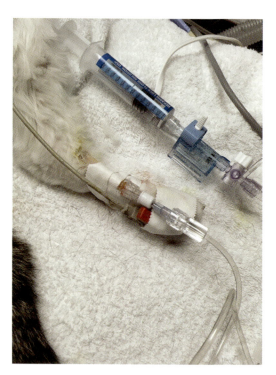

Figure 19.8 Example of a 24-gauge arterial catheter placed in the dorsal pedal artery of a cat, secured with tape, and connected to a pressure transducer.

clinical decision-making, although the auricular artery pressures may be more variable and difficult to interpret (Soares *et al.* 2017).

In cats, the dorsal pedal, femoral and median sacral arteries are commonly catheterized (Figure 19.8). In horses, the lateral dorsal metatarsal, transverse facial and facial arteries are the most commonly used (Figure 19.9), whereas the auricular and femoral arteries are frequently used in ruminants (Figure 19.10). In birds, the deep radial, superficial ulnar, cranial tibial and dorsal metatarsal arteries are acceptable choices (Schnellbacher *et al.* 2014). In other, less common species, arterial catheters may be placed in any palpable peripheral artery, such as the auricular artery in rabbits. For comparison studies, when the NIBP cuff is positioned in the antebrachium of dogs, the best anatomical locations for the IBP measurement were found to be the medial sacral artery (da Cunha *et al.* 2017), where less bias and closer limits of agreement were observed.

19.3.1.9 Cleaning and Asepsis

Since one possible complication associated with the IBP technique is local infection of the arterial site, aseptic techniques should be followed during placement and maintenance of the catheter. Usually, the commercially-

available IBP transducers are disposable; however, to reduce the cost associated with the constant replacement of the transducers, when it is not contaminated

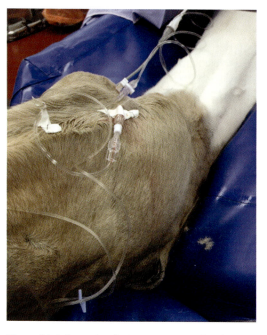

Figure 19.9 Example of a 20-gauge arterial catheter placed in the facial artery in a dorsally recumbent horse. It is attached to non-compliant tubing and a transducer to measure IBP.

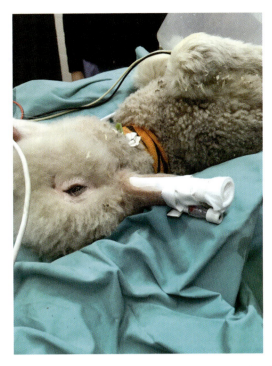

Figure 19.10 Example of an arterial catheter placed in the auricular artery in a dorsally recumbent lamb. It is secured with cotton padding placed inside the ear to act as a "stent" for increased security.

with blood, urine or feces, the IBP transducer can be passively dried and then re-sterilized with ethylene-oxide. A calibration check, as previously described, should be performed after each sterilization.

19.3.2 Non-Invasive BP (NIBP)

Since intra-arterial catheterization for IBP monitoring may be challenging (Wagner and Brodbelt 1997; Mazzaferro and Wagner 2001), especially in hypotensive, hypovolemic or smaller patients (Mishina *et al.* 1997), the non-invasive BP (NIBP) technique may be considered more suitable in anesthetically stable patients (Dyson 1997; Sawyer *et al.* 2004). The NIBP technique depends on the "return-to-flow" principle in which the pressure is detected following occlusion of an artery and subsequent release, allowing return of flow distal to the occluding cuff. However, the accuracy of this technique in veterinary medicine is somewhat disappointing. In general, the techniques available for NIBP monitoring can be subdivided into two major groups: the ultrasonic Doppler flow detector and the oscillometric methods.

19.3.2.1 Ultrasonic Doppler Flow Detector (Doppler)

Since 1977, the ultrasonic Doppler flow detector (Doppler) method has been used in veterinary medicine

for the measurement of BP and is considered inexpensive and easy to use (McLeish 1977; Klevans *et al.* 1979) (Figure 19.11). The Doppler detects blood flow by emitting an ultrasound signal that hits the moving red blood cells located in the arteries. The probe then receives the ultrasound signal back and transduces it into an auditory signal (Kazamias *et al.* 1971). It requires a flat piezoelectric crystal probe (8.2 MHz) that is positioned over an artery after hair clipping and application of ultrasound gel. The gel is essential to improve contact and sound transmission. Ideally, the probe is secured with tape or other wrap (i.e. Vetwrap, 3M Medical, St Paul, MN) directly perpendicular and over the artery to avoid unwanted displacement of the probe during cuff inflation. Then, a cuff with a width of 30–40% of the circumference of the area is applied proximal to the Doppler probe. The cuff is subsequently inflated with a sphygmomanometer to a pressure high enough to cease the pulsating sounds of the arterial blood flow. Then, the cuff is gradually deflated until the first pulsation sound is detected. The sounds of the reappearance of the pulsations during cuff deflation are called the Korotkoff sounds (ANSI/AAMI/SP10:2002/(R) 2008). Korotkoff sounds are a combination of audible frequencies generated by turbulent arterial blood flow distal to the cuff. By definition, the sphygmomanometer pressure correlating to the first Korotkoff sound approximates the SAP

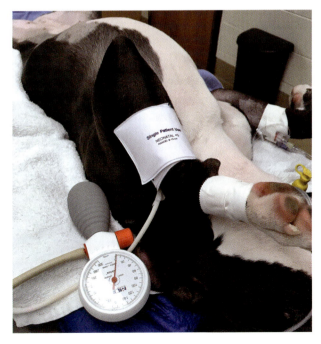

Figure 19.11 Placement of a Doppler blood pressure cuff on the antebrachium of a dog in dorsal recumbency attached to a sphygmomanometer; the crystal is placed on the ventral aspect of the front paw for an audible signal and blood pressure measurements.

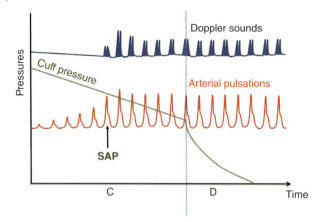

Figure 19.12 Diagram illustrating arterial pulsations and Korotkoff sounds in relation to NIBP cuff pressures. The cuff is deflated over time (C) and subsequently released (D). Doppler sounds reappear when cuff pressure reaches the SAP.

(Figure 19.12). This technique relies on blood flow, therefore states that affect vessel stiffness or reduce peripheral blood flow, such as cardiogenic shock or infusion of vasoconstrictors, can affect readings (Schroeder *et al.* 2015).

The accuracy of Doppler readings in small animals has been questioned (Klevans *et al.* 1979; Grandy *et al.* 1992; Binns *et al.* 1995; Caulkett *et al.* 1998; Acierno and Labato 2005; Henik *et al.* 2005). In anesthetized cats (Binns *et al.* 1995), BP measurements obtained by Doppler offered the highest overall accuracy when compared with an oscillometric method, as indicated by mean error values of less than 10 mmHg. Moreover, others (Caulkett *et al.* 1998) found good correlation between invasively measured SAP and Doppler measurements, but agreement analysis revealed under-estimation of SAP. To improve this relationship, the use of a correction factor to improve the reliability of systolic BPs obtained by the Doppler has been suggested. For example, 14.7 mmHg may be added to the Doppler reading to estimate the SAP in cats (Grandy *et al.* 1992). However, statistical analyses for these results have been questioned (linear regression; Hartnack 2014) and others were unsuccessful in obtaining good agreement when such correction factor was applied (Caulkett *et al.* 1998; da Cunha *et al.* 2014).

In general, results suggest poor agreement between Doppler values and invasively measured BPs in cats; Doppler readings could mislead the veterinary personnel during the diagnosis of systemic BP alterations. Consequently, Doppler readings in cats should be interpreted with caution in a clinical context. Similar results are available for avian species. For example, in red tailed hawks, the Doppler was able to read BPs closer to MAP instead of SAP when the cuff was positioned either on pectoral or pelvic limbs (Zehnder *et al.* 2009). In other species, such as dogs, horses and pigs, Doppler values are used as SAP; however, caution must be used in interpretation, as inaccuracies also exist in these species (Bailey *et al.* 1994; Acierno *et al.* 2008; Johnston *et al.* 2011; Musk *et al.* 2014).

In cats and dogs, the antebrachium is frequently used for the application of the cuff and probe. The cuff is placed proximal to the transducer, in the middle third of the antebrachium and the probe is taped onto the palmar aspect of the carpus, over the superficial palmar artery. For large animals, the ventral tail is recommended; the cuff is applied proximal, approximately 5 cm distal to the perianal area and the probe is applied just proximal to the cuff over the median coccygeal artery.

19.3.2.2 The Oscillometric Blood Pressure (OBP) Method

The oscillometric blood pressure (OBP) method is used in automated NIBP monitors. It requires an inflatable cuff or bladder to first obstruct the blood flow from an area over a major peripheral artery (Figure 19.13). After cuff inflation and a short cuff pressure stabilization, the device deflates the cuff slowly, in a controlled manner, using a stairway deflation strategy that is correlated to the decrease in the pressure applied to the artery over time until the return of normal blood flow (Figure 19.14). When cuff pressure is lower than SAP, the cuff pressure

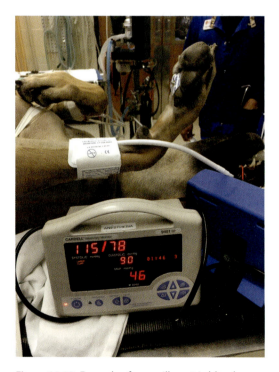

Figure 19.13 Example of an oscillometric blood pressure monitor (Cardell 9401, Paragon Medical, Coral Springs, FL). The cuff is placed on the antebrachium in a dorsally recumbent dog. The SAP = 115, DAP = 78 and MAP = 90 mmHg. The pulse rate is 46 bpm.

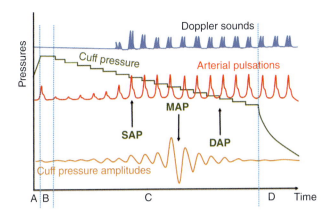

Figure 19.14 Diagram illustrating arterial pulsations and Korotkoff sounds in relation to oscillometric cuff pressures. Doppler sounds disappear during cuff inflation (A) and reappear when cuff pressure reaches the SAP. There is a cuff pressure equilibration period (B) before cuff deflation (C) when the monitor oscillates around the MAP, subsequently calculating the SAP and DAP. The cuff pressure is released at the end of the cycle (D).

amplitude will start to increase until blood flow returns to normal. During deflation, the NIBP board will receive the cuff pressure mechanical signals related to the variation in volume of the area where the cuff is applied (cuff pressure amplitude). This signal is related to the pulse pressure variation associated with the return of normal circulation. Frequently, the greatest cuff pressure amplitude variation is measured as MAP, and then SAP and DAP are calculated by the aid of a proprietary algorithm; results are displayed as BP (Henneman and Henneman 1989; Deflandre and Hellebrekers 2008; Dorsch and Dorsch 2008). Thus, when this technique is used, the SAP and DAP are less reliable than MAP. If pulse detection is not possible, the accuracy will be decreased (Grosenbaugh and Muir 1998). Many different brands of NIBP devices designed for veterinary medicine have been tested in clinical practice; however, questions about the accuracy of each method have been raised (Grandy *et al.* 1992; Binns *et al.* 1995; Branson *et al.* 1997; Caulkett *et al.* 1998; Acierno *et al.* 2010; Garofalo *et al.* 2012).

A few examples (not an exhaustive list) of OBP monitors designed specifically for veterinary use include pet-MAP™ (Ramsey Medical, Inc., Tampa, FL), SunTech Vet20 (SunTech Medical, Inc., Morrisville, NC), Cardell (9401, Paragon Medical, Coral Springs, FL), and HDO VetBP Monitor (Digicare Animal Health, Boynton Beach, FL). For example, the petMAP has "proprietary optimizations" to improve the correlation of readings with arterial pressures and is small and portable. The SunTech 20 also has a veterinary-specific algorithm and a touch screen. Cardell blood pressure monitors similarly have veterinary specific algorithms and are found as individual units or as part of multiparameter monitors.

The HDO VetBP uses new technology based on high definition oscillometry for increased sensitivity and has the advantage of beat-by-beat monitoring. Thus, each different OBP brand and model designed for veterinary species has specific advantages and disadvantages. However, before use, they should be tested clinically within the species in question (Binns *et al.* 1995) and most importantly, results analyzed using the correct statistical technique (Hartnack 2014) and compared to the current standards for validation of NIBP devices (Brown *et al.* 2007; ANSI/AAMI/SP10:2002/(R) 2008). The lack of specific regulations for veterinary equipment testing is hindering the evolution of equipment designed for veterinary patients.

The most important user-specific factors affecting the performance of OBP units are related to cuff size selection and choice of the anatomical location for cuff placement. In general, the current literature recommends the measurement of the circumference of the anatomical location where the cuff will be applied, and the application of cuffs with width of 30–40% of that circumference (Valtonen and Eriksson 1970). If larger cuffs are applied, in general, blood pressure is under-estimated and if smaller cuffs are used, IBP will be over-estimated. In foals, Giguère *et al.* (2005b) observed that agreement of the NIBP readings with IBP was influenced by the brand of OBP; BP in one brand was influenced by cuff location, whereas this relationship was not seen when another brand was used (Giguère *et al.* 2005b). Therefore, it is important for the NIBP user to be well informed of the manufacturer's recommendations and to not treat all monitors as if they were the same.

19.3.2.3 Equipment Testing of NIBP Monitors

The American Association of Medical Instrumentation (AAMI) develops voluntary standards for medical devices, so that manufacturers might provide information on their product and performance criteria that should be considered in qualifying an instrument for clinical use (ANSI/AAMI/SP10:2002/(R) 2008). These standards require that paired NIBP and IBP readings yield measurements with a mean difference of less than or equal to 5 mmHg and a mean ± standard deviation of less than 8 mmHg. Few veterinary BP monitors have met this standard (Bruner *et al.* 1981; Bodey *et al.* 1994, 1996; Binns *et al.* 1995). Due to the difficulty in identifying instruments that meet the AAMI criteria, the American College of Internal Medicine (ACVIM) released a consensus statement in 2007 (Brown *et al.* 2007) regarding the identification, evaluation and management of systemic hypertension in dogs and cats, which also describes a less rigid methodology for testing of NIBP equipment in veterinary medicine. The ACVIM guidelines suggest that good agreement is met when the following is observed:

In general, the criteria and recommendations of the AAMI must be followed. These include recommendations for patient selection, pressure range, number of observers, blinding of observations, and reporting of study findings. N-System efficacy is validated if the following conditions are met:

- The mean difference of paired measurements for systolic and diastolic pressures treated separately is +/- 10 mmHg or less, with a standard deviation of 15 mmHg or less.
- The correlation between paired measures for systolic and diastolic pressures treated separately is ≥0.9 across the range of measured values of BP.
- 50% of all measurements for systolic and diastolic pressures treated separately lie within 10 mmHg of the reference method.
- 80% of all measurements for systolic and diastolic pressures treated separately lie within 20 mmHg of the reference method.
- The study results have been accepted for publication in a referred journal.
- The subject database contains no fewer than 8 animals for comparison with an intra-arterial method, or 25 animals for comparison with a previously validated indirect device.

The ACVIM guidelines lack veterinary specific recommendations for patient selection, blood pressure ranges for a specific experiment, the number of observers, blinding of observations, and reporting technique of study findings; however, it refers the reader to the AAMI guidelines for that information. Noteworthy is that general anesthesia decreased the percentage of error during a comparison study between IBP and NIBP for SAP and increased it for MAP and DAP (Vachon *et al.* 2014). Therefore, comparison studies should consider evaluating NIBP devices in both conscious and anesthetized subjects.

19.3.2.4 Statistical Analysis of Comparison Studies

It is widely accepted that calculation of bias and precision represents the best statistical method for comparing two techniques while measuring the same physiological variable (i.e. BP). For a new method of BP measurement to be used interchangeably with the gold standard, it should rely on the limits of agreements of up to approximately 30%, as described in details by Hartnack (2014). Readers are encouraged to critically evaluate publications centering on the relationship between IBP and OBP in veterinary patients. For example, although good agreement between IBP and NIBP has been shown in cats (Caulkett *et al.* 1998) and dogs (Vachon *et al.* 2014), poor agreement has also been shown in dogs (Acierno *et al.* 2013), horses (Yamaoka *et al.* 2017), camelids

(Aarnes *et al.* 2012) and Hispaniolan Amazon parrots (Acierno *et al.* 2008). Some studies have been criticized for their statistical methodology (Hartnack 2014).

19.3.2.5 Trend Analyses

Serial NIBP measurements, instead of a single measurement, have been proposed as an alternative to IBP for clinical decisions, when the method used for NIBP measurement was associated with poor IBP agreement (Rysnik *et al.* 2013). However, this use is debatable (Acierno *et al.* 2010; da Cunha *et al.* 2016). For example, if the ability to decide on a treatment is based on a BP reading coming from an NIBP monitor that is not able to read BPs in a stable patient, how can one trust the trends generated by that machine? However, if the error is stable and can be calculated, then perhaps the trends generated by that machine could be trusted.

19.3.2.6 Calibration of NIBP Devices

Even if validated, the calibration of an automated NIBP device can drift over time, producing an unrecognized artifactual bias that can lead to false diagnoses. An automatic indirect NIBP measuring device used in clinical practice should be tested to assure accuracy against a standard such as a mercury or aneroid manometer at least twice annually. There are routine methods and standards for testing the accuracy of these devices, and all manufactured NIBP monitors should contain a "test mode" and appropriate instructions for performing this necessary calibration check.

Although many veterinary practices likely will not have a mercury manometer or national pressure standard readily available for use, suitable alternatives include comparing the automatic NIBP device against a second pressure-measuring instrument such as an aneroid manometer. In its simplest form, the NIBP device in question could simply be connected to the pressure manometer and the automatic cuff inflation mode started. The pressures displayed by the NIBP monitor as it inflates and deflates should match the manometer's pressure. A more precise method includes verifying that the static pressure output of the NIBP device matches the static pressure output of the manometer at 10-20 mmHg increments across the clinical useful range of 30-300 mmHg. Similarly, aneroid manometers used in conjunction with yet another indirect device, such as an ultrasonic Doppler system, should also be assessed for accuracy.

19.4 Patient Point of View

In both veterinary medicine (Marino *et al.* 2011) and human medicine (Gorbunov 1997), patients are likely to be stressed in a hospital environment, leading to higher BPs. This is often referred to as "white coat syndrome". Moreover, the ACVIM stated that technical errors associated with lack of personnel experience during BP readings are often the leading cause of BP measurement errors (Brown *et al.* 2007). Therefore, it is recommended that BP measurements be performed routinely to provide adequate training and familiarity with the equipment. In addition, personnel should be skilled in handling animals and aim to provide a calm environment, free of noises and prey–predator interactions, to avoid the white coat syndrome (Henik *et al.* 2005; Brown *et al.* 2007).

19.5 Central Venous Pressure (CVP)

Central venous pressure (CVP) monitoring can also be useful in the critically ill and/or anesthetized patient. A large bore, central venous catheter is aseptically placed into the jugular or femoral vein, with the distal tip located within the intrathoracic cranial or caudal vena cava. Double- or triple-lumen catheters are useful in these situations to not only monitor CVP, but for fluid or drug administration as well. These catheters are then connected to a pressure transducer as described above or to a water manometer to measure CVP (Medex manometer, Smiths Medical, London). If large, rapid fluid boluses are required, large-diameter, short catheters are better suited for this use. Chronic central venous access and long-term CVP monitoring can also be accomplished with long peripherally inserted central venous catheters (PICC lines; multiple manufacturers, e.g. Medical Components, Inc., Harleysville, PA) or through placement of vascular access ports (VAP; Companion Port, Norfolk Vet Products, Skokie, IL; Figure 19.15). Although complications in veterinary patients are rare, in humans, up to 15% experience some type of adverse event associated with central venous pressure monitoring, including vascular injury, respiratory trauma, nerve injury, arrhythmias, thromboembolic issues and site infection (McGee and Gould 2003).

CVP commonly measures the hydrostatic pressure at the junction of the vena cava and right atrium (Mathews 2012; Schroeder *et al.* 2015). In its simplest form, CVP can reflect the filling pressures of the right heart, but relies on both the intravascular blood volume and the capacitance of the vasculature (Kelman 1971). Although not exactly the same, the CVP is related to the volume of blood returning to the right heart (preload) (Marshall *et al.* 2016). Since right heart filling pressures (CVPs) influence stroke volume as dictated by the Frank-Starling principle, CVPs have been used to assess right heart function and adequacy of blood volume expansion

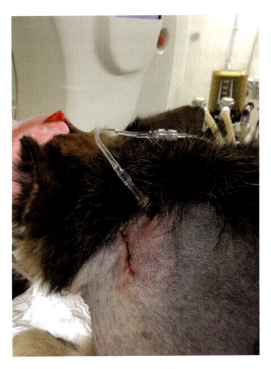

Figure 19.15 One day following VAP placement in a dog undergoing TomoTherapy radiation treatments. The incision required for placement is visible. The catheter tip is located in the intrathoracic vena cava and the access port is placed subcutaneously near the shoulder. A blunt-tipped needle (Huber needle; Norfolk Vet, Products, Skokie, IL) is placed into the VAP for vascular access and fluid administration.

(Cohn 1967). However, current thoughts suggest that CVP measurements are more useful for determining changes in intravascular volume rather than absolute levels. For example, with euvolemia and normal cardiac function, a 2–5 cmH$_2$O increase in CVP is expected following a rapid crystalloid bolus (20 mL/kg), which is expected to return to baseline after 15 minutes. In comparison, in a patient with increased blood volume or reduced cardiac function, the increase in CVP may be more than 5 cmH$_2$O and continues over some time, reflecting the reduced cardiac function and/or fluid overload (Weil and Henning 1979; Mathews 2012).

Normal CVP values (0–10 cmH$_2$O) are slightly above right atrial pressures and single values do not completely predict right heart volumes (Oakley *et al.* 1997; Waddell and Brown 2015). However, increases in CVP values can occur with increased blood volume, decreased cardiac function, increased vascular tone, and increased abdominal and thoracic pressures (positive pressure ventilation). Decreases in CVP can occur with hypovolemia and reduced vascular tone. Rhythmic changes in CVP occur with ventilation and with each heartbeat. Thus, for consistency, CVP should be measured just before inspiration at the lowest diastolic reading. When a transducer is used for

CVP measurement, a waveform is displayed, similar to arterial pressures but quantitatively smaller. Waveform fluctuations should always be present; if absent, the catheter should be adjusted back into the thoracic cavity or manipulated off the vessel wall until fluctuations are seen. The normal CVP waveform consists of three peaks (*a, c* and *v* waves) and two depressions (*x, y* descent) (Figure 19.16). The *a* wave is the most prominent and represents the increase in pressure during atrial contraction. Atrial pressure decreases immediately after as the atrium relaxes. The *c* wave then occurs transiently during isovolumic ventricular contraction as the closed tricuspid valve slightly protrudes into the right atrium. The *x* descent then occurs as pressure falls with ventricular ejection of blood. The *v* wave follows as venous blood flows into the right atrium while the tricuspid valve is still closed. The *y* descent is the decrease in pressure as the blood subsequently flows out of the tricuspid valve and into the right ventricle.

19.6 Cardiac Output Monitoring

Cardiac output is defined as the total blood flow leaving the left ventricle to the systemic vasculature. It is usually indexed to body weight and measured in mL or L/min, or dynes^3/min, where one dyne is the force required to accelerate a 1 g mass at a rate of 1 cm per sec^2 (Shih 2013). Normal cardiac output values vary somewhat between species and are reported as 120–200 mL/kg/min in the dog or cat (Marshall *et al.* 2016) and up to 222 mL/kg/min in 14-day-old foals (Shih 2013). Although cardiac output measurements are not frequently performed in everyday veterinary medicine, these methods are becoming more popular and are often used in some research facilities and tertiary care centers. There are four fundamental methods to measure cardiac output:

1) derivation using the Fick method;

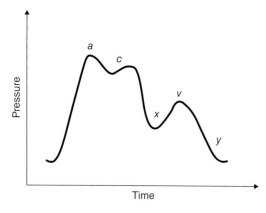

Figure 19.16 Diagram of a normal CVP waveform demonstrating the *a, c* and *v* upstrokes and the *x* and *y* descents.

2) dilution of temperature, lithium, dye or ultrasonic velocity;
3) arterial pulse contour analysis; and
4) ultrasonographic methods.

However, dilution methods are currently the most common technique.

19.6.1 Fick's Method

Cardiac output measured by the Fick's method was the original gold standard proposed by Adolf Fick in 1870; it was subsequently validated in horses in 1890 (Zuntz and Hagemann 1894; Marshall *et al.* 2016). This method requires an intubated patient and blood gas analyses. It relies on the concept that flow is proportional to the rate of uptake/production of a gas such as oxygen, carbon dioxide, nitrous oxide, etc. The original Fick equation is:

$$CO = VO_2 / \left(C_aO_2 - C_vO_2 \right) \quad (19.1)$$

where CO is the cardiac output, VO_2 is the oxygen consumption (calculated as the difference between the inhaled and the expired tidal volume/oxygen concentration), and C_aO_2 and C_vO_2 are the arterial and venous oxygen contents. Although C_aO_2 is not easily measured in clinical practice, oxygen content is calculated from the hemoglobin level (Hb), the hemoglobin oxygen saturation (O_2sat), and the PO_2 from an arterial or venous blood gas; oxygen content = (1.34 × Hb × O_2sat) + (0.003 × PO_2). All values are then inserted into the equation to obtain cardiac output. These measurements are not instantaneous and take multiple minutes as respiratory and blood gas analyses must be performed. In addition, this method is most useful in cardiovascular stable patients, because shunting of blood affects results (Thiele *et al.* 2015).

An extension of Fick's Method relies on carbon dioxide production during a short period of carbon dioxide rebreathing (until the CO_2 level in the breathing circuit plateaus) and has been used in dogs and foals (Gunkel *et al.* 2004; Giguère *et al.* 2005a; Marshall *et al.* 2016). The NICO system (Novametrix Medical Systems Inc., Wallingford, CT) uses a proprietary NICO sensor that adds a rebreathed volume of CO_2 directly to the breathing circuit and provides continual cardiac output monitoring. Cardiac output is proportional to the change in CO_2 production and lung elimination, divided by the change in end tidal CO_2 resulting from a brief rebreathing period (measured every 3 minutes for 35 seconds).

19.6.2 Indicator or Dilution Techniques

19.6.2.1 Indicator Techniques

Indicator or dilution techniques have generally replaced Fick's method for clinical cardiac output monitoring in veterinary medicine (Itami *et al.* 2016). They rely on injection of a premeasured amount of an indicator (cold saline, lithium or a dye such as indocyanine green), which is sampled downstream; a time-concentration curve is generated and cardiac output is subsequently derived using the Stewart–Hamilton principle, as cardiac output is inversely proportional to the area under the curve (Shih 2013). These methods are quite accurate and easy to use but are invasive, require skilled catheter placement, and may have complications such as thromboembolism, infection and vessel damage or rupture.

Transpulmonary Lithium or Dye Techniques A known amount of lithium or dye can be injected into the distal jugular vein or vena cava and concentrations are then measured in a transpulmonary fashion, from a peripheral artery such as the femoral artery. Specifically, lithium dilution techniques (LiDCO, Lake Villa, IL) require hemoglobin and sodium analyses first. Lithium chloride is injected into a large vein and withdrawn from a peripheral artery with flow across a sensor to generate the time–concentration curve from which cardiac output is derived (Shih 2013). Care must be taken in small patients to not remove large quantities of blood. In addition, lithium may accumulate, leading to erroneous values and abnormal behavior (Beaulieu *et al.* 2004).

Thermodilution Techniques In contrast, thermodilution techniques are frequently carried out with a double lumen pulmonary artery catheter (Swan-Ganz), with one port in the right atrium and one in the pulmonary artery; blood does not have to traverse the lungs. Cold isotonic 0.9% saline is injected into the right atrium with a thermistor placed in the pulmonary artery to measure the temperature dilution. Many other cardiac output determinants use the thermodilution method as the standard for comparison (Figure 19.17).

19.6.2.2 Ultrasound Velocity Dilution

The ultrasound velocity dilution technique relies on an arteriovenous loop made with tubing connecting a peripheral artery and central vein to form an extracorporeal circuit; the high resistance of this loop restricts the use of the technique to patients of less than 250 kg (Shih *et al.* 2009a, 2013). An ultrasonic velocity sensor is placed upstream from the venous catheter and another sensor is placed downstream from the arterial catheter. A small amount of isotonic saline is injected into the venous side, resulting in a transient hemodilution and

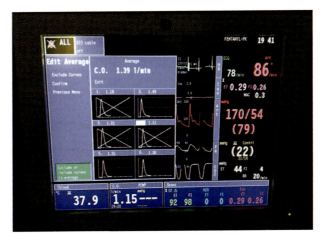

Figure 19.17 An example of a thermodilution cardiac output monitoring system (GE S/5 with thermodilution module, GE Healthcare, Wilmington, MA). Multiple measurements are made and values can be excluded (represented by an "X" over the excluded curves) prior to averaging (photograph courtesy of Dr João Soares, Virginia-Maryland College of Veterinary Medicine, Blacksburg, VA).

changes in the ultrasound velocity in that blood (Shih 2013). Cardiac output is calculated from the volume of injectate and the decrease in ultrasound velocity as the diluted blood passes through a sensor.

19.6.3 Arterial Pulse Contour Analysis

Although stroke volume can be obtained from the area under the arterial waveform until the dicrotic notch, many factors affect this measurement such as vascular resistance and damping (Shih 2013). Thus, dilution techniques have been combined with arterial waveform analysis (Shih 2013; Marshall *et al.* 2016). As a result, cardiac output is measured along with other indices such as stroke volume and pulse pressure variation, providing information pertaining to preload as well. The dilution method is used to calibrate the pulse contour calculation as the waveform is analyzed by propriety software. These measurements can be made using lithium dilution-pulse wave contour techniques (PulseCO; LiDCO, Lake Villa, IL; Figure 19.18) or with thermodilution-pulse wave contour techniques (PiCCO, Pulsion Medical Systems, Munich, Germany) (Shih *et al.* 2009b). Although continuous and relatively non-invasive, they still require an arterial catheter and may not accurately depict cardiac output in all situations (Marshall *et al.* 2016).

19.6.4 Ultrasound Techniques

19.6.4.1 Echocardiography

Echocardiography has frequently been used with Doppler ultrasound to determine stroke volume. All

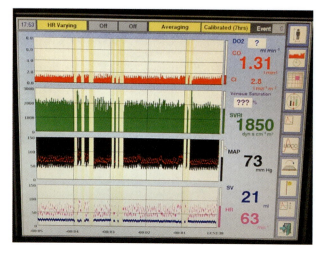

Figure 19.18 Pulse contour analyses used to determine cardiac output (CO) displayed as histograms over time. Periodic calibration with thermodilution or lithium dilution techniques is required. The monitor also displays variables such as cardiac index (CI), systemic vascular resistance index (SVRI), mean arterial pressure (MAP), stroke volume (SR) and heart rate (HR) (photograph courtesy of Dr João Soares, Virginia-Maryland College of Veterinary Medicine, Blacksburg, VA).

ultrasonographic techniques rely on the principle that when Doppler ultrasonic waves hit red blood cells, the waves are reflected back at a differing frequency (i.e. Doppler shift frequency), which is related to the blood flow velocity. When velocity is multiplied by the cross-sectional area of the left ventricular outflow tract, stroke volume is calculated which, when multiplied by heart rate, is the cardiac output. This is a transthoracic method and is completely non-invasive, but requires training in echocardiography to obtain accurate measurements.

Transesophageal Doppler echocardiography can also be used to obtain aortic flow velocity and diameter for cardiac output calculations. The Doppler esophageal probe is placed as close to the direction of flow in the descending aorta as possible (Hemosonic 100™, Teleflex Inc., Wayne, PA). The phase shift in the reflected ultrasound waves as they travel downstream multiplied by the aortic diameter calculates stroke volume and subsequently cardiac output (Marshall *et al.* 2016). Unlike conventional echocardiography, this method requires general anesthesia for correct probe placement and can be less accurate in states of hypovolemia and vasodilation, which decrease and increase the proportion of cardiac output going through the descending aorta respectively.

19.6.4.2 Bioimpedance and Bioreactances

Transthoracic bioimpedance and bioreactance both rely on a high-frequency electric current and four paired electrodes to measure changes in resistance across the chest (bioimpedance) or a shift in the frequency or phase of the current (bioreactance). These are altered during the cardiac cycle with ejection of blood during systole. In bioimpedance techniques, the impedance of the current is affected by changes in intrathoracic blood volume, mainly attributable to blood flow in the aorta. These methods are non-invasive as well, but do not always correlate with thermodilution cardiac output measurements (Marshall *et al.* 2016).

19.7 Conclusion

Accurate BP monitoring in veterinary patients is challenging. Non-invasive equipment should be used only when the technology is tested and approved for the species in question, so that at least the expected errors are known. Invasive techniques are preferred for the situations where monitoring of BP is essential for the clinical assessment of a patient and until a non-invasive technique is identified as reliable.

References

Aarnes, T.K., Hubbell, J.A., Lerche, P. and Bednarski, R.M. (2012) Comparison of invasive and oscillometric blood pressure measurement techniques in anesthetized camelids. *Can Vet J*, 53, 881–885.

Acierno, M.J. and Labato, M.A. (2005) Hypertension in renal disease: diagnosis and treatment. *Clin Tech Small Anim Pract*, 20, 23–30.

Acierno, M.J., da Cunha, A., Smith, J., Tully, T.N., Guzman, D.S. *et al.* (2008) Agreement between direct and indirect blood pressure measurements obtained from anesthetized Hispaniolan Amazon parrots. *J Am Vet Med Assoc*, 233, 1587–1590.

Acierno, M.J., Seaton, D., Mitchell, M.A. and da Cunha, A.F. (2010) Agreement between directly measured blood pressure and pressures obtained with three veterinary-specific oscillometric units in cats. *J Am Vet Med Assoc*, 237, 402–406.

Acierno, M.J., Fauth, E., Mitchell M,A. and da Cunha, A.F. (2013) Measuring the level of agreement between directly measured blood pressure and pressure readings obtained with a veterinary-specific oscillometric unit in anesthetized dogs. *J Vet Emerg Crit Care (San Antonio)*, 23, 37–40.

Acierno, M.J., Domingues, M.E., Ramos, S.J., Shelby, A.M. and da Cunha, A.F. (2015) Comparison of directly measured arterial blood pressure at various anatomic locations in anesthetized dogs. *Am J Vet Res*, 76, 266–271.

ANSI/AAMI/SP10:2002/(R) (2008) Manual, electronic, or automated sphygmomanometers. Arlington, VA: Association for the Advancement of Medical Instruments.

Bailey, J.E., Dunlop, C.I., Chapman, P.L., Demme, W.C., Allen, S.L. *et al.* (1994) Indirect Doppler ultrasonic measurement of arterial blood pressure results in a large measurement error in dorsally recumbent anaesthetised horses. *Equine Vet J*, 26, 70–73.

Bartges, J.W., Willis, A.M. and Polzin, D.J. (1996) Hypertension and renal disease. *Vet Clin North Am Small Anim Pract*, 26, 1331–1345.

Beaulieu, J.M., Sotnikova, T.D., Yao, W.D., Kockeritz, L., Woodgett, J.R. *et al.* (2004) Lithium antagonizes dopamine-dependent behaviors mediated by an AKT/glycogen synthase kinase 3 signaling cascade. *Proc Natl Acad Sci USA*, 101, 5099–5104.

Binns, S.H., Sisson, D.D., Buoscio, D.A. and Schaeffer, D.J. (1995) Doppler ultrasonographic, oscillometric sphygmomanometric, and photoplethysmographic techniques for noninvasive blood pressure measurement in anesthetized cats. *J Vet Intern Med*, 9, 405-414.

Bodey, A.R. and Michell, A.R. (1996) Epidemiological study of blood pressure in domestic dogs. *J Small Anim Pract*, 37, 116–125.

Bodey, A.R., Young, L.E., Bartram, D.H., Diamond, M.J. and Michell, A.R. (1994) A comparison of direct and indirect (oscillometric) measurements of arterial blood pressure in anaesthetised dogs, using tail and limb cuffs. *Res Vet Sci*, 57, 265–269.

Bodey, A.R., Michell, A.R., Bovee, K.C., Buranakurl, C. and Garg, T. (1996) Comparison of direct and indirect (oscillometric) measurements of arterial blood pressure in conscious dogs. *Res Vet Sci*, 61, 17–21.

Branson, K.R., Wagner-Mann, C.C. and Mann, F.A. (1997) Evaluation of an oscillometric blood pressure monitor on anesthetized cats and the effect of cuff placement and fur on accuracy. *Vet Surg*, 26, 347–353.

Brodbelt, D. (2009) Perioperative mortality in small animal anaesthesia. *Vet J*, 182, 152–161.

Brown, S.A. and Henik, R.A. (1998) Diagnosis and treatment of systemic hypertension. *Vet Clin North Am Small Anim Pract*, 28, 1481–1494, ix.

Brown, S., Atkins, C., Bagley, R., Carr, A., Cowgill, L. *et al.* (2007) American College of Veterinary Internal Medicine's guidelines for the identification, evaluation, and management of systemic hypertension in dogs and cats. *J Vet Intern Med*, 21, 542–558.

Bruner, J.M., Krenis, J.L., Kunsman, J.M. and Sherman, A.P. (1981) Comparison of direct and indirect methods of measuring arterial blood pressure, Part III. *Med Instrum*, 15, 182–188.

Caulkett, N.A., Cantwell, S.L. and Houston, D.M. (1998) A comparison of indirect blood pressure monitoring techniques in the anesthetized cat. *Vet Surg*, 27, 370–377.

Cohn, J.N. (1967) Central venous pressure as a guide to volume expansion. *Ann Intern Med*, 66, 1283–1287.

Cooper, E. (2015) Hypotension. In: Silverstein, D.C. and Hopper, K. (eds). *Small Animal Critical Care Medicine*, 2nd ed. Elsevier Saunders, St Louis, MO: pp. 46–50.

da Cunha, A.F., Ramos, S.J., Domingues, M., Beaufrère, H., Shelby, A. *et al.* (2016) Agreement between two oscillometric blood pressure technologies and invasively measured arterial pressure in the dog. *Vet Anaesth Analg*, 43, 199–203.

da Cunha, A.F., Ramos, S.J., Domingues, M., Shelby, A., Beaufrère, H. *et al.* (2017) Validation of noninvasive blood pressure equipment: which peripheral artery is best for comparison studies in dogs. *Vet Anaesth Analg*, doi: 10.1016/j.vaa.2017.07.002.

da Cunha, A.F., Saile, K., Beaufrère, H., Wolfson, W., Seaton, D. and Acierno, M.J. (2014) Measuring level of agreement between values obtained by directly measured blood pressure and ultrasonic Doppler flow detector in cats. *J Vet Emerg Crit Care (San Antonio)*, 24, 272–278.

Davis, P.D., Parbrook, G.D. and Kenny, G.N.C. (1995) Blood pressure measurement. In: *Basic Physics and Measurement in Anaesthesia*. Boston, MA: Butterworth-Heinemann, pp. 219–231.

Deflandre, C.J. and Hellebrekers, L.J. (2008) Clinical evaluation of the Surgivet V60046, a non invasive blood pressure monitor in anaesthetized dogs. *Vet Anaesth Analg*, 35, 13–21.

Dorsch, J.A. and Dorsch, S.E. (2008) Automatic noninvasive blood pressure monitors. In: *Understanding Anesthesia Equipment*. Philadelphia, PA: Wolters Kluwer Health/Lippincott Williams & Wilkins, pp. 905–915.

Dyson, D.H. (1997) Assessment of three audible monitors during hypotension in anesthetized dogs. *Can Vet J*, 38, 564–566.

Gardner, R.M. (1981) Direct blood pressure measurement – dynamic response requirements. *Anesthesiology*, 54, 227–236.

Garofalo, N.A., Teixeira Neto, F.J., Alvaides, R.K., de Oliveira, F.A. *et al.* (2012) Agreement between direct, oscillometric and Doppler ultrasound blood pressures using three different cuff positions in anesthetized dogs. *Vet Anaesth Analg*, 39, 324–334.

Geddes, L.A. (1991) *Handbook of Blood Pressure Measurement*. Clifton, NJ: Humana Press.

Giguère, S., Bucki, E., Adin, D.B., Valverde, A., Estrada, A.H. and Young, L. (2005a) Cardiac output measurement by partial carbon dioxide rebreathing, 2-dimensional echocardiography, and lithium dilution methods in anesthetized foals. *J Vet Intern Med*, 19, 737–743.

Giguère, S., Knowles, H.A. Jr, Valverde, A., Bucki, E. and Young, L. (2005b) Accuracy of indirect measurement of blood pressure in neonatal foals. *Gunke*, 19, 571–576.

Gorbunov, V.M. (1997) The white-coat hypertension syndrome. *Ter Arkh*, 69, 80–83.

Grandy, J.L., Dunlop, C.I., Hodgson, D.S., Curtis, C.R. and Chapman, P.L. (1992) Evaluation of the Doppler ultrasonic method of measuring systolic arterial blood pressure in cats. *Am J Vet Res*, 53, 1166–1169.

Grosenbaugh, D.A. and Muir, W.W. (1998) Accuracy of noninvasive oxyhemoglobin saturation, end-tidal carbon dioxide concentration, and blood pressure monitoring during experimentally induced hypoxemia, hypotension, or hypertension in anesthetized dogs. *Am J Vet Res*, 59, 205–212.

Gunkel, C.I., Valverde, A., Morey, T.E., Hernandez, J. and Robertson, S.A. (2004) Comparison of non-invasive cardiac output measurements by partial carbon dioxide rebreathing with the lithium dilution method in anesthetized dogs. *J Vet Emerg Crit Care*, 14, 187–195.

Hartnack, S. (2014) Issues and pitfalls in method comparison studies. *Vet Anaesth Analg*, 41, 227–232.

Haskins, S. (2015) Monitoring anesthetized patients. In: Grimm, K.A., Lamont, L.A., Tranquilli, W.J., Green, S.A. and Robertson, S.A. (eds). *Veterinary Anesthesia and Analgesia. The Fifth Edition of Lumb and Jones*. Ames, IA: Wiley Blackwell, pp. 86–113.

Hawkins, M.G., Wright, B.D., Pascoe, P.J., Kass, P.H., Maxwell, L.K. and Tell, L.A. (2003) Pharmacokinetics and anesthetic and cardiopulmonary effects of propofol in red-tailed hawks (*Buteo jamaicensis*) and great horned owls (*Bubo virginianus*). *Am J Vet Res*, 64, 677–683.

Henik, R.A., Dolson, M.K. and Wenholz, L.J. (2005) How to obtain a blood pressure measurement. *Clin Tech Small Anim Pract*, 20, 144–150.

Henneman, E.A. and Henneman, P.L. (1989) Intricacies of blood pressure measurement: Re-examining the rituals. *Heart Lung*, 18, 263–271.

Hopper, K. and Brown, S. (2015) Hypertensive crisis. In: Silverstein, D.C. and Hopper, K. (eds). *Small Animal Critical Care Medicine*, 2nd ed. St Louis, MO: Elsevier Saunders, pp. 51–54.

Itami, T., Endo, Y., Hanazono, K., Ishizuka, T., Tamura, J. *et al.* (2016) Comparison of cardiac output measurements using transpulmonary thermodilution and conventional thermodilution techniques in anaesthetized dogs with fluid overload. *Vet Anaesth Anal*, 43, 388–396.

Johnston, M.S., Davidowski, L.A., Rao, S. and Hill, A.E. (2011) Precision of repeated, Doppler-derived indirect blood pressure measurements in conscious psittacine birds. *J Avian Med Surg*, 25, 83–90.

Kazamias, T.M., Gander, M.P., Franklin, D.L. and Ross, J. Jr. (1971) Blood pressure measurement with Doppler ultrasonic flowmeter. *J Appl Physiol*, 30, 585–588.

Kelman, G.R. (1971) Interpretation of CVP measurements. *Anaesthesia*, 26, 209–215.

Klevans, L.R., Hirkaler, G. and Kovacs, J.L. (1979) Indirect blood pressure determination by Doppler technique in renal hypertensive cats. *Am J Physiol*, 237, H720–723.

Littman, M.P. (1994) Spontaneous systemic hypertension in 24 cats. *J Vet Intern Med*, 8, 79–86.

Marino, C.L., Cober, R.E., Iazbik, M.C. and Couto, C.G. (2011) White-coat effect on systemic blood pressure in retired racing greyhounds. *J Vet Intern Med*, 25, 861–865.

Marshall, K., Thomovsky, E., Johnson, P. and Brooks, A. (2016) A review of available techniques for cardiac output monitoring. *Top Companion Anim Med*, 31, 100–108.

Mathews, K.A. (2012) Monitoring fluid therapy and complications of fluid therapy. In: Di Bartola, S.P. (ed.). *Fluid, Electrolyte, and Acid–Base Disorders in Small Animal Practice*, 4th ed. St Louis, MO: Elsevier Saunders, pp. 386–390.

Mazzaferro, E. and Wagner, A.E. (2001) Hypotension during anesthesia in dogs and cats: Recognition, causes and treatment. *Compend Cont Educ Vet*, 23, 728–737.

McGee, D.C. and Gould, M.K. (2003) Preventing complications of central venous catheterization. *N Engl J Med*, 348, 1123–1133.

McLeish, I. (1977) Doppler ultrasonic arterial-pressure measurement in cat. *Vet Record*, 100, 290–291.

Mishina, M., Watanabe, T., Fujii, K., Maeda, H., Wakao, Y. and Takahashi, M. (1997) A clinical evaluation of blood pressure through non-invasive measurement using the oscillometric procedure in conscious dogs. *J Vet Med Sci*, 59, 989–993.

Mooney, A.P., Mawby, D.I., Price, J.M. and Whittemore, J.C. (2017) Effects of various factors on Doppler flow ultrasonic radial and coccygeal artery systolic blood pressure measurements in privately-owned, conscious dogs. *Peer J*, 5, e3101.

Musk, G.C., Costa, R.S. and Tuke, J. (2014) Doppler blood pressure measurement in pigs during anaesthesia. *Res Vet Sci*, 97, 129–131.

Oakley, R.E., Olivier, B., Eyster, G.E. and Hauptman, J.G. (1997) Experimental evaluation of central venous pressure monitoring in the dog. *J Am Anim Hosp Assoc*, 33, 77–82.

Ortega, R., Connor, C., Kotova, F., Deng, W. and Lacerra, C. (2017) Use of pressure transducers. *N Engl J Med*, 376, e26.

Parry, B.W., McCarthy, M.A. and Anderson, G.A. (1984) Survey of resting blood pressure values in clinically normal horses. *Equine Vet J*, 16, 53–58.

Redondo, J.I., Rubio, M., Soler, G., Serra, I., Soler, C. and Gomez-Villamandos, R.J. (2007) Normal values and incidence of cardiorespiratory complications in dogs during general anaesthesia. A review of 1,281 cases. *J Vet Med A Physiol Pathol Clin Med*, 54, 470–477.

Rysnik, M.K., Cripps, P. and Iff, I. (2013) A clinical comparison between a non-invasive blood pressure monitor using high definition oscillometry (Memodiagnostic MD 15/90 Pro) and invasive arterial blood pressure measurement in anaesthetized dogs. *Vet Anaesth Analg*, 40, 503–511.

Sawyer, D.C., Guikema, A.H. and Siegel, E.M. (2004) Evaluation of a new oscillometric blood pressure monitor in isoflurane-anesthetized dogs. *Vet Anaesth Analg*, 31, 27–39.

Scheer, B., Perel, A. and Pfeiffer, U.J. (2002) Clinical review: complications and risk factors of peripheral arterial catheters used for haemodynamic monitoring in anaesthesia and intensive care medicine. *Crit Care*, 6, 199–204.

Schnellbacher, R., da Cunha, A.F., Olson, E.E. and Mayer, J. (2014) Arterial catheterization, interpretation, and treatment of arterial blood pressures and blood gases in birds. *J Exot Pet Med*, 23, 129–141.

Schroeder, B., Barbeito, A., Bar-Yosef, S. and Mark, J.B. (2015) Cardiovascular monitoring. In: Miller, R.D. (ed.). *Miller's Anesthesia*, 8th ed. Philadelphia, PA: Saunders, pp. 1345–1395.

Shih, A.C. (2013) Cardiac output monitoring in horses. *Vet Clin Equine*, 29, 155–167.

Shih, A.C., Giguère, S., Sanchez, L.C., Valverde, A., Bandt, C. *et al.* (2009a) Determination of cardiac output in neonatal foals by ultrasound velocity dilution and its comparison to the lithium dilution method. *J Vet Emerg Crit Care (San Antonio)*, 19, 438–443.

Shih, A.C., Giguère, S., Sanchez, L.C., Valverde, A., Jankunas, H.J. and Robertson, S.A. (2009b) Determination of cardiac output in anesthetized neonatal foals by use of two pulse wave analysis methods. *Am J Vet Res*, 70, 334–339.

Soares,J.H.N., Henao-Guerrero,N., Williamson, A.J. and Pavlisko, N.D. (2017) Blood pressure measured at dorsal pedal, coccygeal, and auricular arteries compared to the pressure abdominal aorta in anesthetized dogs. Abstracts presented at the Association of Veterinary

Anaesthetists Meeting, September 2016, Prague, Czech Republic. *Vet Anaesth Analg*, 44, 389.

Stouffer, G. (2008) Arterial pressure. In: Stouffer, G. (ed.). *Cardiovascular Hemodynamics for the Clinician.* Malden, MA: Blackwell Futura, pp. 57–66.

Thiele, R.H., Bartels, K. and Tong, J.G. (2015) Cardiac output monitoring: contemporary assessment and review. *Crit Care Med*, 43, 177–185.

Touzot-Jourde, G., Hernandez-Divers, S.J. and Trim, C.M. (2005) Cardiopulmonary effects of controlled versus spontaneous ventilation in pigeons anesthetized for coelioscopy. *J Am Vet Med Assoc*, 227, 1424–1428.

Trim, C.M., Hofmeister, E.H., Quandt, J.E. and Shepard, M.K. (2017) A survey of the use of arterial catheters in anesthetized dogs and cats: 267 cases. *J Vet Emerg Crit Care (San Antonio)*, 27, 89–95.

Vachon, C., Belanger, M.C. and Burns, P.M. (2014) Evaluation of oscillometric and Doppler ultrasonic devices for blood pressure measurements in anesthetized and conscious dogs. *Res Vet Sci*, 97, 111–117.

Waddell, L.S. and Brown, A.J. (2015) Hemodynamic monitoring. In: Silverstein, D. and Hopper, K. (eds). *Small Animal Critical Care Medicine*, 2nd ed. St Louis, MO: Elsevier Saunders, pp. 957–962.

Wagner, A.E. and Brodbelt, D.C. (1997) Arterial blood pressure monitoring in anesthetized animals. *J Am Vet Med Assoc*, 210, 1279–1285.

Weil, M.H. and Henning, R.J. (1979) New concepts in the diagnosis and fluid treatment of circulatory shock. *Anesth Analg*, 58, 124–132.

Yamaoka, T.T., Flaherty, D., Pawson, P., Scott, M. and Auckburally, A. (2017) Comparison of arterial blood pressure measurements obtained invasively or oscillometrically using a Datex S/5 Compact monitor in anaesthetised adult horses. *Vet Anaesth Analg*, 44, 492–501.

Valtonen, M.H. and Eriksson, L.M. (1970) The effect of cuff width on accuracy of indirect measurement of blood pressure in dogs. *Res Vet Sci*, 11, 358–362.

Zehnder, A.M., Hawkins, M.G., Pascoe, P.J. and Kass, P.H. (2009) Evaluation of indirect blood pressure monitoring in awake and anesthetized red-tailed hawks (*Buteo jamaicensis*): effects of cuff size, cuff placement, and monitoring equipment. *Vet Anaesth Analg*, 36, 464–479.

Zuntz, N. and Hagemann, O. (1894) Untersuchunger uber den Stoffwechsel des Pferdes bei ruhe und Arbeit. *Landwirtsch Jahrb*, 27, 284–301.

20

Electrocardiography

Tracey Lawrence

Toronto Veterinary Emergency and Referral Hospital, Toronto, Ontario, Canada

20.1 Overview

As the use of anesthetic monitoring equipment has grown in the veterinary industry, electrocardiography has become established as an important monitoring tool. The electrocardiograph (ECG) is the only monitor that allows us to evaluate the electrical function of the heart, as seen through a graphic waveform tracing. ECG abnormalities can manifest during anesthesia and early detection with a monitor can help to prevent potentially fatal arrhythmias, as the anesthetist can perform the appropriate intervention in a timely manner. The use of peri-anesthetic drugs has the potential to alter the electrical properties of the heart muscle and promote arrhythmias. Drugs affecting parasympathetic and sympathetic tone can have a significant arrhythmogenic action (Olshansky *et al.* 2008). The ECG also gives the user an additional tool to help gauge the depth and quality of general anesthesia. For example, when paired with a pulse oximeter, the user can not only record oxygenation and heart rate, but also identify and evaluate cardiac arrhythmias. The ECG is utilized in the diagnosis of structural cardiac disease, electrolyte imbalances and metabolic disease. While the ECG can provide the user with valuable information about the electrical function of the heart, it does not assess the cardiac output of the patient.

20.2 The ECG Machine

The ECG machine consists of a framework that houses power circuitry, a computer microprocessor, signal amplifiers, data recorder and a transmission device. Most monitors will have a screen or oscilloscope to show a real-time digital image of the ECG trace as well as a printer. Electrode cables will attach to the device, of which there may be from 2–10 in number (Figure 20.1).

The ECG machine is programmed to make some electrodes positive and some negative, depending on which lead is being analyzed. Additionally, the device can group two or more electrodes to function as a single electrode, as occurs with the augmented leads.

A lead can be defined as the axis or line of site between a pair of electrodes, not the electrode cable itself or its contact point on the patient as is often done (Tilly 1992). The electrodes are attached to the patient's skin and record the voltage change between a negative and positive electrode. Quality control testing of the ECG machine includes the standardization of input signal ranges, signal filtering, frequency response, accuracy of calibration signal, and recording duration.

Most ECG machines have the capability to run at a variety of speeds. Standard speeds are 25 mm/sec and 50 mm/sec. Some have the option of 12.5 mm/sec, which will provide a very condensed ECG trace, but will allow for a longer recording (using less paper). Employing a slower paper speed will make it easier to identify low amplitude deflections. Utilizing a faster paper speed will stretch out the ECG trace and is beneficial when assessing the ECG morphology, particularly at high heart rates.

The amplitude of the ECG can be adjusted by altering the sensitivity or gain. Using the standard setting for amplitude, 1 mV of input will show as 1 cm of vertical rise on the graph paper. If there is too much amplitude causing the complexes to overlap or leave the paper, the sensitivity can be decreased. Likewise, if the complexes are too small to interpret, the amplitude can be increased.

Advances in ECG technology have led to the development of a wide variety of ECG monitors available to the veterinary practitioner. Single lead, handheld monitors allow real-time and wireless transmission of data. These devices are usually composed of only two electrodes. The device can be placed directly over the heart of the patient or atraumatic clips can be placed to the right and

Veterinary Anesthetic and Monitoring Equipment, First Edition. Edited by Kristen G. Cooley and Rebecca A. Johnson.
© 2018 John Wiley & Sons, Inc. Published 2018 by John Wiley & Sons, Inc.

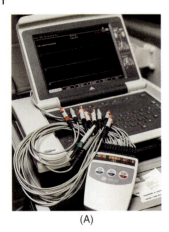
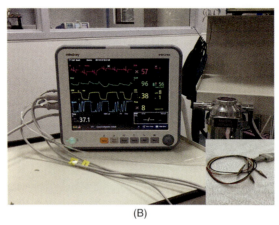

(A)   (B)

Figure 20.1 The ECG machine. (A) A multi-lead ECG is commonly used to provide a diagnostic ECG printout. (B) A three-lead multiparameter monitor is intended for the use of monitoring anesthetized patients as well as the continued monitoring of patients in an intensive-care setting; electrode cables are pictured in the insert at the lower right.

left of the heart, generating an ECG trace for real-time viewing and recording (AliveCor, San Francisco, CA). Other portable units utilize lead wires and electrodes, with snaps or needles placed directly on the patient, to provide a multi-lead ECG trace that is useful for assessing heart rate and rhythm (Figures 20.2A and B).

Some multiparameter anesthesia monitors come equipped with computer software that can screen for irregularities. Algorithms are used to analyze waveform morphology that will trigger an alarm to notify the user of the presence of arrhythmias. These monitors also have the flexibility of allowing the user to set alarm limits and alerts.

20.3 Lead Systems

The ECG works by measuring the voltage change between positive and negative electrodes along a single axis. The heart is a 3-dimensional organ; therefore, in order to accurately evaluate its electrical activity, a multi-

lead system is desirable. This allows for the recording of electrical activity from different axis or *vectors* within the heart. In cats and dogs over the age of 12 weeks, the average direction of electrical activity in the heart is from right to left, cranial to caudal and dorsal to ventral (Côté 2010). If the (net) movement of electrical activity is *towards* a positive electrode, it will result in a *positive* or upward deflection in the ECG waveform. When the (net) movement of electrical activity moves *away* from the positive electrode, the resulting ECG waveform will be *negative* or downward. An isoelectric waveform is created when the positive and negative components are of roughly equal magnitude and the (net) movement of electrical impulses is *perpendicular,* or 90° degrees to the axis of that lead (Figure 20.3).

20.3.1 Bipolar Leads

Bipolar leads use two electrodes, one being negative and one being positive. When using a Lead I system, the

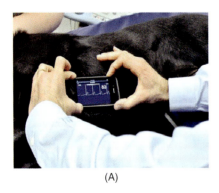
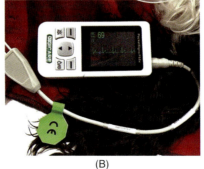
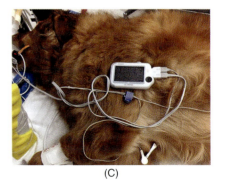

(A)   (B)   (C)

Figure 20.2 Examples of hand-held ECG monitors. (A) AliveCor Monitor, (AliveCor Inc., Mountainview, CA) a smart phone application. (B) The PocketSigns (Digicare, MWI Animal Health, Meridian, ID) hand-held ECG monitor is a portable monitor that is well tolerated by awake or anesthetized patients. (C) The Vetcorder (Sentier, Brookfield, WI) is a two-lead ECG with atraumatic clips or needle attachments.

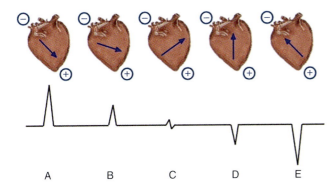

Figure 20.3 Effect of the depolarization wave on the deflections of the ECG waveform. When the electrical movement is traveling in the most direct pathway from negative to positive, the largest positive deflection (A) is created compared to (B). In (C), the electrical movement is perpendicular to the most direct negative to positive pathway (A) and the smallest amount of net deflection is created. When the electrical movement runs from positive to negative (D, E), a negative deflection is created on the ECG (courtesy of Dr M. O'Grady).

electrode placed on the right thoracic limb is negative and the electrode on the left thoracic limb becomes positive. The ECG records the flow of electrical activity between these two points. If the majority of the flow moves toward the positive electrode (in this case from right to left toward the left thoracic electrode) then a positive or upward wave form results. When using Lead II, the right thoracic limb electrode is negative and the left pelvic limb is positive. In Lead III, the left thoracic limb electrode is negative and the left pelvic limb is positive (Figure 20.4). These are the three leads which are most commonly used during anesthetic monitoring.

With ECG placement for large animal species such as equine, bovine and caprine, a base-apex electrode placement is commonly used (modified Lead I). In this set up, the Lead I setting is selected on the ECG monitor. The right arm electrode (negative in Lead I) is attached to the skin at the base of the right side of the dorsal neck, slightly cranial to the withers and scapula. (Figure 20.5) The left arm electrode (positive in Lead I) is attached to

the left side of the thorax, caudal to the elbow and over the apex of the heart (approximately the 5th intercostal space). A third electrode (left leg electrode) acts as a ground and can be placed anywhere on the patient away from the heart. Specialized adhesive electrodes can be attached to the equine patient directly onto an unshaven area. Additional conductive gel can be placed between the patient and electrode, in the case of patients with a long or thick hair coat (van Loon and Patterson 2010; Verheyen *et al.* 2010).

In order to be able to perform diagnostic measurements relating to cardiac function, augmented unipolar limb leads (aVR, aVL, aVF) and unipolar precordial chest leads (CV_5RL or rV_2, CV_6LL or V_2, CV_6LU or V_4, V_{10}) are utilized. Modified or orthogonal lead systems (Lead X, Y, Z) may also be used (Figure 20.6). Multiple leads are recorded simultaneously to provide information about the electrical activity in the heart from many different angles. The use of simultaneous lead recordings also helps to identify artifact. For instance, if a variation in the tracing is not seen in all

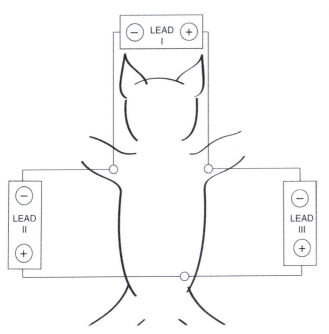

Figure 20.4 Standard bipolar limb leads frequently used in anesthetized patients (I, II, III) (courtesy of Dr R. Wallach).

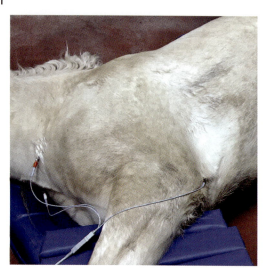

Figure 20.5 The base-apex (modified Lead I) lead arrangement in an anesthetized horse. The right arm lead is placed near the right jugular groove, the left arm lead is near the left cardiac apex, and the third lead is a ground (placed near the left cardiac apex in this photograph). Lead I is selected on the monitor; this arrangement is chosen to accentuate the P wave (photograph courtesy of Dr Rebecca Johnson, University of Wisconsin-Madison, WI).

leads, it may be caused from movement of a limb and therefore would only be viewed in the leads utilizing the electrode attached to that lead (refer to Figure 20.25).

20.3.2 ECG Lead Placement

In addition to obtaining an ECG from electrodes placed on the surface of the patient, an esophageal ECG probe can be used for monitoring the anesthetized patient. This is a guarded and insulated probe containing three electrode cables that is inserted into the esophagus, approximately level with the heart (Figure 20.7). Each electrode cable terminates at a different point along the probe, allowing for measurement of the voltage change between any two of these three points (electrodes). The esophageal probe is closer to the source of electrical activity (the myocardium); therefore, the resulting ECG trace will have a greater amplitude than that obtained with skin-electrode contact. This can improve the accuracy of arrhythmia diagnosis during anesthesia, because the larger P wave is more easily identified, along with the relationship to the QRS complex (Tilley and Smith 2008).

Esophageal ECG probes come in a variety of diameters and lengths, providing slightly different spacing between the electrodes. The middle electrode should be inserted to be level with the heart, but the probe should remain within the thoracic esophagus and not penetrate the gastroesophageal sphincter. If the probe is not inserted to the proper depth, the QRS complex may appear inverted or otherwise abnormal. As with electrodes that are placed on the surface of the skin, the electrodes can act as a ground and create a burn if electrocautery is being utilized without a proper grounding source. Myocardial electrical activity can also be recorded with electrodes placed on the endocardium during cardiac catheterization or epicardium during thoracic surgery.

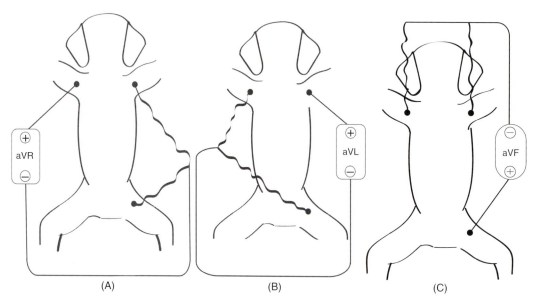

Figure 20.6 Augmented unipolar limb leads. (A) In lead aVR, the left thoracic and left pelvic electrodes combine to function as one negative electrode; the right thoracic electrode is positive. (B) In lead aVL, the right thoracic and left pelvic electrodes combine to function as one negative electrode; the left thoracic electrode is positive. (C) In lead aVF, the right and left thoracic electrodes combine to function as one negative electrode; the left pelvic limb electrode is positive (courtesy of Dr R. Wallach).

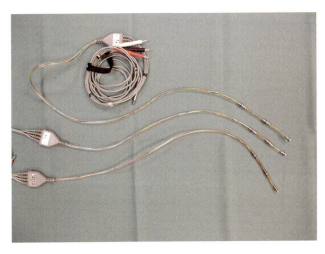

Figure 20.7 Esophageal ECG probes are available in a variety of lengths and diameters (e.g. Midmark Corporation, Dayton, OH).

Table 20.1 Summary of ECG lead placement.

Bipolar Standard Leads	Negative Lead	Positive Lead
Lead I	Right forelimb	Left forelimb
Lead II	Right forelimb	Left hind limb
Lead III	Left forelimb	Left hind limb

Augmented Unipolar Leads	Negative Lead	Positive lead
aVR	Left forelimb and left hind limb	Right forelimb
aVL	Right forelimb and left hind limb	Left forelimb
aVF	Left forelimb and right forelimb	Left hind limb

Unipolar Precordial Chest Leads	Negative Lead	Positive Lead
rV_2	Right forelimb, left forelimb and left hind limb	Fifth right intercostal space between sternum and costochondral junction
V_2	Right forelimb, left forelimb and left hind limb	Sixth left intercostal space between sternum and costochondral junction
V_4	Right forelimb, left forelimb and left hind limb	Sixth left intercostal space at the costochondral junction
V_{10}	Right forelimb, left forelimb and left hind limb	Seventh thoracic dorsal spinous process

Modified Orthogonal Lead Systems	Negative Lead	Positive Lead
Lead X – Lead I	Right	Left
Lead Y – Lead aVF	Cranial	Caudal
Lead Z – Lead V_{10}	Ventral	Dorsal

20.4 Mean Electrical Axis (MEA)

By using the three bipolar leads, a triangle is formed around the frontal plane of the heart. When the left hind limb electrode is moved to the center of the body, an equilateral triangle is formed, known as the Einthoven Triangle. If the sides of the triangle are further transposed to intersect over the center of the heart, a central area of zero electrical potential is indicated (Figure 20.8) (Tilley 1992). When the three unipolar limb leads are superimposed over the heart, the combined chart is known as the hexaxial lead system (Figures 20.9).

The mean electrical axis will point toward the average direction of depolarization of the myocardium in the frontal plane, which is toward the larger left ventricle in the normal heart. It is primarily utilized to detect changes in the size of the ventricles and the presence of intraventricular conduction deficits. Establishing the MEA can be done using different methods.

To find the MEA using the isoelectric method, first locate the isoelectric lead on a six-lead ECG in the frontal plane (Figure 20.10A). The QRS has the least amount of net deflection from the zero baseline in this lead. Next, find the lead that runs perpendicular to the isoelectric lead on the axis chart. The MEA lies along this perpendicular lead. If the net deflection of the QRS in this lead is positive, then the MEA will point to the positive pole. If the net deflection on the ECG is negative, then the MEA will point to the negative pole. This method approximates the MEA.

To find the MEA using the largest net deflection method, identify the lead with the greatest amount of net deflection from zero baseline in the QRS, on a six-lead ECG, in the frontal plane. (Figure 20.10A) The MEA lies along this lead. If the algebraic sum of the deflections is positive, then the MEA points to the positive pole in this

lead. If the algebraic sum of the deflections is negative, then the MEA points to the negative pole in this lead.

A more precise method of locating the MEA is by using the vector method. The net amplitude of the QRS is calculated by subtracting the height of the positive deflection(s) in the QRS from the height of the negative deflection(s) in the QRS in leads I, II or III. This number is plotted on the hexaxial frontal plane chart (Figure 20.10B). The algebraic sum of a second lead is calculated and plotted on the chart. The place where the perpendicular line coming from these two points intersects indicates the ventricular MEA.

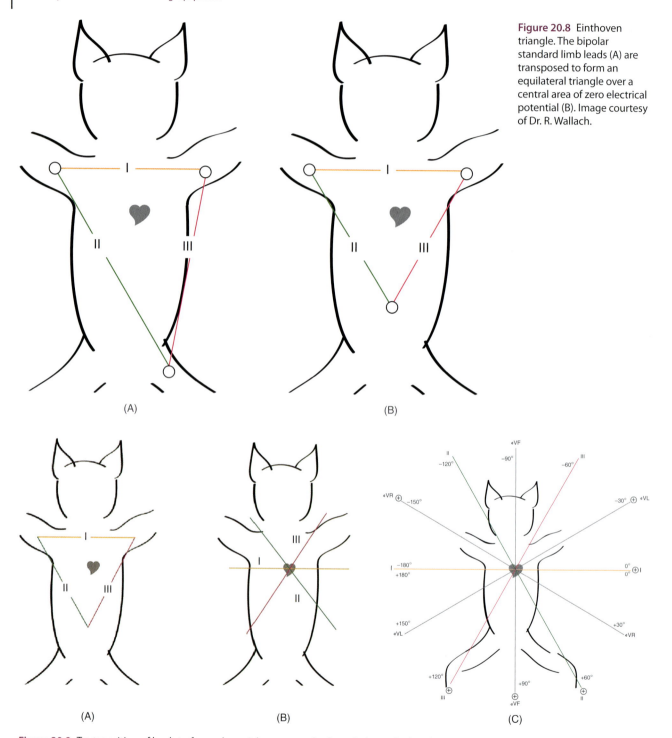

Figure 20.8 Einthoven triangle. The bipolar standard limb leads (A) are transposed to form an equilateral triangle over a central area of zero electrical potential (B). Image courtesy of Dr. R. Wallach.

(A) (B)

(A) (B) (C)

Figure 20.9 Transposition of leads to form a hexaxial system on the frontal plane. The bipolar standard limb leads (A) are further transposed to intersect over a central area of zero electrical potential (B). The augmented limb leads are added to form the hexaxial lead system that is utilized to determine the mean electrical axis (C). Image courtesy of Dr R. Wallach.

20.5 ECG Cycle

A complete ECG cycle consists of a P, Q, R, S and T wave. These waveforms are created as positively charged ions (sodium, potassium and calcium) move across myocardial cell membranes and create a change in voltage leading to the creation of actions potentials. The movement of ions causes the polarized or "charged" cells to depolarize. The resulting coordinated depolarization of myocardial cells creates a contraction of the myocardial muscle.

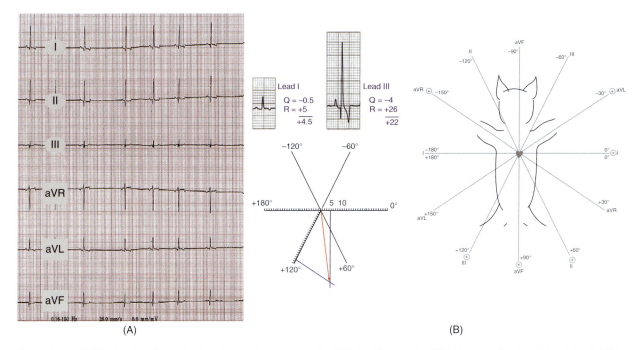

Figure 20.10 (A) The isoelectric method can be used to measure the MEA. In this trace, lead III is the most isoelectric lead. Lead aVR is perpendicular to Lead III on the frontal plane diagram (Figure 20.8). The MEA is approximately +30 degrees. When using the largest net deflection method, in this trace, lead I has the largest net deflection. Therefore, the MEA is estimated at 0 degrees. (B) More accurate, the vector method can also determine MEA. In lead I, the net deflection is +4.5 degrees. This is plotted on the lead I axis. In lead III, the net deflection is +22 degrees. This is also plotted on the lead III axis. The MEA is located at the intersecting point of these lines, between +80 and +85 degrees. Note, the ECG's utilized in (A) and (B) are from different patients and do not have the same MEA (B courtesy of Dr M. O'Grady and Dr R. Wallach).

The electrical conduction system of the heart consists of five main components, the sino-atrial (SA) node, the atrio-ventricular (AV) node, the bundle of His, the left and right bundle branches and the Purkinje fibers (Figure 20.11).

An electrical impulse is generated within the SA node, which initiates cardiac depolarization. The impulse travels through the atria to the AV node, causing atrial contraction. This is represented by the P wave on the ECG tracing or electrocardiogram, which shows as a positive deflection in lead II; the P wave may be notched in large patients due to slightly asynchronous atrial contraction.

After depolarization occurs in the atria, the wave of depolarization slows as it passes through the atrioventricular (AV) node, preventing simultaneous contraction of the atria and ventricles. During this phase, there is no electrocardiographic activity. This is illustrated by the flat-lined PR interval on the electrocardiogram (Miller and Bonagura 1985). The impulse continues through the bundle of His before spreading to the left and right bundle branches. The transmission of the electrical impulse terminates at the end of the Purkinje fibers at the surface of the endocardium. Depolarization and contraction of the left and right ventricles occurs simultaneously and is represented by the QRS waveform on the electrocardiogram (Tilley 2008).

The Q wave is defined as the first negative deflection following the P wave and immediately before the R wave. It is representative of the depolarization of the interventricular septum. The R wave is the first positive deflection occurring after the P wave and indicates depolarization of the ventricular myocardium (from the endocardium to epicardium). The S wave is the first negative deflection immediately following the R wave and occurs during the depolarization of the base of the heart (Figure 20.12). In many small animal patients, the QRS complexes are largely positive in nature. However, when a base-apex lead is used in the large animal patient (see below), ventricular depolarization is often seen as a positive R wave and deep negative S wave with an absence of a Q wave (Verheyen *et al.* 2010) (Figure 20.13).

Repolarization of the atria occurs during ventricular depolarization and is usually masked by the QRS complex. Ventricular repolarization begins at the completion of the QRS complex and is completed by the end of the T wave. The distance between the S wave and the T wave is called the ST segment. Delayed ventricular repolarization will produce a prolonged ST segment (Hillel 2000), possibly indicating myocardial hypoxia, ischemia, or decreased cardiac output.

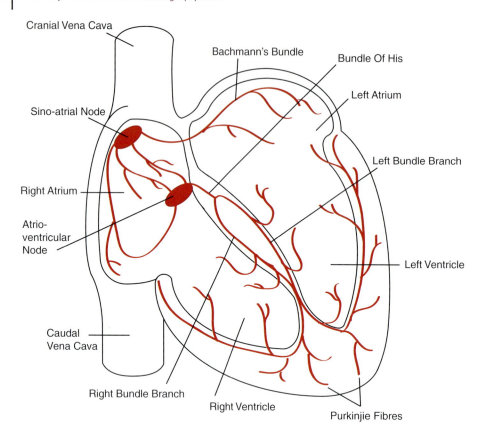

Figure 20.11 The normal electrical conduction through the heart (courtesy of Dr R. Wallach).

Alterations in the size and duration of the P, Q, R, S and T waves can indicate the presence of cardiac disease or electrolyte imbalances. These measurements must be

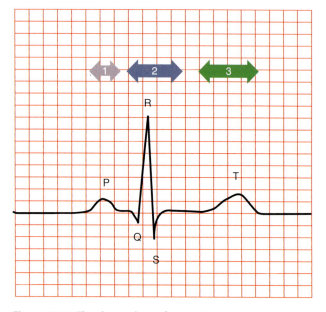

Figure 20.12 The electrical waveform with respect to cardiac depolarization. 1: atrial depolarization/contraction; 2: ventricular depolarization/contraction (atrial repolarization also occurs here); and 3: ventricular repolarization.

taken from an ECG recorded with the patient in right lateral recumbency, in order for the results to be compared to standard normal values in dogs and cats (Table 20.2). Additional diagnostics such as echocardiography and radiography should be utilized, and are preferred, for the diagnosis of structural and functional cardiac disease.

20.6 Electrode Placement

To obtain the ECG, the eupneic small animal patient should be placed on an insulated surface (not metal) in right lateral recumbency (Figure 20.14). This position is required for amplitude measurements of the ECG and is the position from which reference values are standardized (Scalf 2002). If the patient is distressed in this position, the ECG can be done in sternal recumbency or in a standing position (Figure 20.15). When in right lateral recumbency, the limbs should be held parallel to each other and perpendicular to the body. The limbs and electrodes should be prevented from touching one another. The environment should be conducive to maintaining a calm and quiet patient, with limited distractions. The use of electronic equipment should be minimized during ECG recording, as it can cause an electrical interference artifact on the ECG trace (Baranchuk *et al.* 2009).

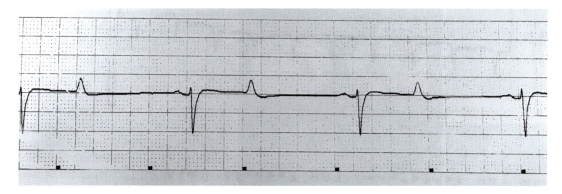

Figure 20.13 The equine electrocardiogram routinely shows a deep negative complex associated with ventricular depolarization.

The electrodes are attached to the patient using blunt/flat alligator clips or metal plates that are strapped to the limbs (Figure 20.16A). A gauze square moistened with alcohol can be placed between the clip and the skin to help alleviate discomfort from pinching. The hinge on

Table 20.2 Normal ECG values in dogs and cats.

Parameter	Canine	Feline
Heart rate (beats per minute)	Puppies: up to 220 Toy breeds: up to 180 Adult: 70–160 Giant breeds: 60–140	100 (asleep) to 240
Heart Rhythm	Normal sinus rhythm Sinus arrhythmia Wandering atrial pacemaker	Normal sinus rhythm Sinus tachycardia
P-wave		
Time	<0.04 sec	<0.04 sec
Amplitude	<0.4 mV	<0.2 mV
P-R Interval	0.06 to 0.13 sec	0.04–0.09 sec
QRS complex (Lead II)		
Time	<0.06 sec	<0.04 sec
Amplitude (R-wave)	<3.0 mV	<0.9 mV
Q-T	0.15 to 0.25 sec	0.12–0.18 sec
S-T (Lead II)	<0.2 mV depression <0.15 mV elevation	No depression or elevation
T-Wave	Positive, negative or biphasic	Positive, occasionally negative or biphasic
MEA (frontal plane)	+40 to +100	0 to +160

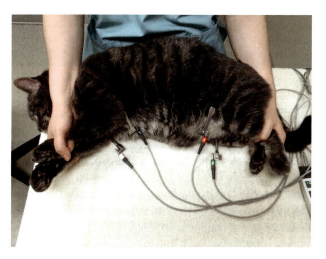

Figure 20.14 Lead placement on a feline patient in right lateral recumbency.

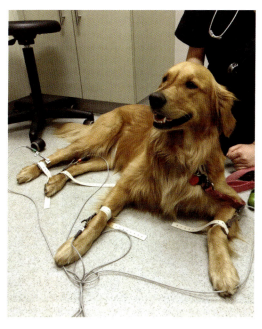

Figure 20.15 Lead placement on a canine patient in sternal recumbency, using metal plates on the limbs.

noise allowing only low frequency signals to pass to the ECG. High frequency artifact can be caused by muscular activity and electrical interference. Muscle movement can produce from 5–50 Hz of activity and 60-cycle interference from an external electrical source can run from 10–60 Hz (Watford 2014).

When looking at cardiac rhythm during routine monitoring, the *monitor mode* filters can be utilized. The monitor mode allows a narrow range of frequencies to pass through to the ECG trace, and produces an ECG with reductions in amplitude. If a high fidelity 12-lead ECG is required, the filters applied are known as *diagnostic mode* filters. In diagnostic mode, the high pass filter is set at 0.05 Hz and the low pass filter at 40, 100 or 150 Hz, which allows for a greater range of frequency to pass through to ECG trace and but may allow for some baseline drift. When filters are used, the R-wave amplitude is significantly altered in the canine and feline patient. This should be taken into consideration when measurements of QRS amplitude are required (Schrope *et al.* 1995; Dvir *et al.* 2002).

20.8   Evaluating the ECG

Standard electrocardiographic recording paper consists of a grid of horizontal and vertical lines spaced at 1-mm intervals. The vertical axis represents amplitude and each 1-mm box is equal to 0.1 mV when the ECG is standardized to 10 mm = 1 mV. One large 5-mm box is equal to 0.5 mV (Figure 20.19). The horizontal axis represents time in seconds and the measurements are variable with paper speed.

20.8.1   Counting Heart Rate

There are a number of techniques utilized to count heart rates; all must be verified with another monitor to ensure cardiac output is present.

For patients with a regular sinus rhythm:

1) Determine how many small 1-mm boxes are equal to 1 min:

   - For a paper speed of 25 mm/sec, 25 mm/sec × 60 sec = 1500 mm/min;
   - For a paper speed of 50 mm/sec, 50 mm/sec × 60 sec = 3000 mm/min.

2) Count the number of small 1-mm boxes between an R-R interval.

3) Heart rate is equal to the paper speed divided by the number of boxes between the R-R interval. In Figure 20.19, there are 21 boxes in the R-R interval. Thus:

   - For 25 mm/sec paper speed: 1500/21 = 71 beats per min (bpm);
   - For 50 mm/sec paper speed: 3000/21 = 143 bpm.

Another method for determining the heart rate involves first counting the number of 1-mm boxes between R-R intervals. In Figure 20.20A, there are 21 1-mm boxes between two R waves:

- For 25 mm/sec, each 1-mm box represents 0.04 sec. 21 boxes × 0.04 sec = 0.84 sec per beat; 60 sec per min/0.84 sec per beat = 71 bpm;
- For 50 mm/sec, each 1-mm box represents 0.02 sec. 21 boxes × 0.02 sec = 0.42 sec per beat; 60 sec per min/0.42 sec per beat = 143 bpm.

A third method for determining heart rate is helpful for ECG printouts showing an irregular heart rhythm. Count the number of R-R intervals in a 3 or 6 second time span and then calculate the rate per minute (Figure 20.20B). Keep in mind, the longer the time counted over, the more accurate the rate will be. By counting the R-R interval, the ventricular rate is determined. The atrial rate can be recorded by counting the number of P-P intervals. The atrial and ventricular rates should be the same with a normal sinus rhythm.

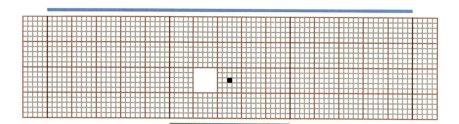

Figure 20.19 An example of ECG paper. At a paper speed of 25 mm/sec, the 1-mm black box represents 0.04 sec in the horizontal axis, therefore the 5-mm white box represents 0.2 sec of time. Five heavily inked boxes (the length of the green line) represent 1 sec of time. The long horizontal blue line represents 3 sec of time. At a paper speed of 50 mm/sec, the 1-mm black box represents 0.02 sec in the horizontal axis, therefore the 5-mm white box represents 0.1 sec of time. The green line represents 0.5 sec of time and the blue line represents 1.5 sec of time. This recording speed is useful when evaluating ECGs with high heart rates, as it is easier to identify the parts of the ECG tracing.

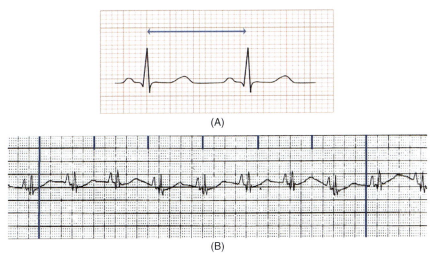

(A)

(B)

Figure 20.20 Example of techniques to calculate heart rate from an ECG. (A) For a regular sinus rhythm, there are 21 small boxes between R waves. For 25 mm/sec paper speed, 1500 sec/21 boxes = 72 bpm or 60 sec per min/0.84 sec per beat = 72 bpm. For 50 mm/sec paper speed, 3000 sec/21 boxes = 143 bpm or 60 sec per min/0.42 sec per beat = 143 bpm. (B) For irregular R-R intervals, at a paper speed of 50 mm/sec, 5 large boxes represent 30 sec. There are 7 complete R-R intervals in 3 sec; therefore, the heart rate is counted as 140 bpm.

20.8.2 Evaluating the Rhythm

A key point when identifying the presence of an arrhythmia is to first identify the P waves and determine if they are each associated with a QRS complex. Then determine if the atrial rate is less than, equal to, or greater than the ventricular rate. The following steps can be followed to help systematically evaluate an ECG printout (Table 20.3):

1) Note the ECG paper speed.
2) Determine the ventricular rate; are the R-R intervals regular?
3) Determine the atrial rate; are the P-P intervals regular?
4) Does every P wave have an associated QRS complex?
    - Are they the same rate?
5) Determine P-R interval:
    - Is the P-R interval of normal width?
    - Is the P-R interval constant or variable?
6) Are there any P waves that are not followed by a QRS complex?
7) Are there any QRS complexes with no P waves?
8) Determine the width of the QRS complexes.
9) Is the rhythm regular or irregular?
10) Are there any premature beats? Note the morphology and duration.
11) Are the P waves positive or negative in lead II?
12) Are the QRS complexes of normal morphology?

20.8.3 Artifact

Artifact is anything that causes a distortion in the ECG trace; the source can be technical or mechanical. The clinician, the machine or the electrodes and cables create technical distortions of the ECG, whereas the patient or patient handler creates mechanical artifact (Tilley and Smith 2008). Artifact is a concern because it can mimic arrhythmias and alter the ECG trace so that it becomes difficult to correctly identify and measure the P-QRS-T complexes (Table 20.4). Variations in ECG morphology or rhythm, such as low amplitude QRS complexes, tall T waves and tachyarrhythmias can affect the ability of the ECG machine to generate an accurate heart rate reading. The user should ensure that they are confirming ECG heart rate readings through manual or alternative methods.

Poor-quality ECG tracings can be produced with even the most conscientiously placed leads. Attention should be paid to the preparation of the patient. Ideally, the area where the electrode is placed should be free of hair and dirt. An exception to this is with the equine patient, where specialized adhesive electrodes are placed on a clean, but unclipped area of skin (Verheyen *et al.* 2010). Isopropyl alcohol is commonly used to clean the surface of the skin and smooth patient hair away from the interface site. This will enhance the conduction of electrical activity between the patient and the electrode and help to produce an ECG trace with minimal artifact.

The skin-electrode interface can produce a large amount of interference, producing a DC component of 200–300 mV. To put this into perspective, the electrical signal generated by the myocardium measures between 0.5 and 2 mV at the skin's surface. The interference seen from this component will be magnified by patient motion (Watford 2014). Periodic addition of conductive gel or alcohol may be required during prolonged periods of recording, especially if a forced air-warming blanket is placed around the patient. Airflow over the electrode contact site will cause an increased rate of evaporation of the alcohol.

Electrodes may become loose or dislodged over time or during patient positioning, resulting in a loss of signal and disruption in the ECG trace. Disruption to the flow of electrical current between the electrode and skin contact point may trigger a "leads-off" warning in the ECG

Table 20.3 Algorithm to identify cardiac rhythm disorders.

Rhythm	Heart Rate	P-Waves Present?	Do QRS Complexes have Associated P-Waves?	Disorders
Regular	Slow	Yes	Yes	Sinus Bradycardia 2nd-Degree Heart Block
			No	3rd-Degree Heart Block
		No		Hyperkalemia Persistent Atrial Standstill
	Normal	Yes	Yes	Normal Sinus Rhythm 2nd-Degree Heart Block Atrial Flutter
			No	Ventricular Tachycardia Hyperkalemia Persistent Atrial Standstill
		No		
	Fast	Yes	Yes	Sinus Tachycardia Supraventricular Tachycardia Atrial Flutter
			No	Ventricular Tachycardia Non-Paroxysmal Junctional Tachycardia
		No		Supraventricular Tachycardia (P-waves present but buried in QRS or T)
Irregular	Slow	Yes	Yes	Sinus Bradycardia Sinus Arrhythmia Sick Sinus Syndrome 2nd-Degree Heart Block
			No	
		No		Slow Atrial Fibrillation
	Normal	Yes	Yes	Sinus Arrhythmia 2nd-Degree Heart Block Atrial Flutter
			No	Ventricular Tachycardia (rhythm is usually regular)
		No		Atrial Fibrillation
	Fast	Yes	Yes	Sinus Tachycardia Atrial Flutter Supraventricular Tachycardia
			No	Ventricular Tachycardia (rhythm is usually regular) Non-paroxysmal Junctional Tachycardia
		No		Atrial Fibrillation

machine. (Gregg *et al.* 2008). Dirty or poorly attached ECG clips will result in similar artifact. If adhesive electrodes are used, ensure that the contact surface of the electrolyte gel is moist and securely placed on the skin surface. This is best done if the skin has been cleaned with soap and water and thoroughly dried. Faulty cables will transmit an inconsistent signal to the monitor, causing artifact. Over time, the insulation surrounding the cable may become damaged, which allows for greater interference from electrical fields in the environment (Hillel and Thys 2000). Damaged electrode cables should be discarded (Figure 20.21).

Poor ECG or patient grounding creates 60-cycle or electrical interference. It appears as a regular sequence of fine, sharp, vertical oscillations on the ECG, which can mimic atrial P waves. With 60-cycle interference, the duration of each oscillation is much shorter than for P waves and the rate of oscillation can be up to 3600 cycles per minute (60 cycles per sec) (Figure 20.22). Equipment using electrical current in close proximity to the ECG can cause interference such as monitors, clippers, lights and electrocautery units (Figure 20.23).

Proper ECG cable and lead shielding will help to minimize artifact. When trying to eliminate 60-cycle interfer-

Table 20.4 Common causes of artifact on the ECG.

Mechanical Artifact	Technical Artifact
Patient movement	Broken cables
- tremors	Dirty, broken or loose cable tips
- voluntary body movements	Improper lead placement or lead reversal
- respiratory patterns	Electrical interference/60 cycle artifact
Movement of patient handler	Damaged or dirty stylus
	Improper paper speed selection

ence, ensure that the power cord for the ECG machine is well inserted into a 3-prong electrical outlet. The patient should be placed on a non-metal surface and the electrodes should be clean and securely attached to the patient as well as the ECG cable. Attention should be given to prevent the electrodes from touching each other by separating the patient's legs. Only enough alcohol or conductive gel sufficient to wet the contact area of the electrodes should be used. Do not soak the patient or the surface they are on, especially if CPR or cardiac defibrillation is imminent. In these cases, only electrolyte gel should be used, as the use of isopropyl alcohol can facilitate burns to the patient if defibrillation is required. Attempt to turn off any electrical equipment or fluorescent lights in the immediate area. Using the battery source feature on the ECG unit can help to reduce 60-cycle artifact, as this will remove the outside electrical circuitry from the system.

Patient movement will cause artifact, as can be seen with panting, muscle tremors/shivering, and purring,

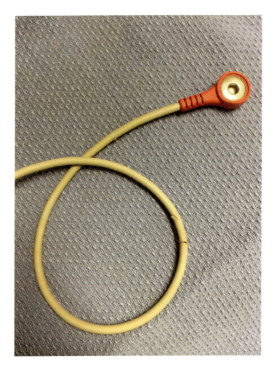

Figure 20.21 A damaged electrode cable where the insulation is peeling away.

manifested as a series of vertical oscillations in the ECG baseline. Electrode placement on a body area with minimal muscle and away from the thoracic movement created during respiration (Figure 20.24) can help minimize this type of artifact. Attempts should be made to quiet the patient and facilitate his/her comfort during recording. The more comfortable the patient, the more likely that movement artifact (Figure 20.25) will be minimized (Miller and Tilley 1988). Decreasing the sensitivity on the ECG monitor may also help improve the trace. With

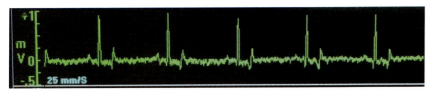

Figure 20.22 Example of an artifact from 60-cycle interference with sharp, fast waves in the baseline.

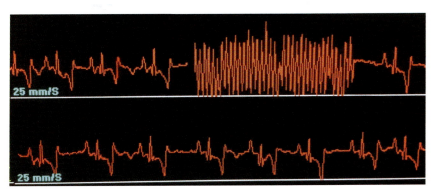

Figure 20.23 Short-lived electrical artifact from electrocautery use (top trace) and return to normal monitoring (bottom trace).

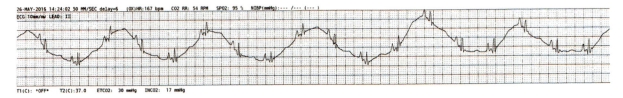

Figure 20.24 Wandering baseline generated from chest wall movement during respiration.

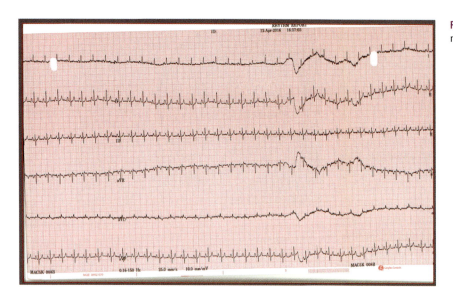

Figure 20.25 Artifact from patient movement of the right forelimb.

dogs that are wide or deep chested, the lungs can create an area of increased electrical resistance that can result in an ECG that is decreased in amplitude (Tilley 1992).

20.9 Equipment Maintenance

ECG machines require minimal maintenance provided they are kept in good working order. Prior to each use, the user should examine the lead wires to check for damage to the wire casing (shield), paying close attention to areas of frequent movement or bending, usually at attachment points. The outer casing of the machine should be kept free of dust and hair and can be wiped down with a damp cloth using a mild detergent. Check that the power cable is securely attached and free of damage. Ensure that the battery is appropriately charged.

After each use, the lead wires and electrode clips can be cleaned with a germicidal solution as required, otherwise a mild detergent is sufficient for cleaning. Electrode clips should be cleaned free of electrode gel and debris. Wires and cables should be stored lying flat or loosely coiled to prevent damage caused by bending. Elevations

in humidity can cause the ECG trace to be inconsistent. To prevent this, store the machine in a dry environment and do not saturate the machine with any liquid. These are general recommendations that apply to most machines; however, always refer to the manufacturer's recommendations for the cleaning and maintenance of the ECG monitor.

Some ECG machines print on thermal paper. This paper has a chemical coating, causing it to react to heat. In the ECG machine, a heated stylus creates the printout of the electrocardiogram. Thermal paper is also reactive to ultraviolet light and moisture and should be stored in a dry and dark environment. Humidity should be between 40 and 65% and the ambient temperature should remain below 26.7°C (80°F) (CDC 1991).

20.10 Summary

The ECG machine can be utilized in a variety of situations in today's veterinary hospital. It is an irreplaceable tool for assessing the electrical function of the heart and is a valuable asset when monitoring the conscious and anesthetized patient.

References

Baranchuk, A., Kang, J., Shaw, C., Campbell, D., Ribas, S. *et al.* (2009) Electromagnetic interference of communication devices on ECG machines. *Clin Cardiol*, 32, 588–592.

Center for Disease Control (CDC) (1991) Electrocardiogram, Available from: https://www.cdc.gov/nchs/data/nhanes/nhanes3/cdrom/nchs/manuals/ecg.pdf [accessed July 2017].

Côté, E. (2010) Electrocardiography and cardiac arrhythmias. In: Ettinger, S.J. and Feldman, E.C. (eds). *Textbook of Veterinary Internal Medicine*, 7th ed. St Louis, MO: Saunders Elsevier, pp. 1159–1167.

Dvir, E., Cilliers, P.J. and Lobetti, R. (2002) Effect of electrocardiographic filters on the R-amplitude of canine electrocardiograms. *Vet Rec*, 150, 171–176.

García-Niebla, J., Llontop-García, P., Valle-Racero, J.I., Serra-Autonell, G., Batchvarov, V.N. and de Luna, A.B. (2009) Technical mistakes during the acquisition of the electrocardiogram. *Anns Noninvas Electro*, 14, 389–403.

Gregg, R.E., Zhou, S.H., Lindauer, J.M., Helfenbein, E.D. and Giuliano, K.K. (2008) What is inside the electrocardiograph? *J Electrocardiol*, 41, 8–14.

Hillel, Z. and Thys, D.M. (2000) Electrocardiography. In: Miller, R.D. (ed.). *Miller's Anesthesia*, 5th ed. Philadelphia, PA: Elsevier Saunders, pp. 1232, 1238.

Miller, M.S. and Bonagura, J.D. (1985) Genesis of the equine electrocardiogram and indications for electrocardiography in clinical practice. *J Equine Vet Sci*, 5, pp. 23–25.

Miller, M.S. and Tilley, L.P. (1988) Electrocardiography. In: Fox, P.R. (ed.). *Canine and Feline Cardiology*. New York: Churchill-Livingston Inc., pp. 46, 47, 50.

Olshansky, B., Sabbah, H.N., Hauptman, P.J. and Colucci, W.S. (2008) Parasympathetic nervous system and heart failure. *Circulation*, 118, 863–871.

Scalf, R. (2002) Electrocardiography. In: Wingfield, W.E. and Raffe, M.R. (eds). *The Veterinary ICU Book*. Jackson, WY: Teton New Media, pp. 241, 245, 253.

Schrope, D.P., Fox, P.R., Hahn, A.W., Bond, B. and Rosenthal, S. (1995) Effects of electrocardiograph frequency filters on P-QRS-T amplitudes of the feline electrocardiogram. *Am J Vet Res*, 56, 1534–1540.

Tilley, L.P. (1992) Generation of the electrocardiogram, In: Cann, C.C. (ed.). *Essentials of Canine and Feline Electrocardiography Interpretation and Treatment*, 3rd ed. Philadelphia, PA: Lea & Febiger, pp. 7, 12, 13, 60, 100.

Tilley, L.P. and Smith, F.W.K. Jr. (2008) Electrocardiography. In: Tilly, L.P. and Smith, F.W.K. Jr. (eds). *Manual of Canine and Feline Cardiography*, 4th ed. St Louis, MO: Saunders Elsevier, pp. 50, 52, 198.

van Loon, G. and Patterson, M. (2010) Electrophysiology and arrhythmiogenesis. In: Marr, C.M. and Bowen, I.M. (eds). *Cardiology of the Horse*, 2nd ed. Edinburgh, Scotland: Elsevier Saunders, pp. 63–66.

Venkatachalam, K.L., Herbrandson, J.E. and Asirvatham, S.J. (2011) Signals and signal processing for the electrophysiologist. Part I: Electrogram acquisition. *Circ Arrhythm Electrophysiol*, 4, 965–973.

Verheyen, T., Decloedt, A., De Clercq, D., Deprez, P., Sys, S.U. and van, Loon, G. (2010) Electrocardiography in horses. Part I: How to make a good recording. *Vlaams Diergeneeskundig Tijdschrift*, 79, 331–336.

Watford, C. (2014) Understanding ECG Filtering. Available from: http://www.ems12lead.com/2014/03/10/understanding-ecg-filtering/ [accessed May 15, 2016].

21

Neuromuscular Transmission Monitoring

Molly Allen[1] and Rebecca A. Johnson[2]

[1] *Lakeshore Veterinary Specialists, Glendale, Wisconsin, USA*
[2] *School of Veterinary Medicine, University of Wisconsin, Madison, Wisconsin, USA*

21.1   Introduction

Neuromuscular blockade (NMB) in veterinary clinical practice is increasingly common due to advancements in surgical procedures and availability of short- to intermediate-acting neuromuscular blocking agents (NMBAs) with minimal adverse cardiovascular effects. These agents may facilitate orthopedic surgery, prevent patient movement during neurologic procedures, ensure a centrally positioned eye during ocular surgery, and facilitate ventilation during cardiothoracic procedures. The level of muscle relaxation required in these circumstances is often only attainable with excessive doses of volatile anesthetic agents, making the NMBAs a valuable adjunct to balanced anesthesia protocols and an attractive option for veterinary specialists.

A detailed description of NMBAs available to the veterinary practitioner is beyond the scope of this chapter and the reader is referred elsewhere (Keegan 2015). However, in veterinary medicine, non-depolarizing neuromuscular blocking agents (e.g. atracurium, vecuronium, pancuronium, etc.) are more commonly used than depolarizing agents (e.g. succinylcholine). This chapter focuses on the requisite equipment for the safe use of NMBAs and monitoring of neuromuscular transmission.

21.2   Neuromuscular Transmission

A short overview of normal neuromuscular transmission is required to understand how equipment functions when monitoring this physiologic response. Briefly, a neural action potential travels down the motor neuron axon and arrives at the axon terminal. Voltage-gated calcium channels open and calcium influx facilitates acetylcholine (ACh) vesicle mobilization and fusion with the terminal cell membrane. ACh is released into the synap-

tic cleft by exocytosis, diffuses across the cleft, and binds to nicotinic ACh receptors on the post-synaptic muscle cell membrane. The ACh receptors undergo a conformational change that allows sodium influx and depolarization of the muscle cell. Propagation of the action potential along the muscle cell causes skeletal muscle contraction. As the ACh molecule disengages from the Ach receptor, acetylcholinesterase (AChE) hydrolyzes it into acetate and choline. Re-uptake by the neuron follows, where choline is combined with another acetate group to reform ACh, which is subsequently repackaged into a vesicle (Martin-Flores 2013).

21.3   Peripheral Nerve Stimulation

A peripheral nerve stimulator (Figure 21.1) is an essential piece of equipment for neuromuscular transmission monitoring. The unit delivers an electrical stimulus near a peripheral nerve and the evoked response of the muscle innervated by that nerve is assessed. The number of muscle fibers activated depends on the current used, with a maximal current being that which activates all muscle fibers innervated by the stimulated nerve and generates the maximal force of contraction (Dorsch and Dorsch 2008). Use of a supramaximal current (10-20% above maximal) is recommended to ensure that maximal stimulation is achieved in the face of increased skin resistance. Submaximal currents may increase the accuracy of visual and tactile monitoring (Brull *et al.* 1990, Brull and Silverman 1991); however, these methods are not reliable for detection of residual NMB and are not recommended over more quantitative techniques (see: Monitoring techniques, Section 21.4).

Peripheral nerve stimulators consist of one positive and one negative electrode. The negative electrode is placed closest to the target nerve and the positive electrode is placed at a site where it is not likely to induce depolarization

Veterinary Anesthetic and Monitoring Equipment, First Edition. Edited by Kristen G. Cooley and Rebecca A. Johnson.
© 2018 John Wiley & Sons, Inc. Published 2018 by John Wiley & Sons, Inc.

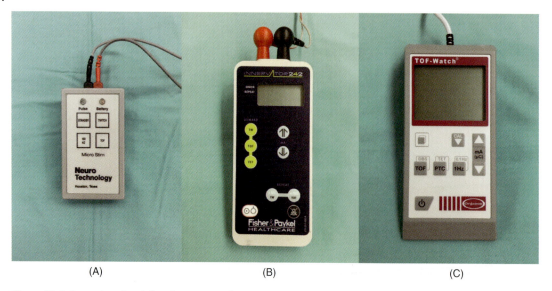

(A)   (B)   (C)

Figure 21.1 Examples of peripheral nerve stimulators. (A) This device has three modes of stimulation: single twitch (TWITCH), tetanus (100 HZ) and train-of-four (TOF). The current is adjusted using a rheostat on the side of the unit (MicroStim; currently available as SunStim, SunMed, Grand Rapids, MI). (B) This device also has three modes of stimulation: single twitch (TW), train-of-four (TOF) and tetanus (TET). The current is adjusted using the mA arrow buttons and the device can be programmed to automatically deliver a stimulus every 1 s for TW or 12 s for TOF. The screen displays the selected current when in use (Innervator 242, Fisher & Paykel, Auckland, New Zealand). (C) This device has five modes of stimulation: train-of-four (TOF), double-burst (DBS), tetanus (TET), post-tetanic count (PTC) and single twitch (TW) (0.1 or 1 Hz). This device can be calibrated to the patient (CAL) and the current is adjusted using the mA arrow buttons. The screen displays the selected current and a measurement of the evoked response (e.g. TOF ratio) when in use (TOF-Watch, MIPM, Mammendorf, Germany).

of another nerve or direct muscle stimulation (Berger *et al.* 1982; Hudes and Lee 1987). To determine the supramaximal current using a device that does not perform this function automatically, single-twitch stimuli (see: Patterns of stimulation, Section 21.3) are delivered at 0.1 Hertz (Hz; 1 Hz = 1 stimulus every second; 0.1 Hz = 1 stimulus every 10 seconds) and the evoked muscle responses noted. The stimulator current is gradually increased until no further increase in evoked response is observed (maximal current), at which point the output is increased a further 10–20 % (Dorsch and Dorsch 2008). Failure to observe a maximal response at 50–70 milliamperes (mA) may be due to inappropriate electrode choice (surface vs. needle electrodes), improper electrode placement, inadequate electrode site preparation, or faulty wire connections.

In most veterinary species, needle electrodes are generally recommended over surface electrodes to ensure a supramaximal stimulus, because their skin tends to be thicker than that of humans, causing increased electrode-skin resistance. Needle electrodes are also recommended if the skin is cold or edematous, or if the patient is obese, hypothyroid or in renal failure (Hunter *et al.* 1985; Miller *et al.* 1989). Conventional 25–22 gauge hypodermic needles are acceptable and should be inserted parallel to the nerve, subcutaneously, and can be held in place with tape, backward-facing needle cap, or a

rubber stopper placed over the needle tip (see: Monitoring techniques, Section 21.4). The stimulator electrode leads should be attached to the needle shafts. Disadvantages of needle electrodes include local irritation, increased risk of direct muscle stimulation or nerve damage, and potential for burns if very high currents are used or if the electrocautery unit has a defective ground (Silverman and Brull 1994a). Direct muscle stimulation due to inappropriate needle electrode placement, and consequent NMBA overdose, has been reported in dogs and can be avoided by placing the negative electrode in close proximity to the target nerve (Jurado *et al.* 2012).

Surface electrodes are generally less effective in veterinary species due to increased electrode-skin resistance. Although increasing the size of the surface electrodes reduces electrode-skin resistance, the larger surface area decreases current density such that a supramaximal stimulus may not be possible, and predisposes to stimulation of multiple nerves (Silverman and Brull 1994a). If surface electrodes are used, the electrode sites must be shaved and dry, and care must be taken to ensure that the electrodes do not overlap or cause stimulation of multiple nerves.

The ideal peripheral nerve stimulator is able to deliver a monophasic, rectangular (square-wave) stimulus lasting 0.2–0.3 milliseconds (ms) at a frequency of 0.1–100 Hz. To ensure a supramaximal current when required, the stimulator should be able to deliver a current of at least

70 mA (Kopman and Lawson 1984; Brull 1996). Newer stimulators are programmed to deliver some or all of the commonly used patterns of stimulation, namely single twitch, train-of-four (TOF), double burst stimulation (DBS), tetanic stimulation and post-tetanic count (PTC).

21.3.1 Patterns of Stimulation

21.3.1.1 Single Twitch
For single-twitch stimulation, single square-wave stimuli are delivered at a frequency between 0.1 and 1 Hz. However, frequencies greater than 0.1 Hz are associated with a progressively diminished response and overestimation of NMB (Dorsch and Dorsch 2008). Frequencies above 0.1 Hz are also associated with augmentation of local blood flow, potentially resulting in faster onset of NMBA action at the stimulation site and overestimation of NMB at other anatomic sites (Curran *et al.* 1987). Use of the single twitch requires that a control is established

prior to administration of the NMBA. After administration of a depolarizing or non-depolarizing NMBA, subsequent twitches are expressed as a percentage of the control twitch, with single twitch depression correlating to the level of NMB (Tw; Figure 21.2). Twitch depression also occurs with decreases in body temperature, which may lead to overestimation of NMB (Heier *et al.* 1990; Eriksson *et al.* 1991; England *et al.* 1994; Young *et al.* 1994).

Single twitch stimulation is useful for establishing a supramaximal current. However, it is relatively insensitive for detecting residual NMB, and full twitch height does not always correlate with full recovery of neuromuscular transmission. During non-depolarizing blockade, the single twitch response is not depressed until 75–80% of the ACh receptors at the neuromuscular junction are occupied, and is abolished only once 90–95% are occupied (Waud and Waud 1972; Silverman and Brull 1994b). This low sensitivity for NMB detection, combined with the need for a control measurement,

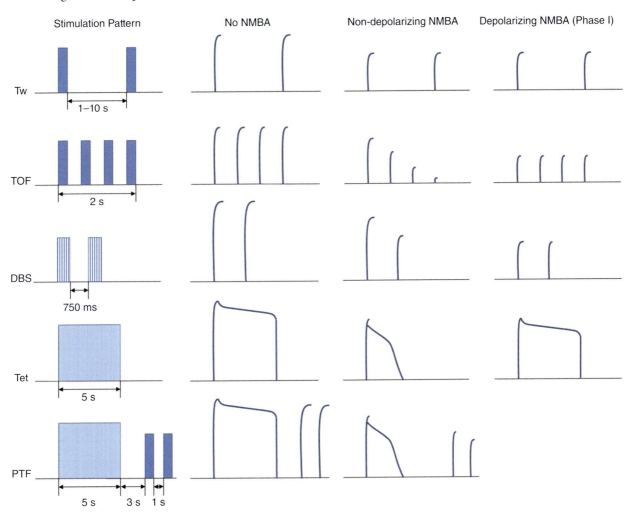

Figure 21.2 Patterns of neuromuscular stimulation and evoked responses without neuromuscular blockade, with non-depolarizing neuromuscular blockade and with depolarizing (Phase I) neuromuscular blockade. Single twitch (TW), train-of-four (TOF), double-burst stimulation (DBS), tetanus (TET) and post-tetanic facilitation (PTF).

makes this pattern of stimulation less desirable than TOF or DBS for neuromuscular transmission monitoring.

21.3.1.2 Train-of-Four (TOF)

The train-of-four (TOF) pattern of stimulation was first described by Ali *et al.* (1970, 1971a, b) and consists of 4 single square-wave stimuli of equal intensity delivered at a frequency of 2 Hz (every 0.5 seconds for 2 seconds), with no less than 10–12 seconds in between trains to allow for recovery of neuromuscular junction function (Ali and Savarese 1980). In the absence of NMB, all four evoked muscle responses (twitches) are of equal amplitude. During partial depolarizing blockade (phase I), all four twitches are depressed, but of equal amplitude. During non-depolarizing blockade, as well as during deep depolarizing blockade (phase II), progressive depression (fade) of each twitch is observed (TOF; Figure 21.2). More specifically, as NMB deepens, the fourth twitch in the train-of-four is eliminated, followed by the third twitch, second twitch, etc., until all four twitches are absent. Thus, counting the number of twitches (TOF count, TOFC) allows for quantitative assessment of non-depolarizing or phase II depolarizing NMB. Likewise, during recovery from NMB, TOFC increases and fade decreases.

Fade during TOF stimulation is observed when 70–75% of ACh receptors at the neuromuscular junction are occupied by a non-depolarizing NMBA (Waud and Waud 1972). Calculating the ratio of the amplitude of the fourth twitch to the amplitude of the first twitch (TOF ratio, TOFR) provides an estimate of the degree of non-depolarizing or phase II depolarizing blockade. TOFR can only be calculated when all four twitches are present (TOFC = 4); TOFR = 1.0 or 100% in the absence of NMB.

The TOF pattern of stimulation is more sensitive than single twitch for detecting residual NMB (Ali *et al.* 1981) and a pre-relaxant control is not required. However, the TOF should be assessed prior to administration of an NMBA to verify stimulator function and correct electrode placement (Dorsch and Dorsch 2008). With TOF, one can distinguish between non-depolarizing and phase I depolarizing blockade, and can detect phase II depolarizing blockade. Importantly, fade (TOFR <1.0 or 100%) cannot be reliably detected using visual or tactile methods (see: Visual and tactile monitoring, Section 21.4.1; Brull and Silverman 1991; Viby-Mogensen *et al.* 1985). A TOFR of more than or equal to 0.9 (90%) is considered sufficient for recovery and extubation in humans with minimal residual NMB present (Gatke *et al.* 2002). Veterinary studies on residual NMB are limited, but it is reasonable to target a TOFR = 0.9–1.0 (90–100%) before patient recovery.

21.3.1.3 Double Burst Stimulation (DBS)

The double burst stimulation (DBS) consists of two short trains of mini-tetanic (50 Hz) stimulation separated by 750 ms (DBS; Figure 21.2). The most common patterns of DBS stimulation are $DBS_{3,3}$ and $DBS_{3,2}$. $DBS_{3,3}$ consists of three 0.2-ms impulses at 50 Hz followed in 750 ms by an identical train of impulses. $DBS_{3,2}$ consists of three 0.2-ms impulses at 50 Hz followed in 750 ms by two 0.2-ms impulses at 50 Hz (Dorsch and Dorsch 2008). Similar to TOF, DBS should be repeated at intervals of no less than 12 seconds to allow for recovery of the neuromuscular junction (Gill *et al.* 1990). DBS is used primarily for detection of residual NMB, where it is superior to TOF when using visual or tactile monitoring, because fade is more readily detectable (Drenck *et al.* 1989; Engbaek *et al.* 1989; Gill *et al.* 1990; Brull and Silverman 1991, 1993; Brull *et al.* 1992). DBS is also used for intraoperative assessment of deep NMB, since the first twitch in DBS can be detected at a deeper level of NMB than the first twitch in TOF (Braude *et al.* 1991). DBS is associated with more discomfort than TOF, but less than that associated with tetanic stimulation (Connelly *et al.* 1990).

21.3.1.4 Tetanic Stimulation

Tetanic stimulation consists of high frequency (50–100 Hz) stimuli, which cause sustained muscle contractions in the absence of NMB. The standard duration of tetanic stimulation is 5 seconds and should be repeated at intervals of no less than 2 minutes (Silverman and Brull 1993). During depolarizing blockade, muscle contractions in response to tetanic stimulation are depressed in amplitude but are sustained. During non-depolarizing blockade, muscle contractions are depressed in amplitude and are not sustained, with fade being observed after 1 to 2 seconds (Tet; Figure 21.2). During very deep NMB, no response may be observed.

With non-depolarizing NMBAs, sustained muscle contractions at 100 Hz require that 50% of ACh receptors at the neuromuscular junction be free of agent (Waud and Waud 1972; Ali and Savarese 1976), whereas a TOFR of 1.0 (or 100%) requires that only 25–30% of receptors be free of agent (Waud and Waud 1972). Halothane-anesthetized horses showed obvious fade during tetanic stimulation at 50 Hz when no fade was detected using TOF stimulation (Klein 1981). Thus, tetanic stimulation at 50 or 100 Hz is a more sensitive indicator of partial or residual NMB compared to TOF stimulation. However, tetanic stimulation is associated with significant discomfort and is not feasible for use in awake patients or patients at light planes of anesthesia (i.e. during the recovery phase when residual NMB is of most concern).

21.3.1.5 Post-Tetanic Count (PTC)

During non-depolarizing blockade, a peripheral nerve stimulus applied after tetanic stimulation of that nerve may result in an increased or exaggerated evoked muscle response, known as post-tetanic facilitation or potentiation (PTF; Figure 21.2) (Brull *et al.* 1991; Silverman and Brull 1993; Saitoh *et al.* 1994). This heightened post-tetanic (compared to pre-tetanic) response is likely due to increased mobilization of ACh at the neuromuscular junction in response to the tetanic stimulus, which outlasts the tetanic stimulus and results in an increased amplitude of subsequent muscle action potentials (Hutter 1952; Viby-Mogensen *et al.* 1981). PTF is maximal at approximately 3 seconds and lasts for up to 2 minutes following a 5-second tetanic stimulation at 50 Hz (Brull *et al.* 1991). PTF is often the first clinical indicator of recovery from NMB, and is useful for estimating the degree of NMB when responses to single twitch, TOF or even tetanic stimulation are absent (Viby-Mogensen *et al.* 1981).

To apply PTF to estimation of NMB, a tetanic stimulus is delivered at 50 Hz for 5 seconds, followed in 3 seconds by single-twitch stimuli delivered at 1 Hz for up to 1 minute, and the number of evoked muscle responses (twitches) to post-tetanic single twitch stimuli are counted (post-tetanic count, PTC). PTC closely correlates with recovery from NMB, such that an inverse relationship exists between PTC and the time to first (pre-tetanic) TOF response (Viby-Mogensen *et al.* 1981; Muchhal *et al.* 1987; El-Orbany *et al.* 2003).

21.4 Monitoring Techniques

Individual patient responses to NMBAs are highly variable and are affected by other drugs, disease states, temperature and acid–base balance. Therefore, the extent and duration of NMB cannot be predicted by dosage or timing of drug administration. Vigilant monitoring of neuromuscular transmission is essential for prevention of inadequate or excessive dosing of NMBAs, resulting in patient movement or post-operative residual curarization (PORC), respectively. PORC is a term used to describe residual NMB during the recovery period, and

may result in hypoxia, tracheal aspiration and upper airway obstruction due to inadequate respiratory muscle function. In humans, the incidence of PORC (TOFR < 0.9) is approximately 45–62% (Debaene *et al.* 2003; Baillard *et al.* 2005). The risk of PORC-related complications is significantly reduced when objective neuromuscular transmission monitoring techniques are used (Eriksson *et al.* 1992, 1997; Murphy *et al.* 2008).

In dogs and cats, neuromuscular transmission monitoring is frequently accomplished using the facial, ulnar and peroneal nerves (Mosing *et al.* 2009). The facial nerve innervates the levator nasolabialis muscle and is palpated over the masseter muscle (Figure 21.3A). The ulnar nerve innervates the carpal and digital flexor muscles and is located on the medial aspect of the olecranon (Figure 21.3B). The peroneal nerve innervates the tarsal flexor and digital extensor muscles and is found just caudal and distal to the head of the fibula (Figure 21.3C).

In horses, neuromuscular transmission monitoring is accomplished at the facial, radial and superficial peroneal nerves (Klein 1981; Mosing *et al.* 2010; Martin-Flores 2013; Keegan 2015). The facial nerve innervates the levator nasolabialis and can be palpated over the masseter muscle (Figure 21.4A). Alternatively, the ventral buccal branch of the facial nerve, which innervates the orbicularis oris muscle, is palpated in a groove caudal and ventral to the commissure of the lip (Mosing *et al.* 2010). The radial nerve innervates the carpal and digital extensor muscles of the thoracic limb and is located distal to the lateral tuberosity of the radius, in the groove between the lateral digital extensor and lateral ulnaris muscles (Figure 21.4B; Mosing *et al.* 2010). The superficial peroneal nerve innervates the digital extensor muscles of the pelvic limb and is palpated caudal to the tibial tuberosity, in the groove between the long and lateral digital extensor muscles (Figure 21.4C; Mosing *et al.* 2010).

Neuromuscular monitoring in sheep and goats is described in the facial and radial nerves, respectively. In

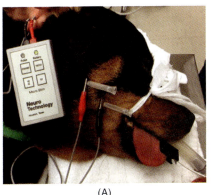 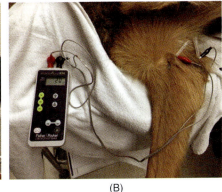 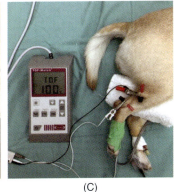

(A)   (B)   (C)

Figure 21.3 Correct lead placement for neuromuscular transmission monitoring at the facial nerve (A), ulnar nerve (B) and peroneal nerve (C) in the dog. Note the needle caps and rubber stoppers used to protect needle tips.

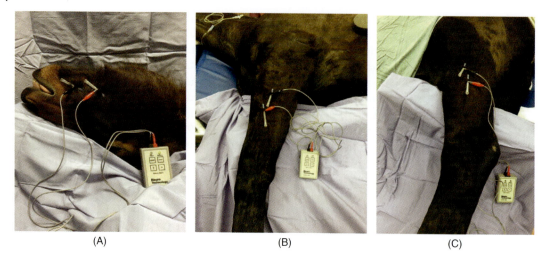

(A)   (B)   (C)

Figure 21.4 Correct lead placement for neuromuscular transmission monitoring at the facial nerve (A), radial nerve (B) and superficial peroneal nerve (C) in the horse.

sheep, the dorsal buccal branch of the facial nerve innervates the levator nasolabialis and can be located approximately 3 cm below the medial canthus of the eye (Clutton and Glasby 2008). In goats, the radial nerve innervates the carpal and digital extensor muscles and can be located in the spiral groove on the lateral aspect of the humerus (Ibebunjo and Hall 1994). Successful use of superficial peroneal nerve stimulation is also described in llamas (Hildebrand and Hill 1993). In pigs, the common peroneal nerve is used. The common peroneal nerve innervates the digital extensor muscles of the pelvic limb and is located over the distal end of the femur (Clutton *et al.* 2013).

In horses, there is good agreement in TOF variables between the superficial peroneal and radial nerves (Mosing *et al.* 2010). However, the facial muscles in this species may be more resistant to NMBAs, and the use of the facial nerve is therefore a less sensitive indicator of NMB (Hildebrand *et al.* 1989; Hildebrand 1990; Mosing *et al.* 2009, 2010; Jones *et al.* 2015). On the other hand, two equine studies suggest that the ocular muscles are more sensitive than the muscles of the extremities (Auer *et al.* 2007b; Auer and Moens 2011). Hence, the most appropriate location for monitoring is still debatable.

In dogs, the facial muscles generally exhibit a faster onset and slower recovery compared to the muscles of the extremities following NMBA administration (McMurphy *et al.* 2004; Auer 2007; Auer *et al.* 2007a; Jones *et al.* 2015). The reason for species and muscle group variations in sensitivity to NMBAs is unclear but may be related to muscle fiber composition, ACh receptor density and local blood flow (Martyn *et al.* 1992; Ibebunjo and Hall 1993; Mosing *et al.* 2010). Overall, the facial muscles are probably less suitable for neuromuscular transmission monitoring compared to the muscles of the extremities.

Regardless of the monitoring technique used, if muscle relaxation is inadequate to complete the given procedure, despite the evoked responses (or lack thereof) indicative of NMB, proper electrode placement, correct wire connections, and appropriate monitor function should be verified before administering additional doses of NMBA.

21.4.1 Visual and Tactile Monitoring

Visual and tactile monitoring involves assessment of twitch strength and presence or absence of fade by observation or palpation, respectively. Tactile monitoring is accomplished by placing the fingertips over the muscle to be stimulated such that a slight preload is imposed at the site, then feeling the strength of contraction during stimulation. Human studies suggest that tactile assessment is more sensitive than visual assessment (Klein 1981; Dorsch and Dorsch 2008). In addition, visual or tactile monitoring using DBS is more sensitive than when TOF or 50-Hz tetanic stimulation is used (Drenck *et al.* 1989; Engbaek *et al.* 1989; Gill *et al.* 1990; Brull and Silverman 1991, 1993; Brull *et al.* 1992; Capron *et al.* 2006).

Visual and tactile methods can predictably identify onset of NMB and be used to determine whether recovery from NMB is sufficient for administration of an antagonist (i.e. whether partial recovery has occurred). TOFC (not TOFR) and PTC can be calculated visually or manually. However, these methods are not reliable for detecting residual NMB and preventing PORC, regardless of whether TOF, DBS or tetanic stimulation is used (Claudius and Viby-Mogensen 2008). Some observers fail to detect visually or manually the presence of fade at a TOFR as low as 0.3–0.4, while others indicate fade at a

TOFR of 0.9–0.95 (Viby-Mogensen *et al.* 1985; Kopman *et al.* 1994). In horses, even the most experienced observers may be unable to visually detect fade at a TOFR as low as 0.5 (Martin-Flores *et al.* 2008). Given that a TOFR of at least 0.9 is required before a patient can be extubated safely, visual and tactile monitoring to determine adequacy of recovery from NMB predispose the patient to complications associated with PORC (hypoxia, aspiration pneumonia, upper airway obstruction, etc.).

21.4.2 Mechanomyography (MMG)

Mechanomyography (MMG) is the measurement of force during isometric muscle contraction, and has been described in dogs (Cason *et al.* 1990), cats (Forsyth *et al.* 1990), horses (Klein *et al.* 1983, Hildebrand and Hill 1994), ponies (Hildebrand and Howitt 1984), llamas (Hildebrand and Hill 1991) and pigs (Clutton *et al.* 2013). Stimulating electrodes are placed over the target nerve and a force-displacement transducer is attached to the part of the body that will move during stimulation (i.e. a paw or hoof), at a right-angle to the direction of contraction. The limb is immobilized and a constant resting tension (preload) of 100–300 g in small animals (Keegan 2015) or at least 1 kg in large animals (Hildebrand and Hill 1994) is applied. A supramaximal stimulus is delivered to the target nerve using single twitch, TOF, DBS or tetanic stimulation. During stimulation, the transducer generates an electrical signal from the mechanical force detected. MMG provides accurate quantification of NMB and is considered the gold standard for neuromuscular transmission monitoring. However, the equipment is cumbersome and setup is elaborate. Careful transducer placement and isometric conditions are required to prevent changes in resting tension and twitch angle. Therefore, MMG is not practical for clinical use in veterinary species and is generally reserved for the research setting.

21.4.3 Electromyography (EMG)

During motor nerve stimulation, a muscle action potential (MAP) is generated in each muscle fiber supplied by that nerve, and electromyography (EMG) records these evoked MAPs. EMG utilizes five electrodes: two stimulating electrodes placed over the target nerve, an active receiving electrode placed over the innervated muscle belly, an indifferent (reference) electrode placed over the insertion site of that muscle, and a ground electrode placed between the latter two electrodes. The EMG device automatically generates the supramaximal stimulus, measures a control response, and then measures evoked responses to stimuli delivered at a preselected interval (Dorsch and Dorsch 2008). During non-depolar-

izing NMB, the amplitude of the MAP is decreased and MAP fade is observed during TOF stimulation. Martinez *et al.* (1998) found no significant difference between EMG and MMG during TOF stimulation in dogs during non-depolarizing NMB. MAP responses during depolarizing NMB are less straightforward and EMG results can be contradictory and less reliable (Donati and Bevan 1984; Weber and Muravchick 1986. 1987).

Compared to MMG, EMG involves less bulky apparatus at the monitoring site and requires less immobilization, since measurements depend on cellular activation rather than movement. However, some fixation or resting tension is needed to minimize motion artifact (Paloheimo 1990; Sakabe and Nakashima 1990). EMG can be used to quantify intense NMB when TOF cannot be detected by other methods (Eisenkraft *et al.* 1986). Disadvantages include susceptibility to electrical interference, time-consuming setup, and the importance of careful electrode placement for obtaining accurate results (Dorsch and Dorsch 2008). The latter issue is especially challenging in smaller species, and more studies are needed to develop standards for EMG use in veterinary species.

21.4.4 Acceleromyography (AMG)

Acceleromyography (AMG), introduced in 1988 (Jensen *et al.* 1988; Viby-Mogensen *et al.* 1988), is currently the best compromise for the veterinary practitioner, allowing objective monitoring that is practical, versatile and reliable (Figure 21.1). AMG is based on Newton's second law ($F = m \times a$), which states that when mass (m) is held constant, acceleration (a) is directly proportional to force (F). Thus, acceleration of an anatomic site during muscle contraction is directly proportional to the force of that contraction. Indeed, a close linear relationship was found between AMG TOFR and MMG TOFR in humans (Viby-Mogensen *et al.* 1988). The AMG monitor generally consists of a peripheral nerve stimulator and a piezo-electric acceleration transducer. The transducer generates a voltage proportional to the acceleration of the moving part, from which an electric signal is created (Claudius and Viby-Mogensen 2008). Unlike MMG and EMG, a preload is not required (Claudius and Viby-Mogensen 2008). Acceleration of the moving part must be free and unopposed, so immobilization is not warranted. However, when an extremity is used for monitoring, the limb should be stabilized proximally because changes in position can affect the results (Keegan 2015).

Currently available AMG monitors are designed for neuromuscular transmission monitoring in people, and default to a reference value for twitch magnitude defined in healthy adult humans. In other words, the preset sensitivity of the acceleration transducer may be too low to produce accurate results in veterinary species. Without baseline calibration of the AMG monitor, results using TOF stimulation were inaccurate and therefore insufficient to determine the adequacy of recovery from NMB in dogs (Martin-Flores *et al.* 2012) and pediatric humans (Driessen *et al.* 2005). Therefore, although the use of TOF stimulation and calculation of a TOFR should theoretically negate the need for a pre-relaxant control twitch, calibration of the AMG monitor prior to NMBA administration is recommended until monitors designed for veterinary use become available.

Martin-Flores *et al.* (2008) demonstrated that AMG detects residual NMB in horses when visual assessment of TOF does not. However, Sakai *et al.* (2015) found that in dogs, an AMG TOFR of 0.9 correlated with an EMG TOFR of 0.47. Similarly, AMG indicates recovery of neuromuscular transmission before EMG in humans (Kopman *et al.* 2005a, b; Liang *et al.* 2013), suggesting that EMG may be a more robust monitor than AMG. Nevertheless, in an extensive human literature review, Claudius and Viby-Mogensen (2008) found that AMG was as useful as MMG and EMG for measuring onset of action of NMBAs and detection of PORC, and was significantly more sensitive than visual/tactile assessment and clinical criteria in detecting PORC. An AMG TOFR of 1.0 correlated with an MMG TOFR of at least 0.9, and predicted with good certainty adequate recovery of the upper airway muscles from NMB.

21.4.5 Kinemyography (KMG)

Kinemyography (KMG) measures the extent of bending and deformation of a piezoelectric sensor due to muscle contraction (Trager *et al.* 2006). KMG is only available through the NMT-Mechanosensor® integrated in the Datex anesthetic machine (NMT-Mechanosensor, Datex Instrumentations Inc., Madison, WI). The sensor is a molded plastic device that is applied in the groove of the thumb and forefinger. Studies showed good agreement between KMG and MMG (Motamed *et al.* 2003; Trager *et al.* 2006), and between KMG and EMG (Gaffar *et al.* 2013), although more recent studies found that KMG underestimates the degree of residual NMB when compared with EMG (Stewart *et al.* 2014; Khandkar *et al.* 2016; Salminen *et al.* 2016). Currently, KMG is only validated and available for human patients.

21.4.6 Phonomyography (PMG)

Phonomyography (PMG) is based on the fact that low-frequency sounds are produced by lateral vibrations in contracting skeletal muscle, the amplitude of which increases linearly with the force of contraction and can

be measured to monitor NMB (Oster and Jaffe 1980; Frangioni *et al.* 1987; Bolton *et al.* 1989; Bellemare *et al.* 2000; Hemmerling *et al.* 2002). These low-frequency sounds, most of which have frequencies of between 2 and 20 Hz, can be recorded with special condenser microphones (Bolton *et al.* 1989; Dascalu *et al.* 1999; Hemmerling *et al.* 2004a). Good correlation between PMG and MMG, EMG, AMG and KMG are found in humans (Dascalu *et al.* 1999; Hemmerling *et al.* 2004a, b; Trager *et al.* 2006). In contrast, PMG measured a slower onset of and faster recovery from NMB compared to MMG (Bellemare *et al.* 2000) and AMG (Hemmerling *et al.* 2002).

The PMG apparatus is simple to set up and can be applied to various muscles of interest, including very small muscles, since this technique depends on vibrations rather than movement. PMG is susceptible to artifacts from vascular pulsations and electrocautery. Accuracy depends on good contact between the microphone and skin surface (Bolton *et al.* 1989), which may be problematic in some veterinary species.

21.4.7 Other Criteria

Clinical criteria, such as negative inspiratory force, tidal volume, reflexes, ability to swallow, etc., cannot be used as surrogates for neuromuscular transmission monitoring with peripheral nerve stimulation. For example, in dogs administered vecuronium for NMB, significant residual NMB was measured with AMG, even when spontaneous ventilation was deemed adequate, as measured by tidal volume, end tidal CO_2, peak inspiratory flow and minute ventilation (Martin-Flores *et al.* 2014). In addition, even "low-dose" NMB with pancuronium in dogs resulted in clinically and statistically significant respiratory depression when adequate eye rotation was present (Lee *et al.* 1998).

In any case, clinical criteria should still be incorporated into any assessment of neuromuscular function in the recovering patient, since the duration of action of some NMBAs can outlast that of the reversal agents, predisposing patients to PORC during the recovery period when peripheral nerve stimulation becomes less practical (Martinez 1999). Furthermore, post-operative upper airway obstruction has been reported with a TOFR of 0.9 as measured with AMG (Eikermann *et al.* 2006). One objective clinical test involves negative inspiratory pressure; negative inspiratory pressure can be used as a measure of respiratory strength and is easily assessed in veterinary species during anesthesia by closing the adjustable pressure limiting (APL) valve and occluding the bag port just before inspiration. The patient should be able to generate at least 15–20 cmH_2O of negative pressure during inhalation (Klein 1981; Hubbell and Muir 2009). In addition, during recovery, respiratory efforts should be strong, thoracic and sustained. Spontaneous respiratory rate and tidal volume should be such that hypoventilation (based on arterial or end-tidal CO_2 levels) is absent to mild. Upon stimulation of the palpebral reflex, the eyelids should close completely. Finally, the patient should demonstrate the ability to swallow prior to extubation. Again, these criteria should not replace neuromuscular monitoring, but could alert the practitioner to PORC in case of monitor failure or inaccuracies.

21.5 Other Equipment

21.5.1 Ventilation

Controlled ventilation, whether with a mechanical ventilator (refer to Chapter 6) or a dedicated staff member, is essential in patients undergoing NMB, because significant hypercarbia, acidosis and hypoxia develop even in the absence of complete respiratory paralysis. An adequate depth of anesthesia should be verified (palpebral reflex, muscle or jaw tone, stable cardiovascular parameters) and controlled ventilation commenced prior to administration of an NMBA. If a mechanical ventilator is to be used, this equipment should be checked for proper function before use (refer to Chapters 6 and 27).

Controlled ventilation settings should be adequate to maintain normocarbia. Respiratory acidosis due to increased arterial CO_2 impedes Hoffman elimination, an important mechanism for atracurium metabolism, such that even mild to moderate increases in CO_2 may result in a prolonged duration of action (Hughes and Chapple 1981). This is especially important in patients with pre-existing acidosis, in which more aggressive ventilation strategies may be indicated for compensation.

21.5.2 Cardiorespiratory Monitoring

Despite newer NMBAs having minimal cardiovascular effects, monitoring of patients undergoing NMB should include blood pressure, electrocardiography (ECG), capnography and (ideally) blood gases. These monitors are important in any patients undergoing anesthesia and are described in Chapters 17–20; however, a brief description of their relevance to NMB is warranted.

ECG monitoring is of particular importance when pharmacologic reversal of NMB is implemented. In horses, reversal with neostigmine or edrophonium is generally recommended, even when responses to TOF and 50-Hz tetanic stimulation have returned to normal, since at least 25–30% of ACh receptors may still be occupied by the

NMBA (Waud and Waud 1972) and even mild muscle weakness can lead to catastrophic injuries during recovery. Pharmacologic reversal is associated with bradyarrhythmias due to sudden increases in ACh levels (Martin-Flores 2013), making ECG monitoring essential in these cases. In some cases, atropine or glycopyrrolate can be administered as well to alleviate the ACh-mediated bradycardia. In these instances, an ECG is essential to detect tachycardia as well as bradycardia or other arrhythmias. Finally, changes in heart rate during NMB can alert the anesthetist to changes in anesthetic depth and adequacy of analgesia.

During NMB, parameters normally used to assess anesthetic depth – eye position, palpebral reflexes, lacrimation, neck muscle tone, jaw tone, anal tone, purposeful movement, and respiratory pattern – are absent. Blood pressure monitoring thus becomes one of the only means by which the practitioner can verify a stable plane of anesthesia and adequacy of analgesia. Prior to adjusting anesthetic depth or re-dosing analgesic drugs, blood pressure should always be evaluated in combination with heart rate, pulse quality, mucous membrane color, capillary refill and end tidal CO_2, to determine whether derangements are related to other causes (volume status, vagal tone, intracranial disease, etc.).

Capnography (end tidal CO_2) and blood gas monitoring are useful during NMB and can help predict the likelihood of a prolonged recovery due to the pH-dependent nature of Hoffman elimination (see above). Changes in blood pH and derangements in CO_2 partial pressure help guide the practitioner with regards to controlled ventilation and acid/base correction, thereby avoiding unpredictable NMBA metabolism and duration of action. In the absence of blood gas monitoring, end tidal CO_2 can be used to estimate arterial CO_2 partial pressure. However, a difference between arterial and alveolar CO_2 (a-A gradient) of 3–6 or 10–15 mmHg is common in anesthetized small and large animals, respectively; alterations in the distribution of ventilation and perfusion during anesthesia and recumbency can exacerbate this difference (Hubbell and Muir 2009; Haskins 2015).

21.5.3 Thermoregulation

Drugs used for anesthetic induction and maintenance impede thermoregulation (Haskins 2015). Active warming equipment should be readily available to prevent hypothermia, not only because hypothermia has negative physiologic consequences for the anesthetized patient, but also because cooling of the neuromuscular monitoring site impairs nerve conduction, resulting in overestimation of NMB (Heier *et al.* 1990; Eriksson *et al.* 1991; England *et al.* 1994; Young *et al.* 1994). Similar to acidosis, hypothermia also impedes Hoffman elimination and therefore prolongs the duration of action of atracurium (Hughes and Chapple 1981).

21.5.4 Drug Delivery Systems

NMBAs have variable durations of action across different veterinary species. For example, atracurium has a duration of 20–35 minutes in dogs and cats (Martinez 1999), 12–15 minutes in horses (Martinez 2002), and only 7 minutes in llamas (Hildebrand and Hill 1993). For procedures that are anticipated to be longer than the duration of action of the NMBA, use of an infusion pump may be desirable so that an NMBA continuous rate infusion can be delivered, avoiding the plasma level peaks and troughs associated with bolus injections and allowing more controlled titration of clinical effect.

21.5.5 Recovery

During the recovery period, adequacy of ventilation and oxygen-hemoglobin saturation should be continuously monitored by capnography and pulse oximetry, respectively, until extubation. Pulse oximetry and visual assessment of respiratory function should also continue after extubation. If an NMBA antagonist was used, monitoring should extend beyond the expected duration of action of the antagonist, and intravenous access should be maintained during this time. Supplies for re-induction of anesthesia and re-intubation should be available in case of PORC resulting in airway failure. Extra induction agent, endotracheal tubes, a laryngoscope, lubricant, lidocaine spray, endotracheal tube ties, a cuff inflation syringe, and a means of ventilation (Ambu bag, anesthesia machine) should be readily available.

References

Ali, H.H. and Savarese, J.J. (1976) Monitoring of neuromuscular function. *Anesthesiology*, 45, 216–249.

Ali, H.H. and Savarese, J.J. (1980) Stimulus frequency and dose-response curve to *d*-tubocurarine in man. *Anesthesiology*, 52, 36–39.

Ali, H.H., Utting, J.E. and Gray, C. (1970) Stimulus frequency in the detection of neuromuscular block in humans. *Br J Anaesth*, 42, 967–978.

Ali, H.H., Utting, J.E. and Gray, C. (1971a) Quantitative assessment of residual antidepolarizing block (Part I). *Br J Anaesth*, 43, 473–477.

Ali, H.H., Utting, H.E. and Gray, C. (1971b) Quantitative assessment of residual antidepolarizing block (Part II). *Br J Anaesth*, 43, 478–485.

Ali, H.H., Savarese, J.J., Lebowitz, P.W. and Ramsey, F.M. (1981) Twitch, tetanus and train-of-four as indices of recovery from non-depolarizing blockade. *Anesthesiology*, 54, 294–297.

Auer, U. (2007) Clinical observations on the use of the muscle relaxant rocuronium bromide in the dog. *Vet J*, 173, 422–427.

Auer, U. and Moens, Y. (2011) Neuromuscular blockade with rocuronium bromide for ophthalmic surgery in horses. *Vet Ophthalmol*, 14, 244–247.

Auer, U., Mosing, M. and Moens, Y.P.S. (2007a) The effect of low dose rocuronium on globe position, muscle relaxation and ventilation in dogs: a clinical study. *Vet Ophthalmol*, 10, 295–298.

Auer, U., Uray, C. and Mosing, M. (2007b) Observations on the muscle relaxant rocuronium bromide in the horse – a dose-response study. *Vet Anaesth Analg*, 34, 75–82.

Baillard, C., Clec'h, C., Catineau, J., Salhi, F., Gehan, G. *et al.* (2005) Postoperative residual neuromuscular block: a survey of management. *Br J Anaesth*, 95, 622–626.

Bellemare, F., Couture, J., Donati, F. and Plaud, B. (2000) Temporal relation between acoustic and force responses at the adductor pollicis during non-depolarizing neuromuscular block. *Anesthesiology*, 93, 646–652.

Berger, J.J., Gravenstein, J.S. and Munson, E.S. (1982) Electrode polarity and peripheral nerve stimulation. *Anesthesiology*, 56, 402–404.

Bolton, C.F., Parkes, A., Thompson, T.R., Clark, M.R. and Sterne, C.J. (1989) Recording sound from human skeletal muscle: technical and physiological aspects. *Muscle Nerve*, 12, 126–134.

Braude, N., Vyvyan, H.A.L. and Jordan, M.J. (1991) Intraoperative assessment of atracurium-induced neuromuscular block using double-burst stimulation. *Br J Anaesth*, 67, 574–578.

Brull, S.J. (1996) Muscle relaxants, what should I monitor and what does it tell me? *ASA Annual Refresher Courses*, New Orleans, LA.

Brull, S.J., Ehrenwerth, J. and Silverman, D.G. (1990) Stimulation with submaximal current for train-of-four monitoring. *Anesthesiology*, 72, 629–632.

Brull, S.J. and Silverman, D.G. (1991) Visual assessment of train-of-four and double burst induced fade at submaximal stimulating currents. *Anesth Analg*, 73, 627–632.

Brull, S.J., Garcia, R.M. and Silverman, D.G. (1992) Visual and tactile assessment of neuromuscular fade. *Anesthesiology*, 77, 352–355.

Brull, S.J., Connelly, N.R., O'Connor, T.Z. and Silverman, D.G. (1991) Effect of tetanus on subsequent neuromuscular monitoring in patients receiving vecuronium. *Anesthesiology*, 74, 64–70.

Brull, S.J. and Silverman, D.G. (1993) Visual and tactile assessment of neuromuscular fade. *Anesth Analg*, 77, 352–355.

Capron, F., Fortier, L.P., Racine, S. and Donati, F. (2006) Tactile fade detection with hand or wrist stimulation using train-of-four, double-burst stimulation, 50-Hertz tetanus, 100-Hertz tetanus, and acceleromyography. *Anesth Analg*, 102, 1578–1584.

Cason, B., Baker, D.G., Hickey, R.F., Miller, R.D. and Agoston, S. (1990) Cardiovascular and neuromuscular effects of three steroidal neuromuscular blocking drugs in dogs (ORG 9616, ORG 9426, ORG 9991). *Anesth Analg*, 70, 382–388.

Claudius, C. and Viby-Mogensen, J. (2008) Acceleromyography for use in scientific and clinical practice. *Anesthesiology*, 108, 1117–1140.

Clutton, R.E. and Glasby, M.A. (2008) Cardiovascular and autonomic nervous effects of edrophonium and atropine combinations during neuromuscular blockade antagonism in sheep. *Vet Anaesth Analg*, 35, 191–200.

Clutton, R.E., Dissanayake, K., Lawson, H., Simpson, K., Thompson, A. and Eddleston, M. (2013) The construction and evaluation of a device for mechanomyography in anaesthetized Gottingen minipigs. *Vet Anaesth Analg*, 40, 134–141.

Connelly, N.R., Silverman, D.G., O'Connor, T.Z. and Brull, S.J. (1990) Subjective responses to train-of-four and double burst stimulation in awake patients. *Anesth Analg*, 70, 650–653.

Curran, M.J., Donati, F. and Bevan, D.R. (1987) Onset and recovery of atracurium and suxamethonium-induced neuromuscular blockade with simultaneous train-of-four and single twitch stimulation. *Br J Anaesth*, 59, 989–994.

Dascalu, A., Geller, E., Moalem, Y., Manoah, M., Enav, S. and Rudick, Z. (1999) Acoustic monitoring of intraoperative neuromuscular block. *Br J Anaesth*, 83, 405–409.

Debaene, B., Plaud, B., Dilly, M. and Donati, F. (2003) Residual paralysis in the PACU after a single intubating dose of non-depolarizing muscle relaxant with an intermediate duration of action. *Anesthesiology*, 98, 1042–1048.

Donati, F. and Bevan, D.R. (1984) Muscle electromechanical correlations during succinylcholine infusion. *Anaesth Analg*, 63, 891–894.

Dorsch, J.A. and Dorsch, S.E. (2008) Neuromuscular transmission monitoring. In: *Understanding Anesthesia Equipment*, 5th ed. Philadelphia, PA: Lippincott Williams & Wilkins, pp. 805–827.

Drenck, N.E., Ueda, N., Olsen, V., Engbaek, J., Jensen, E. *et al.* (1989) Manual evaluation of residual curarization using double burst stimulation. A comparison with train-of-four. *Anesthesiology*, 70, 578–581.

Driessen, J.J., Robertson, E.N. and Booij, L.H. (2005) Acceleromyography in neonates and small infants: baseline calibration and recovery of the responses after neuromuscular blockade with rocuronium. *Eur J Anaesthesiol*, 22, 11–15.

Eikermann, M., Blobner, M., Groeben, H., Rex, C., Grote, T. *et al.* (2006) Post-operative upper airway obstruction after recovery of the train of four ratio of the adductor pollicis muscle from neuromuscular blockade. *Anesth Analg*, 102, 937–942.

Eisenkraft, J.B., Pirak, L. and Thys, D.M. (1986) Monitoring neuromuscular blockade. EMG versus twitch tension. *Anesth Analg*, 65, S47.

El-Orbany, M.I. Joseph, N.J. and Salem, M.R. (2003) The relationship of post-tetanic count and train-of-four responses during recovery from intense cisatracurium-induced neuromuscular blockade. *Anesth Analg*, 97, 80–84.

Engbaek, J., Ostergaard, D. and Viby-Mogensen, J. (1989) Double burst stimulation (DBS). A new pattern of nerve stimulation to identify residual neuromuscular block. *Br J Anaesth*, 62, 274–278.

England, A..J, Wu, X. and Feldman, S.A. (1994) Effect of temperature on the sensitivity of transducers used on human volunteers during neuromuscular stimulating experiments. *Anaesthesia*, 49, 554.

Eriksson, L.I., Lennmarken, C., Jensen, E. and Viby-Mogensen, J. (1991) Twitch tension and train-of-four ratio during prolonged neuromuscular monitoring at different peripheral temperatures. *Acta Anaesthesiol Scand*, 35, 247–252.

Eriksson, L.I., Lennmarken, C., Wyon, N. and Johnson, A. (1992) Attenuated ventilatory response to hypoxaemia at vecuronium-induced partial neuromuscular block. *Acta Anaesthesiol Scand*, 36, 710–715.

Eriksson, L.I., Sundman, E., Olsson, R., Nilsson, L., Witt, H. *et al.* (1997) Functional assessment of the pharynx at rest and during swallowing in partially paralyzed humans: simultaneous videomanometry and mechanomyography of awake human volunteers. *Anesthesiology*, 87, 1035–1043.

Forsyth, S.F., Ilkiw, J.E. and Hildebrand, S.V. (1990) Effect of gentamicin administration on the neuromuscular blockade induced by atracurium in cats. *Am J Vet Res*, 51, 1675–1678.

Frangioni, J.V., Kwan-Gett, T.S., Dobrunz, L.E. and McMahon, T.A. (1987) The mechanism of low-frequency sound production in muscle. *Biophys J*, 51, 775–783.

Gaffar, E.A., Fattah, S.A., Atef, H.M., Omera, M.A. and Abdel-Aziz, M.A. (2013) Kinemyography (KMG) versus electromyography (EMG) neuromuscular monitoring in pediatric patients receiving cisatracurium during general anesthesia. *Egypt J Anaesth*, 29, 247–253.

Gatke, M.R., Viby-Mogensen, J., Rosenstock, C., Jensen, F.S. and Skovgaard, L.T. (2002) Post-operative muscle paralysis after rocuronium: less residual block when acceleromyography is used. *Acta Anaesthesiol Scand*, 46, 207–213.

Gill, S.S., Donati, F. and Bevan, D.R. (1990) Clinical evaluation of double-burst stimulation. Its relationship to train-of-four stimulation. *Anaesthesia*, 45, 543–548.

Haskins, S.C. (2015) Monitoring anesthetized patients. In: Grimm, K.A., Lamont, L.A., Tranquilli, W.J., Greene, S.A. and Robertson, S.A. (eds). *Veterinary Anesthesia and Analgesia. The Fifth Edition of Lumb and Jones.* Ames, IA: John Wiley & Sons, Inc., pp. 86–113.

Heier, T., Caldwell, J.E., Sessler, D.I. and Miller, R.D. (1990) The effect of local surface and central cooling on adductor pollicis twitch tension and core, skin and muscle temperature during nitrous oxide-isoflurane anesthesia in humans. *Anesthesiology*, 72, 807–811.

Hemmerling, T.M., Donati, F., Beaulieu, P. and Babin, D. (2002) Phonomyography of the corrugator supercilli muscle: signal characteristics, best recording site and comparison with acceleromyography. *Br J Anaesth*, 88, 389–393.

Hemmerling, T.M., Michaud, G., Trager, G., Deschamps, S., Babin, D. and Donati, F. (2004a) Phonomyography and mechanomyography can be used interchangeably to measure neuromuscular block at the adductor pollicis muscle. *Anesth Analg*, 98, 377–381.

Hemmerling, T.M., Michaud, G., Trager, G. and Deschamps, S. (2004b) Phonomyographic measurements of neuromuscular blockade are similar to mechanomyography for hand muscles. *Can J Anaesth*, 51, 795–800.

Hildebrand, S.V. (1990) Neuromuscular blocking agents in equine anesthesia. *Vet Clin North Am Equine Pract*, 6, 587–606.

Hildebrand, S.V. and Howitt, G.A. (1984) Dosage requirement of pancuronium in halothane-anesthetized ponies: a comparison of cumulative and single-dose administration. *Am J Vet Res*, 45, 2441–2444.

Hildebrand, S.V. and Hill, T. (1991) Neuromuscular blockade by atracurium in llamas. *Vet Surg*, 20, 153–154.

Hildebrand, S.V. and Hill, T. (1993) Neuromuscular blockade by use of atracurium in anesthetized llamas. *Am J Vet Res*, 54, 429–433.

Hildebrand, S.V. and Hill, T. (1994) Interaction of gentamycin and atracurium in anaesthetised horses. *Equine Vet J*, 26, 209–211.

Hildebrand, S.V., Holland, M., Copland, V.S., Daunt, D. and Brock, N. (1989) Clinical use of the neuromuscular blocking agents atracurium and pancuronium for equine anesthesia. *J Am Vet Med Assoc*, 195, 212–219.

Hubbell, J.A.E, and Muir, W.W. (2009) Monitoring anesthesia. In: Muir, W.W. and Hubbell, H.A.E. (eds)

Equine Anesthesia: Monitoring and Emergency Therapy, 2nd ed. St Louis, MO: Saunders, Elsevier, Inc., pp. 149–170.

Hudes, E. and Lee, K.C. (1987) Clinical use of nerve stimulators in anaesthesia. *Can J Anaesth*, 34, 525–534.

Hughes, R. and Chapple, D.J. (1981) The pharmacology of atracurium: a new competitive neuromuscular blocking agent. *Br J Anaesth*, 53, 31–44.

Hunter, J.M., Kelly, J.M. and Jones, R.S. (1985) Difficulties with neuromuscular monitoring. *Anaesthesia*, 40, 916.

Hutter, O.F. (1952) Post-tetanic restoration of neuromuscular transmission blocked by D-tubocurarine. *J Physiol*, 118, 216–227.

Ibebunjo, C. and Hall, L.W. (1993) Muscle fibre diameter and sensitivity to neuromuscular blocking drugs. *Br J Anaesth*, 71, 732–733.

Ibebunjo, C. and Hall, L.W. (1994) Succinylcholine and vecuronium blockade of the diaphragm, laryngeal and limb muscles in the anaesthetized goat. *Can J Anaesth*, 41, 36–42.

Jensen, E., Viby-Mogensen, J. and Bang, U. (1988) The Accelograph: a new neuromuscular transmission monitor. *Acta Anaesthesiol Scand*, 32, 49–52.

Jones, R.S., Auer, U. and Mosing, M. (2015) Reversal of neuromuscular block in companion animals. *Vet Anaesth Analg*, 42, 455–471.

Jurado, O.M., Mosing, M., Kutter, A.P.N., Boretti, F. and Bettschart-Wolfensberger, R. (2012) Cardiovascular effects of cis-atracurium overdose in a dog following misplacement of neuromuscular monitoring electrodes. *Vet Anaesth Analg*, 39, 555–562.

Keegan, R.D. (2015) Muscle relaxants and neuromuscular blockade. In: Grimm, K.A., Lamont, L.A., Tranquilli, W.J., Greene, S.A. and Robertson, S.A. (eds). *Veterinary Anesthesia and Analgesia. The Fifth Edition of Lumb and Jones.* Ames, IA: John Wiley & Sons, Inc., pp. 260–276.

Khandkar, C., Liang, S., Phillips, S., Lee, C.Y. and Stewart, P.A. (2016) Comparison of kinemyography and electromyography during spontaneous recovery from non-depolarising neuromuscular blockade. *Anaesth Intensive Care*, 44, 745–751.

Klein, L.V. (1981) Neuromuscular blocking agents in equine anesthesia. *Vet Clin North Am Large Anim Pract*, 3, 135–161.

Klein, L.V., Hopkins, K., Beck, E. and Burton, B. (1983) Mechanical responses to peroneal nerve stimulation in halothane-anesthetized horses in the absence of neuromuscular block and during partial non-depolarizing blockade. *Am J Vet Res*, 44, 781–785.

Kopman, A.F. and Lawson, D. (1984) Milliamperage requirements for supramaximal stimulation of the ulnar nerve with surface electrodes. *Anesthesiology*, 61, 83–85.

Kopman, A.F., Mallhi, M.U., Justo, M.D., Rodricks, P. and Neuman, G.G. (1994) Antagonism of mivacuriuminduced neuromuscular blockade in humans. Edrophonium dose requirements at threshold train-of-four count of 4. *Anesthesiology*, 81, 1394–1400.

Kopman, A.F., Chin, W.A. and Moe, J. (2005a) Dose-response relationship of rocuronium: a comparison of electromyographic vs. acceleromyographic-derived values. *Acta Anaesthesiol Scand*, 49, 323–327.

Kopman, A.F., Chin, W. and Cyriac, J. (2005b) Acceleromyography vs. electromyography: an ipsilateral comparison of the indirectly evoked neuromuscular response to train-of-four stimulation. *Acta Anaesthesiol Scand*, 49, 316–322.

Lee, D.D., Meyer, R.E., Sullivan, T.C., Davidson, M.G., Swanson, C.R. and Hellyer, P.W. (1998) Respiratory depressant and skeletal muscle relaxant effects of low-dose pancuronium bromide in spontaneously breathing, isoflurane-anesthetized dogs. *Vet Surg*, 27, 473–479.

Liang, S.S., Stewart, P.A. and Phillips, S. (2013) An ipsilateral comparison of acceleromyography and electromyography during recovery from non-depolarizing neuromuscular block under general anesthesia in humans. *Anesth Analg*, 117, 373–379.

Martin-Flores, M. (2013) Neuromuscular blocking agents and monitoring in the equine patient. *Vet Clin North Am Equine Pract*, 29, 131–154.

Martin-Flores, M., Campoy, L., Ludders, J.W., Erb, H.N. and Gleed, R.D. (2008) Comparison between acceleromyography and visual assessment of train-of-four for monitoring neuromuscular blockade in horses undergoing surgery. *Vet Anaesth Analg*, 35, 220–227.

Martin-Flores, M., Gleed, R.D., Basher, K.L., Scarlett, J.M., Campoy, L. and Kopman, A.F. (2012) TOF-Watch® monitor: failure to calculate the train-of-four ratio in the absence of baseline calibration in anaesthetized dogs. *Br J Anaesth*, 108, 240–244.

Martin-Flores, M., Sakai, D.M., Campoy, L. and Gleed, R.D. (2014) Recovery from neuromuscular block in dogs: restoration of spontaneous ventilation does not exclude residual blockade. *Vet Anaesth Analg*, 41, 269–277.

Martinez, E.A. (1999) Newer neuromuscular blockers: is the practitioner ready for muscle relaxants? *Vet Clin North Am Small Anim Pract*, 29, 811–817.

Martinez, E.A. (2002) Neuromuscular blocking agents. *Vet Clin North Am Equine Pract*, 18, 181–188.

Martinez, E.A., Hartsfield, S.M. and Carroll, G.L. (1998) Comparison of two methods to assess neuromuscular blockade in anesthetized dogs. *Vet Surg*, 28, 127.

Martyn, J.A., White, D.A., Gronert, G.A., Jaffe, R.S. and Ward, J.M. (1992) Up and down regulation of skeletal muscle acetylcholine receptors. Effects on neuromuscular blockers. *Anesthesiology*, 76, 822–843.

McMurphy, R.M., Davidson, H.J. and Hodgson, D.S. (2004) Effect of atracurium on intraocular pressure, eye position and blood pressure in eucapnic and hypocapnic isoflurane-anaesthetized dogs. *J Am Vet Med Assoc*, 65, 179–182.

Miller, L.R., Benumof, J.L., Alexander, L., Miller, C.A. and Stein, D. (1989) Completely absent response to peripheral nerve stimulation in an acutely hypothyroid patient. *Anesthesiology*, 71, 779–781.

Mosing, M., Auer, U., Bardell, D., Jones, R.S. and Hunter, J.M. (2010) Reversal of profound rocuronium block monitored in three muscle groups with sugammadex in ponies. *Br J Anaesth*, 105, 480–486.

Mosing, M., Auer, U., Jones, R.S. and Hunter, J.M. (2009) Comparison of three stimulation sites for neuromuscular monitoring in dogs and ponies. *Br J Anaesth*, 103, 916 p.

Motamed, C., Kirov, K., Combes, X. and Duvaldestin, P. (2003) Comparison between the Datex-Ohmeda M-NMT module and force-displacement transducer for monitoring neuromuscular blockade. *Eur J Anaesthesiol*, 20, 467–469.

Muchhal, K.K., Viby-Mogensen, J., Fernando, P.U.E., Tamilarasan, A., Bonsu, A.K. and Lambourne, A. (1987) Evaluation of intense neuromuscular blockade caused by vecuronium using post-tetanic count (PTC). *Anesthesiology*, 66, 846–849.

Oster, G. and Jaffe, J.S. (1980) Low frequency sounds from sustained contraction of human skeletal muscle. *Biophys J*, 30, 119–128.

Paloheimo, M. (1990) Quantitative surface electromyography (qEMG): applications in anaesthesiology and critical care. *Acta Anaesthesiol Scand Suppl*, 93, 1–83.

Saitoh, Y., Masuda, A., Toyooka, H. and Amaha, K. (1994) Effect of tetanic stimulation on subsequent train-of-four responses at various levels of vecuronium-induced neuromuscular block. *Br J Anaesth*, 73, 416–417.

Sakabe, T. and Nakashima, K. (1990) The Datex relaxograph NMT-100. *Anesthesiol Rev*, 17, 45–51.

Sakai, D.M., Martin-Flores, M., Tomak, E.A., Martin, M.J., Campoy, L. and Gleed, R.D. (2015) Differences between acceleromyography and electromyography during neuromuscular function monitoring in anesthetized Beagle dogs. *Vet Anaesth Analg*, 42, 233–241.

Salminen, J., van Gils, M., Paloheimo, M, and Yli-Hankala, A. (2016) Comparison of train-of-four ratios measured with Datex-Ohmeda's M-NMT MechanoSensor™ and M-NMT ElectroSensor™. *J Clin Monit Comput*, 30, 295–300.

Silverman, D.G. and Brull, S.J. (1993) The effect of a tetanic stimulus on the response to subsequent tetanic stimulation. *Anesth Analg*, 76, 1284–1287.

Silverman, D.G. and Brull, S.J. (1994a) Features of neurostimulation. In: Silverman, D.G. (ed.). *Neuromuscular Block in Perioperative and Intensive Care*. Philadelphia, PA: JB Lippincott, pp. 23–36.

Silverman, D.G. and Brull, S.J. (1994b) Patterns of stimulation. In: Silverman, D.G. (ed.). *Neuromuscular Block in Perioperative and Intensive Care*. Philadelphia, PA: JB Lippincott, pp. 37–50.

Stewart, P.A., Freelander, N., Liang, S., Heller, G. and Phillips, S. (2014) Comparison of electromyography and kinemyography during recovery from non-depolarising neuromuscular blockade. *Anaesth Intensive Care*, 42, 378–384.

Trager, G., Michaud, G., Deschamps, S. and Hemmerling, T.M. (2006) Comparison of phonomyography, kinemyography and mechanomyography for neuromuscular monitoring. *Can J Anaesth*, 53, 130–135.

Viby-Mogensen, J., Howardy-Hansen, P., Chraemmer-Jorgensen, B., Ording, H., Engbaek, J. and Nielsen, A. (1981) Post-tetanic count (PTC): a new method of evaluating an intense non-depolarizing neuromuscular blockade. *Anesthesiology*, 55, 458–461.

Viby-Mogensen, J., Jensen, N.H., Engbaek, J., Ording, H., Skovgaard, L.T. and Chraemmer-Jorgensen, B. (1985) Tactile and visual evaluation of the response to train-of-four nerve stimulation. *Anesthesiology*, 63, 440–443.

Viby-Mogensen, J., Jensen, E., Werner, M. and Nielsen, H.K. (1988) Measurement of acceleration: a new method of monitoring neuromuscular function. *Acta Anaesthesiol Scand*, 32, 45–48.

Waud, B.E. and Waud, D.R. (1972) The relation between the response to "train-of-four" stimulation and receptor occlusion during competitive neuromuscular block. *Anesthesiology*, 37, 413–416.

Weber, S. and Muravchick, S. (1986) Electrical and mechanical train-of-four responses during depolarizing and non-depolarizing neuromuscular blockade. *Anaesthesia*, 40, 146–151.

Weber, S. and Muravchick, S. (1987) Monitoring technique affects measurement of recovery from succinylcholine. *J Clin Monit Comput*, 3, 1–5.

Young, M.L., Hanson, W. III, Bloom, M.J., Savino, J.S. and Muravchick, S. (1994) Localized hypothermia influences assessment of recovery from vecuronium neuromuscular blockade. *Can J Anaesth*, 41, 1172–1177.

22

Temperature Regulation and Monitoring

Caroline Baldo[1] and Darci Palmer[2]

[1] *College of Veterinary Medicine, University of Minnesota, St Paul, Minnesota, USA*
[2] *Southeastern Veterinary Surgery Center, Columbus, Georgia, USA*

22.1 Introduction

The body requires suitable conditions to accomplish physical and chemical reactions effectively. Acid–base balance and ideal core temperature are imperative for such reactions and are tightly regulated by a dynamic, coordinated system of sensors and effectors that regulate homeostasis. Anesthesia-induced hypothermia has received a great deal of attention in the last few years, due to the negative associations with patient outcome and increased hospital stay.

22.2 Heat and Thermodynamics

Heat, or thermal energy, is the kinetic energy of molecules in motion, and is responsible for a system's temperature. Heat can be transferred from one object to another or can be created at the expense of other types of energy (mechanical, electrical, chemical, light or friction). Temperature is the average kinetic velocity of all atoms/molecules in a system and determines whether the substance transfers heat to or accepts heat from another substance (Davis and Kenny 2007). Finally, heat is thermal energy transferred between systems due to temperature difference or created at the expense of other types of energy (mechanical, electrical, chemical, light, friction). Thermodynamics is a branch of science that studies the effects of energy, heat and work on a system, under the premise that these variables are governed by four laws of physics for the transfer of energy:

1) The zeroth law of thermodynamics states that if two separate systems are in thermodynamic equilibrium with a third system, then the two are also in equilibrium with each other. Objects are in thermodynamic equilibrium when they have the same temperature. The zeroth law enabled the creation of thermometers.

2) The first law of thermodynamics states that energy cannot be created or destroyed, it is conserved. In other words, the total amount of energy always remains the same, as it is the sum of its change in form (sometimes by transfer to another object or its surroundings).

3) The second law of thermodynamics states that entropy of a closed system when not in equilibrium will increase over time until equilibrium is reached and entropy is at its maximum. Entropy is a measure of unusable energy and refers to the thermal energy of a system that cannot be converted into mechanical work, often interpreted as the degree of disorder or randomness in the system.

4) The third law of thermodynamics states that as a system approaches absolute zero, all processes stop and entropy is at a minimum. Absolute zero is the temperature at which all processes would stop and it corresponds to $-273.1\,^{\circ}\text{C}$, 0 Kelvin or $-459.67\,^{\circ}\text{F}$.

Laws of energy transfer are equally applicable to the context of biological systems. They are applied to monitoring devices such as thermometers, to thermoregulation and transfer of energy, such as that seen during shivering and panting, and during states like hypothermia and active warming, just to name a few.

22.3 Thermoregulation

Thermoregulation is a neural process that senses the environmental temperature changes and elicits a response to maintain stable internal body conditions (Nakamura and Morrison 2008). Normal thermoregulation is important due to the dependence of chemical and physical reactions on temperature. For example, in many veterinary species, impaired metabolic processes are observable at temperatures below $38\,^{\circ}\text{C}$ ($100.4\,^{\circ}\text{F}$) and while thermoregulation is lost at $34\,^{\circ}\text{C}$ ($93.2\,^{\circ}\text{F}$), cardiac fibrillation and death occurs at $27–29\,^{\circ}\text{C}$ ($80.6–84.2\,^{\circ}\text{F}$)

(Robinson 2013). At the other extreme, high body temperatures are associated with cardiovascular collapse and central nervous system injury, such as that seen with heat stroke (Hemmelgarn and Gannon 2013a, b).

Temperature regulation mechanisms vary between species. For example, fish, reptiles and amphibians are poikilotherms, as their body temperature varies with the environment. Poikilotherms adopt a variety of behaviors to maintain temperature, such as sunbathing or hiding during cold and hot environmental temperatures. Other means of thermoregulation include adjustment of enzyme systems (Somero 2004), use of lipid membranes and/or heat shock proteins (Guschina and Harwood 2006), and modulation of resting metabolic rate (Clarke 2004), to name a few.

Mammals and birds are endothermic homeotherms and maintain a constant internal or core temperature despite external variation. Core temperature (temperature of deep tissues, internal organs and brain), is a dynamic balance between metabolic heat production and environmental losses. Thermoregulatory mechanisms are comprised of a complex system to maintain a core temperature within the inter-threshold range, the core temperature range at which no active compensatory activity such as panting or vasoconstriction occurs. The range of environmental temperatures in which there is no triggering of autonomic effectors is called the thermoneutral zone.

The environmental thermoneutral zone is 20–25 °C (68–77 °F) for dogs, 30–35 °C (86–9 °F) for cats (Hill and Scott 2004), 5–25 °C (41–77 °F) for horses (Morgan 1998), 0–25 °C (32–77 °F) for beef cattle and 4–24 °C (39.2–75.2 °F) for dairy cattle (Hahn 1981). Several physiologic steps are required for an animal to maintain its core temperature, which are likely conserved between mammals and reptiles (Seebacher 2009). The afferent pathway begins with depolarization of TRP (transient receptor potential) channels located in the free nerve endings of A-delta and C somatosensory neurons. Cold stimuli are transmitted via A-delta and warmth via C fibers, whose cells bodies are located in the dorsal or the trigeminal ganglia. TRPs can detect temperature changes from more than 20 °C (68 °F) (TRPA1 for noxious cold, TRPM8 for non-noxious cold) to 52 °C (125.6 °F) (TRPV1 and 2 for noxious warmth, TRPV3 and 4 for non-noxious warmth) in both the periphery and core (Collier and Gebremedhin 2015). A complete description of TRPs can be found elsewhere (Romanovsky 2007).

The periphery exhibits a predominance of cold receptors, approximately 10 times more than central compartments. Central receptors present in the hypothalamus, spinal cord, viscera and great vessels act like pacemaker cells; thermosensitivity is due to currents determining the rate of spontaneous depolarization. They mainly trigger heat defense mechanisms (Romanovsky 2007). These thermoreceptors are present in primary afferent fibers that terminate on Lamina I, where they synapse with secondary fibers. The secondary synapses connect with tertiary fibers at the lateral parabrachial nucleus located at the junction of the midbrain and pons. The tertiary fibers project to the median pre-optic nucleus of the anterior hypothalamus (Morrison and Nakamura 2011). Effectors leave the medial pre-optic area and descend to the dorsomedial hypothalamus and rostral raphe pallidus nuclei to the spinal cord and target organs such as vessels, muscle and brown adipose fat (Nakamura *et al.* 2004; Morrison and Nakamura 2011). In-depth reviews of physiologic responses to hypothermia can be found elsewhere (Clark-Price 2015).

22.4 Types of Heat Loss

Heat can be lost in the form of sensible heat and latent (insensible) heat. Sensible heat is associated with changes in body or surface temperature and depends on a temperature gradient between the animal and environment. It occurs by conduction, convection and radiation. Latent (insensible, evaporative) heat loss occurs by evaporation. The ability of an animal to lose heat from evaporation is related to the animal's ability to use sensible heat for evaporation of moisture (sweat). When the temperature of the skin is equal to that of the environment, sensible losses are absent and evaporative losses are the only way of acquiring thermal comfort (Collier and Gebremedhin 2015). Under normal conditions, approximately 70% of heat is lost primarily through radiation, convection and conduction and, secondarily, by sweating, panting and excretory activity (Redaelli *et al.* 2014) (Figure 22.1).

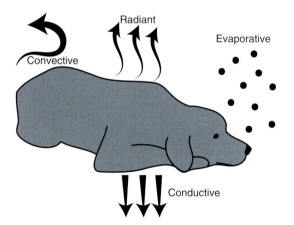

Figure 22.1 Diagram of the common methods of heat loss in veterinary patients (courtesy of Kristen Cooley, University of Wisconsin-Madison, WI).

22.4.1 Radiant

Radiation is a form of heat transfer associated with emission of infrared electromagnetic waves. In animals, radiated heat is lost from internal structures to the subcutaneous vessels to the environment. Short or clipped hair and open body cavities enhance this process. Although radiation is the main source of heat loss in human patients under anesthesia (Diaz and Becker 2010), in normal animals, heat loss is mainly due to convection and conduction (Brodeur *et al.* 2017).

22.4.2 Convective

Convection can be of two types: free or forced. In both, it depends on molecular motion in fluid or air flowing over the animal's skin or open cavity resulting from a temperature gradient. Free convection occurs when temperature varies at the boundary of the skin, promoting changes in the air density and expansion, resulting in convection currents. Forced convection is associated to the use of fans or rooms with laminar airflow, such as in operating rooms (Collier and Gebremedhin 2015).

22.4.3 Conductive

Conduction occurs when two surfaces with different temperatures are in contact; it is a molecular mode of transfer (Collier and Gebremedhin 2015). The temperature gradient and thermal conductivity coefficient of the material in contact with skin will determine the flow of heat exchange. This occurs when an animal is placed on a metal table for anesthetic induction for example.

22.4.4 Evaporative

Latent heat exchange is the evaporative loss of heat by sweating, panting or salivation. Horses and cows tend to sweat, whereas sheep, dogs, cats, swine and birds exchange heat mainly by panting. Both sweating and panting are triggered by the autonomic nervous system in response to skin temperature variation rather than core temperature (Collier and Gebremedhin 2015). Loss of heat by evaporation causes venous blood to be cooler and reduce core temperature once drained into the venous system (Robertshaw 2006). The side effects of panting and sweating are associated with water loss and, in ruminants, loss of bicarbonate and phosphate buffers (Reece 2015). Excessive use of surgical scrub, alcohol, lavage solutions and soaked hair are factors contributing to increased evaporative heat loss (Clark-Price 2015).

22.5 Heat Loss During Anesthesia

One of the main effects of anesthetics is to widen the inter-threshold range by decreasing the lower critical temperature and delaying the onset of autonomic effectors to counteract heat loss. The inter-threshold range increases 10–20 times during general anesthesia, evoking a state of poikilothermia in anesthetized patients (Sessler 2016). The mechanism by which anesthesia widens the inter-threshold range is still unknown. The inhibitory effect of inhalants on TRP receptors (Cornett *et al.* 2008) may be associated with decreased thermal input (Caterina 2007). Anesthesia-induced heat loss has three phases: redistribution, linear and plateau phases. This phasic heat loss has been described for cats (Redondo *et al.* 2012a) and dogs (Redondo *et al.* 2012b; Rose *et al.* 2016) with a decrease of 1.6 °C during the first hour reported in humans (Rose *et al.* 2016).

22.5.1 Redistribution of Heat

During redistribution of heat, centrally mediated vasodilation, more specifically, loss of tonic thermoregulatory vasoconstriction and dilation of arteriovenous shunts, quickly facilitates transfer of heat from the core to the periphery under anesthesia. Even though total heat content is maintained, the core cools and becomes hypothermic as skin is warmed up by heat transfer.

22.5.2 Linear Heat Loss

For the first few hours (˜4 h), heat loss exceeds metabolic heat production in a linear fashion. During surgery, losses are mainly due to radiation and convection with contributions from conduction and evaporation. Factors contributing to intra-operative heat loss are temperature of the operating room, extension of surgical incision, cavity exposure, presence or absence of patient insulation and active warming.

22.5.3 Plateau Phase

Finally, a plateau phase is reached corresponding to the new anesthesia-induced low limit of the inter-threshold range. Vasoconstriction is triggered, limiting core to periphery heat transfer. An intact autonomic nervous system is mandatory; thus, regional anesthesia, neuropathies and spinal shock will impair such response. Heat loss is still ongoing due to peripheral heat transfer to the environment; however, a steady state can be established by the use of external warming or insulation (Sessler 2015).

22.6 Effects of Hypothermia and Hyperthermia

Normal endothermic core body temperatures vary between species and with circadian rhythm, but are typically 38 °C (100.4 °F) (cattle) up to 42 °C (107.6 °F) (birds) (Clark-Price 2015; Reece 2015). A core to skin temperature gradient is present, but is typically small, approximately 2–4 degrees; core temperature is the main trigger for autonomic responses, while skin temperature elicits behavioral mechanisms (Lenhardt *et al.* 1999). Physiologic responses to decreased temperature include increased muscle activity, shivering, release of epinephrine, norepinephrine and thyroid stimulating hormone, increased brown fat metabolism, increased appetite, piloerection, use of countercurrent systems (e.g. carotid rete, etc.), alpha-adrenergic mediated closure of arteriovenous shunts, and changes in body posture and hibernation.

In warmer environments, responses include post ganglionic cholinergic mediated sweating, nitric oxide mediated vasodilation (Kellogg 2006), opening of arteriovenous shunts, increased ventilation and panting, decreased appetite, and decreased motor activity (Reece 2015; Sessler 2016). Each of these responses has a triggering core temperature. Core temperature at the onset of sweating or panting is called the upper critical limit and core temperature at onset of vasoconstriction is called the lower critical limit. As previously mentioned, the range in between is the inter-threshold range in which no homeostatic responses occur. Mammals normally keep their inter-threshold ranges tightly regulated within 0.2 °C, except for camels that may allow core temperature to fluctuate by as much as 10 °C per day (Grimm 2015; Reece 2015).

22.6.1 Hypothermia

Hypothermia occurs once core temperature reaches a value below the lower limit of the inter-threshold range (for review see Clark-Price 2015). On the other hand, hyperthermia is seen when the core temperature is greater than the upper critical limit (i.e. the temperature at which panting and sweating are triggered). Recently, hypothermia in dogs and cats has been established as a core temperature of less than 37.5 °C (99.5 °F) (Rose *et al.* 2016).

Peri-anesthetic hypothermia has an incidence of 83.6% (rectal temperature <36.5 °C (96.7 °F); Redondo *et al.* 2012b) to 88% (rectal temperature <37.5 °C; Rose *et al.* 2016) in dogs. In cats, the incidence (<36.5 °C) is even higher at 97.4% (Redondo *et al.* 2012a). Horses also experience hypothermia and temperature may decline 0.8 ± 0.6 °C/hour during anesthesia (Tomasic 1999; Mayerhofer *et al.* 2005).

Mild to moderate hypothermia is seldom an anesthetic emergency, but it is associated with numerous side effects. For example, significantly increased recovery times (Tomasic 1999; Mayerhofer *et al.* 2005; Pottie *et al.* 2007) are likely due to slower drug clearance (van den Broek *et al.* 2010) and increased solubility of volatile agents in tissue (Regan and Eger 1967). In children, isoflurane MAC decreased 5.1% for every 1 °C drop in core temperature (Liu *et al.* 2001) and at 20 °C (68 °F), isoflurane requirements are negligible in goats (Antognini 1993). Toxicity of anesthetic agents may become more evident during re-warming due to the re-establishment of receptor activity in the face of increased plasma concentrations and prolonged half-life resultant from limited clearance.

Mild hypothermia (33–35 °C/91.4–95.0 °F in humans) increases cardiac output and blood pressure from tachycardia and peripheral vasoconstriction. Anesthetic agents (Wong 1983) counteract these sympathetically mediated effects, thus decreased cardiac output and hypotension may result. Bradyarrhythmias eventually occur (Solomon 1989; Bashour *et al.* 1989; Roscher *et al.* 2001) with associated myocardial depression (Mattheussen *et al.* 1996). Asystole can occur below 24 °C (75.2 °F) and ventricular arrhythmias are more likely to develop below 27–29 °C (80.6–84.2 °F) (Lloyd and Mitchell 1974). Under 30–32 °C (86–89.6 °F), arrhythmias may become unresponsive to atropine, lidocaine or electrical cardioversion (Bjørnstad *et al.* 1991; Thomas and Cahill 2000). There is an initial left shift of the oxygen dissociation curve at 30 °C (86 °F), increasing hemoglobin affinity to oxygen by 5.7%/ °C (Baer 1989; Mallet 2002). However, in profound hypothermia (<28 °C/82.4 °F), this shift may be replaced by a right shift due to hypoxia-induced acid lactic acidosis, reduced lactate clearance by the Cori cycle and respiratory acidosis (Mallet 2002).

Mild hypothermia results in tachypnea (Mallet 2002). However, ventilation is impaired as hypothermia (34 °C/93.2 °F) decreases the sensitivity of the respiratory center to the partial pressure of CO_2, and CO_2 production decreases by 50% as temperatures approach 30 °C/86 °F (Mallet 2002). The left shift in the oxyhemoglobin dissociation curve and capillary blood sludging may predispose to tissue hypoxia; however, since oxygen consumption also decreases, tissue damage is minimized (Armstrong *et al.* 2005; Brodeur *et al.* 2017).

Coagulation disorders of primary and secondary hemostasis and fibrinolysis are associated with increased transfusion needs in human surgical patients (Yoshihara *et al.* 1985; Rajagopalan *et al.* 2008). Blood viscosity and hematocrit increase with hypothermia, compromising tissue perfusion. Increased wound infection occurs in humans (Putzu *et al.* 2007), although in veterinary medicine, surgical time has greater effects than hypothermia on rate of infection (Beal *et al.* 2000).

Hypothermia-induced shivering (De Witte and Sessler 2002) increases intraocular and intracranial pressure, pain and discomfort during anesthetic recovery. Shivering in dogs is triggered at a rectal temperature of approximately 37–37.5 °C (98.6–99.5 °F) (Hammel *et al.* 1960). Heat production during this process is associated with increased oxygen consumption varying from 50–400%, depending on core temperature (Bay *et al.* 1968).

Although frequently an unwanted effect, intentional hypothermia is performed in anesthesia for its beneficial effects in certain situations. For example, therapeutic hypothermia is useful in animals such as swine, mice and dogs undergoing cardiac arrest, cardiopulmonary bypass and neurological interventions (Brodeur *et al.* 2017; Frank and Broessner 2017). Hypothermia in this context usually approaches temperatures of 28–33 °C (82.4–91.4 °F).

22.6.2 Hyperthermia

Unlike hypothermia, hyperthermia is not as common in peri-anesthetic settings and is defined as core body temperatures above the upper critical limit. Patients may have febrile or non-febrile hyperthermia.

22.6.2.1 Febrile Hyperthermia

Fever is defined as an increase in core temperature targeted by the thermoregulatory center with a regulated and adaptive higher hypothalamic thermal threshold established as part of a coordinated host defense. As such, heat loss mechanisms are not initiated unless the new upper critical limit is reached. Febrile hyperthermia is mainly a result of septicemia, endotoxemia, infections, trauma, neoplasia, immune-mediated diseases and transfusion reactions, which will all initiate the synthesis and release of inflammatory cytokines such as IL-1, IL-6 and TNF-alpha. Targeting normothermia in febrile anesthetic patients will trigger heat-producing effectors and unnecessary increases in metabolic rate that are more detrimental than the much milder 13% increase in metabolic rate for every 1 °C increase in core temperature (Roth 2009).

22.6.2.2 Non-Febrile Hyperthermia

Non-febrile hyperthermia can result from overexertion (as in working or zoo animals), drug reactions, thyroid storm, excessively light anesthetic plane, excessive endogenous heat delivery, malignant hyperthermia, central nervous system dysfunction, heat stroke, pheochromocytoma, and anesthetic machine malfunction (Herlich 2013; Luthra *et al.* 2016). If left untreated, moderate to severe hyperthermia triggers a life-threatening syndrome known as heatstroke. Heatstroke can lead to severe dehydration, decreased cardiac output, vasoconstriction, hypoxia, rhabdomyolysis, brain damage, multiple organ failure, disseminated intravascular coagulation and death (Johnson 2006). Excellent reviews on the pathophysiology of hyperthermia can be found elsewhere (Herlich 2013; Hemmelgarn and Gannon 2013a, b; Walter *et al.* 2016).

Although the environment and procedural factors influence the risk of hyperthermia, patient-related risk factors are mainly associated to co-morbidities associated to body composition, color and thickness of fur, higher metabolic rate and work of breathing, and impairment of the thermal central control and effectors. In addition, malignant hyperthermia (MH) is a pharmacogenetic disorder associated with a life-threatening hypermetabolic syndrome involving the skeletal muscle (Hopkins 2011). MH was first described in pigs under halothane anesthesia (Berman *et al.* 1970) and more recently in horses and dogs (for review see Brunson and Hogan 2004). Opioids affect the hypothalamic thermal balance by their agonistic activity on mu, kappa, delta and sigma receptors (Rawls and Benamar 2011), but the global effect can be hypothermia (dogs, rabbit, bird), hyperthermia (cat, horse, goat, sheep), or dose-dependent hyperthermia at low doses and hypothermia at high doses (rat, mouse, monkey) (Adler *et al.* 1988).

22.7 Re-Warming

Re-warming is the primary therapy for hypothermia and should be performed with caution (Brodeur *et al.* 2017). The process of restoring core temperature may counteract the protective effects of therapeutic hypothermia or aggravate its effects. Oxygen consumption (VO_2) and delivery (DO_2) are impaired during re-warming due to changes in metabolic rate, tissue extraction of oxygen, mitochondrial oxidative phosphorylation function, cardiac output, blood flow distribution, blood viscosity, pH and shifts in the oxy-hemoglobin dissociation curve (Scaravilli *et al.* 2012). According to Scaravilli *et al.* (2012), side effects can be minimized if re-warming is performed slowly along with control of pain and shivering and close hemodynamic monitoring including echocardiography and goal-directed hemodynamic optimization, if necessary, along with urinary output measurement and contractility support for left ventricular dysfunction. Ideal rates of re-warming have not yet been described for veterinary clinical settings, but rates vary from 0.1–0.5 °C/h (Schmutzhard *et al.* 2012; Faulds and Meekings 2013). These rates pertain to re-warming following therapeutic hypothermia or hypothermia due to snow and water trauma/accidents, in which the core cools to temperatures far below (<28 °C/82.4 °F). Studies on the re-warming rate after unintentional peri-operative hypothermia are sparse. Nevertheless, re-warming should be carried out slowly and gradually, especially in patients with morbidities compromising oxygen content and delivery or tissue oxygen extraction, such as anemia, cardiomyopathy, pulmonary diseases, sepsis, systemic inflammatory reaction syndrome, and ischemia and reperfusion injury. The metabolic cost of shivering should also be considered and, unless contraindicated, maintaining the patient under anesthesia with active warming devices until core temperature is above the shivering threshold may have great utility.

Overheating is a risk associated to peri-operative control of hypothermia. There are no studies in veterinary medicine demonstrating the ideal core temperature at which removal or adjustment of active re-warming is recommended, but temperatures at which active re-warming techniques are stopped frequently approach 98–99 °F (36.6–37.2 °C) in some institutions. Overheating or rebound hyperthermia is caused by vasodilation, which facilitates transfer of heat from the periphery to the core.

22.8 Temperature Monitoring Devices

22.8.1 Simple (Non-Electrical) Monitors

22.8.1.1 Mercury Thermometers

The oldest and simplest device to measure temperature is the mercury thermometer, which relies on the ability of liquid mercury to expand or contract (high expansion coefficient) when submitted to a wide range of temperatures. Mercury is sealed in a thin glass bulb connected to a capillary tube marked in degrees Celsius or Fahrenheit (Figure 22.2). Heat energy from the skin or mucous membrane is transferred through the thin glass bulb and mercury expands moving up the capillary tube. Equilibration is allowed, and the patient's temperature read at the point where the meniscus is observed.

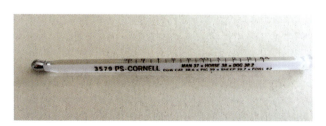

Figure 22.2 A glass mercury thermometer for use in veterinary medicine. The bulb is located at one end with graduated markings (°C). This example is no longer manufactured and has reference values on the back for normal temperatures in veterinary species.

Although this method is cheap and accurate, the display is difficult to read, it is restricted to anesthetized veterinary patients, and is slow (2–3 minutes) and fragile (Davis and Kenny 2007). This device has been banned from many areas due to the potential toxic effects of mercury and has been replaced with safer and faster thermometers. Alcohol may be used instead of mercury in thermometers, which is useful in very low temperatures since mercury solidifies at −39 °C; however, at very high temperatures, alcohol boils and is therefore not useful (78.5 °C) (Davis and Kenny 2007).

22.8.1.2 Dial Thermometers

Dial thermometers use bimetallic strips or a Bourdon gauge. As the temperature rises in a bimetallic strip, two dissimilar metals contract by different amounts, which alter a coil attached to a pointer corresponding to the temperature. Since the Bourdon gauge is a pressure-monitoring device, the temperature-sensing element contains a small cylinder of mercury. As the volume changes, the pressure also changes, and is detected by the gauge, which has units for temperature (Davis and Kenny 2007).

22.8.2 Electrical Monitors

22.8.2.1 Thermistor

A thermistor is a resistor of metal-oxide semi-conductors, most commonly manganese, nickel, cobalt, iron, copper or titanium sintered into a disc, washer, rod, bead or wire (Figure 22.3). Temperature is determined by measuring the change in resistance by applying an electrical current and measuring the voltage output as related by the Ohm's Law ($V = I \times R$; V = voltage; I = current; R = resistance). Thermistors are commonly connected to Wheatstone bridge circuits (Davis and Kenny 2007).

There are two types of thermistors: negative temperature coefficient (NTC) and positive temperature coefficient (PTC). The NTC is commonly applied to the medical field and resistance has an inverse relationship with temperature (higher temperature, lower resistance, and vice-versa). The PTC has a positive temperature–resistance relationship and is mainly used as a fuse

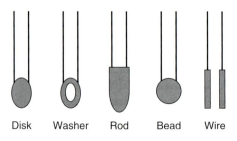

Disk   Washer   Rod   Bead   Wire

Figure 22.3 Common types of thermistor tips.

technology. Although thermistors are highly accurate and sensitive, are small, quick and read continuously, the relationship between temperature and resistance is non-linear. To correct for this non-linearity, mathematical models or added resistances are used; however, they decrease thermistor sensitivity and result in a narrower range of readings.

The digital electronic thermometer is the most common example of a thermistor (Figure 22.4). These use an alkaline battery for power source to ensure a low voltage. The thermistor output is amplified, digitized and the data processed in a module. To allow for rapid steady state and temperature readings, heating circuits preheat the probe when the thermometer is powered on. In addition, a prediction algorithm may be used to predict the temperature at steady state. Both of these in combination may allow readings within 4–6 seconds.

22.8.2.2   Thermocouple Device

Thermocouples combine two metals with different heat conductivities. Thermocouple devices are based on the Seebeck effect, in which a temperature difference between two dissimilar electrical conductors or semi-conductors produces a voltage difference between two substances (Davis and Kenny 2007). Medical thermo-couples use copper-constantan (copper with 40% nickel) junctions, producing small voltages that are measured by amplifiers. Devices have two of the junctions, where one is kept at constant temperature (reference junction) and the other is attached to a probe and exposed to the area being measured (measuring junction). Heat induces the formation of current in each metal which, due to the different conductivities, generates a voltage gradient that is measured and amplified, subsequently generating a temperature reading. Thermocouples are accurate, small, quick and provide continuous readings. However, some can have poor sensitivity and can be affected by interference from nearby electromagnetic fields. Both thermistors and thermocouples are used in hospital settings as surface, tympanic, oral, esophageal and rectal probes.

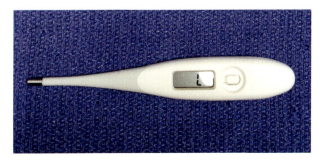

Figure 22.4 Example of a commonly used digital thermometer.

22.8.2.3   Resistance Thermometer

The principle behind the function of a platinum wire thermometer is similar to a thermistor, as the resistance of metal increases linearly with temperature (Davis and Kenny 2007). These probes have to be protected from moisture, as this will render platinum unstable. They can be combined with a digital display to facilitate readings; however, these devices are not very sensitive.

22.8.2.4   Liquid Crystal Thermometers

Liquid crystal thermometers rely on the anisotropic properties of organic compounds exhibited during the transition from solid to liquid state (Bjoraker 1990). Heat will induce a state change and the liquid crystal encapsulated in the form of letters and numbers will scatter the ambient light producing an iridescent light allowing temperature reading. Since these are safe, easily applied, inexpensive and disposable, they are used as skin/contact thermometers in human medicine. However, they have low accuracy, are imprecise and are susceptible to environmental changes. They have no utility in veterinary medicine due to the skin features of our patients (variability in hair, skin thickness, etc.).

22.8.2.5   Infrared Devices

Infrared temperature monitoring devices work according to the principle that an object emits infrared radiation in proportion to its temperature (Davis and Kenny 2007). The tympanic membrane has been used in dogs and cats; however, for accurate readings, the otoscope-like probe has to seal the ear canal from the environment and align with the cranial inferior third of the tympanic membrane. Infrared devices are also used in laboratory species.

The sensor is comprised of a polarized ceramic crystalline material (Davis and Kenny 2007). If the temperature changes with radiation, the polarization changes and an electrical signal is generated. However, the sensor only works with a temperature change, thus a shutter is frequently used to expose the sensor to the infrared radiation at intervals (Davis and Kenny 2007).

22.9   Sites of Temperature Monitoring

The body has two main thermal compartments, the core and periphery. Core temperature refers to deep, vital internal organs and periphery to the shell that insulates the core.

22.9.1   Core Body Temperatures

Temperature of the core compartment is kept higher and in tight regulation compared with the periphery. It is the temperature of clinical interest, especially at sites such as the brain (which has the highest core temperature; Clark-Price 2015) and heart. A telemeter transponder can be implanted (usually in the abdominal cavity, but other places as well) in animals to monitor core temperature, as well as to collect data regarding gross motor activity and heart rate. Transponders can be compact enough to be implanted in animals as small as mice (Mini-Mitter, STARR Life Sciences, Oakmont, PA).

22.9.2 Peripheral Temperature

Thermoregulatory vasomotor control maintains a gradient between core and periphery of 2–4 °C. Thus, peripheral sites may not be accurate descriptors of core body temperature due to the slow rate of core-to-periphery temperature equilibrium. Factors that influence the measurement of temperature at different peripheral sites include local heat production, perfusion, insulation (fat, hair) and ambient factors (Blainey 1974).

Many studies have been designed to correlate peripheral to core temperatures in an attempt to determine the best site of sensitivity and accuracy for reliable readings. Monitoring sites described are the pulmonary artery, esophagus, nasopharynx, urinary bladder, rectum, tympanic membrane, skin, axilla, mouth, trachea, inguinal area and hypopharynx.

22.9.3 Specific Sites

22.9.3.1 Pulmonary Artery

The presence of a thermistor at the end of a pulmonary artery catheter provides the gold standard for core temperature measurement. Correlation has been found with intrathecal and jugular bulb temperatures (Kumar *et al.* 1994; Crowder *et al.* 1996), which is not true for brain temperatures during extreme hypothermia (Stone *et al.* 1995). However, during thoracotomies and cardiopulmonary bypass, this site becomes unreliable due to the connection with ambient environmental conditions.

22.9.3.2 Esophagus

Thermometers used in the esophagus can be a simple temperature probe or a thermistor attached to an esophageal stethoscope or gastric tube. Positioning is key to allow for reliable readings and should be in the distal third of the esophagus, between the heart and the descending aorta. In humans, esophageal stethoscopes with an incorporated ECG lead will help placement by observing a biphasic P wave (mid-atrial level) when attaching the positive lead to the probe and the negative lead to the right shoulder. If too proximal, readings will be lower and if too distal (in stomach) temperatures may be overestimated from liver metabolism or

underestimated due to gastric contents. The presence of gastric contents in the esophagus may cause falsely low readings. In general, esophageal temperatures correlate well with pulmonary artery measurements in children (Robinson *et al.* 1998). Temperature variations are rapidly relayed from esophageal sites and in profound hypothermia, esophageal readings do not correlate with brain temperature (Sarkar *et al.* 2013). This technique is difficult to use in the awake patient and in patients with esophageal abnormalities, esophageal surgery, gastric suctioning and open chests.

22.9.3.3 Nasopharynx

Probes can be placed against the dorsal wall of the nasopharynx, just caudal to the soft palate and fairly close to the hypothalamus. In some experimental studies using dogs, the nasopharyngeal temperature was closely related to brain temperature (Li *et al.* 1988). Advantages of this technique include easy access and inability of inspired gases or gastric suction to affect readings. However, this site is usable only in anesthetized patients and may result in epistaxis.

22.9.3.4 Urinary Bladder

A thermocouple or thermistor built in an indwelling urinary catheter and inserted in the bladder can be used. Although correlations with pulmonary artery and esophageal sites are reportedly positive, the rate of cooling or heating may affect readings in the bladder, as temperature relies on glomerular filtration rate and urinary output.

22.9.3.5 Rectum

Rectal probes are of the thermistor or thermocouple type and can be disposable or reusable with a protective cover or sleeve. Steady-state temperature readings take 2–3 minutes. Readings are influenced by heat producing flora, venous return from limbs and presence of feces; however, readings are not influenced by ambient temperature. This route is not indicated for monitoring temperature during pelvic surgeries or after enemas.

22.9.3.6 Tympanic Membrane

Thermometry using the tympanic membrane can be performed using contact and infrared techniques. This site is located deep within the skull and separated from the internal carotid artery by a narrow air-filled cleft on the middle ear and a thin shell of bone. Another attractive feature is that the tympanic membrane and the hypothalamus share common blood perfusion. The contact technique consists of inserting a probe in the ear canal until it touches the lower rostral quarter of the membrane. Infrared thermometry will give temperatures lower than the core because of the wide shape of the sensing tip, which makes it read not only infrared waves from the tympanic membrane but also from the ear canal (Ducharme *et al.* 1997). Excellent to poor correlation have been associated to other sites and a difference as high as 1.6 °C can be present from one ear to the other. Readings are affected by ambient air, facial cooling, and in animals, the 90-degree angle between the vertical and horizontal ear canal, which impairs accurate detection of infrared waves. This method is not recommended for anesthesia, due to intermittent readings and large variation of temperature readings.

22.9.3.7 Skin

The skin is likely the site with the least clinical application, due to the large gradient with core temperature and interference from factors such as ambient temperatures, warming devices, changes in cardiac output and regional vasoconstriction. The main site for placement of probes (thermistor, thermocouple or liquid crystal types) is the forehead for its rich blood supply and no fat. In animals, the insulating effect of hair and variance in skin thickness are negative factors.

22.9.3.8 Axilla

The axilla temperature probe is placed over the axillary artery and the arm adducted. Reading times may take as long as 15 minutes and measurements are not reflective of core temperature. Readings are influenced by proper contact with probe, skin perfusion, environment exposure and warming devices.

22.9.3.9 Oral or Sublingual

The oral of sublingual probe is placed in either cheek pocket lateral to the frenulum and with the mouth closed to allow equilibration. Correlation with other sites is fair. Mouth breathers, panting and oral surgeries impair the use of this technique and it is difficult in awake animals.

22.9.3.10 Trachea

A thermistor may be attached to the endotracheal tube to measure tracheal temperature. However, readings are influenced by airflow and heat and moisture exchanges.

22.9.3.11 Inguinal Area

The inguinal probe is placed lateral to the femoral artery and the leg adducted. This site is not applicable to clinical settings due to time warranted for readout and variability and animal acceptance.

22.10 Warming Devices

22.10.1 Passive Warming

Passive warming methods rely on the patient's intrinsic ability to produce heat. The use of blankets or material that can provide thermal insulation (i.e. plastic, bubble wrap, drape material or foil blankets) will reduce heat loss through conduction and convection. Adequate results rely on a few pre-requisites; the patient should be dry (water has a high thermal conductivity), placed on an insulated surface and have only mild hypothermia. The presence of shivering makes passive re-warming more efficient (Aslam *et al.* 2006). Interestingly, horses undergoing colic surgery had a reduction in temperature loss compared to other anesthetized horses, despite the abdominal lavage and subsequent wet hair, potentially attributable use of an encompassing disposable surgical drape preventing evaporative heat losses by trapping water vapor between the body and the drape material (Mayerhofer *et al.* 2005).

22.10.2 Active Warming

Active warming works by applying heat to a patient to reduce the difference between the body and the environmental temperatures (Clark-Price 2015). Examples of active warming devices include circulating warm water blankets, forced warm air heating units, infrared heating devices, and resistive polymer electric blankets. Currently, stationary substances such as warm water bottles are not recommended (see below). Some active warming techniques are designed to combat hypothermia by introducing warmth to the core of the body. Examples of this include infrared warming devices, warmed intravenous fluids, warmed/humidified inspired gas, warm abdominal fluid lavage, and extracorporeal re-warming.

22.10.3 Metabolic Warming

Metabolic warming techniques are used by the body to internally generate more heat when exposed to hypothermic conditions (Clark-Price 2015). For example, IV infusion of amino acids is used to stimulate insulin release, which results in protein synthesis in skeletal muscle. This is associated with heat production and may be a therapeutic direction for hypothermia in the future (Clark-Price 2015).

22.11 Active Warming Devices

22.11.1 Surface Re-Warming

22.11.1.1 Forced-Air Warming

Forced-air warming heating units are designed to be used with an approved blanket placed either over or under the patient, which allows warm air to be evenly distributed around the patient. The goal of these blankets is to minimize convective heat loss by trapping warm air around the patient and limiting air flow leaving the patient. Common units used in veterinary medicine include the Bair Hugger® (3M Company, Maplewood, MN), Baja® (Animal Hospital Supply, Flowery Branch, GA), Equator® (SurgiVet, St Paul, MN) and WarmAir® (Cincinnati Sub-Zero, Cincinnati, OH). Disposable, single-use blankets are available for each unit but they are expensive, not intended for reuse, and difficult to clean (Figure 22.5). Reusable blankets (Warming blankets, Jorvet, Loveland, CO; Everlast II, Animal Hospital Supply, Flowery Branch, GA) offer a more economical and environmental friendly option (Figure 22.6). An additional option and one that is more common in situations where means are limited (shelter situation and field techniques, see Chapter 26), is the use of scrub pants knotted at the ankles and cinched around the warm air hose using the waist drawstrings (Figure 22.7). However, many suppliers do not recommend these as they are not commercial products.

It is recommended that forced warm air heating units always be used with a blanket to avoid burns. Placing the hose by or towards the patient may result in skin burns from the direct heat or indirectly by overheating plastic, metal or other objects that may be in contact with the patient. Contamination of operating room air has been associated with the use of forced-air warming units (Clark-Price 2015). This can be reduced by waiting until the patient is completely draped into surgery before turning the unit on. The effectiveness of active warming using forced air devices during the peri-operative period may be variable due to the effect of vasoconstriction on periphery

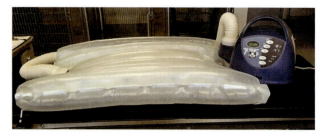

Figure 22.5 Bair Hugger® (3M Company, Maplewood, MN) with a disposable, single-use blanket. Tiny holes on the underside of the blanket are located throughout the length and direct the warm air over the patient.

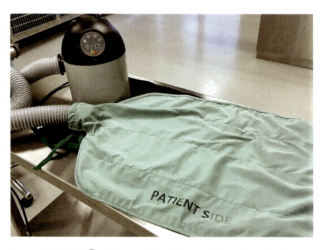

Figure 22.6 Baja® with a reusable blanket (Animal Hospital Supply, Flowery Branch, GA). The reusable blankets have a protective layer on one side that prevents heat from escaping. It is important that the appropriate side of the blanket be placed against the patient to allow heat exchange to occur.

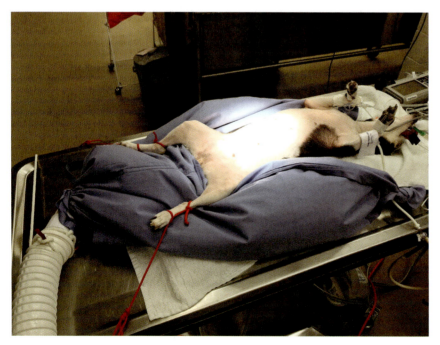

Figure 22.7 Thin scrub pants are connected to the forced warm air unit by cinching the drawstring around the hose. The legs of the pants are knotted at the ankle allowing the pant legs to inflate with warm air. However, these are not approved for use by manufacturers, due to the possibility of unit malfunction.

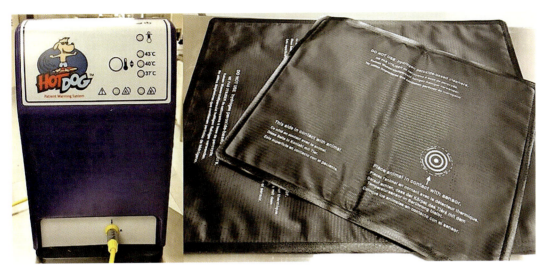

Figure 22.8 HotDog® (Augustine Biomedical & Design, Eden Prairie, MN) with 2 of the 5 sizes of blankets available. The black side of the blanket should be exposed to the patient. It is important that the patient's body meets the sensor located on the blanket. The appropriate size should be selected to ensure the majority of the patient's body is located on the blanket.

to core heat transfer (Ereth *et al.* 1992; Christensen *et al.* 1997).

22.11.1.2   Conductive Fabric Warmers

Resistive polymer heating systems, such as the HotDog® (Augustine Biomedical and Design, Eden Prairie, MN), consist of a control box that attaches to a semi-conductive polymeric blanket (Figure 22.8). The controller delivers a low voltage to the blankets, which warm via electrical resistance. This unit helps prevent conductive heat loss. There are five different sizes of blankets that can be positioned under, over or around the patient (Figure 22.9). The patient should be positioned in contact with the

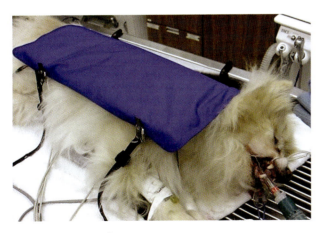

Figure 22.9 HotDog® blanket (Augustine Biomedical & Design, Eden Prairie, MN) wrapped around a patient for a dental procedure. The blankets can be positioned under, over or around the patient. When the blanket can contact the majority of the patient's body, heat exchange is maximized.

heat sensor located on the black side of the blanket. The polymer fibers within the blanket allow heat to be distributed evenly throughout the fabric and the control box monitors and regulates the resistance, allowing for a constant temperature. For best results, the smallest blanket that will completely contact the patient's body should be used. Care should be taken to not use the blanket under the patient if they will be remaining in a single position for a prolonged period of time (>2 hours) or will be placed in a vacuum-activated positioning device, as pressure points can develop that decrease perfusion to certain areas of the skin. Heat energy will accumulate around areas of low blood flow and therefore increase the risk of thermal injury.

22.11.1.3   Circulating Warm Water Blankets

Circulating warm water blankets consist of a pump, water reservoir and a double layer blanket that allows warmed water to circulate through channels located in the pad. Older models consisted of just a heating unit but more contemporary models also have the ability to cool the water. Examples of currently available products include Gaymar T/Pump® (Stryker, Kalamazoo, MI) and Aqua® (Jorvet, Loveland, CO) among others (Figure 22.10). The blankets are available in different sizes and can be placed under or over the patient to help minimize conductive heat loss. For maximum effectiveness, the blanket should cover as much of the patient as possible. The biggest disadvantage to water-filled units is the potential for disconnection or damage to the blankets. If the blanket connections are not secured or a puncture results, it can quickly result in a water-soaked patient. Fortunately, there are products available to

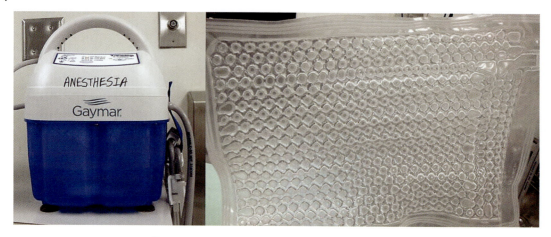

Figure 22.10 Gaymar T/Pump® (Stryker, Kalamazoo, MI) circulating water blanket. Care should be taken to only use these blankets when a patient is sedated or anesthetized to avoid inadvertent blanket puncture due to nails/claws. The water level must be checked regularly to ensure it is at a proper level. Operating the heating unit with little to no water could damage the pump.

minimize damage to the blankets (e.g. Plexiglas sheaths (Hallowell, Pittsfield, MA) and Protect-A-Pad (Jorvet, Loveland, CO).

22.11.1.4 Heated Surgical Tables

Surgery tables can be constructed with a heating element enclosed within the table top, with a control box that allows for the temperature to be adjusted. Heated surgery tables provide a constant heat source, but they lack any type of safety mechanism to detect if the table becomes too hot. Due to the potential risk of thermal injury, it is recommended that a protective barrier such as a towel be placed between the patient and the table. However, if the protective barrier is too thick, then the patient will not benefit from the heat source.

22.11.2 Core Re-Warming

22.11.2.1 Far Infrared Warming Devices

New technology is available (Far Infrared Stasis Technology, FIRs™, Kent Scientific Corporation, Torrington, CT) that promotes patient warming using far infrared light to penetrate into the deep tissues. As cells absorb the light, the energy level of intracellular water increases through resonant absorption, thereby raising body temperature as well (www.kentscientific. com). The unit is battery-operated, less warming is required, no warming of air in between the patient and pad occurs, and re-usable warming pads are available in multiple sizes (Figure 22.11).

22.11.2.2 Inline Intravenous (IV) Fluid Warmers

Delivering warmed intravenous fluids may also help maintain core body temperature. However, fluid delivery rates can be problematic. For example, the effectiveness is dependent on the rate of fluid administration and the distance they are positioned from the patient. If the fluid

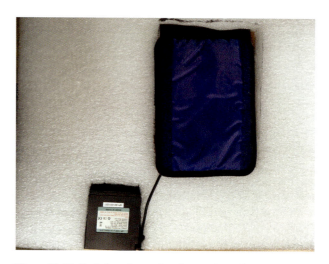

Figure 22.11 Far infrared warming devices (Far Infrared Stasis Technology, FIRst™, Kent Scientific Corporation, Torrington, CT) is a safe and efficient way to warm patients without using warmed air surrounding the patient. Pads are available in three sizes, 6″× 8″, 8″× 10″ and 14″× 14″. This unit is placed on a foam board to hold it and the patient in place during rodent surgery.

rate is too high, then there is inadequate time for the fluid to be heated to the desired temperature. If the fluid rate is too low, then the fluid will likely be cooled back to room temperature before it reaches the patient. A fluid warmer positioned on the IV line too far from the patient will also promote cooling of the fluid before it reaches the patient. In addition, excessive fluid warming may result in damage to blood proteins and should be avoided. Although these limitations exist, inline IV fluid warmers may be more efficacious in regulating core body temperature when used with other warming techniques. Multiple different brands of inline IV fluid warmers are available on the market. Some examples include Animec AM-2S® (FutureMed, Granada Hills, CA), iWarm® (Midmark Corporation, Dayton, OH) and

Jorvet Thermal IV® (Jorgensen Laboratories, Loveland, CO) (Figure 22.12).

22.11.2.3 Warmed/Humidified Inspired Gas

The use of rebreathing circuits (e.g. circle or Universal F systems; Chapter 12), coaxial circuits (e.g. Universal F or Bain systems; Chapters 11 and 12) and heat and moisture exchangers (HME; Chapter 7) are all options that can warm/humidify inhaled air. All of these methods will minimize evaporative heat loss and therefore help maintain current body temperature; however, unless used long term (e.g. long-term mechanically ventilated critical care patient), increases in body temperature are unlikely (Figure 22.13).

When used at acceptable oxygen flow rates, rebreathing systems allow a portion of the exhaled gases to be rebreathed by the patient during inhalation. When the gases pass through the carbon dioxide absorbent canister, a reaction occurs that produces heat and moisture. In a rebreathing system, after the inhalant concentration has reached equilibrium with the patient, oxygen flow rates may be decreased to near 10–30 mL/kg/min to help conserve heat and moisture within the circuit, if applicable to the case.

Coaxial circuits have the inspiratory hose located inside the expiratory hose. The exhaled gases theoretically provide a means to warm the inhaled gases. However, high fresh gas flows required for carbon dioxide removal in the Bain coaxial non-rebreathing system limit the amount of warming that may occur by the expired gas.

HMEs placed between the endotracheal tube and breathing circuit will conserve heat from the exhaled gases and return it to the patient during inhalation. There is a significant increase in mechanical dead space and resistance to breathing when an HME is placed in the circuit, thus they are not suitable for use in all patients.

Commercially available temperature controlled breathing circuits with feedback loops are also an efficient way to heat inspired gases (Darvall Vet, Advanced Anesthesia Specialists, Payson, AZ). Tubes are cleanable, lightweight and fit all standard anesthesia machines. The computer-controlled closed loop feedback precisely controls airway temperature and avoids burns (Figure 22.14). In addition, warming blocks attached to the

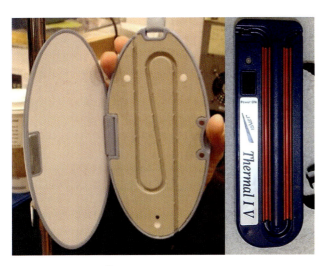

Figure 22.12 iWarm® (Midmark, Dayton, OH, left) and Jorvet Thermal IV® (Jorgensen Laboratories, Loveland, CO, right) inline IV fluid warmers. The effectiveness of these devices depends on the fluid administration rate and the distance they are positioned on the IV line in comparison to the patient.

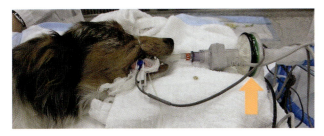

Figure 22.13 ThermoFlo™ System (ARC Medical Inc., Tucker, GA, orange arrow) placed in the breathing circuit to provide humidification of the inspired gases during long-term mechanical ventilation for an ICU patient. Unless used long term, these devices will unlikely contribute to an increase in body temperature.

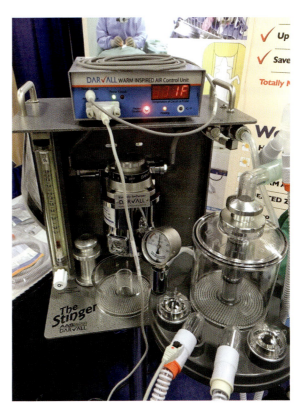

Figure 22.14 A heated breathing circuit with a computer controlled closed loop to safely control warming of inspired gases (Darvall Vet, Advanced Anesthesia Specialists, Payson, AZ). The sensor is placed within the inspiratory limb of the system.

endotracheal tube (ZDS Qubes, Darvall Vet, Advanced Anesthesia Specialists, Payson, AZ; see Chapter 34) are also helpful to warm inspired gases, especially in very small patients.

22.11.2.4 Warm Fluid Lavage

In patients with significant to severe hypothermia, heated fluid lavaged into a body cavity may help in core re-warming. Peritoneal lavage is performed by placing a peritoneal catheter to infuse a warmed isotonic dialysate. The fluid is left in place for 20–30 minutes, then removed and repeated as necessary. Although this procedure is invasive, it allows transfer of heat to a large surface area by contacting the great vessels and abdominal viscera. Peritoneal lavage should be used with caution in patients with current coagulopathies or electrolyte abnormalities. Thoracic lavage via thoracostomy tube may be considered during cardiac arrest, but reports of this method performed in veterinary medicine are sparse. Extracorporeal re-warming via cardiopulmonary bypass or hemodialysis is an option in humans, but is not commonly performed in veterinary patients. Gastric, urinary bladder and colonic lavage are described in veterinary literature as a treatment for significant to severe hypothermia. Unfortunately, these methods are not as effective as once thought, due to the limited surface area that encounters the heated fluid (Todd 2015).

22.12 Other Techniques to Minimize Heat Loss

Because anesthetic agents interfere with normal thermoregulation, pre-operative warming can be beneficial (Roberson *et al.* 2013). Supplemental warming should be used after premedication and continue through induction, surgical prep, procedure and recovery if possible. In humans, approximately 90% of heat loss occurs through the skin (Diaz and Becker 2010). Heat loss through the skin may not be as significant in animals due to their hairy coats. However, if large areas of fur are clipped for the surgical procedure, then convection heat loss may be substantial. Surgical prep solutions (scrub, water or alcohol) can be warmed to body temperature, but evaporative heat loss through use of cool prep solutions is negligible compared to other forms of heat loss (Grimm 2015).

During transport, diagnostic imaging (e.g. CT or MRI), and anesthetic recovery, the patient can be covered in towels/blankets and a reflective blanket (Space All-Weather Blanket, REI, www.REI.com) (Figure 22.15) to help minimize convection heat loss. Gel pads (Blue

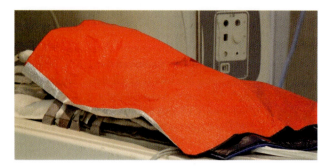

Figure 22.15 Space All-Weather Blanket (REI) is made of a reflective material that helps to conserve body heat. It can be placed over the patient during transport, diagnostic imaging (e.g. CT or MRI) and in recovery to minimize convection heat loss (photograph courtesy of Dr Jacob Johnson).

Diamond®, David Scott Company, Framingham, MA) help provide a layer of insulation to minimize heat loss. They are also safe to use in the MRI and can be placed under or over the patient (Figure 22.16). When maintained above body temperature in a warming cabinet, the gel pads help keep the patient warm during the MRI scan (Figure 22.17). Historically, wrapping the paws (especially in small patients) with plastic wrap and Vetrap® (aluminum foil, rubber gloves, bubble wrap, baby socks, etc.) has been used to minimize heat dissipation. Unfortunately, there is minimal evidence to support that these practices are advantageous for heat loss prevention.

Maintaining an appropriate ambient room temperature in the prep area and operating room is another way to help minimize convection heat loss. The Association of periOperative Registered Nurses (AORN) recommends that the operating room temperature be maintained between 68 and 75 °F (20 and 23.8 °C) (Arndt 1999). Since keeping the operating room temperature at an appropriate level for the patient is often discomforting to the surgeon, external heat sources are mandatory in the operating room.

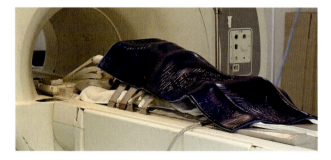

Figure 22.16 Gel pad (Blue Diamond®, David Scott Company) placed on top of a patient during an MRI (photograph courtesy of Dr Jacob Johnson).

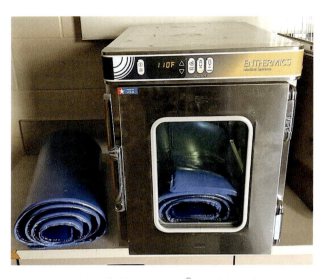

Figure 22.17 Gel pads (Blue Diamond®, David Scott Company) placed in a warming cabinet and kept above body temperature can help keep a patient warm during an MRI. The pads provide a layer of insulation and hold the heat for a few hours once removed from the warming cabinet.

22.13 High-Risk Heating Methods

The use of store bought electric heating pads, microwaved products (e.g. fluid bags, fluid bottles, rice bags, heating discs, etc.) (Figure 22.18) and latex gloves filled with hot water are NOT recommended due to the likelihood of extreme thermal burns if they come into direct contact with the skin (Figure 22.19). The store bought electrical heating pads do not distribute heat evenly over the entire pad and are not intended for use on patients that cannot move away from the heat source (e.g. anesthetized or recumbent patient). They can lead

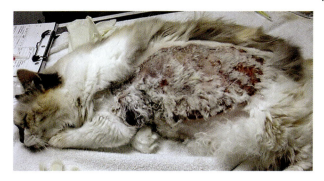

Figure 22.19 Severe thermal burns (other side is burned as well) in a cat after fluid bottles were microwaved, placed in direct contact with the skin and then wrapped tightly in a towel around the patient. This patient presented 10 days after the incident and required 4 reconstructive surgeries and daily bandage changes. Despite all efforts to debride the wounds and manage the pain, the patient developed systemic inflammatory response syndrome (SIRS) and succumbed to the injury.

to steam burns and possible electrocution if they are exposed to large amounts of water. If microwaved fluid items or latex gloves must be used (however not recommended), then ensure that a proper barrier (e.g. several towels or blankets) are placed between the heat source and the patient. It is important to note that as the fluid bag/bottle or glove cools down, it will pull heat away from the patient, resulting in hypothermia. A radiant heat lamp may reduce heat loss through radiation, but this method is difficult to use during a surgical procedure and there is no temperature regulation. In addition, overheating can easily occur if the patient's body temperature is not monitored closely and if too close to an immobile patient, burns may result. Thus, all these devices should be avoided.

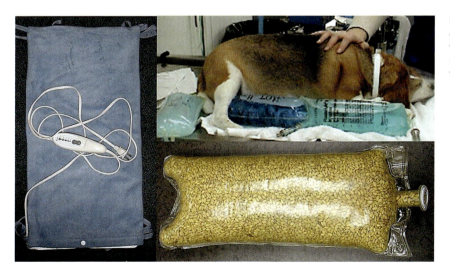

Figure 22.18 The use of store-bought electrical heating pads and microwaved fluid bags/rice bags are NOT recommended as heating sources due to the high risk of thermal burns.

References

Adler, M.W., Geller, E.B., Rosow, C.E. and Cochin, J. (1988) The opioid system and temperature regulation. *Annu Rev Pharmacol Toxicol*, 28, 429–449.

Antognini, J.F. (1993) Hypothermia eliminates isoflurane requirements at 20 degrees C. *Anesthesiology*, 78, 1152–1156.

Armstrong, S.R., Roberts, B.K. and Aronson, M. (2005) Peri-operative hypothermia. *J Vet Emerg Crit Care*, 15, 32–37.

Arndt, K. (1999) Inadvertent hypothermia in the OR. *AORN J*, 70, 204–206.

Aslam, A.F., Aslam, A.K., Vasavada, B.C. and Khan, I.A. (2006) Hypothermia: evaluation, electrocardiographic manifestations, and management. *Am J Med*, 119, 297–301.

Baer, R.W. (1989) Myocardial oxygen transport during leftward shifts of the oxygen dissociation curve by carbamylation or hypothermia. *Adv Exp Med Biol*, 248, 325–333.

Bashour, T.T., Gualberto, A. and Ryan, C. (1989) Atrioventricular block in accidental hypothermia – a case report. *Angiology*, 40, 63–66.

Bay, J., Nunn, J.F. and Prys-Roberts, C. (1968) Factors influencing arterial PO_2 during recovery from anaesthesia. *Br J Anaesth*, 40, 398–407.

Beal, M.W., Brown, D.C. and Shofer, F.S. (2000) The effects of perioperative hypothermia and the duration of anesthesia on post-operative wound infection rate in clean wounds: a retrospective study. *Vet Surg*, 29, 123–127.

Berman, M.C., Harrison, G.G., Bull, A.B. and Kench, J.E. (1970) Changes underlying halothane-induced malignant hyperpyrexia in Landrace pigs. *Nature*, 225, 653–655.

Bjoraker, D.G. (1990) Liquid crystal temperature indicators. *Anesthesiol Rev*, 17, 50–56.

Bjørnstad, H., Tande, P.M. and Refsum, H. (1991) Cardiac electrophysiology during hypothermia. Implications for medical treatment. *Arctic Med Res*, 50, 71–75.

Blainey, C.G. 1974. Site selection in taking body temperature. *Am J Nurs*, 74, 1859–1961.

Brodeur, A., Wright, A. and Cortes, Y. (2017) Hypothermia and targeted temperature management in cats and dogs. *J Vet Emerg Crit Care (San Antonio)*, 27, 151–163.

Brunson, D.B. and Hogan, K.J. (2004) Malignant hyperthermia: a syndrome not a disease. *Vet Clin North Am Small Anim Pract*, 34, 1419–1433.

Caterina, M.J. (2007) Transient receptor potential ion channels as participants in thermosensation and thermoregulation. *Am J Physiol Regul Integr Comp Physiol*, 292, R64–R76.

Christensen, R., Clough, D., Kurz, A., Plattner, O., Sessler, D.I. and Xiong, J. (1997) Thermoregulatory vasoconstriction does not impede core warming during cutaneous heating. *Ann NY Acad Sci*, 813, 827–834.

Clark-Price, S.C. (2015) Inadvertent Perianesthetic hypothermia in small animal patients. *Vet Clin North Am Small Anim Pract*, 45, 983–994.

Clarke, A. (2004) Is there a universal temperature dependence of metabolism? *Funct Ecol*, 18, 252–256.

Collier, R.J. and Gebremedhin, K.G. (2015) Thermal biology of domestic animals. *Annu Rev Anim Biosci*, 3, 513–532.

Cornett, P.M., Matta, J.A. and Ahern, G.P. (2008) General anesthetics sensitize the capsaicin receptor transient receptor potential V1. *Mol Pharmacol*, 74, 1261–1268.

Crowder, C.M., Tempelhoff, R., Theard, M.A., Cheng, M.A., Todorov, A. and Dacey, R.G. Jr. (1996) Jugular bulb temperature: comparison with brain surface and core temperatures in neurosurgical patients during mild hypothermia. *J Neurosurg*, 85, 98–103.

Davis, P.D. and Kenny, G.N.C. (2007) Temperature. In: *Basic Physics and Measurement in Anaesthesia*, 5th ed. New York: Butterworth-Heinemann, pp. 97–105.

De Witte, J. and Sessler, D.I. (2002) Perioperative shivering: physiology and pharmacology. *Anesthesiology*, 96, 467–484.

Diaz, M. and Becker, D.E. (2010) Thermoregulation: physiological and clinical considerations during sedation and general anesthesia. *Anesth Prog*, 57, 25–32.

Ducharme, M.B., Frim, J., Bourdon, L. and Giesbrecht, G.G. (1997) Evaluation of infrared tympanic thermometers during normothermia and hypothermia in humans. *Ann NY Acad Sci*, 15, 225–229.

Ereth, M.H., Lennon, R.L. and Sessler, D.I. (1992) Limited heat transfer between thermal compartments during rewarming in vasoconstricted patients. *Aviat Space Environ Med*, 63, 1065–1069.

Faulds, M. and Meekings, T. (2013) Temperature management in critically ill patients. *Contin Educ Anaesth Crit Care Pain*, 13, 75–79.

Frank, F. and Broessner, G. (2017) Is there still a role for hypothermia in neurocritical care? *Curr Opin Crit Care*, 23, 115–121.

Grimm, K. (2015) Peri-operative thermoregulation and heat balance. In: Grimm, K., Lamont, L., Tranquilli, W., Greene, S. and Robertson, S. (eds). *Veterinary Anesthesia and Analgesia – The Fifth Edition of Lumb and Jones*. Ames, IA: Blackwell Wiley, pp. 372–379.

Guschina, I.A. and Harwood, J.L. (2006) Mechanisms of temperature adaptation in poikilotherms. *FEBS Lett*, 580, 5477–5483.

Hahn, G.L. (1981) Housing and management to reduce climatic impacts on livestock. *J Anim Sci*, 52, 175–186.

Hammel, H.T., Hardy, J.D. and Fusco, M.M. (1960) Thermoregulatory responses to hypothalamic cooling in unanesthetized dogs. *Amer J Physiol*, 198, 481–486.

Hemmelgarn, C. and Gannon, K. (2013a) Heatstroke: clinical signs, diagnosis, treatment, and prognosis. *Compend Contin Educ Vet*, 35, E3.

Hemmelgarn, C. and Gannon, K. (2013b) Heatstroke: thermoregulation, pathophysiology, and predisposing factors. *Compend Contin Educ Vet*, 35, E4.

Herlich, A. (2013) Perioperative temperature elevation: not all hyperthermia is malignant hyperthermia. *Paediatr Anaesth*, 23, 842–850.

Hill, R.C. and Scott, K.C. (2004) Energy requirements and body surface area of cats and dogs. *J Am Vet Med Assoc*, 225, 689–894.

Hopkins, P.M. (2011) Malignant hyperthermia: pharmacology of triggering. *Br J Anaesth*, 107, 48–56.

Johnson, S. (2006) Heatstroke in small animal medicine: a clinical practice review. *J Vet Emerg Crit Care*, 16, 112–119.

Kellogg, D.L. Jr. (2006) *In vivo* mechanisms of cutaneous vasodilation and vasoconstriction in humans during thermoregulatory challenges. *J Appl Physiol*, 100, 1709–1718.

Kumar, M., Murray, M.J., Werner, E. and Lanier, W.L. (1994) Monitoring intrathecal temperature: does core temperature reflect intrathecal temperature during aortic surgery? *J Cardiothorac Vasc Anesth*, 8, 35–39.

Lenhardt, R., Greif, R., Sessler, D.I., Laciny, S., Rajek, A. and Bastanmehr, H. (1999) Relative contribution of skin and core temperatures to vasoconstriction and shivering thresholds during isoflurane anesthesia. *Anesthesiology*, 91, 422–429.

Li, D.M., Mullaly, R., Ewer, P., Bell, B., Eyres, R.L. , Brawn, W.J. and Mee, R.B.B. (1988) Effects of vasodilators on rates of change of nasopharyngeal temperature and systemic vascular resistance during cardiopulmonary bypass in anaesthetized dogs. *Aust NZ J Surg*, 58, 327–333.

Liu, M., Hu, X. and Liu, J. (2001) The effect of hypothermia on isoflurane MAC in children. *Anesthesiology*, 94, 429–432.

Lloyd, E.L. and Mitchell, B. (1974) Factors affecting the onset of ventricular fibrillation in hypothermia. *Lancet*, 2, 1294–1296.

Luthra, A., Dube, S.K., Kumar, S. and Goyal, K. (2016) Intraoperative hyperthermia: Can surgery itself be a cause? *Indian J Anaesth*, 60, 515–517.

Mallet, M.L. (2002) Pathophysiology of accidental hypothermia. *QJM*, 95, 775–785.

Mattheussen, M., Mubagwa, K., Van Aken, H., Wusten, R., Boutros, A. and Flameng, W. (1996) Interaction of heart rate and hypothermia on global myocardial contraction of the isolated rabbit heart. *Anesth Analg*, 82, 975–981.

Mayerhofer, I., Scherzer, S., Gabler, C. and van den Hoven, R. (2005) Hypothermia in horses induced by general anaesthesia and limiting measures. *Equine Vet Educ*, 17, 53–56.

Morgan, K. (1998) Thermoneutral zone and critical temperatures of horses. *J Therm Biol*, 23, 59–61.

Morrison, S.F. and Nakamura, K. (2011) Central neural pathways for thermoregulation. *Front Biosci (Landmark Ed.)*, 16, 74–104.

Nakamura, K., Matsumura, K., Hubschle, T., Nakamura, Y., Hioki, H. *et al.* (2004) Identification of sympathetic premotor neurons in medullary raphe regions mediating fever and other thermoregulatory functions. *J Neurosci*, 24, 5370–5380.

Nakamura, K. and Morrison, S.F. (2008) A thermosensory pathway that controls body temperature. *Nat Neurosci*, 11, 62–71

Pottie, R.G., Dart, C.M., Perkins, N.R. and Hodgson, D.R. (2007) Effect of hypothermia on recovery from general anaesthesia in the dog. *Aust Vet J*, 85, 158–162.

Putzu, M., Casati, A., Berti, M., Pagliarini, G. and Fanelli, G. (2007) Clinical complications, monitoring and management of perioperative mild hypothermia: anesthesiological features. *Acta Biomed*, 78, 163–169.

Rajagopalan, S., Mascha, E., Na, J. and Sessler, D.I. (2008) The effects of mild perioperative hypothermia on blood loss and transfusion requirement. *Anesthesiology*, 108, 71–77.

Rawls, S.M. and Benamar, K. (2011) Effects of opioids, cannabinoids, and vanilloids on body temperature. *Front Biosci (School Ed.)*, 3, 822–845.

Redaelli, V., Tanzi, B., Luzi, F., Stefanello, D., Proverbio, D., Crosta, L. and Di Giancamillo, M. (2014) Use of thermographic imaging in clinical diagnosis of small animal: preliminary notes. *Ann Ist Super Sanita*, 50, 140–146.

Redondo, J.I., Suesta, P., Gil, L., Soler, G., Serra, I. and Soler, C. (2012a) Retrospective study of the prevalence of postanaesthetic hypothermia in cats. *Vet Rec*, 170, 206.

Redondo, J.I., Suesta, P., Serra, I., Soler, C., Soler, G., Gil, L. and Gómez-Villamandos, R.J. (2012b) Retrospective study of the prevalence of postanaesthetic hypothermia in dogs. *Vet Rec*, 171, 374.

Reece, W.O. (2015) Body temperature and its regulation. In: Reece, W.O., Erickson, H.H., Goff, J.P. and Uemure, E.E. (eds). *Dukes' Physiology of Domestic Animals*, 13th ed. Ames, IA: Wiley Blackwell, pp. 149–156.

Regan, M.J. and Eger, E.I. (1967) Effect of hypothermia in dogs on anesthetizing and apneic doses of inhalation agents. Determination of the anesthetic index (Apnea/MAC). *Anesthesiology*, 28, 689–700.

Roberson, M.C., Dieckmann, L.S., Rodriguez, R.E. and Austin, P.N. (2013) A review of the evidence for active pre-operative warming of adults undergoing general anesthesia. *AANA J*, 81, 351–356.

Robertshaw D. (2006) Mechanisms for the control of respiratory evaporative heat loss in panting animals. *J Appl Physiol*, 101, 664–668.

Robinson, J.L., Seal, R.F., Spady, D.W. and Joffres, M.R. (1998) Comparison of esophageal, rectal, axillary, bladder, tympanic, and pulmonary artery temperatures in children. *J Pediatr*, 133, 553–336.

Robinson, N.E. (2013) Thermoregulation. In: Klein, B.G. (ed.). *Cunningham's Textbook of Veterinary Physiology*, 5th ed. St Louis, MO: Elsevier Saunders, pp. 559–568.

Romanovsky, A.A. (2007) Thermoregulation: some concepts have changed. Functional architecture of the thermoregulatory system. *Am J Physiol Regul Integr Comp Physiol*, 292, R37–R46.

Roscher, R., Arlock, P., Sjöberg, T. and Steen, S. (2001) Effects of dopamine on porcine myocardial action potentials and contractions at 37 degrees C and 32 degrees C. *Acta Anaesthesiol Scand*, 45, 42–426.

Rose, N., Kwong, G.P. and Pang, D.S. (2016) A clinical audit cycle of post-operative hypothermia in dogs. *J Small Anim Pract*, 57, 447–452.

Roth, J.V. (2009) Some unanswered questions about temperature management. *Anesth Analg*, 109, 1695–1699.

Sarkar, S., Donn, S., Bhagat, I., Dechert, R.E. and Barks, J.D. (2013) Esophageal and rectal temperatures as estimates of core temperature during therapeutic whole-body hypothermia. *J Pediatr* 162, 208–210.

Scaravilli, V., Bonacina, D. and Citerio, G. (2012) Rewarming: facts and myths from the systemic perspective. *Crit Care*, 16 (Suppl 2), A25.

Schmutzhard, E., Fischer, M., Dietmann, A. and Brössner, G. (2012) Therapeutic hypothermia: the rationale. *Crit Care*, 16(Suppl 2), A2.

Seebacher, F. (2009) Responses to temperature variation: integration of thermoregulation and metabolism in vertebrates. *J Exp Biol*, 212, 2885–2891.

Sessler, D.I. (2015) Temperature regulation and monitoring. In: Miller, R.D. (ed.). *Miller's Anesthesia*, 8th ed. Philadelphia, PA: Elsevier Saunders, pp. 1622–1646.

Sessler, D.I. (2016) Peri-operative thermoregulation and heat balance. *Lancet*, 387, 2655–2664.

Solomon, A., Barish, R.A., Browne, B. and Tso, E. (1989) The electrocardiographic features of hypothermia. *J Emerg Med*, 7, 169–173.

Somero, G.N. (2004) Adaptation of enzymes to temperature: searching for basic "strategies". *Comp Biochem Physiol B Biochem Mol Biol*, 139, 321–333.

Stone, J.G., Young W.L., Smith, C.R., Solomon, R.A., Wald, A. et al. (1995) Do standard monitoring sites reflect true brain temperature when profound hypothermia is rapidly induced and reversed? *Anesthesiology*, 82, 344-351.

Thermodynamics [on line]. Available at: http:// physicsforidiots/physics/thermodynamis [Accessed October 7, 2017].

Thomas, R. and Cahill, C.J. (2000) Successful defibrillation in profound hypothermia (core body temperature 25.6 degrees C). *Resuscitation*, 47, 317–320.

Todd, J.M. (2015) Hypothermia. In: Silverstein, D.C. and Hopper, K.H. (eds) *Small Animal Critical Care Medicine*, 2nd ed. St Louis, MO: Elsevier-Saunders, pp. 789–795.

Tomasic, M. (1999) Temporal changes in core body temperature in anesthetized adult horses. *Am J Vet Res*, 60, 556–562.

van den Broek, M.P., Groenendaal, F., Egberts, A.C. and Rademaker, C.M. (2010) Effects of hypothermia on pharmacokinetics and pharmacodynamics: a systematic review of preclinical and clinical studies. *Clin Pharmacokinet*, 49, 277–294.

Walter, E.J., Hanna-Jumma, S., Carraretto, M. and Forni, L. (2016) The pathophysiological basis and consequences of fever. *Crit Care*, 20, 200.

Wong, K.C. (1983) Physiology and pharmacology of hypothermia. *West J Med*, 138, 227–232.

Yoshihara, H., Yamamoto, T. and Mihara, H. (1985) Changes in coagulation and fibrinolysis occurring in dogs during hypothermia. *Thromb Res*, 37, 503–512.

23

Fluid Regulation and Monitoring

Julie Walker

School of Veterinary Medicine, University of Wisconsin, Madison, Wisconsin, USA

23.1 Overview of Fluid Physiology

Adult animals, like humans, are comprised of approximately 60% water as a portion of lean body mass (Moore *et al.* 1962; Bauer *et al.* 1975; Scheltinga *et al.* 1991; Wamberg *et al.* 2002). Two-thirds of body water is intracellular fluid (ICF) and one-third is extracellular fluid (ECF) (Moore *et al.* 1962; Bauer *et al.* 1975; Wellman *et al.* 2012). Approximately three-quarters of the ECF is the interstitial fluid (ISF), which occupies the space between cells and within connective tissue, whereas the remaining quarter of the ECF makes up the intravascular plasma volume (Figure 23.1) (Moore *et al.* 1962; Bauer *et al.* 1975; Wellman *et al.* 2012).

The intravascular space consists of water, proteins, electrolytes and cells that occupy the blood vessels. In normal fluid balance, the venous circulation stores approximately 70% of the intravascular fluid volume and readily accepts additional volume with minimal changes in pressure (Gelman 2008). Water within the intravascular space is in continuous balance with the interstitial space, and movement of water between these spaces is governed by differences in hydrostatic pressure, oncotic pressure and capillary permeability. In health, fluid movement between these compartments exists in equilibrium, and net fluid movement out of the capillary bed is returned to the circulation by lymphatic drainage.

23.1.1 Euhydration and Fluid Loss

Euhydration exists when there is a neutral fluid balance, with water intake approximately equaling water loss. Hydration becomes abnormal when there is a net loss or gain of body fluid. Dehydration describes a net deficit of total body water ± electrolytes. A water deficit that accompanies electrolyte loss (an isotonic fluid loss)

primarily affects the extracellular (interstitial and intravascular) space. A net loss of pure water (or hypotonic fluid) causes hypernatremia that additionally depletes water from the intracellular space as water is drawn out of the ICF by diffusion until equilibrium of tonicity is reached (Bhave and Neilson 2011).

Hypovolemia describes a fluid deficit of the intravascular space, which may result from hemorrhage or non-hemorrhagic fluid loss. Hypovolemia can occur without concurrent dehydration of the interstitial space, as with healthy patients experiencing acute traumatic or surgical hemorrhage. However, when hypovolemia occurs because of non-hemorrhagic fluid loss, an interstitial fluid deficit is frequently present.

Normal maintenance fluid requirements in animals include the amount of water that is required to balance the daily expected sensible (urinary) and insensible (evaporative, fecal) fluid losses. A fluid deficit develops when fluid loss exceeds fluid intake. Fluid intake is reduced in patients with limited mobility, abnormal mentation, inability to drink or swallow, and confinement or otherwise reduced access to a fresh water source, situations that may be present in the peri-anesthetic patient. Fluid loss can occur by many mechanisms, including those summarized in Table 23.1.

Fluid redistribution occurs to replace intravascular volume deficits following hemorrhagic or non-hemorrhagic fluid losses. Transcapillary shift of fluid from the interstitial space provides a mechanism for recovery of up to 80% of the blood volume within 24 hours (Bhave and Neilson 2011). To replace the total body fluid deficit that exists between the intravascular and interstitial fluid spaces, fluid intake must occur. In nature, water intake occurs most commonly through the enteral route, although alternative routes might be used to administer fluid as part of medical therapy.

Veterinary Anesthetic and Monitoring Equipment, First Edition. Edited by Kristen G. Cooley and Rebecca A. Johnson.
© 2018 John Wiley & Sons, Inc. Published 2018 by John Wiley & Sons, Inc.

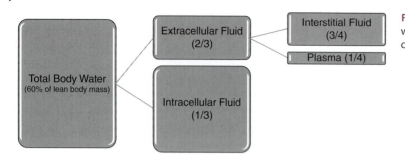

Figure 23.1 Schematic representation of total body water and its distribution in various tissue compartments.

Table 23.1 Differential diagnoses for fluid loss or redistribution.

Sources of Fluid Loss
- Gastrointestinal losses
  - Vomiting
  - Diarrhea
  - Regurgitation
- Renal losses
  - Polyuric acute kidney injury
  - Polyuric chronic kidney disease
  - Conditions involving primary or secondary nephrogenic diabetes insipidus
- Evaporative loss
  - Excessive panting
  - Fever
  - Severe cutaneous burns
  - Thoracic or abdominal surgery
- Third-space loss
  - Pleural effusion
  - Peritoneal effusions
  - Pericardial effusion
  - Retroperitoneal effusion
  - Subcutaneous edema
- Hemorrhage
  - Internal hemorrhage
  - External hemorrhage (e.g. due to trauma, coagulopathy, gastrointestinal hemorrhage, endoparasitism or ectoparasitism).

23.1.2 Fluid Excess

Fluid excess frequently occurs during anesthesia due to endogenous fluid retention, iatrogenic administration, or a combination of these etiologies. Patients conserve water (with or without sodium) due to endogenous release of antidiuretic hormone and upregulation of the renin-angiotensin-aldosterone system. These mechanisms are present in patients with severe chronic anemia, congestive heart failure, and also kidney disease (Lee *et al.* 1983). Pathologically decreased urine output in patients with oligo-anuric kidney injury might also contribute to fluid excess. While prolonged or large-volume fluid administration might independently contribute, patients with pre-existing volume retention or oligo-anuria are at an increased risk of volume overload. Critically ill dogs, and likely other species, are at increased risk of developing fluid overload and have an associated increased mortality rate (Cavanaugh *et al.* 2016).

23.2 Assessment of Fluid Balance

Clues from the patient's medical history, along with physical examination and diagnostic test findings, are used to estimate a patient's fluid balance. Pre-anesthetic assessment is essential to compare changes in fluid balance during and after the anesthetic procedure.

23.2.1 Patient History

The patient's medical history provides insights regarding fluid balance. For example, fluid loss is suspected with recent hemorrhage, repeated vomiting and diarrhea episodes, or recent diuretic treatment (e.g. furosemide). A fluid deficit might also be related to reduced water intake, polyuria or evaporative water loss secondary to excess panting, heat exposure and fever. One must also consider the patient's comorbidities, such as diabetes mellitus, heart failure and chronic kidney disease, as these indicate predispositions toward fluid loss or retention (Greco 1998).

Recent hospitalization and intravenous (IV) fluid loading or at-home subcutaneous fluid administration can contribute to partial or full replacement of the fluid deficit. Recently administered subcutaneous fluids can cause inaccuracy in assessing skin turgor, as fluid that was recently administered might still be in the process of resorption and might give a false (regional) assessment of euhydration.

Trends in body weight from recent hospital visits may be helpful in assessing changes in body composition. Rapid fluctuations in body weight are likely due to fluid gain or loss, whereas long-term decreases or increases in body weight suggest a change in muscle mass or fat stores. Routine body condition score recording with body weight trends can assist the assessment of body composition.

23.2.2 Physical Examination

Physical examination findings may support the presence of hypovolemia, dehydration or fluid overload. However, clinical examination alone does not consistently predict the amount of weight gain following fluid therapy

(Hansen and DeFrancesco 2002). Any one of these findings can be misleading when evaluated as a single feature, but assessment will be more comprehensive when multiple examination parameters and other clinical features are evaluated.

Examination findings suggesting dehydration do not become clinically apparent until the patient is at least 5% dehydrated in small animals (Langston 2012) and even 10% or greater in some larger species such as donkeys (du Toit and Burden 2015). Clinical signs of mild to severe, experimentally-induced dehydration include loss of skin elasticity, sunken eyes, congestion of mucous membranes, coldness of extremities and variable loss of body weight (Sinha and Ganapathy 1967).

23.2.2.1 Integument and Mucous Membranes

Skin turgor/elasticity decreases with dehydration (with reduced skin and subcutaneous tissue water content), aging (loss of collagen) and emaciation (reduced subcutaneous fat stores). Therefore, examiners may overestimate dehydration in patients with advanced age or decreased body condition. Conversely, skin turgor appears increased with overhydration and excess body condition (increased subcutaneous fat content) (DiBartola and Bateman 2012). Patients developing marked fluid excess of the interstitial space may have "gelatinous" integument or pitting edema of the distal limbs. However, these findings might also be present in patients with other conditions such as severe hypoalbuminemia or increased vascular permeability.

Interpretation of mucous membrane moisture assumes that moist mucous membranes indicate patients are likely well hydrated and those with "tacky" or dry mucous membranes are likely dehydrated. However, a dehydrated patient can exhibit moist mucous membranes secondary to ptyalism, hypersalivation or recent drinking, and a euhydrated patient can exhibit dry mucous membranes related to other conditions such as panting (DiBartola and Bateman 2012). In addition, patients with renal failure might have reduced secretion or abnormal composition of saliva (xerostomia) that is not reflective of hydration (Langston 2012). In addition, pharmacologic agents (e.g. atropine or glycopyrrolate) also may affect composition of oral sections independent of hydration status.

Pale mucous membranes can indicate anemia, vasoconstriction and/or hypoperfusion. Capillary refill time is also prolonged by severe vasoconstriction or hypoperfusion. Fast capillary refill time and injected (inappropriately pink or red) mucous membranes can be present with sepsis, anaphylaxis, hyperthermia, and with other causes of vasodilation.

23.2.2.2 Cardiovascular and Respiratory Systems

In dogs, heart rate frequently increases when a fluid deficit causes hypovolemia severe enough to induce compensation by the body. Cats might also demonstrate tachycardia with hypovolemia, but more frequently exhibit bradycardia in moderate to severe hypovolemic shock. Peripherally cool extremities with or without a low rectal temperature might indicate vasoconstriction related to hypovolemia. In addition, larger species such as horses may not demonstrate significant changes in heart rate with hypovolemia (Magdesian et al. 2006).

Respiratory rate and depth of breathing may increase in patients with hypovolemic shock to compensate for metabolic (lactic) acidosis, especially in dogs. Signs such as serous nasal discharge, increased respiratory rate and effort, pulmonary crackles, or decreased lung sounds due to pleural effusion might be observed with moderate to severe fluid excess (Cornelius *et al.* 1978; Langston 2012).

23.2.2.3 Neurologic and Ophthalmic Systems

A decreased level of consciousness (obtundation) occurs in animals with hypoperfusion. In addition, eyes might appear sunken secondary to the effects of dehydration (decreased water content) or emaciation (reduced fat content) on the retrobulbar tissues. Decreased corneal moisture and tear production might also be present with dehydration. Chemosis (conjunctival edema; Figure 23.2) is observed with moderate to severe overhydration.

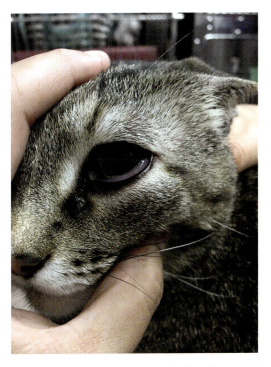

Figure 23.2 Chemosis (conjunctival edema) in an adult cat resulting from overhydration (photograph courtesy of Dr Jennifer Loewen, University of Wisconsin-Madison, WI).

23.2.3 Laboratory Monitoring Techniques

Basic laboratory testing used to monitor hydration status and performed bedside or in the hospital laboratory also provides insights into the assessment of hydration and perfusion.

23.2.3.1 Packed Cell Volume (PCV) and Total Protein (TP)

Packed cell volume (PCV) and total protein (TP) rise with dehydration, unless a patient has a comorbidity causing concurrent anemia or hypoproteinemia (Greco 1998). Blood loss is ultimately reflected by a decrease in PCV and TP, although these changes are reflected following fluid administration or redistribution of water from the interstitial and intracellular spaces as well. Adequate or excessive volume expansion might also cause a decrease in PCV and TP. Indeed, PCV and TP levels decrease with general anesthesia/fluid administration in dogs (Dismukes *et al.* 2010) and TP decreases in horses (Boscan *et al.* 2007). Discordant PCV and TP changes might be present in patients with hemolysis, blood product transfusion, or protein losing disease of the kidney, skin or GI tract. Consideration of baseline PCV and TP measurement and comorbidities are helpful in interpreting day-to-day changes in red blood cell and protein concentrations and changes during or following anesthesia.

23.2.3.2 Albumin

Similar to the trends stated above regarding total protein, albumin concentrations are expected to increase in patients with dehydration and decrease in patients with hemorrhage and/or protein loss with or without IV fluid administration.

23.2.3.3 Blood Urea Nitrogen (BUN) and Creatinine

An increase in blood urea nitrogen (BUN) and creatinine secondary to a fluid deficit and/or poor renal perfusion is known as pre-renal azotemia. Pre-renal azotemia typically is accompanied by decreased urine output and increased urine concentration/osmolality, except in patients with limited urine concentrating ability (e.g. patients with diabetes mellitus, chronic kidney disease and diuretic administration).

23.2.3.4 Lactate

Lactate, a metabolic fuel produced during anaerobic metabolism, most commonly increases in patients when tissue oxygen demand exceeds the oxygen supply (known as type A lactic acidosis). Plasma lactate concentrations increase in patients with conditions of systemic hypoperfusion, most commonly with hypovolemia, even in anesthetized patients (Gillespie *et al.* 2017). Lactate concentrations also increase in patients with other forms of systemic or regional tissue hypoxia (i.e. distributive shock or gastrointestinal ischemia), increased oxygen demand (i.e. seizures or exercise), or even without tissue hypoxia (type B lactic acidosis, such as with various drugs or toxins, neoplasia, or abnormalities of cellular energy metabolism) (Gillespie *et al.* 2017).

If hyperlactatemia is due to hypovolemic shock, serial lactate measurements are expected to decrease as the volume deficit is corrected. Therefore, serial lactate measurements might be helpful in assessing a patient's response to volume resuscitation.

22.2.3.5 Urine Specific Gravity (USG)

In the dehydrated animal with normal renal function, urine specific gravity (USG) and urine osmolality should be increased (Greco 1998) and is expected to decrease as a patient's fluid deficit is corrected. Urine specific gravity is not a helpful indicator of hydration in patients with pre-existing limitations of urine concentrating ability, such as chronic kidney disease.

23.2.4 Other Physiologic Trends in Hospitalized Patients

By reviewing trends in recorded monitoring data, veterinary professionals can gain additional insight regarding a patient's hydration status.

23.2.4.1 Body Weight

Depending on the type of tissue (fat or muscle) catabolized, it is estimated that a 0.1–0.25 kg loss in body mass will occur per 1000 kcal energy deficit. Although long-term trends in body weight likely reflect changes in body tissue composition, day-to-day changes in body weight are usually due to fluid loss and gain. Based on an estimated weight of 1 g per mL of water, body weight changes can be used to estimate fluctuations in hydration status. Body weight changes less accurately reflect changes in interstitial or intravascular fluid compartments in patients with third-space accumulation of fluid (i.e. peritoneal or pleural effusion).

23.2.4.2 Urine Output

In the euhydrated patient, normal urine output is estimated to be between 1 and 2 mL/kg/hour. Decreased urine output (physiologic oliguria) occurs in patients with dehydration and normal urine concentrating abilities. Increased urine output (polyuria) is expected to occur in patients with excess fluid intake. Pathologic conditions (i.e. oligo-anuric or polyuric chronic kidney disease) and drug therapies (i.e. vasopressin or diuretics) also contribute to alterations in urine output. Reduced urine output during some anesthetic protocols commonly occurs in dogs (Boscan *et al.* 2010), whereas urine output generally increases during anesthesia in horses due to the frequent use of alpha-2 adrenergic agonists (Steffey *et al.* 2000).

23.2.4.3 "Ins" versus "Outs"

A patient's net fluid balance is estimated by comparing fluid intake to fluid loss. To estimate fluid intake accurately, all sources of water administration and voluntary consumption must be accounted for. Fluid loss should be measured when possible, yet some sources of water loss, known as insensible losses (including water lost by evaporation or in saliva and feces) must be estimated. While comparing "ins" versus "outs" in a clinical setting remains an estimate, consideration of all sources and comparing changes in body weight are helpful to understand whether a patient has a net gain or loss of water. Inclusion of seemingly small-volume fluid administration (i.e. intermittent IV catheter flushing) is particularly important in small patients in which several, 1-mL flushes throughout the anesthetic procedure might account for a sizeable percentage of the total fluid administered. Table 23.2 summarizes common sources of water loss

Table 23.2 Common sources of water loss and gain and calculation of fluid balance.

Sources of Water Intake (INS)
- Parenteral
  - IV crystalloid fluids
  - Blood product transfusions
  - Drugs administered by constant rate infusion
  - Drugs diluted in 0.9% NaCl or 5% Dextrose
  - Parenteral nutrition
  - Subcutaneous fluid or drug administration
- Enteral
  - Enteral tube feedings
  - Enteral tube flush
  - Voluntary food and water intake

Sources of Water Loss (OUTS)
- Urine output
  - Closed collection system
  - Voided urine
- Gastrointestinal
  - Vomiting and regurgitation
  - Gastric residual volume removal via enteral feeding tube
  - Diarrhea
- Effusions
  - Pleural fluid removed via thoracocentesis or thoracic drainage catheter
  - Peritoneal fluid removed via abdominocentesis or peritoneal drain
  - Closed suction wound drains
- Insensible loss
  - Insensible loss is approximated as 1/3 of the patient's maintenance fluid requirement at rest.
  - Insensible losses increase with exercise, fever, panting, and severe compromise of the skin barrier

Fluid balance = INS – OUTS

Note: This comparison should occur over fixed (6–24 hour) time intervals. A positive value indicates a net fluid gain. Conversely, a negative value indicates net fluid loss. The net fluid balance should be compared to the change in body weight over the same time interval.

and gain that should be included in the calculation of fluid "ins" and "outs".

When a patient is treated for hypovolemia and/or dehydration, a net gain of water is expected. A patient undergoing treatment for congestive heart failure or overhydration is expected to have an initial net negative fluid balance. However, when the goal is to maintain a neutral (zero) net fluid balance, comparison of "ins" versus "outs" and change in body weight allows the veterinarian to identify sources of overestimation or underestimation of fluid gain/loss and adjust the fluid plan accordingly.

23.3 Advanced Fluid Balance Monitoring Techniques

23.3.1 Blood Pressure

Because of the pharmacologic effects of inhalants and some injectable anesthetic drugs, blood pressure can be dynamic throughout the anesthetic period in healthy and critically ill animals. Patients experience hypotension under anesthesia for numerous reasons, such as blood loss, dehydration, vasodilation, reduced cardiac contractility and arrhythmias. In patients anesthetized with inhalant anesthetics, blood pressure is a poor predictor of fluid responsiveness. For example, while hypotension caused by hypovolemia is expected to resolve following IV fluid resuscitation, administration of IV fluid boluses to patients that are hypotensive due to inhalant anesthetics does not predictably cause an increase in blood pressure (Muir *et al.* 2014).

Since patients are commonly receiving an inhalant anesthetic when concurrently experiencing surgical blood loss or other physiologic causes of hypotension, blood pressure is not always a predictable means of estimating the patient's fluid deficit. However, if a patient is hypotensive prior to anesthesia, one should anticipate that hypotension would worsen when the patient is maintained under general anesthesia. Techniques for blood pressure measurement are described in Chapter 19.

23.3.2 Central Venous Pressure

Central venous pressure (CVP) is measured using a pressure transducer or water manometer that is attached to a catheter inserted into a patient's cranial vena cava (Figure 23.3). Most commonly, the catheter is placed percutaneously into the jugular vein and is also used for central venous administration of drugs and for blood sampling. The measurement of CVP represents right atrial pressures and has been used as an estimate of the filling pressures of the circulatory system.

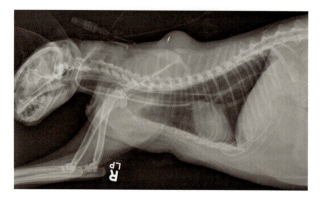

Figure 23.3 Lateral thoracic radiograph of a cat, confirming placement of a central venous catheter (thick radiopaque tube) in the jugular vein, extending to the cranial vena cava, just cranial to the heart. A nasogastric feeding tube is also apparent in this radiograph (thin radiopaque tube).

Historically, CVP measurement is used as an endpoint of resuscitation for fluid administration in human patients with septic shock. While protocol-driven fluid resuscitation strategies, in which IV fluid boluses were given until CVP exceeded 8 mmHg, was found to improve survival (Rivers *et al.* 2001), recent evidence no longer supports the use of CVP measurement to guide volume expansion. Baseline CVP, trends in CVP over time, and change in CVP following an IV fluid bolus, do not correlate with fluid responsiveness (Marik *et al.* 2008). However, of these three measurements, the magnitude of the change in right atrial pressure (estimated by change in CVP) in response to an IV fluid bolus shows the most promise in predicting fluid responsiveness (Michard and Teboul 2002). Additional information regarding CVP waveforms can be found in Chapter 19.

23.3.3 Central Venous Oxygen Saturation

Another benefit of central venous catheter placement is having immediate access to central venous blood for measurement of oxygen saturation. While arterial oxygen saturation (SaO_2) is used to assess lung function, measurement of central venous oxygen saturation ($ScvO_2$), which is normally greater than 65%, provides an assessment of blood flow. If a patient's arterial blood has normal hemoglobin and dissolved oxygen concentrations and oxygen saturation, $ScvO_2$ reflects the difference between oxygen delivery and oxygen consumption (Prittie 2006). Since patients under anesthesia should not have fast fluctuations in tissue oxygen consumption, a rapid decline in $ScvO_2$ suggests decreased oxygen delivery due to low cardiac output. Indeed, $ScvO_2$ measurements in septic dogs with pyometra were found to be significantly lower in non-survivors than in surviving patients (mean $ScvO_2$ 62.4% vs. 74.6%), with a higher $ScvO_2$ at admission associated with a lower probability of death (Conti-Patara *et al.* 2012).

23.3.4 Dynamic Indices of Intravascular Volume

In spontaneously breathing healthy patients, the diaphragm contracts during inspiration, causing the intrathoracic pressure to become more negative, which allows movement of air into the lungs. With negative intrapleural pressures, the large intrathoracic vessels are minimally compressed, supporting venous return to the heart and leading to an increase in cardiac output during inspiration. With positive pressure ventilation, air moves into the lungs because positive pressure is applied at the patient's airway during inspiration. Therefore, with positive pressure ventilation there is an increase in intrapleural pressure, which causes compression of the large intrathoracic vessels, reducing venous return and cardiac output. In a patient with normal intravascular volume status, the magnitude of these changes throughout the respiratory cycle is small. However, this variation in cardiac performance and arterial pressure throughout the respiratory cycle is exaggerated in patients with hypovolemia and volume-responsive changes in cardiac output (Gomez and Pinsky 2013).

On an arterial blood pressure tracing or measurement, pulse pressure is the difference between systolic and diastolic pressures. Mechanical ventilation causes cyclic increases in systolic blood pressure and pulse pressure that is more profound in patients with hypovolemia than in patients with normal volume status. For patients with a high amount of respiratory variation in arterial pulse pressure, increasing blood volume decreases pulse pressure variability, whereas blood loss or other volume depletion, enhances the changes. Measurements of pulse pressure variation are valuable and becoming the standard for the prediction of fluid responsiveness (Michard 2005). Several techniques employ this phenomenon, including arterial pulse pressure variation, systolic pressure variation, stroke volume variation and pulse oximeter signal variation (Figure 23.4 here).

23.3.4.1 Pulse Pressure Variability (PPV) and Systolic Pressure Variability (SPV)

Pulse pressure is the difference between systolic and diastolic arterial blood pressures. The percent variation in pulse pressure throughout the respiratory cycle in mechanically ventilated patients is termed the pulse pressure variability (PPV). Similarly, the percent change in systolic arterial blood pressure throughout inspiration and expiration is known as the systolic pressure variability (SPV). When connected to a peripheral arterial

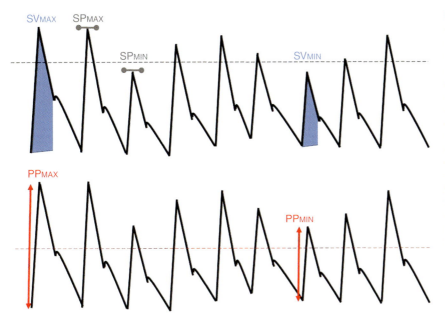

Figure 23.4 Drawing representing arterial blood pressure waveforms and the measurements used in the calculation of stroke volume variation (SVV), pulse pressure variability (PPV) and systolic pressure variability (SPV). Maximum stroke volume (SVMAX) and minimum stroke volume (SVMIN), estimated through measurement of the area under the curve of the systolic arterial blood pressure tracing, are used to calculate SVV. The maximum systolic blood pressure (SPMAX) and the minimum systolic blood pressure (SPMIN) are used to calculate SPV. Maximum pulse pressure (PPMAX) and minimum pulse pressure (PPMIN) are used to calculate pulse pressure variability (PPV).

catheter, a multiparameter monitor (e.g. DX-2020, Dixtal Biomedical, Sao Paulo, Brazil) is used to calculate and display PPV and SPV (Figure 23.4).

PPV and SPV allow accurate prediction of fluid responsiveness in human patients with acute circulatory failure due to sepsis (Michard *et al.* 2000). In this setting, PPV had improved accuracy in detecting fluid responsiveness, compared to SPV. In mechanically ventilated, isoflurane anesthetized dogs undergoing orthopedic surgery, PPV accurately predicted fluid responsiveness (Fantoni *et al.* 2017). In addition, anesthetized dogs with experimentally-induced hemorrhage had significantly higher PPV than baseline (pre-hemorrhage) values (Diniz *et al.* 2014; Klein *et al.* 2016), except in dogs concurrently receiving dexmedetomidine via constant rate infusion (Diniz *et al.* 2014).

One drawback to PPV and SPV is that patients must be mechanically ventilated, without spontaneous ventilatory efforts, and instrumented with a peripheral arterial catheter, limiting this technology to intubated patients undergoing general anesthesia. In addition, the patient must have a regular pulse rhythm with heart rate between 40 and 140 beats per minute (Fantoni *et al.* 2017).

23.3.4.2 Stroke Volume Variation

The systemic arterial pulse pressure is directly proportional to the left ventricular stroke volume. The FloTrac/Vigileo system (Edwards Lifesciences, Irvine, CA) is an arterial blood pressure sensor, transducer and monitor combination that uses an arterial blood pressure waveform and software algorithm to estimate stroke volume. This system's software reports stroke volume variation (SVV), which is calculated based on the amount of

variation in arterial waveform amplitude throughout the respiratory cycle in a patient receiving positive pressure ventilation (Figure 23.4; Taguchi *et al.* 2011).

Clinical experience with the FloTrac/Vigileo system is limited in veterinary species. While the FloTrac/Vigileo monitor has been found to overestimate cardiac output with high relative error (Valverde *et al.* 2011), experimental studies demonstrate that SVV significantly increases in dogs undergoing moderate hemorrhage, compared to baseline values (Kawazoe *et al.* 2015). SVV appears to be sensitive enough to detect an 8 mL/kg or greater change in blood volume (Taguchi *et al.* 2011). SVV has also been estimated using electrical velocimetry (Aesculon monitor, Osypka Medical, La Jolla, CA), a technology that relies on analysis of electrical conductivity of aortic blood flow throughout the cardiac cycle. Despite limited clinical and research experience with this monitor, initial data supports the use of electrical velocimetry to predict fluid responsiveness in dogs (Sasaki *et al.* 2017).

Similar to other monitors, measurement of SVV requires a patient to be mechanically ventilated and instrumented with an arterial catheter. Arrhythmias or poor signal quality reduce the accuracy of SVV calculations.

23.3.4.3 Plethysmography Variability Index (PVI)

The plethysmography variability index (PVI) measures the average change in the pulse oximetry waveform amplitude (perfusion index) between inspiratory and expiratory values over two respiratory cycles (Figure 23.5). As internally calculated by the pulse oximeter (Rad-7, Masimo Corporation, Irvine, CA), PVI has been found to have reasonable sensitivity and

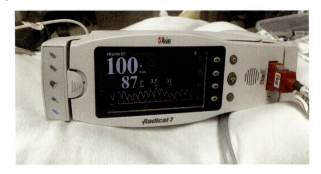

Figure 23.5 Photograph of a pulse oximeter (Radical 7, Masimo Corporation, Irvine, CA) demonstrating perfusion index (PI) and the calculated value for plethysmography variability index (PVI). The variability in the pulse oximetry waveform during the respiratory cycle in this mechanically ventilated dog is clearly visible.

specificity to predict fluid responsiveness in mechanically ventilated human patients undergoing surgery or ICU hospitalization (Fu *et al.* 2012; Sandroni *et al.* 2012; Chu *et al.* 2016). In anesthetized, mechanically ventilated dogs, hypotension-inducing hemorrhage was found to cause significantly increased PVI and PPV; both PPV and PVI decreased to pre-hemorrhage values after volume replacement, which suggests that these measurements might non-invasively predict volume responsiveness in dogs (Klein *et al.* 2016).

As with measurement of PPV and SVV, patients must be mechanically ventilated to evaluate changes in PVI. However, the measurement of PVI does not require arterial catheter placement, as plethysmographic measurements are made with transcutaneous or transmembranous sensors of arterial blood flow. The accuracy of PVI measurements is limited by interference from spontaneous breathing, movement, skin pigmentation, arrhythmias, and low peripheral perfusion (Chu *et al.* 2016).

23.3.5 Ultrasound Techniques

23.3.5.1 Vena Caval Measurements

In humans, bedside ultrasound is used to measure the diameter of the inferior vena cava (dIVC) in a standardized location caudal to its junction with the hepatic vein. Measurements of dIVC are made on inspiration and expiration, which are expected to differ throughout the respiratory cycle, due to changes in pressure within the thorax and abdomen. The raw measurements of inspiratory and expiratory dIVC are lower in patients with hypovolemia (Zengin *et al.* 2013). The calculated percent change in dIVC between inspiration and expiration, known as the "collapsibility index", is expected be greater in patients with blood loss and fluid-responsive shock (Sefidbakht *et al.* 2007). The

change in these measurements appears sensitive enough to detect blood loss as little as 450 mL in volunteer blood donors (Lyon *et al.* 2005). The ability of the collapsibility index to predict fluid responsiveness is supported by data collected from both spontaneously breathing (Sefidbakht *et al.* 2007) and mechanically ventilated (Feissel *et al.* 2004; Zhang *et al.* 2016) humans with shock.

The collapsibility index appears to be more reliable than measurement of CVP (Zhang *et al.* 2016), but is still inferior to PPV (de Oliveira *et al.* 2016) to predict fluid responsiveness. These measurements of dIVC and collapsibility index cannot be interpreted in patients with right-sided heart failure or severe tricuspid regurgitation due to the effects of these conditions on pressure within the inferior (caudal) vena cava (Sefidbakht *et al.* 2007).

In hypotensive, anesthetized dogs, the ratio of caudal vena cava (CdVC) to descending aorta (Ao) diameters (CdVC:Ao ratio) increased following fluid resuscitation and that correlated well with systolic pressure variation (used to predict fluid responsiveness) (Meneghini *et al.* 2016). However, the measurements in this study were made during a brief period of suspended ventilation. The utility of ultrasonographic measurements of respiratory variation in CdVC diameter for prediction of fluid responsiveness in animals is presently unknown.

23.3.5.2 Bedside Echocardiography

In human intensive care units, transthoracic echocardiography is valuable because of its portability, availability and ability to provide information rapidly. The kinetics and size of the cardiac chambers can provide immediate information to the experienced operator. When decreased, measurement of parameters such as left ventricular end-diastolic area can suggest hypovolemia, although this finding does not necessarily indicate fluid responsiveness (Beaulieu 2007). Bedside echocardiography is used to demonstrate transient concentric left ventricular remodeling, or pseudohypertrophy, which is commonly seen during hypovolemia (Di Segni *et al.* 1997). The pleural and pericardial spaces can also be evaluated for effusion while performing bedside echocardiography.

Despite the growing use of echocardiographic evaluation in human intensive care units, the utility of this practice performed in animals by non-cardiologists is unknown. Echocardiography findings in clinically normal dogs before and after experimentally-induced fluid deficit demonstrated a significant reduction in left ventricular end-diastolic volume (LVEDV; Fine *et al.* 2010). Trends in measurement of left ventricular end-diastolic diameter (LVEDD) might indicate an increase or decrease in preload. However, measurement of the left atrium:aorta ratio (an indicator of left atrial enlargement), and shortening fraction (an estimate of left ventricular contractility), are more likely to have a high degree of variability in operators that are not extensively trained (Chetboul *et al.* 2004). Despite its growing use in humans, the diagnostic utility of measuring selected transthoracic echocardiography values by non-cardiologists in animals is unknown.

23.3.5.3 Other Applications of Point-of-Care Ultrasound

By identifying cavitary effusions in patients in the perianesthetic period, one can quickly detect and qualitatively assess the severity of blood and other fluid losses. Identification of pleural, pericardial, peritoneal and retroperitoneal effusions is accomplished using brief point-of-care ultrasound examinations of the thorax and abdomen. These systematic techniques, named thoracic and abdominal focused assessment with sonography for trauma (TFAST and AFAST, respectively) are performed in less than 10 minutes and can be performed by clinicians with experience levels ranging from novice (undergoing a brief 2-hour training session) to expert (Boysen *et al.* 2004; Lisciandro 2011). Because these examinations are now broadly used in both traumatized and non-traumatized patients, it has been suggested that the last "T" in AFAST and TFAST should stand for trauma, triage and tracking (monitoring) (Lisciandro 2011; Figure 23.6).

Another rapidly performed point-of-care transthoracic ultrasound technique, called the veterinary bedside lung ultrasound exam (Vet BLUE), has been used to detect cardiogenic edema and other lung infiltrates in dogs and cats with acute dyspnea (Rademacher *et al.* 2014; Ward *et al.* 2017). While this technique is useful for predicting the presence of cardiogenic pulmonary edema (Rademacher *et al.* 2014), Vet BLUE is unable to differentiate pulmonary edema from other pulmonary parenchymal disease (Ward *et al.* 2017). Based on its overlapping pathophysiology with cardiogenic pulmonary edema, one would expect that use of the Vet BLUE exam should be helpful in identifying early signs of fluid overload. The reader is directed to the Lisciandro reference (2014) for detailed descriptions of these ultrasound techniques.

23.4 Fluid Therapy

Although in-depth physiologic considerations underlying the development of a fluid therapy plan is beyond the scope of this chapter, when developing a fluid therapy

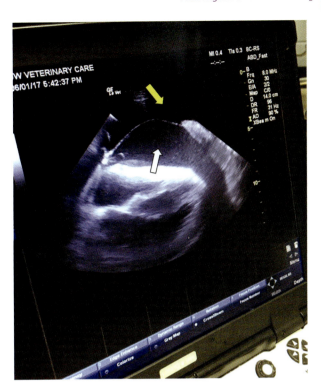

Figure 23.6 Bedside thoracic ultrasound is used here (TFAST) to identify pericardial effusion (hypoechoic space near white arrow) and pleural effusion (hypoechoic space near yellow arrow) using a TFAST (thoracic focused assessment with sonography for trauma/triage) technique.

plan for a patient, the following questions should be considered:

- Is the patient hypovolemic?
- Are there known ongoing losses of water/fluid or blood?
- Is the patient dehydrated?
- Is there a volume excess?
- Is the patient at an increased risk for complications with liberal fluid administration?

Historically recommended anesthetic rates for IV fluids at 10 mL/kg/hour are not evidence-based. Recent AAHA guidelines (Davis *et al.* 2013) suggest starting with an initial anesthetic fluid rate of 3 mL/kg/hour in cats and 5 mL/kg/hour in dogs. Lower fluid rates are used in patients with cardiovascular disease. The administration rate is gradually decreased if the anesthetic time lasts for more than 1 hour and fluid loss is not excessive. A typical guideline would be to reduce fluid rate by 25% per hour until maintenance rates are reached if the patient remains hemodynamically stable (Davis *et al.* 2013). Adjustments to these values should be made if patients have underlying disease states (e.g. renal disease) and the type of fluids should be chosen based on patient assessment and monitoring (Davis *et al.* 2013).

For example, cats have a smaller blood volume, lower metabolic rate, and higher incidence of occult heart disease, and their fluid rate and type should be adjusted accordingly. Readers are directed to other references for more detailed information (DiBartola 2012; Silverstein and Hopper 2014).

23.5 Equipment for Fluid Therapy

Other than by voluntary enteral water intake, fluids can be administered by enteral feeding tubes and parenteral (e.g. IV, intraosseous, intraperitoneal and subcutaneous) routes. Intravenous and intraosseous fluids are the most relevant and predictable routes by which fluids are administered to patients in the peri-anesthetic period.

23.5.1 IV Catheters

Fluid and drug delivery in hospitalized and/or anesthetized patients is commonly accomplished using an IV catheter. Based on a patient's vascular integrity and concurrent needs, the venous catheter is placed into a peripheral vessel or in a central vein. Skin integrity must be considered when choosing a site of catheter placement, as entry through wounded or infected skin might promote entry of bacteria into circulation. In addition, strategic bandaging or splinting might be required when a catheter must be placed in a high-motion area such as over the tarsus or carpus, as catheter displacement is more likely in these regions.

23.5.1.1 Peripheral Venous Catheters

Peripheral venous catheters are commonly placed in the cephalic vein and the medial and lateral saphenous veins in cats and dogs. Other sites that are used less commonly in small animal species include the dorsal common digital vein and auricular vein. In general, peripheral venous catheters range from small to large bore (24–12 gauge), are of shorter lengths (0.75–2 inches), and are for short-term use (usually up to 96 hours). They are typically placed without sedation or general anesthesia (see Chapters 29–37 for more species specifics).

Benefits of peripheral catheters include their low cost, wide availability and rapid placement without the need for special training or equipment. The short length allows rapid fluid administration in patients requiring volume resuscitation. While short-term sampling can be performed by aspirating blood from peripheral catheters (Elliott *et al.* 2010), blood collection is accomplished more reliably using central venous catheters. Blood collection through small-bore peripheral catheters is prone to hemolysis, which might affect blood test results (Kennedy *et al.* 1996).

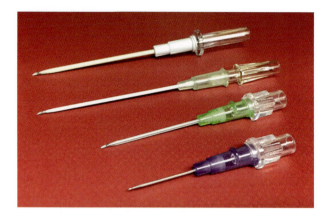

Figure 23.7 Examples of peripheral over-the-needle catheters of various sizes and materials. Pictured from top to bottom: 16-gauge, 1.88-inch fluorinated ethylene propylene polymer catheter (Angiocath, Becton Dickinson, Sandy, UT); 18-gauge, 2-inch ethylene tetrafluoroethylene catheter (Terumo Medical Products, Somerset, NJ); 18-gauge, 1.25-inch polyurethane catheter (Monoject, Covidien, Mansfield, MA); 26-gauge 0.75-inch polyurethane catheter (Monoject, Covidien, Mansfield, MA).

Percutaneous placement of an over-the-needle catheter is most commonly used for peripheral venous catheterization, although a variety of catheter designs, sizes and materials are available. Catheters can be made from a variety of plastic materials, such as polyvinyl chloride, polyurethane, fluorinated ethylene propylene or ethylene tetrafluoroethylene (Figure 23.7). These plastics vary in stiffness, tissue reactivity and thrombogenicity. In general, catheters made of stiff materials are easier to tunnel through subcutaneous tissues, but may be more likely to kink and irritate the vessel wall. Further detail regarding catheter types, materials and placement techniques are published elsewhere (Hansen 2012).

23.5.1.2 Central Venous Catheters

Central venous catheters are typically long, small-bore catheters that are available in single-or multiple-lumen configurations. These catheters, placed with the distal end within the jugular vein, cranial or caudal vena cava (depending on species), offer several advantages over peripheral catheters. For example, they allow measurement of central venous pressure, frequent blood sample collection and long-term vascular access. These catheters also allow administration of hyperosmolar drugs or other drugs likely to induce phlebitis in a peripheral vessel and, when a multiple-lumen catheter is used, concurrent administration of fluids and/or medications that are chemically or physically incompatible (Figure 23.8).

Central venous catheters are placed by percutaneous insertion of a needle or IV catheter introducer into the external jugular vein or possibly through the medial or lateral saphenous vein. A guidewire is inserted through the introducer, followed by removal of the introducer,

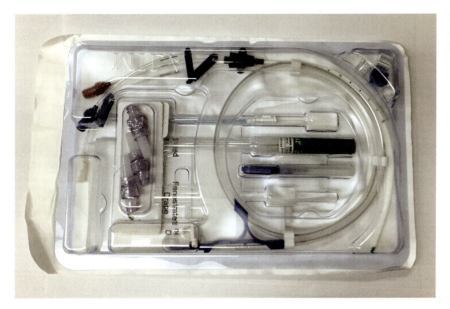

temporary passage of a venous dilator, and placement of a long, flexible catheter over the guidewire as modified from the technique initially described by Seldinger (1953). Other central venous catheter styles exist, which involve placement of a catheter through a needle or peel-away introducer catheter. In addition, central catheters, such as peripherally inserted central catheters (PICC catheters) and vascular access ports (VAPs), may also be used to provide central venous access (see Chapter 19). Further details regarding catheter types, materials and placement techniques have been previously published (Hansen 2012); readers are also directed to the species-specific chapters in this book (Chapters 29–37).

23.5.2 Intraosseous Catheters

An intraosseous catheter is a vascular access device that is inserted into the bone marrow cavity. Because the catheter must penetrate cortical bone to reach the medullary canal, intraosseous catheters are rigid, metallic catheters that typically have an integrated stylet for use during placement. A range of catheter types are used for intraosseous access. Hypodermic needles and spinal needles can be used in neonates and other animals with thin cortical bone, while more specialized catheters are required for use in adult animals. An Illinois bone marrow needle (Figure 23.9), traditionally used for bone marrow aspirates, can be placed manually for infusion of IV fluids and medications. Alternatively, two automatic devices are available, including the EZ-IO intraosseous vascular access system (Teleflex, Morrisville, NC; Figure 23.10), which utilizes a rotational power driver to insert the intraosseous catheter, and the Bone Injection Gun (Vet BIG, WaisMed Ltd., Houston, TX), which

drives the catheter into place using a spring-loaded impact mechanism. Descriptions of intraosseous catheter placement have been published and are found in the manufacturer's instructions (Campbell and Macintire 2012; Hansen 2012). Briefly, the site should be surgically clipped and prepared before catheter placement. Correct

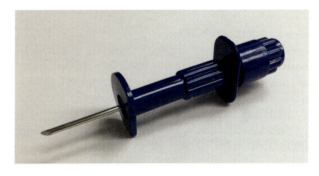

Figure 23.9 An Illinois bone marrow aspiration needle (CareFusion, Vernon Hills, IL) can be used for intraosseous infusion of IV fluids.

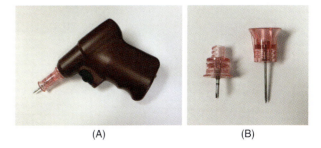

(A)   (B)

Figure 23.10 (A) The EZ-IO intraosseous power driver (Teleflex, Morrisville, NC) with an intraosseous catheter loaded on the driver and with the catheter and stylet separated (B).

placement should be verified and the catheter secured with sterile dressing.

When success rates, ease of placement, and speed of placement were compared between the EZ-IO device, the Vet BIG, and a manually placed bone marrow needle in feline cadavers, the EZ-IO device was fastest and easiest to use, but all techniques had similar success rates (Bukoski *et al.* 2010). The EZ-IO technique and jugular venous cut-down were found to have similar success rates in achieving vascular access in canine cadavers, although the intraosseous catheter placement was significantly faster (Allukian *et al.* 2017).

Fluid and drugs infused into the medullary canal quickly reach central venous circulation. Intraosseous fluid administration is an option for fluid resuscitation in patients in which vascular access is difficult to establish in a timely manner, such as neonates, very small patients, or those with hypovolemia, hypotension or cardiac arrest. Common placement sites in small animals include the proximal humerus, tibial tuberosity, wing of the ilium and the trochanteric fossa of the femur (Figure 23.11). Intraosseous catheter placement sites for birds include the distal ulna and proximal tibiotarsal bone (Jenkins 2016). Pneumatic bones, which communicate with gas exchange surfaces of the air sacs, must be avoided when selecting a site for intraosseous catheterization in birds.

23.5.3 Fluid Containers and Administration Sets

23.5.3.1 Fluid Containers

Fluids for intravenous administration are available in assorted sizes of flexible plastic bags. IV fluid containers and tubing have been classically produced from polyvinylchloride (PVC). Concerns with leaching of plasticizers, such as di(2-ethylhexyl)-phthalate (DEHP) from PVC into IV solutions, which is suspected to contribute to conditions such as testicular dysgenesis syndrome in male neonates (Kaul *et al.* 1982; Sampson and de Korte 2011), have resulted in the use of other plastics. For example, current manufacturers are using polypropylene or polyethylene (collectively called polyolefin plastics) and non-DEHP containing PVC, which are associated with reduced leaching of plasticizers (Trissel *et al.* 2006). Polyolefin plastic fluid bags are also associated with reduced adsorption of drugs compared with PVC containers (Aloumanis *et al.* 2009; Trissel *et al.* 2001).

IV fluid bags range in size from 50–5000 mL. Actual volumes present in these bags are slightly greater than what is labeled on each package. The purpose of this overfill is to account for the loss of water that can occur due to permeability of the plastic container and relate to storage conditions and surface area-to-volume ratios of the containers (Cohen and Smetzer 2014). One manufacturer's overfill volumes range from 2.4–30 mL of extra fluid, for fluid containers with sizes ranging from 50–1000 mL (Freeflex, Fresenius Kabi, Lake Zurich, Illinois). While the relative amount of overfill (~3–5%) seems minimal, this overfill might affect the concentration of drugs that are added to an IV fluid container.

IV fluid containers should be clearly labeled with the patient's information and with the details (name, concentration, date) of any drug additives. The compatibility of the drugs should be verified before combining multiple drugs in the same fluid container. After medications are added, the fluid bag should be inverted 3–5 times to ensure thorough mixing and avoid high drug concentrations in the bottom of the bag (Hoehne *et al.* 2015).

A burette integrated into the fluid path can be used for convenience and safety in small patients (Figure 23.12). Burettes contain up to 150 mL of fluid per aliquot for use, with or without fluid additives, and are integrated into a fluid line or can be added to an existing bag and line system (Burette Set, Hospira, Lake Forest, IL; Buretrol, Baxter Healthcare, Deerfield, IL). In small

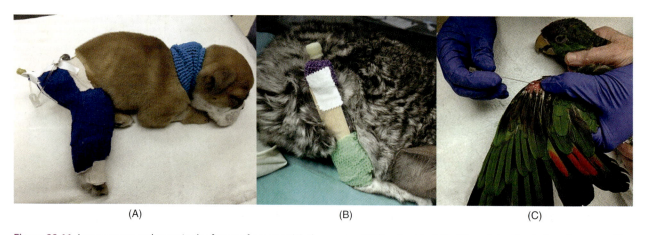

(A) (B) (C)

Figure 23.11 Intraosseous catheters in the femur of a puppy (A), the proximal tibia of a chinchilla (B), and the distal ulna of a parrot (C).

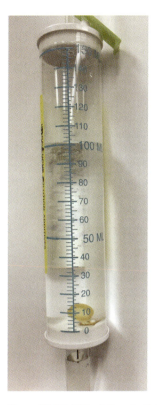

patients, fluid burettes can be used to verify precise volume delivery and to limit unintentional bolus delivery. In addition, the use of a burette allows medications to be mixed into smaller total volumes of fluids and to reduce drug waste in patients in which fluid additives will likely be changed frequently (e.g. patients with electrolyte disturbances or refractory hypoglycemia).

23.5.3.2 Administration Sets

Fluid administration sets are available in a variety of configurations from several manufacturers. A fluid administration set consists of a spike adapter, which is inserted into the outlet port of the IV fluid bag, drip chamber, tubing, clamps, injection ports or needless connector hubs, and a luer lock adapter that connects to the patient's catheter or t-connector (Figure 23.13A). Each brand comes with a different number of drops per mL and attention should be paid to these differences (e.g. 10, 12, 15 or 60 drops/mL). In addition, burettes (mentioned above) may be integrated directly into the fluid line for careful delivery of fluids or drugs. Additional components are available in some administration sets, such as filters with various pore sizes intended to remove bacteria, crystallized medication (e.g. mannitol), or micro-aggregates of cells or fibrin from blood transfusion products (Figures 23.13B and C). Fluid lines made specifically for

Figure 23.12 150-mL Burette Set (Hospira, Lake Forest, IL) with integrated microdrip fluid set (60 drops = 1 mL).

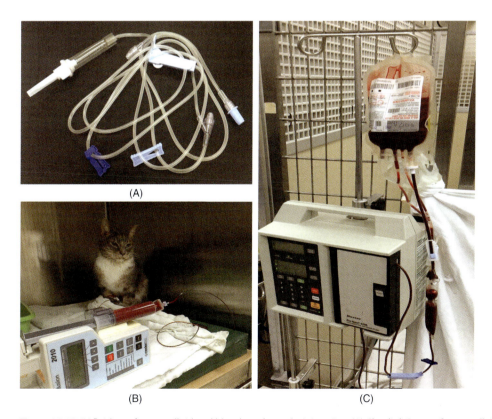

(A)

(B)

(C)

Figure 23.13 IV fluid sets for crystalloid and blood product administration. (A) Clearlink System for crystalloid administration (Baxter Healthcare Corporation, Deerfield, IL). (B) Hemo-Nate 18 micron blood filter (Utah Medical Products, Midvale, UT). An in line filter can also be added to filter syringe administered transfusions. (C) Interlink System for blood administration (Baxter Healthcare Corporation, Deerfield, IL).

delivery of large volumes are also manufactured. For example, some large animal sets are patented and deliver up to 28 L/hr by gravity when connected to two bags (Large Animal Rapid Infusion Set, International WIN, Ltd., Kennett Square, PA). When selecting and purchasing fluid administration sets, care should be used to ensure that the fluid line is correct for the intended purpose (e.g. blood transfusion vs. crystalloid fluid administration) and compatible with the infusion pump that will be used.

23.5.4 Manual and Automatic Fluid Delivery

Intravenous fluids can be administered via manual techniques, which include fluid administration using gravity-dependent or pressure-assisted flow. Alternatively, veterinary professionals commonly use automatic (pump) delivery methods to regulate and monitor fluid administration.

23.5.4.1 Gravity-Assisted Flow

With gravity-dependent flow, fluid flows from the bag through a calibrated drip chamber that allows the caregiver to determine and adjust the fluid rate. Drip chambers are model and manufacturer specific, ranging from 10–60 drops per mL. The fluid administration rate is estimated based on the number of drops per unit time that are passing through the drip chamber. An example

calculation is provided below (Text Box 23.1). Since the rate of gravity-dependent flow is dependent on the difference in pressure between the bag and the patient's IV catheter, several factors will increase or decrease the flow rate. Raising the height of the fluid bag with respect to patient height will increase the flow rate of IV fluids, while lowering the bag will decrease the flow rate. Partial obstructions due to clot formation, changes in limb or body position, or catheter extravasation might also decrease flow. Relief of catheter obstruction or repositioning of the patient's limb may increase flow. Therefore, it is important to closely monitor the drip rate over time when administering fluids by gravity-dependent flow, as the actual rate delivered can change over time.

23.5.4.2 Pressure-Assisted Flow

To deliver fluids rapidly, a bag can be placed inside a pressurized infusion system, which consists of a netting or plastic sleeve to hold the fluid bag against an inflatable bladder and an attached inflation bulb and pressure gauge (Figure 23.14). These bags are manually inflated and are usually pressurized up to 300 mmHg, to achieve the desired fluid flow. Since there is no automated air detector and clamp as part of this system, all fluid boluses delivered using a pressure infusion bag should be closely monitored to avoid delivery of the residual air that remains within the IV fluid bag. Alternatively,

---

Text Box 23.1

Example Calculations for Fluid Administration via Gravity Flow

Fluid calculations for a large dog and a small cat are presented here. The hourly rate is first calculated in mL/hour, then converted to drops per second. If the value (drops per second) is not a whole number, this value can be multiplied by a number of seconds (e.g. 2–15 seconds) to enable counting of drops per unit time.

Case #1

Patient: 2-year-old spayed female Labrador retriever
Body weight: 30 kg
Fluid Delivery Rate: 5 mL/kg/hour
Calibration of Fluid Set: 10 drops/mL

30 kg × 5 mL/kg/hour = 150 mL/hour

150 mL/hour × 1 hour/60 minutes × 1 minute/60 seconds × 10 drops/mL = 0.42 drops/second

= 0.42 drops/second × 5 seconds

= 2.1 drops per 5 seconds

→ rounded to 2 drops per 5 seconds = 144 ml/hour (actual amount delivered)

Case #2

Patient: 6-month-old intact male domestic shorthaired cat
Body weight: 2.8 kg
Fluid Delivery Rate: 5 mL/kg/hour
Calibration of Fluid Set: 60 drops/mL

2.8 kg × 5 mL/kg/hour = 14 mL/hour

14 mL/hr × 1 hour/60 minutes × 1 minute/60 seconds × 60 drops/mL = 0.23 drops/second

= 0.23 drops/second × 10 seconds	= 0.23 drops/second × 4 seconds
= 2.3 drops per 10 seconds	= 0.92 drops per 4 seconds
→ Rounded to 2 drops per 10 seconds	→ 1 drop per 4 seconds
actual amount delivered = 12 ml/hr	actual amount delivered = 15 ml/hr

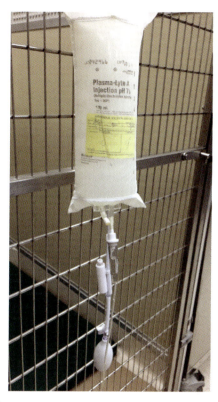

Figure 23.14 Mesh pressure infusion bag used to rapidly deliver intravenous fluids (Infu-Stat, Mason Tayler Medical Products, Buffalo, NY).

the air can be carefully expressed from the IV fluid bag before the infusion has been started. Pressure sleeves are available from more than 10 manufacturers.

23.5.4.3 Fluid Pumps

There are two main designs of pumping action used to control fluid movement by electronic intravenous infusion pumps: peristaltic and volumetric. Peristaltic pumps use a mechanism that squeezes the fluid line from proximal to distal, moving fluid forward using an action that resembles the biological process of peristalsis (Figure 23.15). A volumetric pump uses a unique style of administration set that incorporates a reservoir chamber (Willis 1995) into a cassette design (Figure 23.16). Volumetric pumps alternate between filling the chamber from the bag and pushing fluid out of the cassette to the patient (Hansen 2012).

Syringe pumps are also used to deliver drugs and fluids at low infusion rates (Figure 23.17). A syringe (up to a volume of 60 mL) is directly connected to an IV line or connected to a patient's catheter by extension tubing. Syringe pumps securely hold the syringe barrel and flange and apply pressure to control plunger movement. After a syringe is loaded and the pump is started, there is a variable start-up delay until the volume delivered is equal to the set rate. Start-up delay duration is related to several factors, including spatial gaps around the syringe, engagement of the syringe pump mechanics, and inertia within the syringe. This delay is further increased by the use of compliant infusion lines, lower flow rates and larger syringes (Schmidt *et al.* 2010). Start-up delay is an important consideration when small fluctuations in fluid delivery affect patient stability (e.g. vasopressors) or when a syringe pump requires frequent re-loading.

Intravenous fluid pumps and syringe pumps are generally set to deliver a desired volume per unit time (e.g. mL per hour). Most pumps display essential information including the fluid administration rate, total volume delivered, and volume to be infused. Depending on software, pumps might also calculate the delivery rate when the patient's weight and dose (e.g. in µg/kg/min,

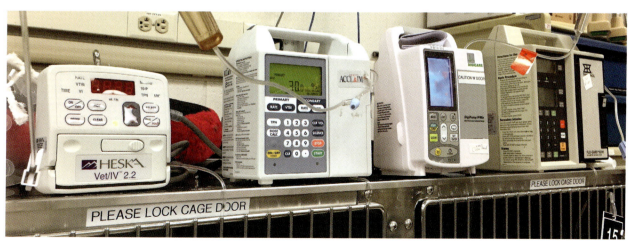

Figure 23.15 Peristaltic intravenous infusion pumps which squeeze fluid through the line (from left to right: Vet/IV 2.2 Infusion Pump, Heska, Loveland, CO; Acclaim encore, Abbott Laboratories, North Chicago, IL; DigiPump IP88x, Digicare Biomedical Technology, Boynton Beach, FL; Flo-Gard, Baxter Healthcare Corporation, Deerfield, IL).

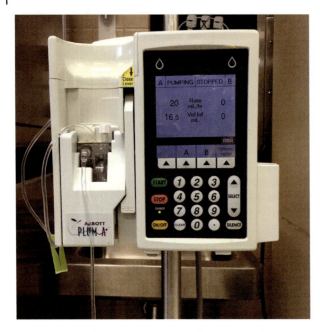

Figure 23.16 Volumetric intravenous infusion pump that uses a manufacturer-specific cassette for fluid administration (Plum A+, Abbott/Hospira, Lake Forest, IL) (photograph courtesy of Dr Meghan Fick, North Carolina State University).

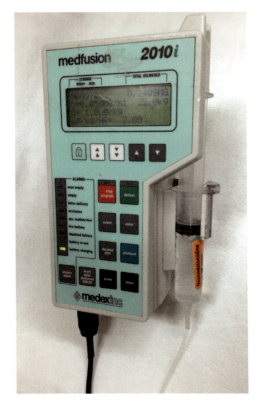

Figure 23.17 Syringe infusion pump used to deliver small volumes or precise quantities of drugs (Medfusion 2010i Infusion Pump, Medex, Duluth, GA).

μg/kg/hour, mg/kg/hour) are entered. To reduce medical errors, newer "smart pumps" (Figure 23.18) are equipped with pre-programmed therapy libraries that operate within set concentration and dose range limits based on the drug delivered (Harding 2011; see Chapter 24).

Electronic infusion pumps are often equipped with a set of alarms that alert the operator to the presence of air, increased pressure and occlusions within the system. Additionally, safety features like "keep vein open" (KVO) might be displayed after completing infusion of the set volume, which means that a slow fluid rate (e.g. 0.1–2 mL/hour) will be delivered until the pump has been reset, with the goal of maintaining catheter patency.

Although a pump appears to be functioning properly, one cannot assume 100% accuracy for fluid delivery using automatic pumps. Several factors can increase or decrease the actual amount of fluid received by the patient. Care providers are reminded to use administration sets that are deemed compatible by the manufacturer of the specific fluid pump in use, as use of wrong materials could promote inaccurate fluid delivery. High tubing compliance (distention of the tubing when pressure is applied) and downward displacement of the fluid pump (lowering the position on a pole or shelf) tend to decrease actual fluid delivery. For syringe pumps, the plunger can occasionally become stuck to the inner aspect of the syringe barrel, leading to pump obstruction and undetected drug boluses. These inaccuracies are magnified for patients receiving slow flow rates (Van der Eijk *et al.* 2013). Caregivers should manually verify volume delivered and investigate pump inaccuracies if actual volumes delivered differ from what is displayed on the pump.

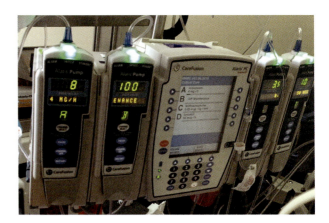

Figure 23.18 "Smart" intravenous infusion pump with pre-programmed libraries (Alaris Infusion System with Guardrails Safety Software, CareFusion, San Diego, CA).

23.5.5 Flushing Venous Catheters

It is standard practice to administer a small bolus of fluid into an unused IV catheter lumen to maintain catheter patency. Flushing with normal saline (0.9%) versus heparinized (1–10 units/mL) saline every 4–8 hours appears to be equally effective for maintaining short-term patency of central and peripheral venous catheters (Ueda *et al.* 2013; Lopez-Briz *et al.* 2014). Lines should also be flushed after administering each dose of drug, to prevent mixing of incompatible drugs in the administration tubing and catheter to ensure that the patient has received the entire dose of medication.

23.6 Summary

Fluid monitoring and administration are integral parts of daily veterinary medicine. Accurate techniques in fluid therapy monitoring are advancing rapidly and are becoming affordable and practical in the clinical setting. Use of fluid delivery equipment is now commonplace and allows for improved patient care and management.

References

Allukian, A.R., Abelson, A.L., Babyak, J. and Rozanski, E.A. (2017) Comparison of time to obtain intraosseous versus jugular venous catheterization on canine cadavers. *J Vet Emerg Crit Care*, 27, 506–511.

Aloumanis, V., Ben, M., Kupiec, T.C. and Trissel, L.A. (2009) Drug Compatibility with a new generation of VISIV Polyolefin infusion solution containers. *Int J Pharm Compd*, 13, 162–165.

Bauer, J.H., Willis, L.R., Burt, R.W. and Grim, C.E. (1975) Volume studies II: Simultaneous determination of plasma volume, red cell mass, extracellular fluid, and total body water before and after volume expansion in dog and man. *J Lab Clin Med*, 86, 1009–1017.

Beaulieu, Y. (2007) Bedside echocardiography in the assessment of the critically ill. *Crit Care Med*, 35, S235–S249.

Bhave, G. and Neilson, E.G. (2011) Volume depletion versus dehydration: how understanding the difference can guide therapy. *Am J Kidney Dis*, 58, 302–309.

Boscan, P., Pypendop, B.H., Siao, K.T., Francey, T., Dowers, K. *et al.* (2010) Fluid balance, glomerular filtration rate, and urine output in dogs anesthetized for an orthopedic surgical procedure. *Am J Vet Res*, 71, 501–507.

Boscan, P., Watson, Z. and Steffey, E.P. (2007) Plasma colloid osmotic pressure and total protein trends in horses during anesthesia. *Vet Anaesth Analg*, 34, 275–283.

Boysen, S.R., Rozanski, E.A., Tidwell, A.S., Holm, J.L., Shaw, S.P. and Rush, J.E. (2004) Evaluation of a focused assessment with sonography for trauma protocol to detect free abdominal fluid in dogs involved in motor vehicle accidents. *J Am Vet Med Assoc*, 225, 1198–1204.

Bukoski, A., Winter, M., Bandt, C., Wilson, M. and Shih, A. (2010) Comparison of three intraosseous access techniques in cats. *J Vet Emerg Crit Care*, 20, 393–397.

Campbell, M.T. and Macintire, D.K. (2012) Catheterization of the venous compartment. In: Burkitt Creedon, J.M. and Davis, H. (eds). *Advanced Monitoring and Procedures for Small Animal Emergency and Critical Care*. Ames, IA: Wiley-Blackwell, pp. 51–68.

Cavanaugh, A.A., Sullivan, L.A. and Hansen, B.D. (2016) Retrospective evaluation of fluid overload and relationship to outcome in critically ill dogs. *J Vet Emerg Crit Care*, 26, 578–586.

Chetboul, V., Athanassiadis, N., Concordet, D., Nicolle, A., Tessier, D. *et al.* (2004) Observer-dependent variability of quantitative clinical endpoints: the example of canine echocardiography. *J Vet Pharmacol Therap*, 27, 49–56.

Chu, H., Wang, Y., Sun, Y. and Wang, G. (2016) Accuracy of pleth variability index to predict fluid responsiveness in mechanically ventilated patients: a systematic review and meta-analysis. *J Clin Monit Comput*, 30, 265–274.

Cohen, M.R. and Smetzer, J.L. (2014) Understanding and managing intravenous container overfill: potential dose confusion. *Hosp Pharm*, 49, 221–226.

Conti-Patara, A., de Araújo Caldeira, J., de Mattos-Junior, E., de Carvalho Hda, S., Reinoldes, A. *et al.* (2012) Changes in tissue perfusion parameters in dogs with severe sepsis/septic shock in response to goal-directed hemodynamic optimization at admission to ICU and the relation to outcome. *J Vet Emerg Crit Care*, 22, 409–418.

Cornelius, L.M., Finco, D.R. and Culver, D.H. (1978) Physiologic effects of rapid infusion of Ringer's lactate solution into dogs. *Am J Vet Res*, 39, 1185–1190.

Davis, H., Jensen, T., Johnson, A., Knowles, P., Meyer, R. *et al.* (2013) AAHA/AAFP fluid therapy guidelines for dogs and cats. *J Am Anim Hosp Assoc*, 49, 149–159.

de Oliveira, O.H., Freitas, F.G., Ladeira, R.T., Fischer, C.H., Bafi, A.T. *et al.* (2016) Comparison between respiratory changes in the inferior vena cava diameter and pulse pressure variation to predict fluid responsiveness in post-operative patients. *J Crit Care*, 34, 46–49.

Di Segni, E., Preisman, S., Ohad, D.J., Battier, A., Boyko, V. *et al.* (1997) Echocardiographic left ventricular remodeling and pseudohypertrophy as markers of hypovolemia. An experimental study on bleeding and volume repletion. *J Am Soc Echocardiogr,* 10, 926–936.

DiBartola, S.P. (2012) *Fluid, Electrolyte, and Acid-Base Disorders in Small Animal Practice,* 4th ed. St Louis, MO: Saunders/Elsevier.

DiBartola, S.P. and Bateman, S. (2012) Introduction to fluid therapy. In: DiBartola, S.P. (ed.). *Fluid, Electrolyte, and Acid-Base Disorders in Small Animal Practice,* 4th ed. St Louis, MO: Saunders/Elsevier, pp. 331–350.

Diniz, M.S., Teixeira-Neto, F.J., Candido, T.D., Zanuzzo, F.S., Teixeira, L.R. *et al.* (2014) Effects of dexmedetomidine on pulse pressure variation changes induced by hemorrhage followed by volume replacement in isoflurane-anesthetized dogs. *J Vet Emerg Crit Care,* 24, 681–692.

Dismukes, D.I., Thomovsky, E.J., Mann, F.A. and Middleton, J.R. (2010) Effects of general anesthesia on plasma colloid oncotic pressure in dogs. *J Am Vet Med Assoc,* 236, 309–311.

Du Toit, N. and Burden, F. (2015) Donkey colic. In: Sprayberry, K.A. and Robinson, N.E. (eds). *Robinson's Current Therapy in Equine Medicine,* 7th ed. St Louis, MO: Elsevier Saunders, p. 333.

Elliott, K.F., Fleeman, L.M. and Rand, J.S. (2010) Using 20-gauge percutaneous peripheral catheters to reliably collect serial 4-ml blood samples from conscious dogs. *Aust Vet J,* 88, 215–221.

Fantoni, D.T., Ida, K.K., Gimenes, A.M., Mantovani, M.M., Castro, J.R. *et al.* (2017) Pulse pressure variation as a guide for volume expansion in dogs undergoing orthopedic surgery. *Vet Anaesth Analg,* 44, 710–718.

Feissel, M., Michard, F., Faller, J.P. and Teboul, J.L. (2004) The respiratory variation in inferior vena cava diameter as a guide to fluid therapy. *Intens Care Med,* 30, 1834–1837.

Fine, D.M., Durham, H.E., Rossi, N.F., Spier, A.W., Selting, K. and Rubin, L.J. (2010) Echocardiographic assessment of hemodynamic changes produced by two methods of inducing fluid deficit in dogs. *J Vet Intern Med,* 24, 348–353.

Fu, Q., Weidong, M. and Zhang, H. (2012) Stroke volume variation and pleth variability index to predict fluid responsiveness during resection of primary retroperitoneal tumors in Hans Chinese. *BioSci Trends,* 6, 38–43.

Gelman, S. (2008) Venous function and central venous pressure: a physiologic story. *Anesthesiology,* 108, 735–748.

Gillespie, I., Rosenstein, P.G. and Hughes, D. (2017) Update: clinical use of plasma lactate. *Vet Clin North Am Small Anim Pract,* 47, 325–342.

Gomez, H. and Pinsky, M.R. (2013) Effect of mechanical ventilation on the heart–lung interactions. In: Tobin, M.J. (ed.). *Principles and Practice of Mechanical Ventilation,* 3rd ed. Chicago, IL: McGraw Hill, pp. 821–849.

Greco, D.S. (1998) The distribution of body water and general approach to the patient. *Vet Clin North Am Small Anim Pract,* 28, 473–482.

Hansen, B. (2012) Technical aspects of fluid therapy In: DiBartola, S.P. (ed.). *Fluid, Electrolyte, and Acid-Base Disorders in Small Animal Practice,* 4th ed. St Louis, MO: Saunders/Elsevier, pp. 351–358.

Hansen, B. and DeFrancesco, T. (2002) Relationship between hydration estimate and body weight change after fluid therapy in critically ill dogs and cats. *J Vet Emerg Crit Care,* 12, 235–243.

Harding, A.D. (2011) Use of intravenous smart pumps for patient safety. *J Emerg Nurs,* 37, 71–72.

Hoehne, S.N., Hopper, K. and Epstein, S.E. (2015) Accuracy of potassium supplementation of fluids administered intravenously. *J Vet Intern Med,* 29, 834–839.

Jenkins, J.R. (2016) Critical care of pet birds. *Vet Clin North Am Exot Anim Pract,* 19, 501–512.

Kaul, A.F., Souney, P.F. and Osathanondh, R. (1982) A review of possible toxicity of di-2-ethylhexylphthalate (DEHP) in plastic intravenous containers: effects on reproduction. *Drug Intell Clin Pharm,* 16, 689–692.

Kawazoe, Y., Makashima, T., Iseri ,T., Yonetani, C., Ueda, K. *et al.* (2015) The impact of inspiratory pressure on stroke volume variation and the evaluation of indexing stroke volume variation to inspiratory pressure under various preload conditions in experimental animals. *J Anesth,* 29, 515–521.

Kennedy, C., Angermuller, S., King, R. and Noviello Walker Warden Vang, J. (1996) A comparison of hemolysis rates using intravenous catheters versus venipuncture tubes for obtaining blood samples. *J Emerg Nurs,* 22, 566–569.

Klein, A.V., Teixeira-Neto, F.J., Garofalo, N.A., Lagos-Carvajal, A.P., Diniz, M.S. and Becerra-Velásquez, D.R. (2016) Changes in pulse pressure variation and plethysomographic variability index caused by hypotension-inducing hemorrhage followed by volume replacement in isoflurane-anesthetized dogs. *Am J Vet Res,* 77, 280–287.

Langston, C. (2012) Managing fluid and electrolyte disorders in renal failure. In: DiBartola, S.P. (ed.) *Fluid, Electrolyte, and Acid-Base Disorders in Small Animal Practice,* 4th ed. St Louis, MO: Saunders/Elsevier, pp. 544–556.

Lee, J.C., Fagenholz, S.A. and Downing, S.E (1983) Cardiac dimensions in severely anemic neonatal pigs. *Am J Vet Res,* 44, 1940–1942.

Lisciandro, G.R. (2011) Abdominal and thoracic focused assessment with sonography for trauma, triage, and monitoring in small animals. *J Vet Emerg Crit Care,* 21, 104–122.

Lisciandro, G.R. (2014) *Focused Ultrasound Techniques for the Small Animal Practitioner.* Ames, IA: Wiley-Blackwell.

Lopez-Briz, E., Ruiz Garcia, V., Cabello, J.B., Bort-Marti, S., Carbonell-Sanchis, R. and Burls, A. (2014) Heparin versus 0.9% sodium chloride intermittent flushing for prevention of occlusion in central venous catheters in adults. *Cochrane Database Syst Rev*, 10, CD008462.

Lyon, M., Blaivas, M. and Brannam, L. (2005) Sonographic measurement of the inferior vena cava as a marker of blood loss. *Am J Emerg Med*, 23, 45–50.

Magdesian, K.G., Fielding, C.L., Rhodes, D.M. and Ruby, R.E. (2006) Changes in central venous pressure and blood lactate concentration in response to acute blood loss in horses. *J Am Vet Med Assoc*, 229, 1458–1462.

Marik, P.E., Baram, M. and Vahid, B. (2008) Does central venous pressure predict fluid responsiveness? A systematic review of the literature and the tale of seven mares. *Chest*, 134, 172–178.

Meneghini, C., Rabozzi, R. and Franci, P. (2016) Correlation of the ratio of caudal vena cava diameter and aorta diameter with systolic pressure variation in anesthetized dogs. *Am J Vet Res*, 77, 137–143.

Michard, F. (2005) Changes in arterial pressure during mechanical ventilation. *Anesthesiology*, 103, 419–428.

Michard, F., Boussat, S., Chemla, D., Anguel, N., Mercat, A. et al. (2000) Relation between respiratory changes in arterial pulse pressure and fluid responsiveness with acute circulatory failure. *Am J Resp Crit Care*, 162, 134–138.

Michard, F. and Teboul, J.L. (2002) Predicting fluid responsiveness in ICU patients. *Chest*, 121, 2000–2008.

Moore, F.D., Muldowney, F.P., Haxhe, J.J., Marczynska, A.W., Ball, M.R. and Boyden, C.M. (1962) Body composition in the dog. Part I: Findings in the normal animal. *J Surg Res*, 2, 245–253.

Muir, W.W., Ueyama, Y., Pedraza-Toscano, A., Vargas-Pinto, P., Delrio, C.L. et al. (2014) Arterial blood pressure as a predictor of the response to fluid administration in euvolemic nonhypotensive or hypotensive isoflurane-anesthetized dogs. *J Am Vet Med Assoc*, 245, 1021–1027.

Prittie. J. (2006) Optimal endpoints of resuscitation and early goal-directed therapy. *J Vet Emerg Crit Care*, 16, 329–339.

Rademacher, N., Pariaut, R., Pate, J., Saelinger, C., Kearney, M.T. and Gaschen, L. (2014) Transthoracic lung ultrasound in normal dogs and dogs with cardiogenic pulmonary edema: a pilot study. *Vet Radiol Ultrasound*, 55, 447–452.

Rivers, E., Nguyen, B., Havstad, S., Ressler, J., Muzzin, A. et al. (2001) Early goal-directed therapy in the treatment of severe sepsis and septic shock. *New Eng J Med*, 345, 1368–1377.

Sampson, J. and de Korte, D. (2011) DEHP-plasticised PVC: relevance to blood services. *Transfus Med*, 21, 73–83.

Sandroni, C., Cavallaro, F., Marano, C., Falcone, C., De Santis, P. and Antonelli, M. (2012) Accuracy of plethysmographic indices as predictors of fluid responsiveness in mechanically ventilated adults: a systematic review and meta-analysis. *Intens Care Med*, 38, 1429–1437.

Sasaki, K., Mutoh, T., Mutoh, T., Kawashima, R. and Tsubone, H. (2017) Electrical velocimetry for noninvasive cardiac output and stroke volume variation measurement in dogs undergoing cardiovascular surgery. *Vet Anaesth Analg*, 44, 7–16.

Scheltinga, M.R., Helton, W.S., Rounds, J., Jacobs, D.O. and Wilmore, D.W. (1991) Impedance electrodes positioned on proximal portions of limbs quantify fluid compartments in dogs. *J Appl Physiol*, 70, 2039–2044.

Schmidt, N., Saez, C., Seri, I. and Maturana, A. (2010) Impact of syringe size on the performance of infusion pumps at low flow rates. *Pediatr Crit Care Med*, 11, 282–286.

Sefidbakht, S., Assadsangabi, R., Abbasi, H.R. and Nabavizadeh, A. (2007) Sonographic measurement of the inferior vena cava as a predictor of shock in trauma patients. *Emerg Radiol*, 14, 181–185.

Seldinger, S.I. (1953) Catheter replacement of the needle in percutaneous arteriography; a new technique. *Acta Radiol*, 69, 368–376.

Silverstein, D.C. and Hopper, K. (2014) *Small Animal Critical Care Medicine*, 2nd ed. St Louis, MO: Saunders/Elsevier.

Sinha, R.P. and Ganapathy, M.S. (1967) Studies on experimental dehydration in canines, with particular reference to clinical picture, hemoglobin concentration, hematocrit, specific gravity of the plasma, and plasma sodium concentration. *Indian Vet J*, 44, 127–136.

Steffey, E.P., Pascoe, P.J., Woliner, M.J. and Berryman, E.R. (2000) Effects of xylazine hydrochloride during isoflurane-induced anesthesia in horses. *Am J Vet Res*, 61, 1225–1231.

Taguchi, H., Ichinose, K., Tanimoto, H., Sugita, M., Tashiro, M. and Yamamoto, T. (2011) Stroke volume variation obtained with Vigileo/FloTrac system during bleeding and fluid overload in dogs. *J Anesth*, 25, 563–568.

Trissel, L.A., Xu, Q.A. and Baker, M. (2006) Drug compatibility with new polyolefin infusion solution containers. *Am J Health Syst Pharm*, 63, 2379–2382.

Ueda, Y., Odunayo, A. and Mann, F.A. (2013) Comparison of heparinized saline and 0.9% sodium chloride for maintaining peripheral intravenous catheter patency in dogs. *J Vet Emerg Crit Care*, 23, 517–522.

Valverde, A., Gianotti, G. and Hathaway, A. (2011) Comparison of cardiac output determined by arterial pulse pressure waveform analysis method (FloTrac/Vigileo) versus lithium dilution method in anesthetized dogs. *J Vet Emerg Crit Care*, 21, 328–334.

Van der Eijk, A.C., van Rens, R.M., Dankelman, J. and Smit, B.J. 2013. A literature review on flow-rate variability in neonatal IV therapy. *Paediatr Anaesth*, 23, 9–21.

Wamberg, S., Sandgaard, N.C.S.F. and Bie, P. (2002) Simultaneous determination of total body water and plasma volume in conscious dogs by the indicator dilution principle. *J Nutr*, 132, 1711S–1713S.

Ward, J.L., Lisciandro, G.R., Keene, B.W., Tou, S.P. and DeFrancesco, T.C. (2017) Accuracy of point-of-care lung ultrasonography for the diagnosis of cardiogenic pulmonary edema in dogs and cats with acute dyspnea. *J Am Vet Med Assoc*, 250, 666–675.

Wellman, M.L., DiBartola, S.P. and Kohn, C.W. (2012) Applied physiology of body fluids in dogs and cats. In:

DiBartola, S.P. (ed.). *Fluid, Electrolyte, and Acid-Base Disorders in Small Animal Practice*, 4th ed. St Louis, MO: Saunders/Elsevier, pp. 2–25.

Willis, J. (1995) Infusion devices: volumetric and peristaltic pumps. *Prof Nurse*, 10, 433–435.

Zengin, S., Behcet, A..I, Genc, S., Yildirim, C., Ercan, S. *et al.* (2013) Role of inferior vena cava and right ventricular diameter in assessment of volume status: a comparative study. *Am J Emerg Med*, 31, 763–767.

Zhang, X., Feng, J., Zhu, P., Luan, H., Wu, Y. and Zhao, Z. (2016) Ultrasonographic measurements of the inferior vena cava variation as a predictor of fluid responsiveness in patients undergoing anesthesia for surgery. *J Surg Res*, 204, 118–122.

24

Anesthetic Records

Thomas Riebold

College of Veterinary Medicine, Oregon State University, Corvallis, Oregon, USA

24.1   Introduction

Anesthetic records were originally developed by Codman and Cushing in 1894 to improve patient safety (Kheterpal 2011). Since then, anesthetic records have continued to develop and become more detailed, as additional variables have been added due to availability of improved monitoring techniques. Even in their most rudimentary form, they allow the user to refer to earlier hand-plotted vital signs data, draw conclusions regarding anesthetic depth and response to anesthetic drugs and/or administration of ancillary drugs, and adjust current administration rates of those drugs. All of this allows the anesthesia provider to make rational decisions regarding anesthetic management and provide benefit and safety to the patient.

24.2   Maintaining Anesthetic Records

Maintaining an anesthetic record, while anesthetizing animals, is a very important part of case management. In addition to allowing one to observe trends in vital signs and record changes made in anesthetic drug and ancillary drug administration, the anesthetic record also serves as a legal document and serves as a component of the patient's medical record. An accurate anesthetic record allows one to verify duration of anesthesia and the procedure(s) performed, to document anesthetic drugs administered to the animal, to record the animal's responses to those drugs, to document supportive therapy that is delivered, and to document participation of personnel involved in the procedure. An accurate anesthetic record provides the user with the opportunity to determine the cause of complications should they occur, so that future potential complications can be recognized sooner and better prevented; thus, it is a valuable adjunct to increase safety of

anesthesia. Completed anesthetic records also serve as reference points when animals are anesthetized for subsequent procedures and allow one to perform retrospective studies to assess efficacy and safety of anesthetic protocols. Finally, if litigation occurs as a result of an anesthetic related complication, the anesthetic record serves to verify the events that occurred with the animal's care and conveys the veterinary team's commitment to delivering a high level of care.

24.3   Monitoring Recommendations

The American College of Veterinary Anesthesia and Analgesia (ACVAA) formulated guidelines for monitoring anesthesia in 1994 and again in 2009 (American College of Veterinary Anesthesia and Analgesia 2009). Those guidelines include sequential assessment of circulation, oxygenation, ventilation and temperature.

The ACVAA also recommends that an anesthetic record be maintained and that it includes the amount, route and time of all drugs administered during anesthesia, including whether unanticipated reactions occurred with drug administration. Additionally, it is recommended that the data from all available monitored vital signs be recorded, preferably at 5-minute intervals, and at no greater than 10-minute intervals. Other components of the anesthetic record should include the owner's name, patient identification number, patient signalment (species, breed, name, age, weight, sex and physical status), the premedication, induction and maintenance drug(s) used, supportive therapy administered, personnel involved and the reason for anesthesia.

State veterinary licensing boards often do not require what are traditionally considered anesthetic records to be maintained. Their requirements are often met by recording the amounts of drugs used, their concentration, and time and route of administration in the animal's

Veterinary Anesthetic and Monitoring Equipment, First Edition. Edited by Kristen G. Cooley and Rebecca A. Johnson.
© 2018 John Wiley & Sons, Inc. Published 2018 by John Wiley & Sons, Inc.

medical record. Licensing boards often require documentation that the patient was observed until it recovered from anesthesia. Taking the additional step of maintaining a thorough anesthetic record that includes the patient's physiological responses to administration of anesthetic drugs and supportive medication is valuable, as it conveys an impression of the level of care delivered to the patient and the practice's commitment to patient safety as well as its attention to detail.

24.4 Paper Anesthetic Records

Traditional paper records (Figure 24.1) have been maintained for decades during delivery of veterinary anesthesia. There are numerous versions of paper records, many of which are unique to the user, but they have many common features. As previously mentioned, they should include various fields for entry of the owner's name, patient identification number, patient signalment (species, breed, age, weight, gender and physical status), the personnel involved, the procedure, drugs used, supportive therapy administered, information regarding recovery, and incidence of intra-operative and post-operative complications. Many also include a grid to record values for the physiological variables recorded at 5-minute intervals by use of different characters for each variable. This method allows for trend monitoring at a glance. Some basic monitoring sheets are not graph-based and require the anesthetist to record actual values at intervals (Figure 24.2). Additionally, space is available on the record to note remarks pertinent to the case as free text. There is also some variety in the record, as some are designed to allow the user to record salient portions of blood gas analysis results, pre-operative hematology and chemistry data, etc., while other records do not have those features.

Many paper records are customized for their location, either by purchase or by obtaining a suitable record and superimposing the letterhead of the veterinary clinic or hospital on it. One can also use commercially available software (e.g. InDesign®, Adobe Systems Incorporated, San Jose, CA) to create custom forms that can be used as anesthesia records. The record is printed either as a single sheet form or printed on multiple page NCR (No Carbon Required) paper.

Paper anesthetic records have distinct advantages, such as their simplicity and ability to hold much data in a succinct format. A well-designed form can prompt the user to complete the fields, facilitating training of new personnel. Printing the record on NCR paper enables multiple copies to automatically be made, allowing the user to place one copy in the patient's medical record and to save the others in multiple places. Proper record use allows the user to plot the patient's physiological data at 5-minute intervals and observe the trends as they begin to form on the graph, and thus adjust drug administration or intervene when necessary.

In contrast, paper anesthetic records also have disadvantages. If NCR paper is used, the user must press firmly with their pen to insure transfer of the information to the other sheets. With time, written information can fade. The record is also susceptible to physical damage from liquid spills while it is being compiled or after. While paper records allow accurate completion of the fields, they are inherently imprecise with vital signs data. Their completion is dependent on the user's diligence in recording the data points accurately on the graph, because the scale on the vertical axis is often in large increments. Retrospectively, the user can have trouble differentiating values; for example, discerning 83 heartbeats per minute from 82 or 84 beats per minute. In many instances, that level of precision is not needed unless the record is being maintained as part of a prospective research study or one is performing a retrospective study where accuracy of data is important. Non-graphic monitoring forms have the advantage when accuracy is required, because the actual value is recorded rather than a symbol on a graph. The use of a paper record is prone to errors of omission, in that gaps in the data occur because of lack of user attention or distraction when the next set of vital signs data is due. Lastly, when a retrospective study is performed, the pertinent data must be extracted individually from each record, a laborious process.

24.5 Electronic Anesthetic Records

The influence of computers on our personal and business lives has extended to the medical profession. The last two decades have seen a transition from paper medical records to electronic medical record-keeping in human healthcare. Interested individuals have utilized the power and utility of computers and software to develop an area of anesthesia called Anesthesia Informatics, with textbooks (Stonemetz and Ruskin 2008; Kheterpal and Tremper 2011) and chapters within textbooks devoted to that subject (Dorsch and Dorsch 2008; Kheterpal 2011; Ruskin 2013; St Jacques and Berry 2013). The efforts of those interested individuals, in conjunction with software developers, have produced commercial Anesthesia Information Management Systems (AIMS) for use during anesthesia of people in community hospitals and referral centers.

☐ External defibrillation
☐ Internal defibrillation
☐ Do Not Resuscitate

ANESTHETIC RECORD

Patient ID _____ Body weight _____ Case No._____ Cage/Stall No._____ ☐ Out-Patient

Preanesthetic Medication				
Physical status (circle) I II III IV V Emergency Heart Rate _____ Respiratory Rate _____ Comments _____	Lab Results	Sedation Present None Moderate Mild Marked	Procedure	Recumbency (circle) Sternal Dorsal Left lateral Right lateral Other _____

Time	:00	15	30	45	:00	15	30	45	:00	15	30	45
Vaporizer Setting (%)												
Expired Agent (%)												
Oxygen (L/M)												

Anesthesia
START STOP

Procedure
START STOP

CODE

• Pulse rate
o Respiratory rate
V Systolic pressure
∧ Diastolic pressure
+ Mean arterial pressure
☐ Carbon dioxide
∆ Oxygen saturation

MONITORS USED
☐ Direct BP
☐ Indirect BP
　☐ Doppler
　☐ Oscillometric
　Cuff Size ____
☐ ECG
☐ Blood gas analysis
☐ $ETco_2$ / F_iO_2
☐ Pulse oximetry
☐ ET Agent
☐ Temperature
☐ Other
　_____
　_____

(graph y-axis values: 200 190 180 170 160 150 140 130 120 110 100 90 80 70 60 50 40 30 20 10 0)

Surgeon _____ Staff
Anesthetist _____ Staff
Surgeon _____ Student
Anesthetist _____ Student

ANESTHETIC AGENTS
a. Induction _____
_____
b. Maintenance _____
_____

E/T Tube ☐ Nasal ☐ Oral
　☐ Tracheotomy Size _____
Endobronchial ☐ Right ☐ Left
　Size _____

ANESTHETIC SYSTEM
a. Induction
　☐ Inhalation ☐ IV _____
b. Maintenance _____
　☐ Semiclosed circle Amount discarded
　☐ Closed circle
　☐ Nonrebreathing
　☐ IV _____

IV Fluids Yes _____ No _____
Catheter Sites
_____
_____

Complications ☐ No
　☐ Yes _____
Duration of Anesthesia / Recovery
_____
Recovery Quality _____

Dobutamine / Dopamine Given	Total Fluids Given

REMARKS: Medication, Fluids, Amount, Route; Blood Gas Analysis, etc.

Anesthetist _____ Date _____
(Signature)

ANESTHETIC RECORD

Rev 11/06 (press firmly when writing) White copy--case record Canary--anesthesiology

Figure 24.1 An example of a graph-based paper anesthetic record.

Anesthesia Monitoring Form

TRUE VETERINARY CARE

PATIENT ID STICKER

Date:_____ Dr:_____ CVT:_____

Weight in Lb:_____ Weight in kg:_____ Anesthesia Risk Score:_____

Procedure(s):_____

Preoperative Vitals: T:_____   P:_____   R:_____

Premedication:_____

Premed Route: IM Time:_____ Sedation:_____ Rebreathing / Non-rebreathing

IVC gauge:_____   Location:_____ Fluid type:_____   Fluid Rate Range:_____

Propofol 4mg/kg:_____   Draw:_____   Amount Given:_____   Waste:_____

ET Tube size:_____   Fit:_____   Intubated/Iso Start:_____   Iso Off:_____   Extubated:_____   Eyes Lubed:____

Nail Trim:_____Total Fluids:_____   Anesthesia Maint:___Iso/Oxygen___   Before Pic:___ After Pic:___

Notes:

Time																			
O_2 L																			
ISO%																			
HR																			
CO_2																			
RR																			
SPO_2																			
BP S																			
BP D																			
MAP																			
Temp																			
IVF																			

Figure 24.2 An example of a tabular format anesthetic record (record courtesy of True Veterinary Care, Verona, Wisconsin-Madison, WI).

These products have both a hardware and software component. Hardware components of these systems include a server, and network and multiple workstations present in locations where patients are anesthetized. The software component can include several phases of patient care, beginning with pre-operative care and including anesthetic management and post-anesthetic care. By interfacing with the patient's electronic medical record, information can be obtained about health history, current medications, laboratory results and imaging results, allowing anesthetic risk to be assessed and case classification to be assigned.

Components of AIMS while the patient is anesthetized include an interface with patient multi-parameter monitors and display of the data for those variables on a computer/screen mounted on or near the anesthesia machine, and automatic transfer of that data to the patient's anesthetic record. Correction of artifacts in the transferred data must also be provided, as well as provision for recording information that cannot be obtained from patient monitors; for example, color of mucous membranes, perfusion time, palpebral and/or ocular reflexes, response to peripheral nerve stimulation, name, amount and route of drugs administered, alterations in patient position, and other interventions.

It is also preferable that the software interfaces with the anesthesia machine and ventilator for automatic transfer of information regarding carrier gas flow rate, vaporizer setting and ventilator settings (rate, tidal volume, inspiratory:expiratory ratio and inspiratory pressure). The software should also continue to gather information during the recovery phase following the patient's transfer to the post-anesthetic care unit.

These systems are very sophisticated and fulfill a number of purposes. Foremost, they generate an anesthetic record. They also aid hospital administrative functions by generating billing information and by allowing tracking of number of cases managed by individual providers. The software aids the academic and research mission of the institution by providing records of individual cases that can be used for training purposes or collectively for generation of retrospective studies. Lastly, their use provides convenience and accuracy, and generates a very thorough and comprehensive anesthetic record (Shah *et al.* 2011).

24.5.1 Advantages of AIMS

Advantages of AIMS are accuracy and legibility of the anesthetic record, timeliness, the option for performing retrospective studies and outcome assessment studies, quality assurance, decreased paper use, accessibility of the patients' previous anesthesia records, convenience and use for administrative purposes (scheduling, room usage, billing, etc.). Another advantage is decision support. For example, anesthetic software interfaced with hospital information software can allow the user to access the patient's record to determine results of clinical pathology examinations, presence of drug sensitivities, etc., which help make timely bedside patient decisions (Shah *et al.* 2011).

24.5.2 Disadvantages of AIMS

Disadvantages of AIMS include the potential for recording artifacts as true data from the patient monitors. In addition, space and accommodations for computers, display screens and keyboards in locations where anesthesia is performed are required. Interfacing the various software products in the hospital and with the various types of patient monitors can be challenging. User attitude and acceptance, training, security and lack of standardization between programs also pose difficulties (Shah *et al.* 2011). The cost of AIMS is considerable, estimated to be up to $30,000 per anesthesia location, not including purchase of the multi-parameter patient monitor to interface with it (Sorci 2016). Thus, the equipment cost of AIMS plus the required IT support makes adoption of these systems in veterinary medicine unlikely.

24.5.3 Examples of AIMS Software

Examples of these systems include Innovian® Anesthesia (Dräger Inc., Teford, PA), Centricity® (GE Healthcare, Madison, WI), OpTime OR Management System® (Epic Systems Corporation, Verona, WI), SurgiNet® Anesthesia Management (Cerner Corporation PTY Limited, North Sydney, Australia), Metavision® (iMDsoft, Dusseldorf, Germany), Picis Anesthesia® (Picis, Wakefield, MA), CompuRecord® (Phillips Healthcare, Highlands Heights, OH), SIS Anesthesia® (Surgical Information Systems, Alpharett, GA) and Anesthesia Touch® (Plexus Technology Group, Birmingham, AL) (Figure 24.3).

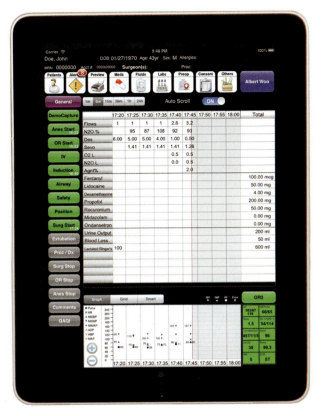

Figure 24.3 An example of AIMS technology, specifically the Anesthesia Touch, Plexus Anesthesia Information Management Systems digital anesthetic record-keeping software (photograph courtesy of Plexus Technology Group, Birmingham, Alabama).

24.6 Transitioning from Paper to Electronic Medical Records

The transition from paper to electronic medical records is also occurring in veterinary medicine. Veterinary software has evolved from practice management (scheduling, reminder cards, inventory, billing, etc.) to also include more and more of the patient's medical record. It is logical that paperless anesthetic record systems be developed to interface with electronic medical records. Much progress has been made in monitoring technology and it has become available or adaptable for use in anesthetized veterinary patients. That progress has outpaced the methods used to record the information. Various methods of digital anesthesia record-keeping are starting to be developed, as the progression of electronic veterinary medical records continues.

At this time, most anesthetic records in veterinary practices, when kept, are paper records. Some veterinarians are using commercial spreadsheet software (e.g. Microsoft Excel®) to record data in tabular form. Use of spreadsheet software to record vital signs data in anesthetized animals creates a permanent record. It has the advantage of being customizable for the user, as the user can create rows for the variables that are monitored in anesthetized animals and columns for time. Data from spreadsheet software is also available to the user while anesthesia is ongoing. The disadvantage is that the data are presented in tabular format and not in graphical format. Trend formation is more difficult to quickly ascertain during critical situations when the data are presented in tabular format, particularly if many variables are monitored and the case is lengthy.

24.7 Specific Types of Anesthetic Monitoring Software

24.7.1 SurgiVet Veterinary Data Logger®

One veterinary anesthesia vendor, SurgiVet (Smiths Medical, Dublin, Ohio), manufactures a multi-parameter monitor (Advisor®) that accepts a data logger (only Data Logger® compatible Advisor® monitors) (Figure 24.4). The purpose of this product is to reduce human error associated with manually transcribed data. It records patient vital signs at regular intervals and has the capability to capture screen shots and primary ECG tracings that can later be uploaded into the patient's medical record.

The Data Logger® utilizes an SD card for data transfer to a personal computer to be integrated into the medical record, emailed or printed out. The user has a choice between a basic or detailed anesthetic record (Figure 24.5). After downloading the data to either of the two anesthesia forms, the user is able to enter comments about the case, and record amounts of drugs administered, results of pre-operative hematology and chemistry examinations, amount of intravenous fluids

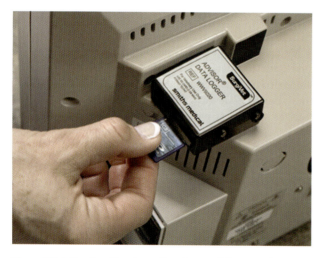

Figure 24.4 Surgivet Veterinary Data Logger (photograph courtesy of Smiths Medical, Dublin, Ohio).

administered, etc. The user does not have access intra-operatively to the record to add notes or record information as it occurs. The anesthetist must wait until anesthesia is completed and use their notes to accurately compile the record. After the record is completed, it can be attached to the clinic/hospital's hospital information software.

24.7.2 Morpheus® Electronic Anesthesia Sheet

Another veterinary product is the Morpheus® Electronic Anesthesia Sheet, part of Smart Flow® Sheet's suite of products (Veterinarium Corp., Etobicoke, Ontario). Smart Flow® software works alongside all types of practice management software and can integrate easily into any hospital to help optimize patient care.

Morpheus® is an iPad® application that allows the user to work up and monitor an anesthetic case from intake through recovery, as well as record vital signs, test results and events during an anesthetic event. The user is able to fully tailor the anesthetic monitoring sheet to match what is currently being used (Figure 24.6). It offers the option to include drug dosages and calculations as well as fully customizable templates for common types of procedures. The information on the sheet can be as basic or as detailed as each clinic sees fit. The application will interface with some brands of anesthetic monitors, such as Cardell (Midmark Corporation, Versailles, Ohio), Digicare (Digicare Animal Health, Boynton Beach, Florida), Bionet (Bionet America, Tustin, California), DRE (DRE Healthcare, Louisville, Kentucky), Vetland (Vetland Louisville, Kentucky) and SurgiVet (Smiths Medical, Dublin, Ohio), to automatically populate the monitoring sheet with patient vital signs at regular intervals.

Morpheus® allows for the use of color-coding, which can be used to highlight changes in trending data or to draw attention to specific events or interventions (addition of adjunctive medications, change in anesthetic depth, etc.), also allowing for the sheet to be manually updated in the application during a case (Figure 24.7). It also permits entry of oxygen flow rate, vaporizer settings, and will calculate duration of anesthesia and surgery. Finally, the application can be used offline if the Internet connection is compromised. The data is then automatically updated once the software comes online again. This is helpful in areas where WiFi is not available, such as in an MRI area.

24.7.3 Veterinary Digital Anesthesia Record Keeping

Another application, Veterinary Digital Anesthesia Records (VetDAR,® Dimple Hill Software, Corvallis, Oregon) is software that can be loaded on an individual

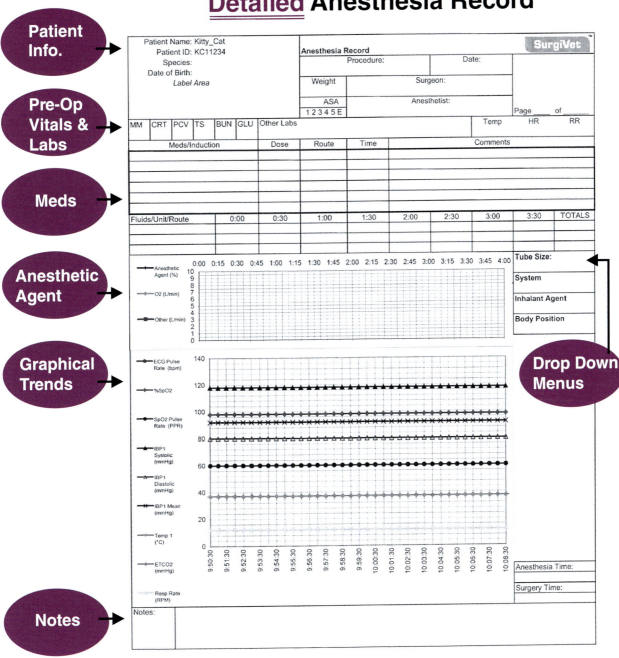

Figure 24.5 Surgivet Veterinary Data Logger Detailed Anesthesia sheet (courtesy of Smiths Medical, Dublin, Ohio).

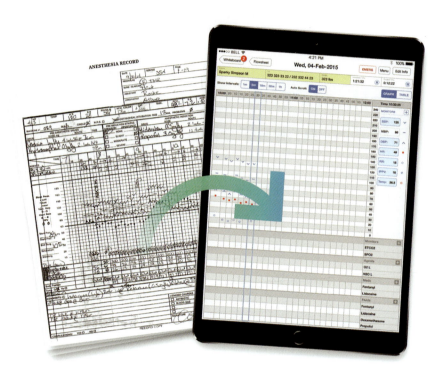

Figure 24.6 Smart Flow's Morpheus® electronic anesthetic record allows the user to transfer all of the information from a paper record onto their iPad based digital record (image courtesy of Veterinarium Corp, Etobicoke, Ontario).

notebook, tablet or MacIntosh located where anesthesia is administered or installed on a server for use with multiple individual workstations (Figure 24.8). It has many distinct advantages over some other products. For example, VetDAR® allows the user to record pre-operative information, document their pre-operative patient assessment, formulate an anesthetic plan, select and record drugs, and select the monitors used during anesthesia. It has a built-in formulary and can automatically calculate patient-specific drug doses, as well as an emergency formulary containing emergency drugs, fluid rates and ventilator settings. It prompts the user to record intra-operative information, and graphs vital signs, flowmeter settings and vaporizer data. It also records remarks following administration of medications, mechanical ventilator settings, other interventions and other pertinent comments (Figure 24.9).

VetDAR® can record post-operative information and vital information during recovery. It summarizes the duration of anesthesia, all entered procedures, mechanical ventilation information, and the amounts of drugs administered and discarded. It also provides veterinary anesthesiologists with remote access via the Internet to ongoing cases, which helps with prompt decision support to individuals anesthetizing cases in other areas. While the anesthetic record can be attached to the patient's medical record, VetDAR® retains all the anes-

thetic records in a separate, secure database, rather than dispersing them to the individual case records for easy record retrievability for training, demographic or research use.

24.8 Patient Management and Digital Records

Case management is improved with electronic monitoring products, because the software will record the data in tabular format and display the data in graphical format in real time, allowing the user to see a display similar to that of a traditional paper anesthesia record. Having the data graphed allows the user to quickly identify subtle trends in vital signs and intervene when needed to decrease the incidence of complications. Additionally, most software prompts the user at defined intervals (e.g. every 5 minutes) to re-evaluate the patient and enter the current data for vital signs. Entry of vital signs data by the person responsible for monitoring anesthesia virtually eliminates the likelihood of artifactual data being recorded and helps the anesthetist to remain on task if they are multitasking during the anesthetic event.

These applications reduce the likelihood of mistakes by providing decision support. For example, in some applications, when the user enters in the species and

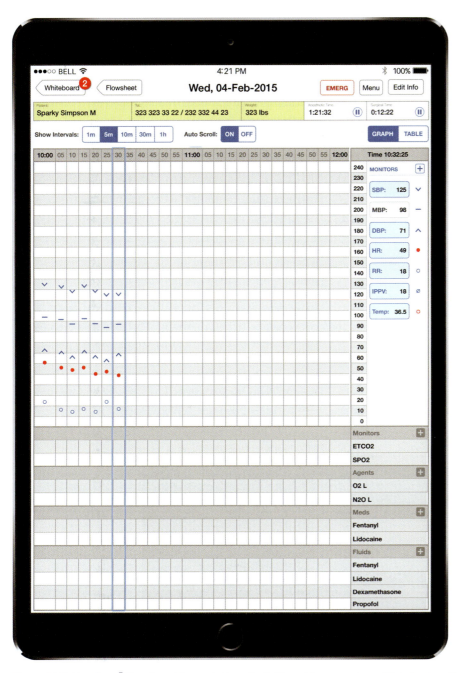

Figure 24.7 Morpheus® Veterinary Electronic Anesthetic Sheet (sheet courtesy of Veterinarium Corp, Etobicoke, Ontario).

weight of the patient, a number of calculations are made. Some brands (VetDAR® and Morpheus®) provide a formulary to populate the dosage range for anesthesia-related drugs (sedatives, tranquilizers, induction agents, ancillary drugs, emergency drugs, etc.) and calculate doses. VetDAR® specifically provides users with anesthetic, analgesic and ancillary drug doses for multiple species including dogs, cats, horses, cattle, sheep, goats, camelids and swine. In addition to calculating the dose of anesthetics, some software also calculates the volume of

emergency drugs appropriate for the patient as previously mentioned.

Alterations in vital parameters produce automatic alerts with these systems. Specifically, the entry of species allows the VetDAR® software to calculate normal limits for species–specific vital signs. Morpheus® relies on the parameter alarms built into the anesthetic monitor as does the Data Logger®. When values for vital signs fall outside the normal range, an alarm sounds or that field is highlighted on the screen, attracting the users'

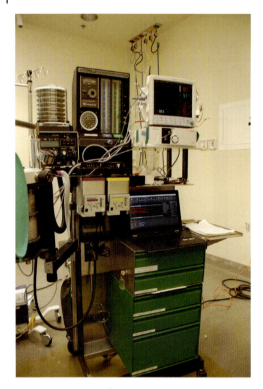

Figure 24.8 VetDAR® laptop based software shown integrated into an anesthesia workstation (photograph courtesy of VetDAR®, Corvallis, Oregon).

attention. In the VetDAR® software, when data for vital signs changes by more than 20% between successive readings, but are still within the normal range, that field is highlighted in yellow, conveying to the user that even though the data point is within the normal range, a significant change has occurred and increased vigilance is warranted.

The use of handwritten anesthesia records has done much to improve patient management. Anesthetic record-keeping software will allow one to incorporate the anesthetic record into the patient's electronic medical record and continue the transition to electronic medical records in veterinary medicine. The currently available electronic anesthetic record products for veterinary use have a variety of features, but none of them have all of the features of the AIMS products available for use with anesthetized persons. It is expected that currently available and future veterinary products will continue to mature and provide additional patient safety and convenience to veterinarians. The reader is directed to the websites of the individual companies for more current information as additional features are added to those applications. Implementation of these applications is dependent on cost, benefit, IT infrastructure requirements, ease of use, customer service, etc. and is a decision left to the practice owner(s). Use of these applications

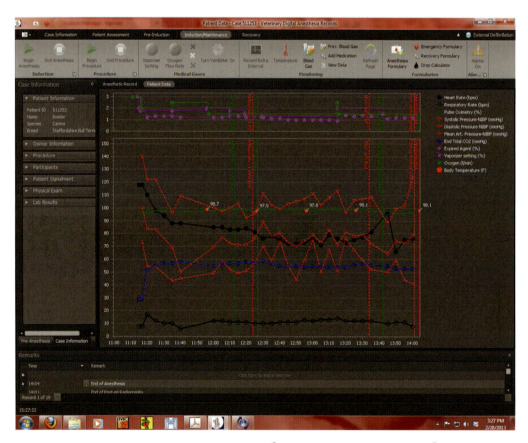

Figure 24.9 Detailed anesthetic record from the VetDAR® system (sheet courtesy of VetDAR®, Corvallis, Oregon).

will provide availability of more comprehensive anesthetic records that will allow the user and others to have a better opportunity to determine the cause of complications when they occur during and after anesthesia and will allow further improvement in patient safety with retrospective studies of anesthesia records.

24.9 Automated Dispensing Systems and Record Keeping

Automated dispensing systems are designed to quickly dispense and accurately record all agents and supplies removed from them, including scheduled or controlled substances. These systems use computers to inventory all anesthetic supplies within them (as well as other hospital supplies), thus improving controlled substance regulation, record keeping, inventory management and client billing. The secure, locked systems are accessed by personal keycode or fingerprint and are configured in many useable designs (Figure 24.10). After gaining entrance into the system, the patient's record number (or name) is obtained and all supplies are directly removed and recorded specifically under their identifying file. Although many manufacturers are available, two are frequently used in veterinary medicine, OmniCell® (Mountainview, CA) and Cubex (Therian Animal Care Solutions, Ashmore, Australia). Although they sometimes dispense only in preset amounts (e.g. 5 mL of midazolam, 10 mL of propofol), multiuse vials can be placed inside and used as well. In these instances, the specific desired amount is typed into the unit and withdrawn by anesthesia personnel. To help keep track of these agents, VetDAR® has a space where the dispensed amount can be entered in the case where the amount

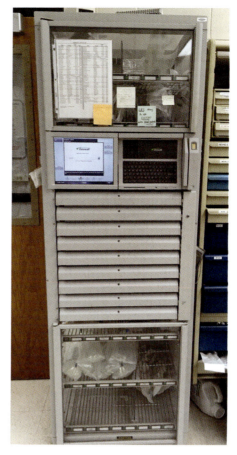

Figure 24.10 The OmniCell® automatic dispenser system. All controlled substances are kept within the drawers and are automatically recorded to the patient.

dispensed is more than the amount used for the patient. All substances are thereby accounted for automatically, reducing human error in drug usage records.

References

American College of Veterinary Anesthesia and Analgesia (2009) Recommendations for monitoring anesthetized veterinary patients. Available from: http//www.acvaa.org/docs/smallanimal [accessed September 9, 2016].

Dorsch, J.A. and Dorsch, S.E. (2008) *Understanding Anesthesia Equipment*, 5th ed. Philadelphia, PA: Lippincott Williams & Wilkins.

Kheterpal. S. (2011) Anesthesia information management systems. In: Sandberg, W.S., Urman, R.D. and Ehrenfeld, J.M. (eds). *The MGH Textbook of Anesthesia Equipment.* Philadelphia, PA: Elsevier Saunders, pp. 283–296.

Kheterpal, S. and Tremper, K.K. (2011) Information technology applied to anesthesiology. In: *Anesthesiology Clinics*, vols 29-3. Philadelphia, PA: Elsevier Saunders.

Ruskin, K.J. (2013) Computing and the internet in clinical practice. In: Ehrenwerth. J., Eisenkraft, J.B. and Berry,

J.M. (eds). *Anesthesia Equipment: Principles and Applications*. Philadelphia, PA: Elsevier Saunders, pp. 424–433.

Shah, N.J., Tremper, K.K. and Kheterpal, S. (2011) Anatomy of an anesthesia information management system. *Anesthesiol Clin*, 29, 355–365.

Sorci, M. (2016) Anesthesia equipment supply. *Black Diamond, WA: personal communication.*

Stonemetz, J. and Ruskin, K. (2008) *Anesthesia Informatics.* Verlag, London: Springer.

St Jacques, P. and Berry, J.M. (2013) Perioperative informatics. In: Ehrenwerth, J., Eisenkraft, J.B. and Berry, J.M. (eds). *Anesthesia Equipment: Principles and Applications*. Philadelphia, PA: Elsevier Saunders, pp. 434–447.

25

Equipment for the Magnetic Resonance Imaging System

Kris Kruse-Elliott

AnimalScan SF, Redwood City, California, USA

25.1 Basic Principles of Magnetic Resonance Imaging

Magnetic resonance imaging (MRI) systems are becoming increasingly common in veterinary medicine. For veterinary patients, MRI is particularly useful for imaging the central nervous system and musculoskeletal system, as well as occasional imaging of the cardiovascular system, other major organs, peripheral nerves and miscellaneous body regions (Labruyere and Schwarz 2013). Many consider MRI safer than imaging modalities that use ionizing radiation (conventional radiography, computed tomography [CT], fluoroscopy). However, MRI does present rather unique challenges to patient care and safety, due to the environment of very powerful stagnant magnetic fields and radiofrequency energy used to produce images. Scanning times for MRI are usually a minimum of 30 minutes and are frequently greater than an hour, during which patients must be free of motion. On the other hand, CT scans can take just a few minutes (Labruyere and Schwarz 2013). Consequently, general anesthesia is usually required for veterinary MRI. Functional and safe anesthesia and monitoring of the anesthetized patient requires specialized MRI compatible equipment. This equipment must be tested and certified safe and is, unfortunately, significantly more expensive and difficult to obtain than conventional veterinary anesthesia equipment.

25.1.1 MRI Classification

25.1.1.1 Low Field MRI

MRI systems are classified as low or high field, depending on the strength of the static magnetic field. Low field MRI scanners commonly have field strengths of 0.2–0.4 Tesla (T) and are either permanent or resistive magnets (Bushong 2003b; Westbrook *et al.* 2011b). Permanent magnet low field MRI systems result when

ferromagnetic material is exposed to an external magnet and becomes permanently magnetized. Permanent magnets consist of a flat magnet above and below an open space, with a table for the patient between the two magnets (Figure 25.1). They are extremely heavy (5000–40 000 kg), but have almost no fringe field (see below) beyond more than a meter in any direction. They also have an open gantry, which makes for easy patient access. Permanent magnets have a limited but fixed magnetic field that is always present.

In contrast, resistive low field MRIs are more common than permanent magnet MRI systems. Resistive MRIs require significant current passing through coiled wire to generate the magnetic field (Westbrook *et al.* 2011b). Resistive magnets have very high power requirements and need a water cooling system; however, they can be turned off and the magnetic field shut down by cutting power to the magnet. The field strength of a resistive magnet MRI is usually 0.2–0.5 T.

While low field MRIs are relatively less expensive to operate than a high field superconducting MRI, the images from low field MRI systems may be of lesser quality, depending on the body region being imaged. In addition, scans can take substantially longer than with a high field, superconducting magnet. Regardless, while they are described as low field magnets, they still pose the hazard of a powerful magnetic field and require considerable considerations for personnel safety and the required selection of compatible anesthesia equipment (Bushong 2003d).

25.1.1.2 High Field MRI

High field or superconducting MRIs generate a powerful static magnetic field at strengths from 1.0–3.0 T, with some research scanners having field strengths up to 9 T (Bushong 2003b; Westbrook *et al.* 2011b; Labruyere and Schwarz 2013). For perspective, the strength of Earth's magnetic field is somewhat less than 1 Gauss (G),

Veterinary Anesthetic and Monitoring Equipment, First Edition. Edited by Kristen G. Cooley and Rebecca A. Johnson.
© 2018 John Wiley & Sons, Inc. Published 2018 by John Wiley & Sons, Inc.

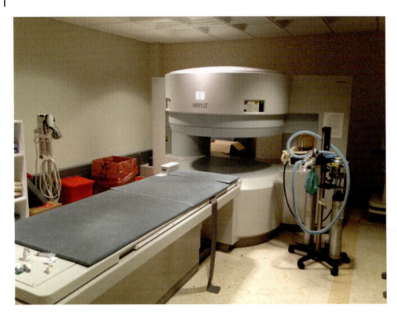

Figure 25.1 Example of a low-field permanent magnet used for MRI. Note the flat magnets that reside above and below the patient area with a table that moves between the two for scanning (photograph courtesy of Jim Stuppino, CEO, AnimalScan LLC, Easton, PA).

depending on your location. One T is equivalent to 10 000 G, therefore a 1-T MRI has a static magnetic field that is 10 000 times that of the Earth; the static magnetic field of a 3-T MRI is 30 000 times the Earth's magnetic field.

High field MRI scanners are constructed with alloy coils that allow superconductivity when cooled below a critical temperature of 4 Kelvin (−269 °C or −450 °F), usually with liquid helium or occasionally with liquid nitrogen. While electrical current is initially required to create the magnetic field, once the magnet is ramped up to full strength, the magnetic field is always present, regardless of power supply to the coils. Consequently, the dangers associated with these extremely powerful magnets are a constant concern, even when the scanner is not in use for imaging patients (Bushong 2003d; Westbrook *et al.* 2011b). Failure to limit access to the MRI suite and the "always on" state of these magnets has resulted in several accidents with significant injury, especially since the magnetic field makes no sound to warn of its presence (Chen 2001; Gosbee and Gosbee 2003; Zimmer *et al.* 2004; Miller 2005; Joint Commission 2008; Tan *et al.* 2014).

25.1.2   Image Generation

While a complete discussion of image generation is beyond the scope of this chapter, a brief overview of the basics helps in understanding the nature and hazards of the working environment when anesthetizing patients for MRI. The interaction of atomic nuclei with the magnetic field is exploited in generating images (Menon *et al.* 1992; Bushong 2003a; Westbrook *et al.* 2011a; Labruyere and Schwarz 2013). Within the nucleus of an atom,

individual protons and neutrons spin about their axis. In nuclei with odd mass numbers, there is a net spin or angular momentum; these are magnetic resonance active nuclei.

MRI uses the magnetic property of protons, in particular hydrogen ion protons, which are present in abundance in water found throughout body tissues. When a patient is placed within the bore of a MRI scanner, the static magnetic field causes these normally randomly orientated nuclei to align relative to the magnetic field. Thus, all the individual magnetic moments of nuclei are aligned with the external static field of the MRI.

Using radiofrequency (RF) pulses, a secondary magnetic field is created, which changes the alignment of protons within the static magnetic field. When this RF pulse is discontinued, the nuclei realign to the magnetic field, thus releasing energy (which is called relaxation). This generates an RF signal proportional to the difference between the energized magnetic resonance state of the nucleus and its original alignment in the magnetic field. Radiofrequency receiver coils detect these low-level RF signals; they are amplified and processed to create images. Realignment rates (relaxation times) vary, depending on the body tissue. This creates the observed contrast between various tissues in MRI. By varying the combination of RF pulses and magnetic fields during the scan, different tissue contrasts can be created and imaged.

In order to prevent interference from outside stray RF waves, the entire MRI suite is shielded with copper from the walls to the windows. Paging systems, radio systems, television transmitters, etc. can all interfere with image acquisition and create artifacts on MRI images that render the images unable to be interpreted. Similarly, any

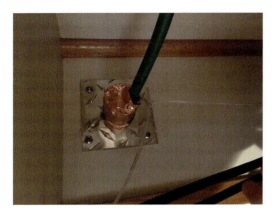

Figure 25.2 Copper shielded wave-guides can be placed during MRI suite construction and are shown here with an oxygen line and sampling tubing running through.

anesthesia equipment must have shielding to prevent RF interference. This is part of the requirement for MRI compatible equipment (Peden *et al.* 1992; McBrien *et al.* 2000; Joint Commission 2008; Reddy 2012; Henrichs and Walsh 2014). As discussed below, when anesthesia equipment cannot be housed in the MRI suite due to incompatibility, it can be kept just outside and adjacent to the room. A wave-guide or copper-shielded pipe (Figure 25.2) is used to pass cables and tubing into the room and maintain the integrity of the RF shielding (Miller 2005).

25.2 Regulations

In the US, federal safety standards, guidelines and regulations governing MRI are managed through the Division of Radiological Health within the Food and Drug Administration (FDA) (Delfino 2015). The FDA oversees and regulates the manufacture, repackaging, labeling and re-labeling, and import of devices such as MRI equipment. MRI systems are FDA Class II devices and are subject to performance standards, special labeling requirements, premarket data requirements, and other FDA-defined general controls (Delfino 2015). The actual installation and use of MRI equipment is regulated by various federal or state agencies, as well as by any accreditation bodies and institutional regulations.

In the EU, there are directives published as legislative acts from 2013, which spell out the goals for health and safety requirements for exposure to electromagnetic fields that EU members are expected to achieve. However, it is up to the individual countries to implement these directives and the European Society of Radiology has published diagnostic imaging standards that include MRI safety guidelines (Directive 2013/35/EU 2016, European Society of Radiology 2016). The Royal

Australian and New Zealand College of Radiologists have guidelines for quality and safety, which include quality assurance activities for MRI (Royal Australian and New Zealand College of Radiologists 2016). Their website includes an MRI resource list with information on accreditation, as well as links to MRI safety guidelines for the region. In general, most international and US regulations incorporate similar safety standards and guidelines.

In veterinary medicine, MRI equipment installation and use is variably regulated among localities. This is particularly true concerning repurposed, refurbished, older MRI equipment that migrates from the human medical facilities into veterinary practices. This happens through a variety of vendors of used equipment with variable knowledge and understanding of MRI. Even in human medicine, there can be some variation in facility preparedness for performing MRI on anesthetized patients (McBrien *et al.* 2000). Awareness of the need for safety standards has steadily increased, with heightened interest in performing interventional procedures in the MRI suite (Henrichs and Walsh 2014; Apfelbaum *et al.* 2015). For anesthesia in the MRI suite, the American Society of Anesthesiologists has a practice advisory regarding patient care that is regularly updated and a resource on patient and personnel hazards and recommendations regarding anesthesia equipment for MRI (Apfelbaum *et al.* 2015).

25.3 MRI Hazard Classification

The American Society for Testing and Materials (ASTM) sets the standards for how devices are marked for MRI safety. They classify MRI hazards as either direct or indirect (ASTM International 2013; Delfino 2015). Direct hazards can be classified as mechanical, electromagnetic and acoustic. Strong magnetically-induced displacement forces, torque and vibration create mechanical hazards (Bushong 2003c; Gilk and Kanal 2013; Kanal *et al.* 2013; Westbrook 2011b). Electromagnetic hazards include induction (heating and stimulation) and discharge (spark gap). Noise during scanning caused by switching of the gradient magnetic field creates an acoustic hazard to personnel working in the environment. In addition, with non-MRI compatible monitors, anesthesia machines, pumps or other equipment malfunction, an indirect hazard is produced with the potential for patient harm due to equipment failure; this also includes implantable programmable devices such as pacemakers.

The ASTM also defines how items should be labeled with regard to their use (Woods 2007, ASTM International 2013, Gilk and Kanal 2013, Bell 2016). Three categories of standardization are MRI Safe, MRI

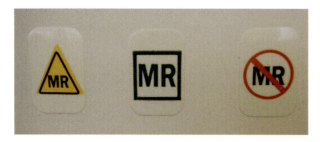

Figure 25.3 ASTM labeling for MRI equipment compliance. The yellow triangle on the left indicates MRI Conditional, the green square indicates MRI Safe, and the red circle indicates MRI Unsafe.

Conditional, and MRI Unsafe (Figure 25.3). MRI Safe items are non-magnetic and non-conducting, for example, plastic parts on an anesthesia machine or plastic tubing. MRI Conditional items do not pose a hazard in the MRI environment, as long as their use is within specified parameters. For example, items that must be kept a minimum distance from the bore of the magnet, such as some monitoring equipment and fluid pumps. MRI Unsafe items are not allowed in the MRI suite at any time, as they are known to pose a hazard in any MRI environment.

25.4 Types of Metal

Ferromagnetic items, such as traditional oxygen cylinders, scissors, laryngoscopes, hoof picks, standard stethoscopes, clippers, or any other item that may be attracted to the magnetic field can become a hazardous projectile object when brought into the MRI suite (Colletti 2004; ASTM International 2013; Kanal *et al.* 2013). Figure 25.4 demonstrates the forces attracting a standard pair of

bandage scissors into the bore of a 1.5T MRI. Unrestrained, this item would become a projectile if brought into the MRI suite, as it is classified as MRI Unsafe.

Any ferromagnetic object is a hazard in the MRI environment, whereas non-ferromagnetic metals do not pose a hazard in the presence of the magnetic field. Iron, cobalt and nickel are ferromagnetic, whereas aluminum, brass, titanium and copper are non-ferromagnetic. However, given the common mixing of ferromagnetic and non-ferromagnetic metals in a variety of manufactured items and materials, the safety of an item or device is not obvious to the naked eye. Stainless steel is a good example of something that may or may not be ferromagnetic, since it is a mix of ingredients that vary with manufacturer. A hand-held magnet can be used to demonstrate and determine ferromagnetic properties of items or equipment, such as MRI Unsafe laryngoscope handles (Figure 25.5).

Trained individuals, generally the MRI technologist, must screen personnel or patients entering the MRI suite beforehand. In addition, a ferromagnetic detection device can be used to determine if a person is magnetically unsafe, as recommended by the American College of Radiology and the Joint Commission (Joint Commission 2008; Gilk and Kanal 2013; Kanal *et al.* 2013).

25.5 Gauss Lines and Safety Zones

The static magnetic field of the MRI strays outside the bore (sometimes referred to as the iso-center) of the magnet in three dimensions and is known as the "fringe field". The fringe field will extend through conventional

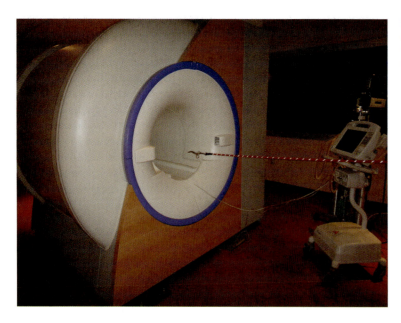

Figure 25.4 Demonstration of the static magnetic field in a 1.5-T MRI and the force pulling a pair of MRI Unsafe bandage scissors into the magnet bore toward the center of the magnetic field.

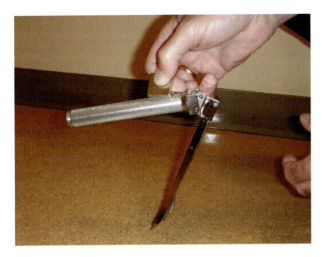

Figure 25.5 Demonstration of using a magnet to test ferromagnetic properties of a laryngoscope handle indicating significant ferromagnetic material and an item that is MRI Unsafe.

doors, walls, ceilings and floors, and can thus expose those outside the MRI suite to the static magnetic field (Bushong 2003b, d; Westbrook *et al.* 2011b). In general, the critical fringe field is the 5G line (equivalent to 0.0005 T or 0.5 mT) (Figure 25.6). As the distance from the magnet increases, the intensity or strength of the fringe field decreases. Requirements to exclude a device or person from the MRI depend on the intensity of the fringe field and associated distance from the magnet. For example, persons or animals with cardiac pacemakers or similar implanted devices should not be allowed any closer to the MRI than the 5G line (Bushong 2003d; Woods 2007; Joint Commission 2008; Westbrook *et al.* 2011b).

In general, exposure to static magnetic field strengths in excess of 5G should be limited to screened personnel and equipment that is considered MRI Safe. Because the fringe field or 5G line represents the most significant

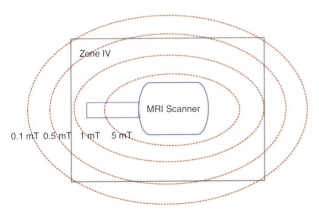

Figure 25.6 Diagram of the fringe field extent and Zone IV safety zone. The 5G (or 0.5 mT) line delineates the area where personnel and equipment may not enter until screened.

hazard area around a magnet, active shielding (as previously mentioned) is built into the design of the MRI system and used to confine the fringe field to the smallest area possible. Location of MRI scanners is limited by the 3-dimension extension of the fringe field and the need to prevent its inadvertent interaction with personnel, patients and equipment.

Safety zones are recommended by the American College of Radiology and the Joint Commission that restrict access to the static magnetic field (Bushong 2003d; Joint Commission 2008; Westbrook *et al.* 2011b; Gilk and Kanal 2013; Kanal *et al.* 2013). Zone I is the area where the public can have unrestricted access. Zone II is where patients and non-MRI personnel have initial contact with MRI staff and is often the reception area where initial screening occurs. In Zone III, there is the possibility of exposure to some level of fringe field from the MRI. Access to this area by non-MRI personnel, ferromagnetic materials, or equipment is severely restricted. In Zone III, patients and equipment undergo final safety screening before entering the MRI suite or Zone IV. Zone IV is where the MRI unit is housed and entrance to Zone IV must be clearly marked as to the presence of an extremely strong and hazardous magnetic field.

With the exception of resistive systems, which can be turned off when not in use, there should be signage indicating that the magnet is ALWAYS ON. For resistive systems, a light that indicates when the magnet is on versus off is required. Any time the MRI is not in use or MRI trained personnel are not present, the door to Zone IV should remain locked.

25.6 Specific Hazards

Objects with ferromagnetic materials that come into proximity with the static magnetic field are subjected to both translational (attractive) and rotational forces (Bushong 2003d; Woods 2007; Westbrook *et al.* 2011b; Tan *et al.* 2014). For example, rotational forces of the magnetic field may create twisting of an aneurysm clip; consequences of such an event can be severe with the potential for intracranial hemorrhage and death. In addition, as ferromagnetic items are brought closer to the magnet bore, the translational forces exerted by the static magnetic field increase exponentially. An object may become an airborne projectile that can result in the item being violently and rapidly pulled into the bore of the magnet at high speed and velocity (Chen 2001; Farling *et al.* 2003; Colletti 2004; Zimmer *et al.* 2004). For example, oxygen cylinders taken into the MRI suite have become projectile missiles, resulting in significant personnel injury and patient mortality (Chen 2001; Colletti 2004).

In addition to injury or the cost of human life, damage to the MRI can be significant. In these instances, the magnet must often be quenched (with release of the liquid helium) in order to power down the magnetic field and remove the items drawn into the magnet (Colletti 2004). Due to the exponential increase in magnetic force as one approaches the MRI, items will be rapidly pulled away at forces far exceeding the person's ability to maintain control of the item.

Thermal injuries are also a significant hazard in MRI (Dempsey *et al.* 2001). Magnetic and radiofrequency fields can cause heating of monitoring cables. Thermal injury can happen when electrically conductive material encounters the patient, particularly if a conductive loop is formed with either the cable itself or the patient. In addition, long lengths of cable can have an antenna effect, resulting in heating at the end of the cable; these situations are further discussed below.

In addition to the ASTM, the Institute for Magnetic Resonance Safety, Education and Research has a website that provides a resource for those using MRI (Shellock 2016). Safety, bioeffects, patient management, up-to-date results of MRI equipment compatibility testing and other information are readily available on the website. In particular, there is a regularly updated list of MRI compatible and incompatible implants with specifics, regarding their use in different magnetic field strengths.

25.7 Compatible MRI Equipment

For equipment to be considered MRI Safe, it must not be affected by the magnetic field and it should not interfere with imaging (Miller 2005; Olive 2005; Woods 2007; Reddy *et al.* 2012; Bell 2016). Since every MRI scanner is different, it is important to know the extent of the fringe field, the location of the 5G line surrounding the MRI, and that all equipment has been tested and proven MRI Safe in an identical magnetic field environment.

Equipment that has been tested and considered MRI Safe for a 1.5 T MRI cannot be assumed safe around a 3.0 T MRI, unless tested and cleared. Items should be labeled with the rating that describes safe placement. MRI Safe equipment can be readily placed in the MRI suite (Zone IV), and there are no known concerns or hazards for such devices. MRI Conditional equipment poses no hazard if used according to specific conditions. However, there may be limits to how MRI Conditional equipment can be configured, how close it can be placed to the bore of the magnet and the 5G line, what types of RF fields it can be used in, etc.

25.8 Anesthetic Machines

MRI Safe anesthesia machines have ferromagnetic components replaced with non-ferromagnetic materials. For example, MRI Safe oxygen E tanks made of aluminum (Figure 25.7) must be used within the MRI and are readily available from most medical gas suppliers. Wheel castors for machines, all bolts, supporting structures, etc. should be composed of non-ferromagnetic material. Long rebreathing tubing or long fresh gas supply hoses for non-rebreathing systems must be used in order to accommodate the requirement of keeping a particular anesthesia machine outside the 5G line or in order to reach the patient within the magnet bore. Most circle system and non-rebreathing system components are plastic or non-ferromagnetic and so of minimal concern; however, any metal components on breathing systems must be tested with a magnet.

Fortunately, several companies make anesthesia machines for large and small animal patients that are labeled as MRI Safe in both 1.5 T and 3.0 T MRI environments (Figure 25.8). If no MRI Safe anesthesia machine is available, a machine can be bolted to the wall or otherwise placed outside the 5G line, either in the MRI suite or outside in the control room (Zone III). If the machine is placed far from the bore of the MRI, long breathing circuits are can be used to connect the

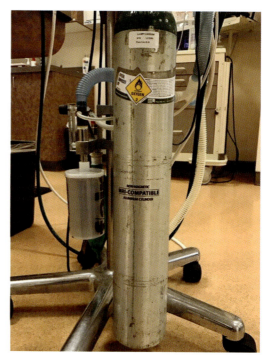

Figure 25.7 Example of an MRI compatible aluminum oxygen E tank. Note that the tank is clearly labeled "MRI compatible".

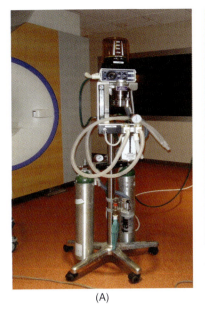
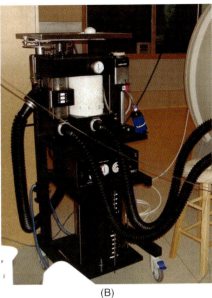

(A)   (B)

Figure 25.8 MRI-compatible small animal (A) and large animal (B) anesthetic machines, with MRI-compatible small and large animal ventilators.

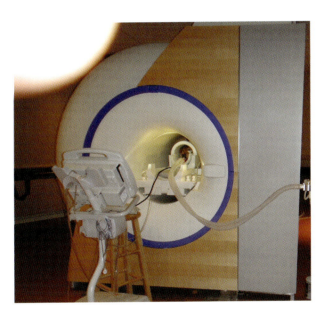

Figure 25.9 Example of using long rebreathing hoses to allow the anesthesia machine to be placed further from the MRI bore.

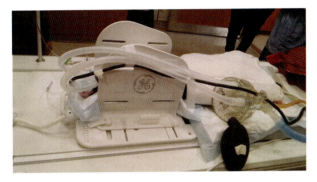

Figure 25.10 Example of a pediatric circle system for use on the MRI table. In this system, the fresh gas tubing enters in the back; the "pop off" valve is located near the top.

25.9 Vaporizers

While vaporizers do contain small amounts of ferromagnetic material, many modern vaporizers are safe as they are bolted to the anesthesia machine. However, if a vaporizer is detached from the machine, it can become a projectile object (Zimmer *et al.* 2004); machine and vaporizer servicing must be done outside the MRI suite. While testing with a hand-held magnet may not demonstrate significant ferromagnetic material in a vaporizer, the temperature compensation module of many vaporizers contains ferromagnetic material. No vaporizer should be allowed into the MRI suite if not attached firmly to an MRI compatible anesthesia machine, regardless of designation of the vaporizer as MRI Safe or MRI Conditional (Figure 25.11).

patient (Figure 25.9). When machines are placed outside the MRI suite, a wave-guide is required to pass the tubing through the MRI shielding (Figure 25.2). For smaller patients, a non-rebreathing circuit with a long fresh gas hose can easily be used. Alternatively, for larger patients, an all-plastic pediatric circle system (King Systems Corporation, Noblesville, IN) can be placed near the patient in the scanner (Figure 25.10). The fresh gas supply hose can again be long enough to reach the anesthesia machine bolted to the distant wall or through the wave-guide and outside Zone IV.

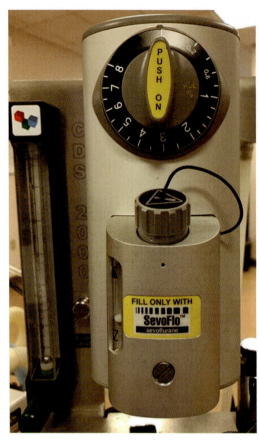

Figure 25.11 An MRI Conditional sevoflurane vaporizer. While it is considered safe to use in the environment of up to a 3.0-T MRI, it is not safe unless firmly attached to the anesthesia machine or bolted to the wall due to the small, but significant amount of ferrous metal within.

25.10 Ventilators

Electronically controlled ventilators and those powered by electricity that are not MRI Safe will often not work well in an MRI. They may also create RF interference and imaging artifacts. Most stand-alone, non-MRI compatible ventilators contain significant ferromagnetic material and electronics that will not work accurately or may cause image artifact (Williams *et al.* 1999; Olive 2005). Fortunately, pneumatically powered small and large animal ventilators are available that work well in MRI (Figure 25.8). These ventilators use compressed gas to power fluidic logic units that then control timing valves for inspiration and expiration (Olive 2005). Any ventilator used in MRI should be validated in the MRI environment (Williams *et al.* 1999; Olive 2005) to insure accurate tidal volume, respiratory rate, manometer accuracy, inspiratory pressure setting, inspiratory and expiratory time or ratios, and positive end-expiratory pressure (Williams *et al.* 1999).

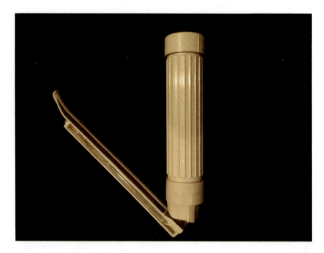

Figure 25.12 An example of a plastic laryngoscope.

25.11 Laryngoscopes

Standard laryngoscopes are not MRI-compatible and should not be taken into the MRI. Patients that require airway examination or replacement of an endotracheal tube should be moved outside Zone IV or the 5G line for treatment. MRI-compatible laryngoscopes and blades are available that are composed of little-to-no ferromagnetic material (Figure 25.12). They are plastic, require low-magnetic potential batteries, and are often more expensive than standard laryngoscopes.

25.12 Endotracheal Tubes and Airway Devices

Endotracheal tubes are generally MRI Safe and contain little to no ferromagnetic materials, with the exception of the small spring in most cuff pilots (Figure 25.13). While this is of minimal patient concern, it can cause artifact when scanning the head region (Figure 25.14). For this reason, care must be taken to be sure the cuff pilot is moved away from the region of interest. Endotracheal tubes with built in wire (guarded or spiral imbedded) should not be used due to potential for heating and image artifact. With the exception of some reinforced laryngeal masks, most supraglottic airway devices are generally safe to use. However, the proximity of the cuff pilot to the patient head can make it difficult to eliminate artifact from the small amount of ferromagnetic material in the spring (Olive 2005).

25.13 Monitors

Monitoring anesthetized patients presents a particular challenge when working around any MRI unit (Olive 2005). MRI-compatible monitoring systems are readily

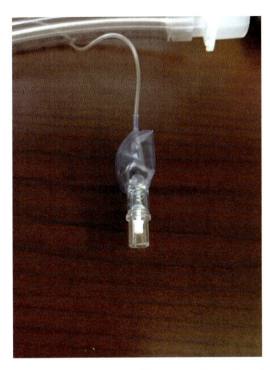

Figure 25.13 The spring within the standard endotracheal tube cuff pilot may cause image artifact if not moved away from the head during scanning.

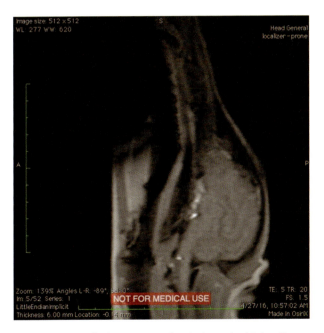

Figure 25.14 Cuff pilot image artifact is shown in this localizer sequence, where the lower jaw has been blacked out due to the artifact from the cuff pilot spring.

available in human medicine, but no veterinary-specific MRI compatible monitors currently exist. Fortunately, used monitors are often available. Manufacturers vary depending on the country; however, commonly used

brands include Medrad Inc. (Bayer Healthcare LLC, Warrandale, PA), Invivo (Invivo Corp, Royal Philips, Gainesville, FL) and GE (GE Healthcare, Madison, WI), among other worldwide manufacturers. Each monitor must be approved for use in the specific MRI environment. For example, a monitor that is approved for use with a 1.5 T MRI may not necessarily be safe in a 3.0 T MRI environment (Medical Advisory Secretariat 2016; Shellock 2016).

Regardless of manufacturer, most MRI monitors are listed as, and should be labeled as, MRI Conditional with specific use restrictions (Olive 2005). The user's manual will detail the restrictions on how close they can be placed relative to the fringe field strength, and monitors have been drawn into the magnet bore when recommendations have not been followed (Farling *et al.* 2003). Thus, MRI compatible monitors are restricted to being kept outside the 5G (or 0.5 mT) line. While some may work in this environment, they will frequently experience battery or electronic issues with prolonged exposure to a magnetic field.

25.13.1 MRI-incompatible Monitors

The potential for patient burns exists when MRI-incompatible pulse oximeters or electrocardiograms (ECGs) are used on patients (Bashein and Syrovy 1991; Dempsey *et al.* 2001; Reddy *et al.* 2012; Bell 2016). These burns are likely a result of resonant circuits in loops created in interaction with RF pulses used during imaging (Dempsey *et al.* 2001). Resonant circuits are those that have very low impedance at certain frequencies, such as the radiofrequencies used in MRI. This creates a response in loops that resonate when the peak frequency is reached with resultant heating and the possibility of patient burns (Dempsey *et al.* 2001). Similar resonance with RF pulses can occur with long lengths of cables, causing an antennae-resonance effect and subsequent burns as well (Dempsey *et al.* 2001). In the case of the antennae effect, burns are most likely at the tip of the wire, for example at the end of an incompatible MRI temperature probe or the end of any length of wire embedded in other cables.

Although not recommended, MRI-incompatible monitors can be used in the MRI. However, they need to be placed outside the MRI suite and require modifications. Wave-guides in the shielding will be required to pass cables and tubing into the MRI area (Figure 25.2). For example, MRI-incompatible pulse oximeters have been used when passed through a wave-guide, have no magnetic components, and have cable shielding (possibly with aluminum foil) to prevent RF interference (Peden *et al.* 1992; Tang *et al.* 2006). However, the risk of patient burns by the probe and cable looping (Figure 25.15) and

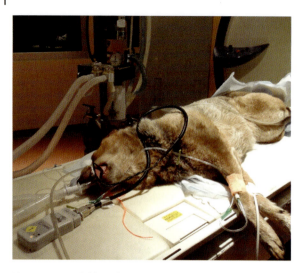

Figure 25.15 Cables of any kind should never be looped as shown here with this pulse oximeter cable (in black). Prior to scanning, this cable must be straightened to prevent potential patient burns.

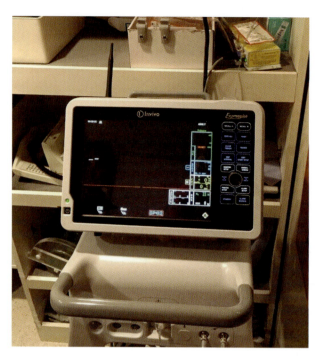

Figure 25.16 Example of one telemetered MRI-compatible monitor. Note the antenna located on the left rear of the machine.

the potential interference with imaging limit their use (Bashein and Syrovy 1991; Peden *et al.* 1992; Reddy *et al.* 2012).

Use of standard MRI-incompatible ECG monitoring is not recommended. ECG leads and electrodes often contain ferromagnetic components and low impedance conductors that are likely to cause burns when interacting with the RF fields (Peden *et al.* 1992; Niendorf *et al.* 2012; Reddy *et al.* 2012). In addition, the lengths of cable used with standard ECG monitors can cause heating and burns due to an antenna effect associated with the electrical component of the RF fields (Dempsey *et al.* 2001). Mainstream end-tidal CO_2 systems also cannot be used in MRI, as the sensors are not MRI-compatible; end-tidal CO_2 monitoring in MRI is limited to sidestream systems.

25.13.2   MRI-Compatible Monitors

MRI-compatible monitoring systems are usually telemetric and battery-powered, with an isolated power source to charge the batteries (Olive 2005; Reddy *et al.* 2012) (Figure 25.16). Because most batteries are ferromagnetic, they usually are placed at a defined distance from the 5G line. Cables or tubing for ECG, pulse oximetry, end-tidal CO_2 and direct arterial pressure measurement will all need to be longer than usual, to accommodate the distance of the monitor from the patient.

Most MRI-compatible pulse oximeter cables are fiber-optic and the sensors are non-magnetic, to reduce patient burns and maximize image quality (Olive 2005; Bell 2016) (Figure 25.15). MRI-compatible oscillomet-

ric blood pressure monitors are used, but are usually designed for optimal function with human patients; however, most have a pediatric option that works reasonably well for small animal patients. For arterial pressure measurement, the added tubing length may affect accuracy due to damping of the waveform in the tubing (Reddy *et al.* 2012). There are no MRI-compatible Doppler blood pressure monitoring systems and they cannot be taken into the MRI. During end-tidal CO_2/ anesthetic gas measurement, the long tubing will increase the lag time significantly, up to 10–20 seconds or more, depending on tube length. Even when using MRI Safe monitoring equipment, it is important that cords and cables not be in direct contact with the patient and that loops are not created in cables, as either may cause burns (Figure 25.15; Bashein and Syrovy 1991).

MRI-compatible ECG monitors use short non-ferromagnetic leads and non-metal electrodes to mitigate these hazards (Figure 25.17). However, ECG recordings during MRI are challenging to interpret, as there are significant signal artifacts during scanning (Olive 2005). Some of the artifact is related to changes associated with ECG voltage signals induced by the static magnetic field that increases as the magnetic field strength increases. In particular, T-wave and S-T segment changes have been observed in humans and may mimic pathology that is not truly present (Peden *et al.* 1992; Olive 2005).

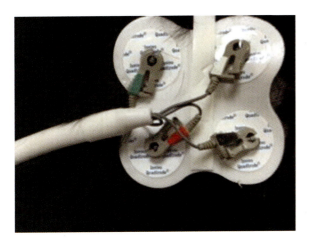

Figure 25.17 The standard MRI-compatible ECG setup with a single 4-lead patient patch.

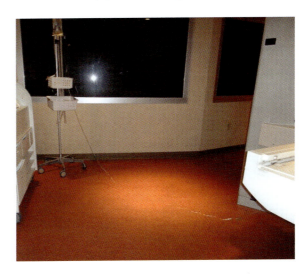

Figure 25.18 An MRI-intravenous (IV) fluid pump that is not MRI-compatible is being used and kept outside the 5G line to prevent interference. Long intravenous tubing is then used to connect to the patient. The pump is secured to an MRI-compatible IV pole and basket for added security.

Shortening the ECG lead length and placement of the electrodes closer together and as close as possible to the center of the magnetic field (iso-center of the MRI), can help to reduce ECG waveform artifacts (Peden *et al.* 1992; Niendorf *et al.* 2012). Consequently, traditional use of limb leads in veterinary patients is not an option and most veterinary patients will need to be shaved over a small area of the chest in order to get all MRI-compatible electrodes in good contact with the skin (Figure 25.17).

25.14 Miscellaneous Items

Fluid pump use in the MRI is challenging, since MRI-compatible pumps are expensive and MRI-incompatible pumps have ferromagnetic components (Olive 2005; Joint Commission 2008). However, some smaller portable pumps can be used with care and caution in the MRI suite if placed outside the 5G line, as far away from the magnet as possible and not in direct site line of the bore to prevent image distortion (Figure 25.18). However, they will frequently experience battery or electronic issues over time with prolonged exposure to the magnetic field. Alternatively (and more desirable for safety and to preserve function of the unit), they can be placed outside the MRI suite and the tubing passed through a wave-guide. In either case, access to the patient intravenous (IV) catheter requires long infusion tubing sets or multiple sets connected in series (Figure 25.18). Injections of anesthetic drugs and contrast agent will require access to a port closer to the IV catheter to reduce transit time in the tubing. Accuracy of pump delivery should be tested, as the effect of the magnetic field on pump delivery is not predictable (Joint Commission

2008). While MRI Conditional fluid pumps are available, they often must also be outside the 5G line and can be expensive.

Gurneys and large animal tables must also be non-ferromagnetic. Large animal Shank's tables (Shank's Veterinary Equipment, Milledgeville, IL) are available that are designed for use in 1.5 and 3.0 T MRIs and have a pneumatic drive using compressed air to position table height appropriately, which eliminates the need for a power source. MRI-compatible gurneys use either all aluminum and other non-ferromagnetic components, or even PVC tubing and non-ferromagnetic wheels and bolts (Figure 25.19). MRI Safe PVC gurneys can be purchased at a reasonable price and hold up to 200 kg on average.

IV fluid poles and baskets must also be non-ferromagnetic (Figure 25.18). MRI Conditional versions are readily available that are generally safe outside the 5G line, with some units allowed closer to the MRI bore (made of aluminum), depending on manufacturer guidelines (Figure 25.20). Care must be taken to ensure that movement of equipment between departments does not result in an MRI Unsafe IV pole setup being taken into the MRI.

Standard stethoscopes are not MRI Safe and will be pulled into the bore of the MRI. MRI Safe and compatible stethoscopes are readily available and recommended. Similarly, standard equipment for measuring body temperature is not MRI Safe; however, MRI Safe temperature probes come with many modern MRI-compatible anesthesia monitoring systems.

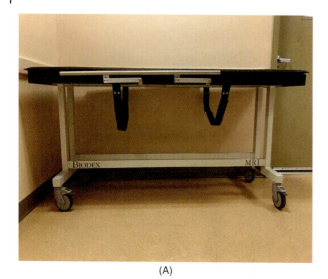

(A)

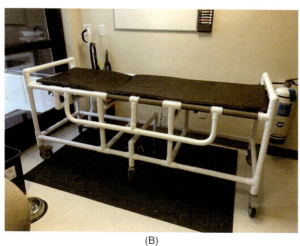

(B)

Figure 25.19 Two examples of MRI-compatible gurneys that may be used to transport patients in the MRI suite. They are composed of either aluminum (A) or PVC pipe (B).

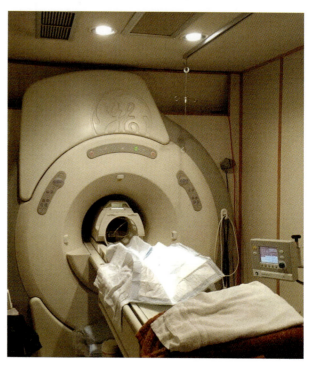

Figure 25.20 Example of an aluminum IV pole located close to the MRI scanner.

25.15   Summary

MRI Safe equipment is essential in the MRI unit, for personnel as well as patient safety. Some standard equipment that can be brought into the MRI is used daily in anesthetic practices (e.g. standard tracheal tubes). However, many devices are ferromagnetic (machines and monitors). However, specific MRI safe equipment is commercially available and affordable for the practitioner.

References

Apfelbaum, J.L., Singleton, M.A., Ehrenwerth, J., Bell, C., Connis, R.T. et al. (2015) American Society of Anesthesiologists Committee on Standards and Practice Parameters: *Practice Advisory on Anesthetic Care for Magnetic Resonance Imaging. Anesthesiology*, 122, 495–520.

ASTM International. Standard Practice for Marking Medical Devices and Other Items for Safety in the Magnetic Resonance Environment (2013) Available from: 10.1520/F2503 [accessed July 2016].

Bashein, G. and Syrovy, G. (1991) Burns associated with pulse oximetry during magnetic resonance imaging. *Anesthesiology*, 75, 382–383.

Bell, C. (2016) Anesthesia in the MRI Suite. Under Resources – Clinical Safety. Anesthesia Patient Safety Foundation. Available from: http://www.apsf.org/resources_safety_suite.php [accessed July 2016].

Bushong, S.C. (2003a) An overview of magnetic resonance imaging. In: Bushong, S. and Clarke, G. (eds). *Magnetic Resonance Imaging, Physical and Biological Principles*, 3rd ed. St Louis, MO: Mosby, pp. 3–17.

Bushong, S.C. (2003b) Purchase decision and site selection. In: Bushong, S. and Clarke, G. (eds). *Magnetic Resonance Imaging, Physical and Biological Principles*, 3rd ed. St Louis, MO: Mosby, pp. 156–170.

Bushong, S.C. (2003c) Biological effects of magnetic resonance imaging. In: Bushong, S. and Clarke, G. (eds). *Magnetic Resonance Imaging, Physical and Biological Principles*, 3rd ed. St Louis, MO: Mosby, pp. 393–409.

Bushong, S.C. (2003d) Managing a magnetic resonance imaging system. In: Bushong, S. and Clarke, G. (eds). *Magnetic Resonance Imaging, Physical and Biological Principles*, 3rd ed. St Louis, MO: Mosby, pp. 410–429.

Chen, D.W. (2001) Boy, 6, dies of skull injury during MRI. *New York Times. July* 31, 2001, B1–5.

Colletti, P.M. (2004) Size "H" oxygen cylinder: accidental MR projectile at 1.5 tesla. *J Magn Reson Imaging*, 19, 141–143.

Delfino, J.G. (2015) US federal safety standards, guidelines and regulations for MRI systems: An overview. *Appl Radiol*, 44, 20–23.

Dempsey, M.F., Condon, B. and Hadley, D.M. (2001) Investigation of the factors responsible for burns during MRI. *J Magn Reson Imaging*, 13, 627–631.

Directive 2013/35/EU. Directive of the European Parliament and of the Council. *Official Journal of the European Union* 2004 *L179/1*. Available from: http://eur-lex.europa.eu/legal-content/EN/TXT/?uri=celex%3A32013L0035. [accessed November 2015].

European Society of Radiology. Clinical Standards and Audit Templates. Available from: http://www.myesr.org/sites/default/files/ESR_Basic_Patient_Safety_Standards_Templates.pdf [accessed November 2016].

Farling, P., McBrien, M.E. and Winder, R.J. (2003) Magnetic resonance compatible equipment: read the small print! *Anaesthesia*, 58, 86–87.

Gilk, T. and Kanal, E. (2013) Interrelating sentinel event alert #38 with the ACR guidance document of MR safe practices. *An MRI accreditation safety review tool. J Magn Reson Imaging*, 37, 531–543.

Gosbee, J. and Gosbee, L.L. (2003) Flying Object hits MRI. *Patient Safety Network of Agency for Healthcare Research and Quality*. Available from: https://psnet.ahrq.gov/webmm/case/4 [accessed July 2016].

Henrichs, B. and Walsh, R.P. (2014) Intra-operative MRI for neurosurgical and general surgical interventions. *Curr Opin Anesthesiol*, 27, 448–452.

Joint Commission (2008) Sentinel Event Alert Issue 38: Preventing accidents and injuries in the MRI suite. Available from: https://www.jointcommission.org/sentinel_event_alert_issue_38_preventing_accidents_and_injuries_in_the_mri_suite [accessed July 2016].

Kanal, E. Barkovich, A.J., Bell, C., Borgstede, J.P., Bradley, W.G. Jr. et al. (2013) ACR guidance document on MR safe practices. *J Magn Reson Imaging*, 37, 501–530.

Labruyere, J. and Schwarz, T. (2013) CT and MRI in veterinary patients. An update on recent advances. *In Practice*, 35, 546–563.

McBrien, M.E., Winder, J. and Smyth, L. (2000) Anaesthesia for magnetic resonance imaging: a survey of current practice in the UK and Ireland. *Anaesthesia*, 55, 737–743.

Medical Advisory Secretariat. Patient monitoring system for MRI: an evidence-based analysis. Ontario Health Technology Assessment Series 2003. Available from: https://www.ncbi.nlm.nih.gov/pmc/articles/PMC3387746/pdf/ohtas-03-16.pdf [accessed November 2016].

Menon, D.K., Peden, C.J., Hall, A.S., Sargentoni, J. and Whitwam, J.G. (1992) Magnetic resonance for the anesthetist. Part I: Physical principles, applications, safety aspects. *Anaesthesia*, 47, 240–255.

Miller, M.G.A. (2005) Anaesthesia for MRI: child's play? *South Afr J Anaesth Analg*, 11, 28–31.

Niendorf, T., Winter, L. and Frauenrath, T. (2012) Electrocardiogram in an MRI environment: Clinical needs, practical considerations, safety implications, technical solutions and future directions. In: Mills, R. (ed.). *Advances in Electrocardiograms – Methods and Analysis*. Available from: http://wwwintechopen.com/books/advances-in-electrocardiograms-methods-and-analysis/electrocardiogram-in-an-mri-environment-clinical-needs-practical-considerations-safety-implications [accessed July 2016].

Olive, D. (2005) Don't get sucked in: anaesthesia for magnetic resonance imaging. *Australas Anaesth*, 85–97.

Peden, C.J., Menon, D.K., Hall, A.S., Sargentoni, J. and Whitwam, J.G. (1992) Magnetic resonance for the anesthetist. Part II: Anesthesia and monitoring in MR units. Anaesthesia, 47, 508–517.

Reddy, U., White, M.J. and Wilson, S.R. (2012) Anaesthesia for magnetic resonance imaging. *CEACCP*, 12, 140–144.

Royal Australian and New Zealand College of Radiologists. Magnetic Resonance Imaging Registration for Accreditation. Available from: http://www.ranzcr.edu.au/quality-a-safety/radiology/practice-quality-activities/mri-accreditation [accessed November 2016].

Shellock, F.G. (2016) Institute for Magnetic Resonance Safety, *Education and Research*. Available from: www.mrisafety.com [accessed November 2016].

Tan, J.K.T., Tan, T.K., Goh, J.P.S. and Ghadiali, N.F. (2014) Prospective review of safety incidents reported in the iMRI OT (Intra-operative magnetic resonance imaging operating theatre). *Proceedings of Singapore Healthcare*, 23, 273–281.

Tang, A.M., Kacher, D.F., Wong, K.K. and Yang, E. (2006) MRI-compatible ultrasound for image guided therapy. *Proc Intl Soc Mag Reson Med*, 14, 1414.

Westbrook, C., Roth, C.K. and Talbot, J. (2011a) Basic principles. In: *MRI in Practice*, 4th ed. West Sussex, UK: Wiley-Blackwell, pp. 1–20.

Westbrook, C., Roth, C.K. and Talbot, J. (2011b) MRI safety. In: *MRI in Practice*, 4th ed. West Sussex, UK: Wiley-Blackwell, pp. 341–371.

Williams, E.J., Jones, N.S., Carpenter, T.A., Bunch, C.S. and Menon, D.K. (1999) Testing of adult and paediatric ventilators for use in a magnetic resonance imaging unit. *Anaesthesia*, 54, 969–974.

Woods, T.O. (2007) Standards for medical devices in MRI: present and future. *J Magn Reson Imaging*, 26, 1186–1189.

Zimmer, C., Janssen, M.N., Treschan, T.A. and Peter, J. (2004) Near-miss accident during magnetic resonance imaging by a "flying sevoflurane vaporizer" due to ferromagnetism undetectable by handheld magnet. *Anesthesiology*, 100, 1329–1330.

26

Equipment for Environmental Extremes and Field Techniques

David Brunson and Kristen G. Cooley

School of Veterinary Medicine, University of Wisconsin, Madison, Wisconsin, USA

26.1 Environmental Extremes

Basic requirements for anesthetic delivery are access to the animal, safe drug delivery, and availability of oxygen and medical support. The first step in anesthesia delivery in an environmentally extreme situation is to determine the details of the location of the animal(s), such as the ambient temperature, altitude and locally available equipment. Anesthesia is normally performed in controlled environments, where temperature is within 65–75 °F (18–24 °C) and atmospheric pressure is close to approximately 1 atmosphere or 760 mmHg (sea level; Dorsch and Dorsch 2008). In addition to the needs for preparation in the planning of the animal capture and medical care, it is necessary to understand the effect that altitude and ambient temperature has on anesthetic equipment function.

Anesthetic medications are typically delivered to the animal as an injection or as gas inhalation. Inhalation anesthesia is advantageous as the dose can be titrated to effect and anesthetic recovery is rapid. One disadvantage of this approach is that special equipment is required. Gas anesthetics are appropriate for many species, but are of limited use when the animal is greater than 1000 kg in body weight or in areas where equipment is not available. However, gas anesthesia can be easily delivered in remote locations such as onboard a boat, at high altitudes, or in field locations (Heath 1997; Gales 1998). The necessary equipment for gas anesthetic delivery includes a gas source, a flowmeter to control gas delivery, and an anesthetic vaporizer (Figure 26.1). The breathing circuit must be selected based on the animal's lean body weight, the available carrier gas, and the type of anesthetic delivery system. Lightweight disposable rebreathing circuits can be used for animals of less than 70 kg in body weight (Figure 26.2).

26.2 Temperature

26.2.1 Oxygenation

The oxyhemoglobin dissociation curve shifts to the left if the patient is hypothermic. These shifts should be reflected in the pulse oximetry values, as left shifts increase the affinity of hemoglobin for oxygen; the function of the pulse oximeter should not be affected.

26.2.2 Pharmacologic Agents

The stability of a drug is ordinarily evaluated at temperatures between 65 and 75 °F (18 and 24 °C), because these are normal for hospital situations (as previously mentioned). If medications are to be used when environmental temperatures are above 100 °F, drugs should be stored in temperature-controlled containers to prevent exposure to the high ambient temperature.

26.2.3 Vaporizers and Inhalant Anesthetics

Gas anesthetics are delivered at precise concentrations to ensure safe and effective anesthesia. At this time, only two anesthetics (isoflurane and sevoflurane) are commonly in use in veterinary anesthesia, although desflurane is used in some institutions. The physical and chemical characteristics of isoflurane and sevoflurane (Table 26.1) require that they are delivered from precision vaporizers that compensate for both total flow rate and environmental temperature. An understanding of the normal vaporizer capabilities is essential and additional information can be found elsewhere (see Chapter 5; Dorsch and Dorsch 2008; Boumphrey and Marshall 2011).

The saturated vapor pressure of current anesthetics at 68 °F (20 °C) will result in a maximal concentration at 1 atmosphere, equaling approximately 31.5% for isoflurane

Veterinary Anesthetic and Monitoring Equipment, First Edition. Edited by Kristen G. Cooley and Rebecca A. Johnson.
© 2018 John Wiley & Sons, Inc. Published 2018 by John Wiley & Sons, Inc.

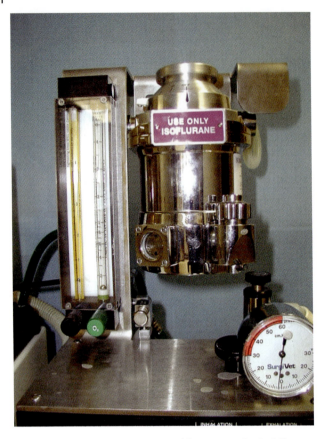

Figure 26.1 The equipment required for gas anesthetic delivery in remote situations. A flowmeter and vaporizer are shown here.

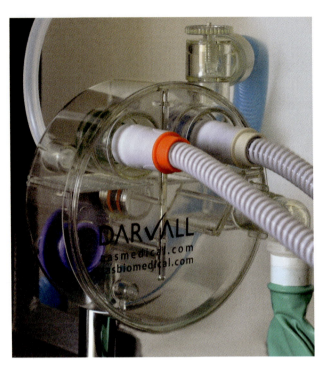

Figure 26.2 Example of a disposable rebreathing circuit for use in smaller patients (Darvall Vet, Advanced Anesthesia Specialists, Payson, AZ).

and approximately 21.0% for sevoflurane. These concentrations are far too high for clinical anesthesia, so they must be administered by means of a precision, temperature compensated vaporizer to deliver usable anesthetic concentrations. Anesthetic vaporizers used in environmental extremes outside of the normal temperature controlled hospital environment may not deliver the anesthetic concentration indicated on the vaporizer dial. For example, the gas anesthetic temperature directly affects the saturated vapor pressure within the vaporizer. Although temperature compensates over a large range, as the temperature increases significantly (>95 °F/35 °C), commonly-used, precision vaporizers in field situations may produce higher anesthetic concentrations, and the opposite will occur as the ambient temperature decreases considerably (<68 °F/20 °C) (Dosch and Tharp 2016).

Additionally, under no circumstances should a vaporizer be used if the environmental temperature is reaching the agent's boiling pressure (isoflurane = 119 °F [48.5 °C]; sevoflurane = 137 °F [58.5 °C]). It is important to note that these boiling points drop with altitude, and in some locations, the boiling point can approach environmental temperatures.

It is recommended to use an anesthetic agent gas analyzer to provide correct information on the inspired and expired concentrations, especially in environmental extremes. However, since most non-hospital situations do not have access to an anesthetic agent monitor, one can assume the vaporizer-delivered concentrations are not accurate at the temperature extremes previously discussed. Each drug has a specific vapor pressure that correlates to the ambient environmental temperature (Figure 26.3). In cold environments, a heating source such as an electric heating blanket can be used to keep the anesthetic vaporizer within the normal working temperature range.

Table 26.1 Physical and chemical properties at 20 °C.

Anesthetic gas	Saturated Vapor Pressure (mmHg)	Maximal % at 20 °C and 1 atm	Boiling Point (°C)	Minimum Alveolar Concentration (MAC) canine
Isoflurane	240	31.5	49	1.28
Sevoflurane	160	21.0	59	2.36

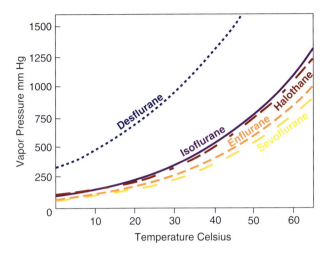

Figure 26.3 Graph depicting how inhalant vapor pressure increases as ambient temperature increases. Note how the curve associated with desflurane is shifted from the others.

26.3 Atmospheric Pressure

26.3.1 Oxygenation

The composition of ambient air is always fixed and is independent of altitude. For example, oxygen always comprises approximately 20.9% of air. However, as atmospheric pressure decreases with altitude, the partial pressure of oxygen (PO_2) decreases as well, as dictated by the alveolar gas equation:

$$PAO_2 = FiO_2 \left(Pb - PH_2O\right) \\ - \left(PaCO_2 / RQ\right) \tag{26.1}$$

where PAO_2 = alveolar partial pressure of oxygen, FiO_2 = inspired oxygen fraction, Pb = barometric pressure, PH_2O = partial pressure of water, $PaCO_2$ = arterial partial pressure of CO_2 and RQ = respiratory quotient. For example, at 5000 ft of elevation, the Pb is 632 mmHg, PAO_2 is approximately 81 mmHg, and SaO_2 is 95%, whereas at 10 000 ft, Pb is 522 mmHg, the inspired partial pressure of oxygen is 111 mmHg, PAO_2 is approximately 59–65 mmHg, and SaO_2 is 84% (James *et al.* 1984; Sutton *et al.* 1988). Pulse oximeter readings should reflect these changes and inspired oxygen levels must remain high to ensure the patient is not hypoxemic during anesthesia. At altitude, since patients are hypoxemic, the hypoxic ventilatory response causes them to hyperventilate as well. Thus, $PACO_2$ (and $PaCO_2$) can be quite low (as determined by blood gas analysis or capnometry); at 5000 ft, $PaCO_2$ is approximately 36 mmHg and at 10 000 ft $PaCO_2$, is approximately 34 mmHg (James *et al.* 1984).

26.3.2 Vaporizers and Inhalant Anesthetics

Modern Tec-type vaporizers (isoflurane and sevoflurane) are agent specific, temperature compensated, and deliver a specific partial pressure of anesthetic due to a variable bypass design for a standard carrier gas flow rate. The saturated vapor pressure is specific to each inhalant and mainly depends on temperature; it is relatively unaltered by ambient pressure changes. However, the percentage delivered from the vaporizer may be altered.

Although traditionally the vaporizer dial setting is referred to as a percent of the anesthetic in the carrier gas, it is actually the partial pressure of the total gas pressure. Dalton's law states that the total pressure is equal to the sum of the partial pressures of all the gases in the system. Since only oxygen and anesthetic vapor are present in the anesthetic vaporizer, and the vaporizer is designed to deliver a specific partial pressure of the anesthetic, the vaporizer output will be the partial pressure of the total pressure changes that occur at different altitudes (James *et al.* 1984).

Similarly, anesthetic effects are related to the partial pressure of the anesthetic gas (defined as the minimal alveolar concentration [MAC]). Thus, MAC remains the same at different altitudes, but the vaporizer output will change. For example, the vaporizer is designed to deliver a consistent anesthetic partial pressure of the total operating pressure. If the barometric pressure significantly decreases (altitude increases) outside the compensation zone for the vaporizer, then the anesthetic output from the vaporizer will also decrease and the vaporizer setting will not match the actual percent output of the anesthetic vaporizer (although the partial pressure of the total atmospheric pressure will remain the same; Steffey 2015).

The following formula can be used to determine the vapor output from the carrier gas flow rate and the ambient temperature (Stanton 2013). The saturated vapor pressure can be determined from the temperature versus vapor pressure graph. The environmental temperature will be the primary determinant of the maximum vaporization of the anesthetic (Figure 26.3):

$$VO = (CG \times SVP) / (Pb - SVP) \tag{26.2}$$

where VO = vapor output (mL), CG = carrier gas flow (mL/min), SVP = saturated vapor pressure (mmHg) at room temperature, and Pb = barometric pressure (mmHg).

26.3.3 Flowmeters

Anesthetic gas flowmeters are calibrated at a standard temperature and at 1 atmosphere Pb. Although gas flows will change as temperature and Pb increases or decreases, the changes will not affect the ability to deliver gases to the patient. Thus, standard fresh gas flows and vaporizer settings should be used in extreme environmental situations.

26.4 Drug Delivery Systems

Planning and execution of capture of exotic animals is well detailed in several textbooks that are specifically oriented to delivery of drugs and management of wild animals (Kreeger 1999; Nielson 1999; West *et al.* 2014). Drug delivery systems may also be needed in domesticated animals that are unable to be caught or restrained sufficiently. Multiple manufacturers of remote drug delivery equipment are currently available. Appropriately used, these systems provide non-traumatic delivery of chemical immobilization drugs. The systems have the potential to injure or kill an animal if the incorrect impact velocity or inappropriate injection site is chosen. Injury is directly related to the impact force and the location of impact on the animal. Remember that energy or force is equal to the product of velocity and mass (weight) of the syringe dart. Comprehensive training coupled with routine practice is a mandatory requirement for safe and effective delivery of anesthetics with remote delivery equipment.

26.4.1 Hypodermic Syringe

The hypodermic syringe is the simplest method of drug delivery. When hand-injected, the drug is delivered accurately and with no risk of impact trauma. Hand-injection does require physical restraint of the animal during the injection and this may pose high potential for injury to either the animal or the veterinary personnel. When the animal can be safely handled, hand-injection is the most reliable and safest method for drug injection. When hand-injecting difficult animals, always use syringes with a luer-lock hub and a large-gauge needle. This insures that the drug can be delivered rapidly and with less risk of detachment or breakage where the needle attaches to the syringe. Even for small dogs and cats, an 18–22-gauge needle is recommended. The trauma of the needle puncture is small compared to repeated attempts to restrain and inject an animal with a smaller-gauge needle. Very large-gauge needles (16–14 gauge) are recommended for larger animals or when large volumes are being administered to wild or fractious animals.

26.4.2 Pole Syringe

The pole syringe is simply a standard syringe with a long plunger (Figure 26.4). These are commercially available from several companies (e.g. Valley Vet Supply,

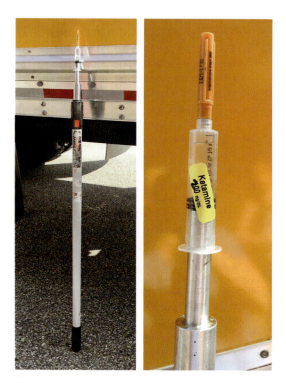

Figure 26.4 Two views of a pole syringe used to deliver injectable anesthetic agents. The syringe with luer-lock tip at the top of the pole is filled with the agent. A large-gauge needle is used to ensure complete injection.

Marysville, KS). They can also be made by modifying the end of a plastic, wood or metal rod to accept the rubber plunger from a syringe. The rod should be as large as possible and still fit inside the syringe barrel. This will provide greater stability and is less likely to break or jam when pushing on the plunger. A shroud should be placed over the outside of the syringe barrel. The shroud protects the hub of the needle and helps to prevent breakage of the syringe barrel if the animal moves during the injection. The best shrouds cover the entire length of the syringe barrel, but still enable visualization of the contents within the syringe. Many homemade and commercial pole syringes are difficult to use in a sterile manner. Thus, a new sterile syringe should be used each time the pole syringe is used. Lastly, the pole syringe should fit easily between the bars of standard animal cages. Opening the cage door to inject an aggressive animal may result in injury to the animal or escape of the animal.

The proper method to use a pole syringe includes positioning the animal where it cannot turn or move forward. Place the needle as close to a large muscle area as possible. This is typically either the shoulder or the hip. With one strong forward push of the pole, drive the drug into the animal's muscle while pushing the animal away from you. Keep pushing until the entire contents of the syringe have been delivered. Do not thrust or jab with the pole syringe.

26.4.3 Syringe Darts

When hand-injection and pole syringes are not possible or appropriate, immobilization drugs can be delivered by syringe darts. These modified syringes are designed to deliver drugs over distances, ranging from less than 1 m to over 50 m. All syringe-darts have four component parts: the needle or cannula, a medication compartment, a discharge mechanism, and a stabilizer or tailpiece. (Figure 26.5) The first section contains the needle and in some cases a plug that prevents the drug from being prematurely injected. The immobilization drug is placed in the medication component. The discharge mechanism creates the force that injects the drug into the animal. The stabilizer or tailpiece controls the flight trajectory of the dart.

26.4.3.1 Commercial Syringe Darts

Syringe darts can be distinguished by their discharge mechanism. The two principal types of discharge mechanisms are air/gas pressure and explosive charge. The discharge mechanism in the air/gas pressure darts is atmospheric air or butane. The gas is loaded through a one-way valve into the rear of the dart, pressurizing the system. Gas inject darts typically have a closed end (pencil point) with holes on the side of the needle. A rubber sleeve is placed over these holes to keep the drug in the chamber even after the dart has been pressurized. On impact with the animal's skin, the sleeve slides back allowing the drug to exit the dart through the needle side-holes as the compressed gas in the rear chamber of the dart expands, and the drug is injected into the animal. This type of injection occurs relatively slowly, caus-

ing less tissue damage due to the injection. In addition, the slow injection time and the side release of medication reduce the tendency for the dart to be pushed out of the animal. This reduced force means that only a small barb is required on the needle to keep it in the animal during injection. This type of system is effective for all types of animals. The gentler injection and lighter-weight darts are especially suited for smaller animals of less than 12 kg. Several companies market darts of this type, including Pneu-Dart, Inc. (Williamsport, PA), Paxarms (Cheviot, New Zealand), Daninject (Borkop, Denmark) and Telinject (Aqua Dulce, California).

In an explosive discharge dart, the discharge mechanism is an explosive charge set inside the dart. Upon impact, the dart stops suddenly causing the firing pin to move forward and ignite a gunpowder charge. This charge creates a small explosion inside the syringe dart that drives the plunger forward and injects the drug into the animal. The injection time for an explosive discharge dart is a fraction of a second. This short injection time creates greater tissue damage. Because of this damage, explosive discharge darts should only be used on animals that weigh more than 12 kg. Because an explosive discharge dart uses a front injecting, wide-bore needle, a large wire barb is recommended to prevent the syringe dart from being pushed out during the injection. Without a large barb, the needle will be forced out of the animal ("reverse jet action"), which reduces the chance for a complete injection. Cap-Chur (Palmer) darts (Powder Springs, Georgia), Daninject (Bokop, Denmark), Disinject (DeChaleons, France) and Pneudart (Williamsport, PA) darts use explosive discharge mechanisms.

26.4.3.2 Handmade Syringe Darts

To make handmade darts, start with two-3 mL syringes; luer-lock are preferred as the needle is less likely to break

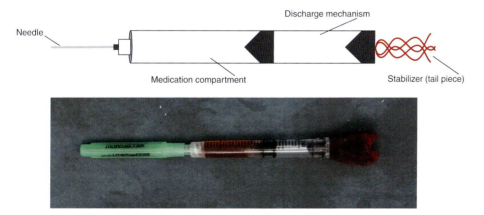

Figure 26.5 Schematic showing the essential pieces of a dart including the needle, a medication compartment, a discharge mechanism, and a tailpiece (top). A red dye is used to show the location of the medication compartment in an actual dart (bottom).

off the syringe at the time of impact. Monoject™ brand syringes have a rubber plunger that has a larger hollow opening that is useful for securing the tailpiece with silicone. Pull back on the plunger until it is in the back of the syringe barrel. Cut off the finger flanges and the plastic plunger shaft (Figures 26.6 and 26.7). Leaving the plastic inside the rubber plunger helps to prevent deformation of the moveable plunger during drug injection. Some syringes allow the rubber end to be peeled off the plunger shaft easily (Figure 26.7); if this is the case, remove the rubber end and discard the plastic (Figures 26.6 and 26.7). If this is not the case, you will need to use a small coping saw or scalpel blade or other knife (box cutter) to cut the end off. Use a sturdy box cutter or similar to remove the finger flanges from the end of the syringe as well. Using a file, make sure that all rough edges are removed from the dart to ensure its smooth travel through the projector (Figure 26.8). It is necessary to place the rubber plunger back inside the syringe barrel. A long needle or paper clip can be used to place the plunger where it allows for filling of the syringe with the appropriate volume of drug (Figure 26.9).

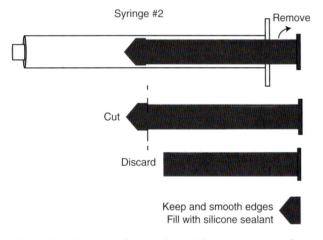

Figure 26.6 Schematic showing the initial steps in creation of handmade darts.

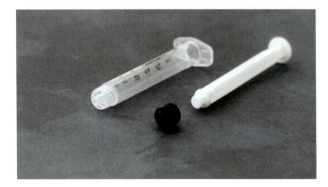

Figure 26.7 Removal of the rubber end of the plunger shaft.

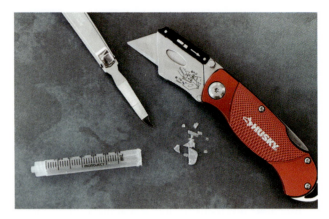

Figure 26.8 Removal of all the extra, sharp pieces of the dart for personnel safety and to ensure easy travel through the projection system.

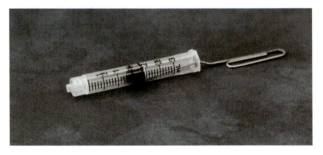

Figure 26.9 A paper clip is used to push the rubber end to its desired location within the dart.

Remove the rubber plunger from the second syringe and fill the plunger with silicone sealant. This will become the tailpiece. At the same time, create a strip of silicone that will be used to plug the needle. The tailpiece of the syringe dart is made by tying a knot into 3–4 loops of brightly colored yarn; the knot is then pushed into the silicone sealant (Figure 26.10). Let the tailpiece silicone and the silicone strip cure overnight before placing the tailpiece into the back end of the previously-made dart syringe (Figure 26.11). The tailpiece is secured into the syringe dart by cross-pinning with 22- or 21-gauge needles (Figure 26.12). Make sure that both of the rubber tailpiece O-rings are inside the syringe dart. Cross-pinning needles should be placed so that they are between the plunger sealing O-rings and at 90 degrees to each other for greater strength of the tailpiece.

Check to make sure that the outside of the syringe dart is smooth and that the needles do not extend on the outside of the syringe dart. Remove any projections that might drag against the blowpipe barrel and alter the dart's trajectory. To charge the dart, cover the side and end holes of the needle with a piece of silicone. Fill a second syringe with air and slide the needle through the

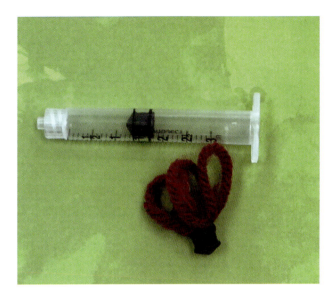

Figure 26.10 Yarn is glued to another rubber end to create a tailpiece.

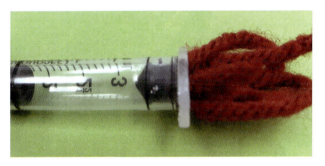

Figure 26.11 The tailpiece is placed into the end of the dart.

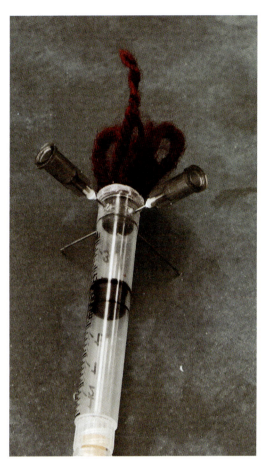

Figure 26.12 The tailpiece is secured using two cross-pinned hypodermic needles.

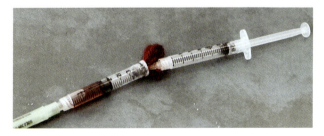

Figure 26.13 The dart is filled with drug (red liquid) into the anterior chamber and air is placed into the posterior chamber to "charge" the dart.

tailpiece and into the back chamber of the syringe dart (Figure 26.13). Carefully fill that space with air to pressurize the dart.

26.4.3.3 Needles

Needles intended for use with syringe darts are commercially available (Figure 26.14) (Teledart, Broomfield, CO). In addition, they can also be made. A triangular file or a small grinding wheel like a Dremel™ tool can be used to make a small hole in the side of a needle. This side-hole will allow the drug to exit the needle when the pressurized dart hits the target. Choose the largest needle size appropriate for the animal to be immobilized. The end-hole in the needle must be plugged so that only the side-hole will allow drugs to be administered to the animal. The silicone sealant used when making the tailpiece can be used to fill the end of the needle. Allow the silicone to harden overnight. Make sure that the side-hole that was created in the needle is not plugged.

26.4.4 Projectors

There are different types of projectors ranging in technology, from lung-powered blowpipes to 0.22-caliber blank cartridge powered projectors.

26.4.4.1 Blowpipes

Classical blowpipes or blow tubes are limited to the distance and force that a person can generate with a single expiration. Thus they are gentle, are limited to less than 3 mL, and distances of less than 15 m.

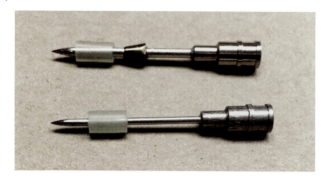

Figure 26.14 Examples of commercially-available collared (top) and non-collared (bottom) dart needles.

26.4.4.2 Carbon Dioxide-Modified Blowpipe

The second class of projectors is comprised of a modified blowpipe that uses carbon dioxide (CO_2) cartridges (caplets) as the source of power to propel the syringe darts to the animal. These projectors can reach farther and hit the animal with greater force. The inclusion of a precision pressure gauge enables controlled release of compressed CO_2. These systems are widely used in zoos and are very reliable for distances of up to 35–40 m.

26.4.4.3 Powder-Charged Projectors

The third class of projectors uses powder cartridges (0.22 caliber) to power these projectors. They propel the dart by a controlled explosion of gunpowder. The greater force enables these systems to reach the farthest distances and generate the highest velocity. Without a built-in velocity control, 0.22-caliber blank cartridge projectors have a high potential to produce severe trauma or death. Systems without velocity controls should be used with extreme caution and only for very large animals.

26.4.5 Safety Concerns and System Selection

26.4.5.1 Safety

Before attempting to use any equipment, be sure to read and understand all instructions carefully and completely. Personnel should:

1) practice all the various steps relating to the operation of equipment;
2) practice frequently so that one feels confident with the equipment;
3) practice loading and test darts with sterile water; practice darts are available for use in target shooting; and
4) seek out supervised help if there are any doubts about the ability to safely handle the equipment.

Before using a piece of equipment, make sure to be fully informed about that equipment. If the user does not take the time to learn about the equipment, they will find themselves in situations where the capabilities of the equipment are not suited to the task. Critical specifications of equipment include the potential range, accuracy, safety, dart drug volume, dart velocity and maintenance record. In addition, great care should be exercised not to contaminate the outside of the syringe or blow pipe with any pharmaceutical, biological, or other agent that may be harmful if it enters the mouth where it can be absorbed through mucous membranes.

26.4.5.2 System Selection

Selection of the system best suited for each situation requires one to consider the present needs and the future needs of the organization, as well as the experience level and abilities of the people who will be using the system. With proper maintenance and handling, a good-quality tranquilizer system will last for many years, even with daily use. Cheaper systems, which lack safety and velocity controls, often pose a greater risk to the public and to the animals being tranquilized. The following is a list of general considerations for purchasing a remote drug delivery system. Select a system that will:

1) be safe and uncomplicated to operate;
2) be easy to service and maintain;
3) be practical and relatively fast to use in the field;
4) be able to accurately deliver the dart within a predetermined distance;
5) provide trouble-free performance;
6) be versatile for use in different species and under varying conditions; and
7) cause minimum dart impact trauma, injection damage and aggravation to the target animal.

For more information on selecting immobilization equipment, refer to the manufacturer's equipment literature or contact the manufacturer's representative in your area.

26.5 Monitoring Equipment

Equipment for patient monitoring must provide information on the ability of the animal's heart to perfuse the vital organs, insure proper ventilation and enable assessment of the depth of anesthesia. The only routinely available device capable of assessing all three areas is a trained person attending the animal. This is why many clinicians believe that if a nurse or technician is watching the animal, then new "complicated" or "fancy" equipment is not needed.

26.5.1 Hands-On Monitoring and Simple Equipment

Hands-on monitoring is the basis of good monitoring, but the use of additional equipment will provide more complete information and make the care of the anesthetized animal easier. As previously mentioned, the three essential pieces of information are blood flow (perfusion), gas exchange in the lungs (ventilation) and assessment of the depth of drug depression. To accomplish these goals, many simple devices have been manufactured and many simply use the anesthetist themselves. For example, manual pulse palpation provides indication of blood flow, the force of blood movement in the peripheral artery, and information about the heart rate and rhythm. Thus, keeping ones' hands on an artery is an essential part of basic monitoring.

Auscultation with a stethoscope will provide similar information. The use of an esophageal probe is often used to make auscultation easier during anesthesia and surgery (Figure 26.15). Devices such as the Doppler flow probe placed over a peripheral artery will provide heart rate, rhythm and even an estimate of blood pressure (Figure 26.16). Visualization of pink mucous membranes and capillary refill time of less than 2 seconds enable the monitoring person to assess blood flow to the periphery and provides a gross estimate of the oxygenation of the capillary blood. Hands-on monitoring cannot be overemphasized, especially in a remote situation.

Evaluation of the depth of anesthetic effect is an art based on experience. Assessment of muscle tone and reflex activity is one way to evaluate the degree of relaxa-

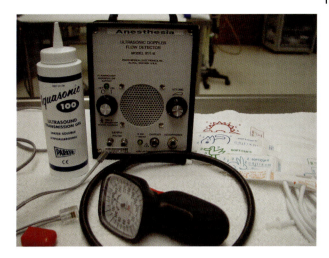

Figure 26.16 An Ultrasonic Doppler Flow Detector used over a peripheral artery to determine pulse rate and rhythm; blood pressure can also be obtained with a sphygmomanometer.

tion and the ability of the animal to make both spontaneous and reflex movement. For example, evaluation of the ease of opening the animal's mouth (jaw tone) is beneficial. During anesthesia, there is normally some resistance to opening the animal's mouth, but active resistance by the animal should not occur. If tone is completely absent, then the animal is likely too deep. Other areas of muscle tone (e.g. neck, limb, etc.) and reflexes (e.g. palpebral, corneal, etc.) are also used in a similar manner to determine depth.

26.5.2 Advanced Equipment

In addition to hands-on monitoring, modern monitoring equipment is often suitable for remote or extreme environmental situations (Figure 26.17). Small battery-operated monitors are available that will work for multiple hours before recharging of the battery is necessary. When working in remote or unusual situations, it is essential to have backup batteries or the ability to recharge the battery in the monitoring equipment used to evaluate blood flow and ventilation.

Portable pulse oximeters, electrocardiograms and end-tidal CO_2 monitors should be used to ensure that the animal is physiologically stable at an adequate depth of anesthesia (West *et al.* 2014). Monitors that are small and lightweight are preferred over those that are large and bulky. The Ultrasonic Doppler Flow Detector (Parks Medical Electronics, Inc., Las Vegas, NV) is a useful, portable monitor that works on virtually every species, to hear and evaluate blood flow. In some species, and with the right equipment, you can also use it to measure blood pressure.

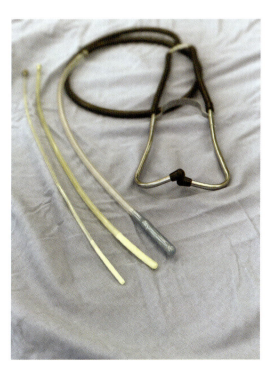

Figure 26.15 Example of an esophageal stethoscope used to detect heart rate and arrhythmias during anesthesia.

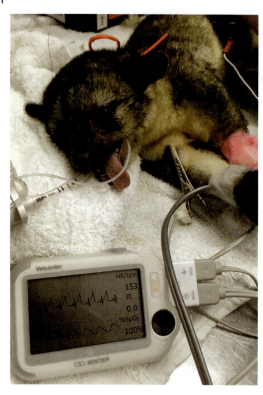

Figure 26.17 Use of a portable monitoring unit showing ECG and pulse oximetry (Sentier Health Connect, LLC, Brookfield, WI). The heart rate is 153 bpm and hemoglobin oxygen saturation is 100% in this anesthetized lemur.

In remote locations, the ability to support breathing of large animals can be challenging. A venturi high flow ventilator has been developed that has the capacity to mechanically ventilate animals larger than 1000 kg (In Case of Anesthesia, Wildlife Veterinary Specialists, La Jolla, CA; Elephant Ventilator, Mallard Medical, Inc., Redding, CA). Large body weight animals are anesthetized with injectable drugs that may depress normal ventilation. These animals need CO_2 monitoring and intermittent positive pressure ventilation to maintain lung function of oxygen delivery and CO_2 elimination (Figure 26.18; Hendrickson 2014). In addition, oxygen concentrators may be used to supplement inspired oxygen levels in remote locations; however, these have limitations to maximal flow and oxygen concentrations (see Chapter 2).

26.6 Field Techniques

The term "field techniques" can refer to remote capture of wild or zoo animals in an open area or performing anesthesia in any area outside of the traditional veterinary hospital. This includes rural areas, underdeveloped countries, farms and animal shelters, which may have limited access to equipment.

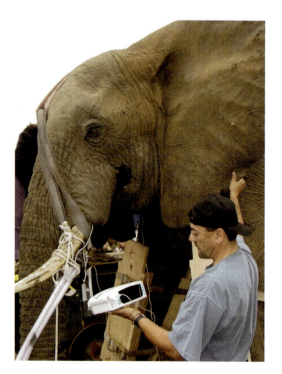

Figure 26.18 Anesthetized elephant depicting use of a capnometer and pulse palpation as monitoring tools in the field (photograph courtesy of Dr Jeff Zuba, San Diego Wild Animal Park, San Diego, CA).

26.7 Anesthesia for Situations with Limited Means

First, it is important to be prepared when performing anesthesia in the field, especially in geographical areas where use of modern anesthetic machines and equipment is limited. Anticipation of issues and the ability to "roll with the punches" is essential. Patients should be evaluated by performing a physical examination; however, this is not always possible, as some animals may be wild or fractious. In lieu of an otherwise dangerous hands-on physical exam, the patient should be evaluated through observation of body condition, hair coat quality, clearness of the eyes, respiratory rate and pattern and energy level. Consider their environment and quality of nutrition. Many street animals (urban free-ranging domestic animals) have a poor-quality diet and will likely have internal and external parasites, making the remote evaluation of their health status difficult. Animals that appear healthy can be assumed to be healthy and the pros and cons of going ahead with surgery should be weighed accordingly (Smith 2016).

Most field situations utilize injectable anesthetic protocols to achieve a surgical plane of anesthesia. It is important to the safety of the animal and the volunteers, that the protocol is adequate and provides proper analgesia. Patients that are under-anesthetized or whose pain is inadequately managed, will likely require more "top of" drugs during the procedure. If the anesthetic time is significantly increased, post-operative morbidity may also increase (Brodbelt 2008; Torrente *et al.* 2017), although more studies are needed to verify specific correlation between anesthetic time and injectable anesthetic procedures. Local and regional anesthetic techniques are a highly effective way to control pain and reduce the need for additional anesthetics. These techniques should be employed whenever possible.

Intravenous catheters can greatly improve quality of care through the administration of intravenous (IV) fluids and the addition of anesthetics and analgesics as constant (continual) rate infusions (CRIs). One bag of IV fluids can be spiked with appropriate drugs and dripped in a pre-determined rate based on body weight. The infusion rate can and should be increased or decreased in order to maintain the patient at an anesthetic level appropriate to the procedure. As a last resort, this mixture can potentially be used between multiple patients if sterile technique has been followed in preparation, and contact with blood and cross-contamination is avoided; the administration set or t-port should be changed between patients to decrease disease transmission and blood contamination between patients, while maintaining excellent patient care.

Endotracheal intubation is a vital part of safe anesthetic practice. Many veterinary hospitals dispose of single-use polyvinyl chloride endotracheal (ET) tubes after one use. However, these tubes may be cleaned and re-sterilized for repeated use in field anesthesia if necessary and done appropriately. To facilitate intubation, if a laryngoscope is not available, one can be fashioned out of a tongue depressor and penlight (Figure 26.19) and the ET tube can be secured with used IV lines. Oxygen masks can be made from empty plastic bottles (Figure 26.20). The opening of the bottle is 22 mm and will readily accept the larger end of the non-rebreathing adapter, a standard end-tidal CO_2 adapter, and the patient end of

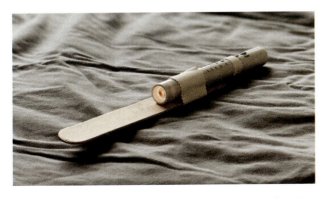

Figure 26.19 Example of a handmade laryngoscope, made with a penlight and tongue depressor.

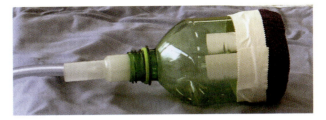

Figure 26.20 Example of an oxygen mask made out of an empty plastic bottle.

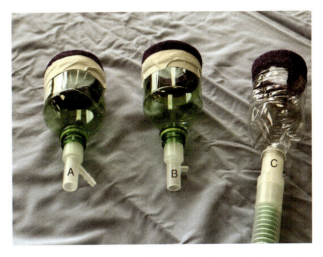

Figure 26.21 Bottle openings frequently adapt to the larger end of non-rebreathing adapters (22 mm), standard end-tidal CO_2 adapters, and the patient end of breathing hoses.

breathing hoses (Figure 26.21). Homemade masks are not ideal for inhalant delivery, as they do not form a seal and therefore allow waste anesthetic gas to escape and contaminate the environment. If inhalants are used, the patient should be intubated if possible.

Animals under anesthesia can experience hypoxemia and respiratory depression. Portable aluminum E or D cylinders of oxygen can be used with a good-quality regulator and flowmeter, or a portable oxygen concentrator can be commissioned (Fahlman *et al.* 2012). Facilities fortunate enough to have an anesthesia machine and an oxygen source can easily deliver fresh oxygen to 4–6 patients at a time using only one machine (Figure 26.22A). Facilities without an anesthesia machine can use this technique with just a portable oxygen concentrator. This "oxygen bar" can easily be made from old anesthetic circuits and adapters. Masks can be made from disposable plastic bottles or patients can be intubated (Figure 26.22B).

To make an "oxygen bar", multiple pieces are required. For example, tubing (silicone tubing or fresh gas tubing from a modified Jackson-Reese non-rebreathing system or oxygen tubing), Y or T (Y/T) tubing connectors (aquarium supply stores), patient adapters from

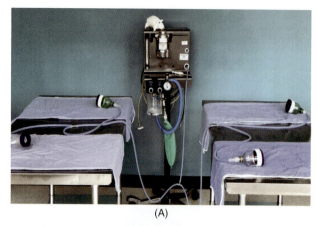

(A)

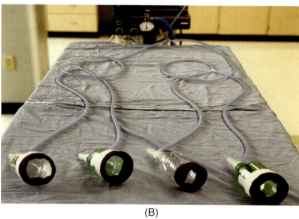

(B)

Figure 26.22 (A) The "oxygen bar" that can deliver oxygen to many patients at once (4 in this instance). (B) The use of masks at the end of the tubing.

modified Jackson-Reese non-rebreathing systems (MJR NRB) and ET tube adapters are used (Figure 26.23). Cut a piece of tubing to a (~12 inches) length and insert an ET adapter into one end of the tube; this end will fit into

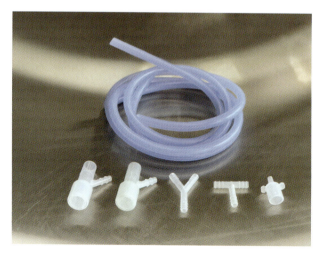

Figure 26.23 Examples of hosing and adapters required to create an "oxygen bar".

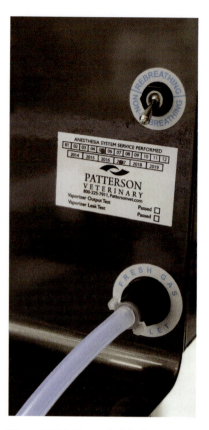

Figure 26.24 The end of the "oxygen bar" fits into the common gas outlet of an anesthesia machine.

the common gas outlet on the anesthesia machine (Figure 26.24). The ideal tubing to use is the blue-tinted silicone tubing used in modern anesthesia machines (Patterson Veterinary Supply, Waukesha, WI). A 4.0-, 4.5- or 5.0-mm ET tube adapter will form a seal with this product; tubing from MJR NRB takes 5.5-, 6.0- and possibly 6.5-mm adapters. A 7.5-mm adapter will fit into the end of suction tubing. A bit of trial and error may be necessary to find a secure and leak-free combination. Place a Y/T tubing connector (aquarium supply) into the other end and connect two more lengths of tubing (Figure 26.25). If only two stations with oxygen are needed, patient adapters can be fit into the ends of this tubing or, if four stations are required, another Y/T tubing adapter can be added into the end and finished off with the patient adapters. Six stations may be attempted by continuing to branch the tubing using the Y/T tubing connectors. In lieu of the tubing adapter shown here, an end-tidal CO_2 adapter will work, but likely with the silicone tubing only. It is possible to use other tubing, as long as a seal can be formed (connections that leak will waste oxygen). Both ends will fit either inside the opening of a bottle or mask, or around the outside of an endotracheal tube adapter (Figure 26.26).

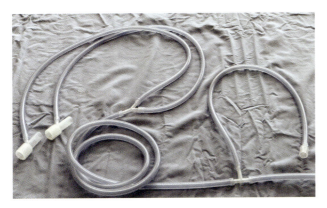

Figure 26.25 Splitting the tubing can create multiple stations on the "oxygen bar".

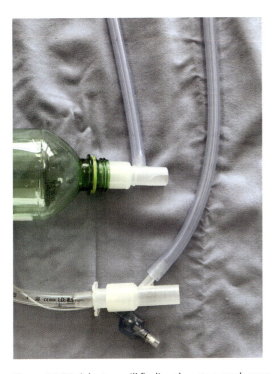

Figure 26.26 Adapters will fit directly onto a mask or an endotracheal tube.

There are limitations to this oxygen delivery system. If delivering oxygen to 4 stations, the fresh gas flow will be split into 4 streams; thus, the flow rate needs to be sufficient to accomplish this. For example, if the fresh gas flow is 4 L/min, each station will receive 1 L/min (assuming resistance is similar between stations). If the patient's facemask is tightly fitting, the patient would receive 100% oxygen (if 100% oxygen is the carrier gas). However, if the facemasks are not completely tight to the muzzle, an enriched oxygen mixture will be delivered. Fresh gas can be diverted from the machine to one station by clamping off the unneeded tubing.

It is important to note that intubated patients connected to the "oxygen bar" need to be able to expire with minimal resistance. The choice of adapters is intentional, because they allow for expired gases to escape through the open end. However, this set-up is not very efficient, as constantly flowing fresh gas only enters the patient as they inspire, with the excess wasted. It is not recommended that inhalant be used with this system, due to the risk of waste anesthetic gas contaminating the work area, resulting in waste gas exposure to personnel; repeated injectable drug dosing or increasing the constant rate infusions of agents can help keep animals in a surgical plane of anesthesia.

Temperature management is important in performing field anesthesia. Some patients lose body heat once sedated and may continue to lose heat well into recovery, whereas some patients may be hyperthermic. Inexpensive ambient thermometers may be placed into the esophagus if more sophisticated temperature devices are unavailable (Figure 26.27). Some field operations require that most or all of the required supplies are hauled into the area, making space and weight of equipment a concern. Although a forced-air heating unit is advantageous, it may not always be feasible. As such, there are other ways to help maintain body temperature in patients that may become hypothermic. Patients should always be placed on an insulated surface such as a mat, pad or towel to avoid conductive heat loss (Figure 26.28A). Yoga mats work well for a variety of uses; they can be cut up for padding the sur-

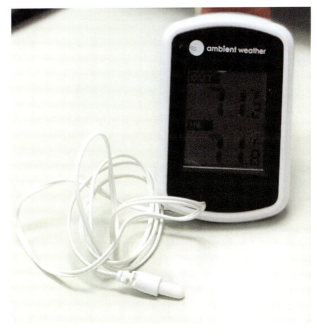

Figure 26.27 An inexpensive ambient thermometer that can be placed in the esophagus to measure body temperature in field situations (Ambient Weather, Chandler, AZ).

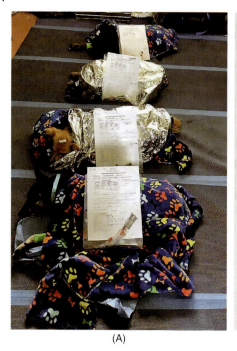

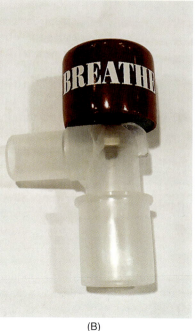

Figure 26.28 (A) Yoga mats placed underneath dogs to aid in warming. In addition, fleece blankets and space blankets are used to wrap dogs to reduce heat loss. (B) An audible monitor used to hear when a patient breathes to detect apnea.

(A)

(B)

gery table or rolled out for recovery. Other inexpensive insulation devices include the use of a space blanket-type of cover, or foil covered bubble wrap (Figure 26.29). Fleece fabric is superior to hauling heavy towels, especially if working in a humid environment. Fleece is warm and lightweight and it dries quickly when washed.

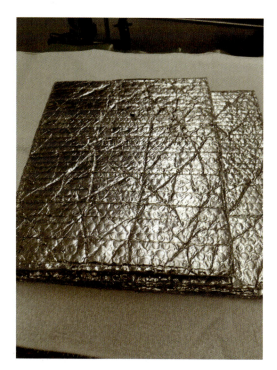

Figure 26.29 Example of foil covered bubble wrap.

Emergency thermal blankets or space blankets are small, compact and work well to retain body heat when placed on or around a patient. Athletic socks filled with rice and heated up in a microwave and warming discs (Snuggle Safe, purchased from many web sites) work relatively well in warming the patient. However, do not allow the rice socks or heating disc to come into direct contact with the patient, as they can easily cause burns. Residual respiratory depression is often a concern in recovery. A respiratory monitor can be connected to a mask or endotracheal tube during recovery. These tiny apnea monitors have a highly sensitive microprocessor that offers an audible sound when even the smallest breath passes through (Figure 26.28B; Vetamac, Rossville, IN).

In some situations, hyperthermia is a concern. Fans, ice packs or water can be used for patient cooling. Supplemental oxygen and intravenous fluids are also advantageous in patient cooling.

26.8 Stress

Anesthesia under extreme environmental situations requires understanding of the particular temperament of the species. It is important to seek out experienced people that have knowledge of the specific situation and species. Minimization of the animal's level of stress has been demonstrated to improve overall care and effective delivery of the anesthetic (Heath 1997; Gales 1998)

26.9   Summary

The use of anesthetic equipment under extreme environmental situations builds on the anesthetic practices that are the current standard of care. Equipment designed for hospital situations are generally useable in remote locations. It is imperative that a thorough understanding of equipment be the foundation of equipment utilization in unusual environments. In addition, remote drug delivery may be necessary. Homemade syringe darts can be fabricated and are readily useable by veterinary personnel or commercially available products may be used.

References

Boumphrey, S. and Marshall, N. (2011) Understanding vaporizers. *Cont Ed Anes Crit Care Pain*, 1, 199–203.

Brodbelt, D. (2009) Peri-operative mortality in small animal anaesthesia. *Vet J*, 182, 152–161.

Dorsch, J. and Dorsch, S. (2008) *Understanding Anesthetic Equipment*, 5th ed. Philadelphia, PA: Lipincott Williams & Wilkins.

Dosch, M.P. and Tharp, D. (2016) The Anesthesia Gas Machine. Available from: https://healthprofessions. udmercy.edu/academics/na/agm/05.htm [accessed October 2017].

Fahlman, A., Caulkett, N., Arnemo, J.M., Neuhaus, P. and Ruckstuhl, K.E. (2012) Efficacy of a portable oxygen concentrator with pulsed delivery for treatment of hypoxemia during anesthesia of wildlife. *J Zoo Wildl Med*, 43, 67–76.

Gales, N. (1998) Fast, safe, field-portable gas anesthesia for ottarids. *Marine Mam Sci*, 14, 355–361.

Heath, R.B., DeLong, R. and Jameson, V. (1997) Isoflurane anesthesia in free ranging sea lion pups. *J Wildl Dis*, 33, 206–210.

Hendrickson, D., Stetter, M., Zuba, J. and Marais, H. (2014) Laparoscopic vasectomy in African elephants (*Loxodonta africana*). *Vet Surg*, 43, 507–514.

James, M.F.M. and White, J.F. (1984) Anesthetic consideration at moderate altitude. *Anesth Analg*, 63, 1097–1105.

Kreeger, T.J. (1999) General principles. *In: Handbook of Wildlife Chemical Immobilization*, 3rd ed. Laramie, WY: International Wildlife Veterinary Services, pp. 12–14.

Nielsen, L. (1999) Considerations and principles. In: *Chemical Immobilization of Wild and Exotic Animals*. Ames, IA: Iowa State University Press. pp. 17–34.

Smith, L. (2016) Patient evaluation. *In: Questions and Answers in Small Animal Anesthesia*. Ames, IA: Wiley Blackwell, p. 3.

Stanton, K. (2013) Vaporizer output calculation. Physics, monitoring and anesthetic delivery. In: Modak, R.K. (ed.). *Anesthesiology Keywords Review*, 2nd ed. Philadelphia, PA: Lippincott Williams & Wilkins, p. 598.

Steffey, E., Mama, K. and Brosnan, R. (2015) Inhalation anesthetics. In: Grimm, K.A., Lamont, L.A., Tranquilli, W.J., Greene, S.A. and Robertson, S.A. (eds) *Veterinary Anesthesia and Analgesia: The Fifth Edition of Lumb and Jones*. Ames, IA: Wiley-Blackwell, pp. 297–331.

Sutton, J.R., Reeves, J.T., Wagner, P.D., Groves, B.M., Cymerman, A. *et al.* (1988) Operation Everest. *Part II: Oxygen transport during exercise at extreme simulated altitude. J Appl Physiol*, 64:1309–1321.

Torrente, C., Vigueras, I., Manzanilla, E.G., Villaverde, C., Fresno, L. *et al.* (2017) Prevalence of and risk factors for intra-operative gastroesophageal reflux and post-anesthetic vomiting and diarrhea in dogs undergoing general anesthesia. *J Vet Emerg Crit Care (San Antonio)*, 27, 397–408.

Vaporizer output at altitude. Available from: http://www. openanesthesia.org/vaporizer_output_at_altitude [accessed October 2017].

West, G., Heard, D. and Caulkett, N. (2014) *Zoo Animal and Wildlife Immobilization and Anesthesia*, 2nd ed. Ames, IA: Blackwell.

27

Equipment Checkout and Maintenance

Molly Allen[1] and Lesley Smith[2]

[1] *Lakeshore Veterinary Specialists, Glendale, Wisconsin, USA*
[2] *School of Veterinary Medicine, University of Wisconsin, Madison, Wisconsin, USA*

27.1 Introduction

Equipment issues may be a source of serious anesthetic-related morbidity and mortality; therefore proper inspection and regular maintenance of all components are essential (Chopra *et al.* 1992; Langford *et al.* 2007; Cassidy *et al.* 2011). Studies indicate that anesthetic equipment checkout practices require considerable improvement (Barthram and McClymont 1992; Armstrong-Brown *et al.* 2000; Langford *et al.* 2007). For example, significant observations involving unsafe anesthetic practices over an 18-month period showed most were due to lack of vigilance and failure to check equipment (Chopra *et al.* 1992). Additionally, only 5% of a select group of anesthetists performed a complete check of the equipment before use (Langford *et al.* 2007). A working understanding of the various types of anesthetic machines, circuits, ancillary equipment and monitors available for veterinary use is essential before one can perform the checks and safety procedures necessary for each component (Mosley 2015). Anesthetists should not attempt to use anesthetic equipment until trained and competent to do so. Included in this chapter are recommendations for checking and maintaining veterinary anesthetic and monitoring equipment, and safety protocols applicable to all levels of veterinary practice.

27.2 Daily Checks

All new equipment should be initially assembled and checked by a representative of the manufacturer, then checked by anesthesia personnel before use. The most reliable way to prevent equipment-related complications is to inspect all components in regular use prior to each anesthesia session (e.g. daily). However, some components (i.e. breathing hoses, bags, endotracheal tubes) should also be checked just prior to each case. For most anesthetic equipment, a user manual is provided by the manufacturer. Some modern anesthesia machines guide the user through a series of electronic checks. The following recommendations should not replace those provided by the manufacturer; instead, a combination of the user manual and a standard anesthesia checklist incorporating the following recommendations should be employed (Hartle *et al.* 2012). To assist in routine checkout procedures, a simplified checklist sheet may be attached to each machine (Figure 27.1).

Some anesthesia machines and most anesthesia monitors require a power source to function, or have batteries that must be fully charged prior to use. Therefore, prior to commencing the checkout procedures, the user should connect and verify the power supply. If the anesthesia machine has a master switch, this should be turned on. Backup batteries should be charged and have at least 30 minutes of backup power available prior to use (Goneppanavar and Prabhu 2013).

27.2.1 High- and Intermediate-Pressure Systems

The high- and intermediate-pressure systems receive gas at high pressures from individual cylinders, a central pipeline supply, or both, and must be checked to ensure adequate gas supply. The high-pressure system includes the hanger yoke, cylinder pressure indicator (gauge) and pressure reducing device (regulator). The intermediate-pressure system includes the pipeline inlet connections, pipeline pressure indicator (gauge), master switch, oxygen fail-safe system, oxygen pressure failure alarm, oxygen flush and flow control valve.

27.2.1.1 Gas Cylinders

All cylinders should be inspected for the appropriate gas (i.e. by color and label) and secure mounting in their

Anesthesia Equipment Checklist		
High- and Intermediate-pressure systems		
Oxygen cylinder	❏	Appropriate gas & adequate supply
	❏	Correct mounting & no audible leaks
	❏	Backup oxygen supply available
Pipeline supply	❏	Connected to supply ("tug test")
	❏	Adequate pressure (55–65 psi)
	❏	Backup oxygen supply available, cylinders off
Oxygen fail-safe	❏	Disconnect O_2 with all flowmeters on
Oxygen failure alarm	❏	Disconnect O_2 with O_2 flowmeter on
Low-pressure system		
Flowmeter	❏	Minimum mandatory flow rate, if applicable
Vaporizer	❏	Dial function
	❏	Properly mounted, locking mechanism engaged
	❏	Fill to maximum fill line
	❏	Filler cap closed & drain valve tight
Leak test	❏	Negative pressure test
	❏	Positive pressure test
	❏	Test with vaporizer on and off
Scavenging system		
Active scavenging	❏	Proper connections
	❏	Vacuum source connected & flow adjusted
Passive scavenging	❏	Waste gas transfer tubing appropriately directed
	❏	Active charcoal canister not exhausted (check weight)
APL valve	❏	Leak check (50 cm H_2O)
	❏	Verify function
Closed scavenging	❏	Check air intake valve
	❏	Check positive pressure relief
Open scavenging	❏	Check negative pressure relief
Breathing circuit		
Oxygen monitor	❏	Check low oxygen alarm with room air
	❏	Verify function with oxygen flush
Status check	❏	CO_2 absorbent canister mounted correctly
	❏	CO_2 absorbent not exhausted
	❏	No cracks or foreign bodies in circuit
Leak check	❏	Acceptable leak ≤ 300 ml/min at 30 cm H_2O
Bain circuit	❏	Inner tube occlusion test
Unidirectional valves	❏	Breathing method
	❏	Pressure method
	❏	Domes screwed on tightly
Ventilator	❏	Leak test
	❏	Low-pressure & high-pressure alarms
	❏	Safety-relief valve
Other equipment	❏	Airway equipment
	❏	Drug delivery systems
	❏	Monitors
	❏	Warming devices
	❏	Padding
	❏	Extension cords & hoses

Figure 27.1 Example of an anesthesia equipment checklist, which may be placed directly on the machine for reference.

respective hanger yolks. A yolk plug should be present in each empty yoke to prevent retrograde leaks. To check an individual cylinder, the cylinder is opened by turning the valve slowly counterclockwise and verified to contain enough gas to complete the intended procedure; generally, the tank should be at least half-full, provided the cylinder size is appropriate for patient size and anticipated flow rates (Figure 27.2). For example, an E cylinder of oxygen with a pressure gauge reading at 1000 psi (full tanks read ~2200 psi and contain ~700 L of gas) should provide around 5 hours of use, assuming oxygen flow rates of approximately 1 L/min, while a G cylinder at 1000 psi (full tanks should ready ~2200 psi and contain ~5000 L of gas) should provide around 7 hours of use, assuming oxygen flow rates of approximately 5 L/min; if oxygen from the cylinder is also used to drive a ventilator, significantly more will be consumed and a larger supply required. Ventilator consumption of oxygen varies with the type of ventilator, driving gas mixture, mode of ventilation, tidal volume and patient compliance, but can range anywhere from 2–16 L/min (Szpisjak *et al.* 2005, 2008; Szpisjak and Starrett-Keller 2014). After checking the cylinder, the cylinder valve is closed and the pressure gauge observed to check for high pressure leaks, indicated by an obvious decrease in pressure. Inadequate tightening of the yoke screw into the tank stem or plug is a common source of high pressure system leaks. After the cylinder is closed and no leaks identified, the oxygen

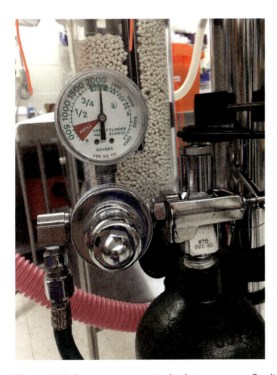

Figure 27.2 Pressure gauge attached to an oxygen E cylinder reading full at 2000 psi. The pressure will decrease proportionately as the gas is used.

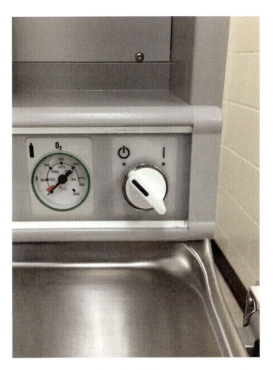

Figure 27.3 Example of a cylinder pressure gauge located on an anesthesia machine. The cylinder is not connected and the gauge is appropriately reading 0 psi.

flush valve is depressed to release pressure from the machine piping before checking the central pipeline supply, if present. Note that some cylinders do not have hanger yokes *per se* (e.g. H cylinders) and must be checked by turning on the anesthesia machine to which they are connected and observing the cylinder pressure gauge (Figure 27.3).

27.2.1.2 Central Pipeline Supply

If central gas pipelines are used, they must be checked as well. To check the central pipeline supply, the machine hoses are connected to the supply at the terminal unit and the fittings checked for audible leaks. Pulling on each hose individually ("tug test") ensures correct insertion of the hoses into the sockets (Hartle *et al.* 2012). The pipeline pressure gauge (Figure 27.4) is checked for a supply pressure of between 55 and 65 psi (380–450 kPa) (Dorsch and Dorsch 2007; Bednarski 2009; Hartle *et al.* 2012). Some veterinary anesthesia machines, especially those used for transport, do not include a pipeline pressure gauge; the pressure must be determined from the area pressure gauge on the area alarm system, which may be located upstream or downstream of the area shutoff valve (Figure 27.5). Alternatively, the pressure may be checked on the gauge installed in the main supply line.

Whether an individual oxygen cylinder or a central pipeline supply is used, a backup oxygen cylinder should

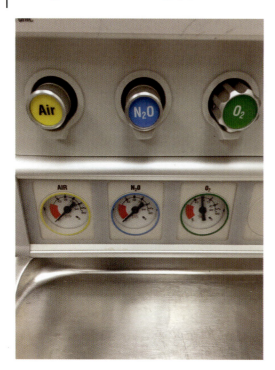

Figure 27.4 Example of a pipeline pressure gauge located on an anesthesia machine. The pipeline is connected and the gauge is appropriately reading ~55 psi.

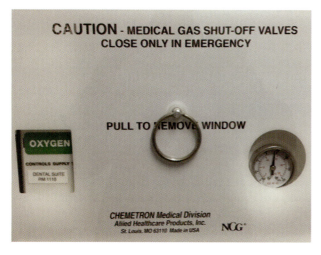

Figure 27.5 Example of a pipeline pressure gauge with area shutoff valve located in a structure wall. Line pressure is ~55 psi.

be available and tested at the same time. After the high-pressure system is checked, the oxygen supply should be turned on by either opening the oxygen cylinder or connecting the machine hoses to the central pipeline supply. If only cylinders are in use, any backup oxygen cylinders should be turned off until their use is required. If a central pipeline supply is connected, one backup oxygen cylinder should remain connected in case of pipeline supply failure.

27.2.1.3 Oxygen Fail-Safe System and Pressure Failure Alarm

If multiple gases are used (e.g. air, nitrous oxide), the oxygen fail-safe system is checked by turning on all gases to the machine (cylinders or pipeline supply) and all flowmeters, then turning off or disconnecting only the oxygen supply. The flowmeter floats of all gases should fall to zero if the oxygen fail-safe system is functioning properly, and should return to their previous location in the tube when the oxygen source is turned on again (Dorsch and Dorsch 2007; Goneppanavar and Prabhu 2013).

An oxygen failure alarm is present on many current anesthesia machines. A defective or absent alarm was a common fault identified in a study of anesthesia machine checks in one teaching hospital (Barthram and McClymont 1992). This alarm is checked by disconnecting or turning off the oxygen source while the oxygen flowmeter is on. An audible alarm indicating a lack of oxygen supply should be activated. Checks of the oxygen fail-safe system and oxygen pressure failure alarm may be simultaneous and should be performed on a weekly basis (Hartle *et al.* 2012).

27.2.2 Low-Pressure System

The low-pressure system is located downstream of the flow control valves and includes the flow indicator within the flowmeter, vaporizer, low-pressure piping and common gas outlet.

27.2.2.1 Flowmeter

The oxygen flowmeter is checked (the master switch must be on, if applicable) by turning the flow control valve on (counterclockwise) and off (clockwise) while observing the float or bobbin, which should rise and fall smoothly within the flowmeter tube. The float should return to a close-to-zero or zero position when the valve is turned off. If the machine has a minimum mandatory flow, the flowmeter should not drop below 50–200 mL/min (Dorsch and Dorsch 2007; Goneppanavar and Prabhu 2013).

27.2.2.2 Vaporizer

The vaporizer is turned off by turning the dial completely clockwise and checked for correct mounting on the machine with locking mechanisms engaged. The vaporizer is filled to the maximum fill indicator line and the filler cap closed tightly. The drain valve should also be checked for tightness.

27.2.2.3 Low-Pressure System Leak Checks

The low-pressure system, including all components between the flowmeter valve and the common gas outlet, is a common source of leaks due to multiple fragile parts. Furthermore, leaks in this system are difficult to detect, as they are usually inaudible. Therefore, the low-pressure system should be checked separately from the breathing circuit to prevent complications such as hypoxia, patient awareness and hypercarbia. The negative pressure test *and at least one* of the positive pressure tests of the low-pressure system should be performed before the breathing circuit is assembled.

Negative Pressure Test (Dorsch and Dorsch 2007; Goneppanavar and Prabhu 2013) To perform the negative pressure test, the flowmeter and vaporizer are turned off (the master switch must be turned off if the machine has a mandatory minimum flow) and the fresh gas hose disconnected from the common gas outlet. A suction bulb is attached to the common gas outlet and the bulb squeezed until fully collapsed, creating negative pressure in the machine (Figure 27.6). If the bulb remains collapsed for at least 10 seconds, no significant leak is present. This test is repeated with the vaporizer turned on to check for internal vaporizer leaks. The vaporizer is then turned off and the fresh gas hose reconnected to the fresh gas outlet.

Positive Pressure Tests If the machine is equipped with a check valve at the common gas outlet, the user may fail to detect a significant leak in the low-pressure system upstream of the check valve using a positive pressure test

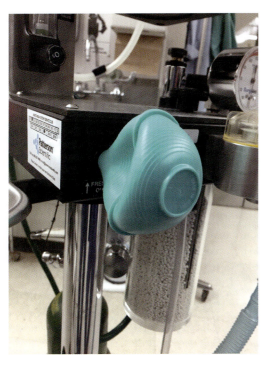

Figure 27.6 A suction bulb is attached to the common gas outlet, demonstrating the proper technique used during the negative pressure test of the low pressure system. The bulb should remain deflated for at least 10 seconds to ensure no significant leaks are present.

(Somprakit and Soontranan 1996). Therefore, unless the user can verify the absence of a check valve at the common gas outlet, the negative pressure test should be performed first, followed by one of the following positive pressure tests:

- *Pressure gauge test* (Somprakit and Soontranan 1996; Dorsch and Dorsch 2007): To perform the pressure gauge test, the flowmeter and vaporizer are turned off (the flowmeter may be set to the mandatory minimum flow) and the fresh gas hose disconnected from the common gas outlet. A pressure gauge (i.e. from a standard sphygmomanometer) is attached to the common gas outlet and the flowmeter slowly turned on until the pressure gauge reads 30 cmH$_2$O (22 mmHg). The flowmeter is then turned down or off to maintain a pressure of 30 cmH$_2$O. The oxygen flow rate at which the pressure remains steady at 30 cmH$_2$O indicates the size of the leak in the low pressure system and should be less than approximately 50 mL/min. This test is repeated with the vaporizer turned on to check for internal vaporizer leaks.
- *Elapsed time test* (Myers *et al.* 1997; Dorsch and Dorsch 2007): If the machine does not have a flowmeter that reads as low as 50 mL/min, the pressure gauge test can be performed by turning the flowmeter completely off when the pressure gauge reads 30 cmH$_2$O (22 mmHg). If the time required for the pressure to decrease to 20 cmH$_2$O (15 mmHg) is greater than 10 seconds, there is not a significant leak in the low-pressure system. Again, this test should be performed with the vaporizer in the off and on positions.
- *Fresh gas line occlusion test* (Myers *et al.* 1997; Dorsch and Dorsch 2007): To perform the occlusion test, the flowmeter and vaporizer are turned off. The fresh gas hose is occluded by kinking the hose and the flowmeter is turned on to 50 ml/min or the minimum mandatory flow rate. If there is no leak in the low-pressure system, the flowmeter indicator should move downward in the tube. This test is repeated with the vaporizer turned on to check for internal vaporizer leaks.

27.2.3 Scavenging System

No direct association has been made between chronic exposure to trace inhalant anesthetic gas and overt toxicity. However, some studies have demonstrated an increased risk of spontaneous abortion and genotoxicity in operating room personnel exposed to varying levels of inhalant anesthetic gas (Armstrong and Spence 1993; Sessler and Badgwell 1998; Shuhaiber *et al.* 2002; Gauger *et al.* 2003; Nilsson *et al.* 2005; Dorsch and Dorsch 2007; El-Ebiary *et al.* 2013; Otaki *et al.* 2013; Yilmaz and Calbayram 2016). Therefore, all efforts should be made to minimize exposure of personnel to trace gas concentrations and a thorough check of the scavenging system responsible for removing waste gas is merited. The adjustable pressure limiting (APL) valve and ventilator (if intended for use) should be properly connected to the scavenging system interface by corrugated waste gas transfer tubing. If active scavenging is used, the vacuum source is connected and the vacuum flow adjusted at the interface. If passive scavenging is used, the waste gas transfer tubing is verified to be going:

1) through a wall to the outdoors;
2) to the air intake of a portable wall air conditioner;
3) to a room ventilation intake duct that is past the point of recirculation; or
4) to an active charcoal canister that is not exhausted.

Note that active charcoal canisters are not practical for large animal systems in which high fresh gas flows are required (Bednarski 2009).

27.2.3.1   Adjustable Pressure Limiting (APL) Valve

The adjustable pressure limiting (APL) valve is most easily checked after assembling the breathing circuit (reservoir bag, breathing hoses and Y-piece). The APL valve is closed, the Y-piece occluded, and the system pressurized to approximately 50 cmH_2O using the oxygen flush. The pressure should hold within the system. The APL valve is then opened, after which a gradual decrease in pressure indicates a properly functioning APL valve and patent waste gas transfer tubing.

27.2.3.2   *Closed Scavenging System* (Dorsch and Dorsch 2007)

Check of the Air Intake Valve   With the APL valve open, the Y-piece occluded, and the oxygen flow rate set to a minimum, suction is applied to the scavenging system (i.e. using the central pipeline vacuum) to check the air intake valve. The bag attached to the scavenging interface should collapse and the reservoir bag in the breathing circuit may also collapse, at which point the breathing system manometer should indicate a pressure of no more than a few cmH_2O negative pressure if the air intake valve on the scavenging interface is functioning properly.

Check of the Positive Pressure Relief Valve   With the APL valve open and the Y-piece occluded, the oxygen flush is activated, during which time the breathing system manometer should indicate a pressure of no more than 10 cmH_2O if the positive pressure relief valve on the scavenging interface is functioning properly.

27.2.3.3   *Open Scavenging System* (Dorsch and Dorsch 2007)

With the APL valve open, the Y-piece occluded, and the flowmeter off, suction is applied to the scavenger interface

to check the open scavenging system. The breathing system manometer should indicate a pressure of $0 \pm 2\,cmH_2O$ if there is adequate negative pressure relief.

27.2.4   Breathing Circuit

27.2.4.1   Oxygen Monitor

Some newer machines are equipped with an oxygen monitor (analyzer). In a study of machine checks in one teaching hospital, poor oxygen monitor reliability was the most common fault identified in the machines checked (Barthram and McClymont 1992). Some oxygen monitors require daily calibration, while others self-calibrate. If the oxygen monitor is separate from the multi-parameter (physiologic) monitor, the sensor can be removed from the breathing system and exposed to room air. The low oxygen alarm is checked by setting the low oxygen alarm limit above the measured oxygen concentration (i.e. the oxygen concentration of room air, or 21% at sea level) and verifying that an audible signal is generated. The sensor is then replaced in the machine and its function verified by repeated activation of the oxygen flush as the reading approaches 90% (Dorsch and Dorsch 2007; Goneppanavar and Prabhu 2013). If the oxygen monitor is part of a multi-parameter monitor and the sensor is not easily removable, the function can be verified by sampling room air and observing a reading of approximately 21% and by adhering to the instruction manual for calibration recommendations (at sea level; Venticinque and Andrews 2015).

27.2.5   Circuit Status Check

Prior to performing leak checks of the breathing circuit, all components (reservoir bag, breathing hoses, Y-piece, CO_2 absorber, CO_2 sampling line if present) should be checked individually for damage, kinks or foreign material. The bag-ventilator selector switch, if present, should be set to "bag" and the breathing system manometer should read zero. The CO_2 absorbent canister should be correctly mounted and filled to within 0.5–1 inch from the top of the canister. The color and texture of the absorbent should be checked and the absorbent changed if indicated by color or texture. If an absorber bypass is present, it should be in the off position (no bypass permitted).

27.2.6   Rebreathing Circuit Leak Check

The rebreathing circuit should be checked for leaks before every use. To do so, breathing hoses, Y-piece and reservoir bag are firmly connected to the machine and all flowmeters turned off. The APL valve is closed, the Y-piece occluded, and the circuit pressurized to 30 cmH_2O using the oxygen flush (Figure 27.7). If the pressure does not remain at 30 cmH_2O for at least 10 seconds, the leak

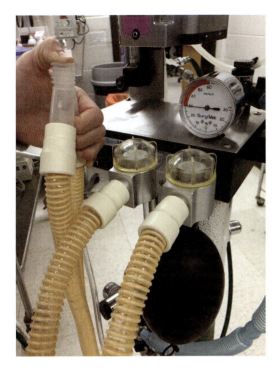

Figure 27.7 Correct technique used to leak test a rebreathing circuit. The APL valve is closed, the patient end is occluded and the system is pressurized to 30 cmH$_2$O. The pressure should hold if no leaks are present.

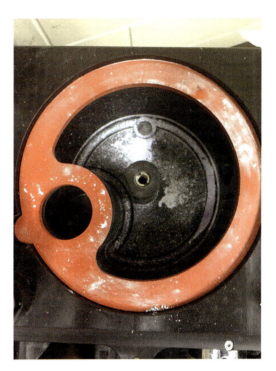

Figure 27.8 CO$_2$ absorbent debris on bottom gasket of CO$_2$ absorbent canister base. This is a common source of leaks within a rebreathing circuit.

can be quantified by adjusting the flowmeter to achieve the minimum oxygen flow rate at which the pressure remains steady at 30 cmH$_2$O (Dorsch and Dorsch 2007). A leak of less than or equal to 300 mL/min at a pressure of 30 cmH$_2$O is acceptable (American Society for Testing and Materials 2005). The APL valve should be opened and a decrease in pressure observed before the Y-piece is released; this allows the user to check APL valve function and waste gas tubing patency, and also prevents absorbent dust from entering the breathing circuit (Dorsch and Dorsch 2007; Goneppanavar and Prabhu 2013).

The most common sites of leaks are loose connections (Y-piece, hoses), worn rubber components (hoses, reservoir bag), loose unidirectional valve dome fittings, or an incomplete seal at the CO$_2$ absorbent canister due to worn gaskets or debris between the gasket and canister (Bednarski 2009) (Figure 27.8).

27.2.7 Bain System Leak Check

Most non-rebreathing circuits can be leak checked in a similar manner to the rebreathing circuit; more specific details concerning leak check procedures for non-rebreathing circuits can be found in Chapter 11. One notable exception is the Bain modification of the Mapleson D circuit. The Bain circuit requires that the internal and external tubes of the coaxial system are intact. After performing the leak check for the external

tube as described above, the internal tube is checked using one of the two methods described below.

27.2.7.1 Inner Tube Occlusion Test

The oxygen flowmeter is set at 2 L/min flow, the APL valve closed, and the patient end of the inner tube occluded using a pencil or syringe plunger to test the patency of the inner tube. If the inner tube is intact, the oxygen flowmeter indicator should fall (Foex and Crampton-Smith 1977; Szypula *et al.* 2008). This test will detect holes in the inner tube as small as 1 mm (Dorsch and Dorsch 2007).

27.2.7.2 Oxygen Flush Test (Pethick Test)

The APL valve is closed, the patient port occluded and the oxygen flowmeter turned on until the reservoir bag is full to begin the oxygen flush test. The oxygen flowmeter is then turned off and the patient port released. When the oxygen flush valve is activated, the reservoir bag should deflate slightly due to the Venturi effect (Pethick 1975; Szypula *et al.* 2008). Both tests of the inner tube of the Bain system are highly specific; however, the inner tube occlusion test is more sensitive than the oxygen flush test for detecting faulty breathing systems (Szypula *et al.* 2008).

27.2.8 Unidirectional Valves

The unidirectional valves of the rebreathing circuit should be properly seated and free of cracks. During a case, watching the valves during inhalation and exhalation can verify that they open, but a failure to close completely may be more difficult to detect. Improper valve function can result in dangerously high levels of inspired CO_2 from rebreathing of expired gases and should be identified before starting a case, to prevent severe hypercarbia, by using one of the three methods below (Baxter *et al.* 1991).

27.2.8.1 Breathing Method (Dorsch and Dorsch 2007)

To test the unidirectional expiratory valve, the inspiratory limb of the breathing circuit is detached from the absorber and occluded. With the APL valve closed, the tester should be able to exhale through the Y-piece, but not inhale. The same test is repeated for the unidirectional inspiratory valve by disconnecting and occluding the expiratory limb of the breathing circuit; the tester should be able to inhale through the Y-piece but not exhale (Figure 27.9).

27.2.8.2 Pressure Method (Dorsch and Dorsch 2007)

To check the unidirectional expiratory valve, a leak-tested reservoir bag is attached to the expiratory outlet and a length of corrugated tubing connected to the bag mount. The inspiratory outlet is occluded while applying positive pressure to the corrugated tube. No gas should flow into

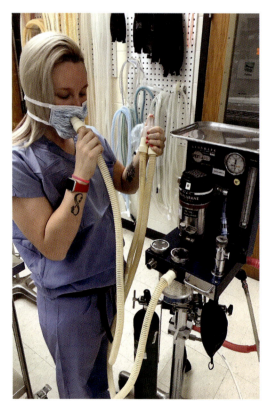

Figure 27.9 Demonstration of the correct technique used during the breathing method for testing unidirectional valves. Note that personnel should wear masks to avoid inhaling particulates and the opposing unidirectional port is occluded during this test.

the tube and the reservoir bag should not inflate. To check the inspiratory valve, a reservoir bag is attached to the bag mount and a length of corrugated tubing connected to the inspiratory outlet on the absorber. The expiratory outlet is occluded while applying positive pressure to the corrugated tube. No gas should flow into the tube and the reservoir bag should inflate.

27.2.8.3 Pressure Decline Method (Kitagawa *et al.* 1994; Dorsch and Dorsch 2007)

To check the unidirectional expiratory valve, a leak-tested reservoir bag is attached to the bag mount and the inspiratory outlet is occluded while pressurizing the system to 30 cmH$_2$O. Since an intact expiratory valve prevents antegrade flow (i.e. flow out of the machine), pressure should be maintained at 30 cmH$_2$O if no leak is present. To check the inspiratory valve, a leak-tested reservoir bag is attached to the inspiratory outlet and the bag mount is occluded while inflating the bag using the oxygen flush valve. Since an intact inspiratory valve prevents antegrade flow (i.e. flow into the machine), the bag should remain inflated if no leak is present.

27.2.9 Ventilators

27.2.9.1 Ventilator Leak Test

The ventilator bellows and ventilator hose can be leak tested by attaching a reservoir bag to the Y-piece and, with the APL valve closed (or isolated by adjusting the bag-ventilator selector switch), filling the bellows and reservoir bag using the oxygen flush valve. The ventilator is turned on and adjusted to approximate settings appropriate for the next patient. During each expiratory phase, the bellows should refill completely (Dorsch and Dorsch 2007). This test may fail to detect a leak in a ventilator with descending bellows due to entrainment of room air through the leak; see recommendations below for descending bellows.

Ascending Bellows   An ascending bellows ventilator can also be checked by closing the APL valve, connecting the bellows to the breathing system, occluding the Y-piece, then filling the bellows using the oxygen flush. If the bellows descend after filling, a leak is present (Dorsch and Dorsch 2007; Bednarski 2009). Note that unlike a descending bellows ventilator, an ascending bellows ventilator can often be checked without an electric supply.

Descending Bellows   A descending bellows ventilator is checked by closing the APL valve, connecting the bellows to the breathing system, allowing the ventilator to cycle until the bellows are almost completely empty (compressed), then occluding the Y-piece and shutting off the ventilator. If the bellows falls, a leak is present

(Dorsch and Dorsch 2007; Bednarski 2009). Holes in the bellows can entrain air from the surrounding cylinder, leading to higher than expected airway pressures (Klein and Wilson 1989).

27.2.9.2   Ventilator Safety Checks

To check the ventilator low-pressure alarm, the ventilator is allowed to cycle with the Y-piece open. The loss of pressure should cause the low-pressure alarm to be activated (Campbell *et al.* 1996). To check the safety-relief valve, the Y-piece is occluded as the ventilator continues to cycle. The pressure in the breathing system should not exceed the safety-relief pressure, usually 65–80 cmH$_2$O (Dorsch and Dorsch 2007). Some ventilators also have an adjustable high-pressure alarm, which should become activated when the pressure inside the ventilator exceeds a preset value (usually 20–30 cmH$_2$O on small animal machines).

27.3   Other Equipment

Prior to starting a case, all other equipment that is intended for use during the anesthetic procedure should be checked. This will vary depending on the species to be anesthetized. Importantly, the anesthetist should identify and check all equipment that might be used, whether by plan or in an emergency (power failure, equipment failure, etc.).

27.3.1   Airway Equipment

Maintaining a patent airway and ability to ventilate is an essential component of anesthesia, as even a short period of hypoxemia can result in brain injury or death (Benumof 1991). A self-inflating manual ventilation device (e.g. AMBU bag) should be available in case of ventilation equipment failure (Hartle *et al.* 2012). Endotracheal tubes of and around the intended size should be inspected for foreign material, and the cuffs inflated and observed for no less than one minute to check for leaks. Khalid and El-Gammal (2010) published a case of partial airway obstruction in a patient due to a plastic meniscus at the distal end of a new endotracheal tube, highlighting the importance of vigilance in checking all equipment, new and used. Laryngoscopes should be checked to verify an adequate connection between blade and handle, and a working light source. Ancillary intubation equipment, including stylets and ties for securing the endotracheal tube in place, should also be available. Whether for pre-oxygenation, anesthesia maintenance, or oxygen supplementation after extubation, an appropriately sized mask that is free of cracks should be available. Oxygen insufflation or demand valve equipment, if applicable, should

be checked for function and is of particular importance during recovery from anesthesia, especially in large species such as horses and cattle.

27.3.2   Drug Delivery Systems

Drug and fluid delivery systems (infusion pumps, syringe pumps, etc.) should have adequate power supplies. Dosage settings should be double-checked in case of calculation errors. A backup means of drug and fluid delivery should be available in case of power failures. Extra breathing hoses, Y-piece and reservoir bag are advisable.

27.3.3   Monitors

Monitors should be turned on to verify proper function. When applicable, monitors can be tested on oneself before use (e.g. pulse oximeter, capnograph, Doppler). If a loss of power supply would interfere with monitors intended for use, battery-operated backup monitors such as portable pulse oximeters, capnographs and blood pressure monitors, should be charged and available.

27.3.4   Additional Equipment

Active warming devices such as heated water blankets and forced air warmers should be ready for use. Padding appropriate for the patient should be readily available; this is of particular importance for large animal species. Equipment for moving the patient, such as hoists for large animal species, should be tested and positioned in the appropriate location. Other transport means (gurney, cart, forklift, etc.) may be required and should be readily available. Extension power cords and pipeline hoses should also be present if anesthesia in a location remote to the hospital induction or operating room is anticipated.

27.4   End of Case

At the end of a case, cylinders should be shut off to prevent depletion of gas through small leaks. Hoses to the central pipeline supply may or may not be disconnected from terminal units for the same reason, depending on practice policies. After the oxygen supply is turned off, the flowmeter should be turned on until the pressure gauge reads zero, and then turned off. If a master switch is present on the anesthesia machine, it should be switched off to prevent oxygen depletion due to the minimum mandatory flow rate; this is especially important if pipeline hoses are not disconnected from the terminal unit.

The anesthesia machine and breathing circuit are disassembled for cleaning, drying and/or reprocessing. The unidirectional valve domes and valves can be removed to allow for air drying of the inner components. The CO_2 absorbent canister is a significant source of moisture and should be wiped down and allowed to dry after proper disposal of exhausted absorbent. The endotracheal tube, mask, reservoir bag, breathing hoses, Y-piece and ventilator hose should be cleaned then disinfected. Cleaning may be performed by hand or in an ultrasonic cleaner to remove macromolecular contamination. Disinfection may be performed by techniques such as pasteurization, by spraying with accelerated hydrogen peroxide products, or by soaking in glutaraldehyde, the only methods that are bactericidal, sporicidal, fungicidal and virucidal (Steffey *et al.* 1984; Accel® TB package insert, Virox Technologies Inc., Oakville, ON). Use of aldehydes, however, may be associated with skin irritation, environmental effects and incomplete disinfection. A more efficient, albeit expensive, option is the use of automated washer-disinfector machines that perform cleaning, disinfection, rinsing and drying in a single process (Geiss 1995; Lewis and McIndoe 2004). Sterilization is generally not necessary given that breathing circuit components do not enter sterile tissues or the vascular system (Geiss 1995; Lewis and McIndoe 2004). Furthermore, gas sterilization of breathing circuit components with ethylene oxide may result in severe respiratory tract burns due to incomplete aeration and should therefore be avoided unless a minimum of one week of aeration is possible (Dorsch and Dorsch 2007; Bednarski 2009).

27.5   Preventative Maintenance

All anesthetic equipment in use should undergo service at regular intervals. Many components of the anesthesia machine deteriorate with use and over time. Continued use of anesthesia equipment with faulty components (worn gaskets, damaged valves, cracked hoses, etc.) may necessitate early replacement of entire machines, which may have been avoided by replacing less expensive parts. Administration of inhalant gases through a vaporizer that is past due for calibration may lead to unpredictable drug delivery and an unstable plane of anesthesia. Many manufacturers of anesthesia machines and monitors offer preventative maintenance as part of a service contract. For equipment not covered by a service contract, the manufacturer or other anesthesia equipment provider should be contacted to determine appropriate service intervals and options. Equipment-specific user manuals or manufacturer web sites should be consulted for more information.

References

American Society for Testing and Materials (2005) *Standard Specification for Minimum Performance and Safety Requirements for Anesthesia Breathing Systems F1208-89 (2005)*. ASTM, West Conshohocken, PA.

Armstrong, P.J. and Spence, A.A. (1993) Toxicity of inhalational anaesthesia: long-term exposure of anaesthetic personnel – environmental pollution. *Bailliere Clin Anaes*, 7, 915–935.

Armstrong-Brown, A., Devitt, J.H. and Kurrek, M. (2000) Inadequate pre-anesthesia equipment checks in a simulator. *Can J Anaesth*, 47, 974–979.

Barthram, C. and McClymont, W. (1992) The use of a checklist for anaesthetic machines. *Anaesthesia*, 47, 1066–1069.

Baxter, G.M., Adams, J.E. and Johnson, J.J. (1991) Severe hypercarbia resulting from inspiratory valve malfunction in two anesthetized horses. *J Am Vet Med Assoc*, 198, 193–195.

Bednarski, R.M. (2009) Anesthesia equipment. In: Muir, W.W. and Hubbell, L.A.E. (eds). *Equine Anesthesia: Monitoring and Emergency Therapy*, 2nd ed. St Louis, MO: Saunders, pp. 315–331.

Benumof, J.L. (1991) Management of the difficult adult airway. With special emphasis on awake tracheal intubation. *Anesthesiology*, 75, 1087–110.

Campbell, R.M., Sheikh, A. and Crosse, M.M. (1996) A study of the incorrect use of ventilator disconnection alarms. *Anaesthesia*, 51, 369–370.

Cassidy, C.J., Smith, A. and Arnot-Smith, J. (2011) Critical incident reports concerning anaesthetic equipment: analysis of the UK National Reporting and Learning System (NRLS) data from 2006–2008. *Anaesthesia*, 66, 879–888.

Chopra, V., Bovill, J.G., Spierdijk, J. and Koornneef, F. (1992) Reported significant observations during anaesthesia: a prospective analysis over an 18-month period. *Br J Anaesth*, 68, 13–17.

Dorsch, J.A. and Dorsch, S.E. (2007) Equipment checkout and maintenance. In: *Understanding Anesthesia Equipment*, 5th ed. Philadelphia, PA: Lippincott Williams & Wilkins, pp. 931–954.

El-Ebiary, A.A., Abuelfadl, A.A., Sarhan, N.I. and Othman, M.M. (2013) Assessment of genotoxicity risk in operation room personnel by the alkaline comet assay. *Hum Exp Toxicol*, 32, 563–570.

Foex, P. and Crampton-Smith, A. (1977) A test for co-axial circuits. *Anaesthesia,* 32, 294.

Gauger, V.T., Voepel-Lewis, T., Rubin, P., Kostrzewa, A. and Tait, A.R. (2003) A survey of obstetric complications and pregnancy outcomes in paediatric and nonpaediatric anaesthesiologists. *Paediatr Anaesth,* 13, 490–495

Geiss, H.K. (1995) Reprocessing of anaesthetic and ventilator equipment. *J Hosp Infect,* 30, 414–420.

Goneppanavar, U. and Prabhu, M. (2013) Anaesthesia machine: checklist, hazards, scavenging. *Indian J Anaesth,* 57, 533–540.

Hartle, A., Anderson, E., Bythell, V., Gemmell, L., Jones, H. *et al.* (2012) Checking anaesthetic equipment 2012: Association of Anaesthetists of Great Britain and Ireland. *Anaesthesia,* 67, 660–668.

Khalid, S. and El-Gammal, K. (2010) Endotracheal tube defects: hidden causes of airway obstruction. *Saudi J Anaesth,* 4, 108–110.

Kitagawa, H., Sai, Y., Nosaka, S., Amakata, Y. and Oku, S. (1994) A new leak test for specifying malfunctions in the exhalation and inhalation check valve. *Anesth Analg,* 78, 611.

Klein, L.V. and Wilson, D.V. (1989) An unusual cause of increasing airway pressure during anesthesia. *Vet Surg,* 18, 239–241.

Langford, R., Gale, T.C. and Mayor, A.H. (2007) Anaesthetic machine checking guidelines: have we improved our practice? *Eur J Anaesthesiol,* 24, 1050–1056.

Lewis, S. and McIndoe, A.K. (2004) Cleaning, disinfection and sterilization of equipment. *Anaesth Intensive Care,* 5, 360–363.

Mosley, C.A. (2015) Anesthesia equipment. In: Grimm, K.A., Lamont, L.A., Tranquilli, W.J., Greene, S.A. and Robertson, S.A. (eds). *Veterinary Anesthesia and Analgesia. The Fifth Edition of Lumb and Jones.* Ames, IA: John Wiley & Sons, pp. 23–85.

Myers, J.A., Good, M.L. and Andrews, J.J. (1997) Comparison of tests for detecting leaks in the low-pressure system of anesthesia gas machines. *Anesth Analg,* 84, 179–184.

Nilsson, R., Bjordal, C., Andersson, M., Björdal, J., Nyberg, A. *et al.* (2005) Health risks and occupational exposure to volatile anaesthetics – a review with a systematic approach. *J Clin Nurs,* 14, 173–186.

Otaki, K., Yashima, N., Kato, F., Oda, S. and Kawamae, K. (2013) The genotoxicity of occupational exposure to sevoflurane in anesthesiologists: 9AP2-9. *Eur J Anaesth,* 30, 145.

Pethick, S.L. (1975) Correspondence. *Can Anaesth Soc J,* 22, 115.

Sessler, D.I. and Badgwell, M. (1998) Exposure of post-operative nurses to exhaled anesthetic gases. *Anesth Analg,* 87, 1083–1088.

Shuhaiber, S., Einarson, A., Radde, I.C., Sarkar, M. and Koren, G. (2002) A prospective-controlled study of pregnant veterinary staff exposed to inhaled anesthetics and X-rays. *Int J Occup Med Environ Health,* 15, 363–373.

Somprakit, P. and Soontranan, P. (1996) Low pressure leakage in anaesthetic machines. *Anaesthesia,* 51, 461–464.

Steffey, E.P., Hodgson, D.S. and Kupershoek, C. (1984) Monitoring oxygen concentrating devices (letter to the editor). *J Am Vet Med Assoc,* 184, 626–638.

Szpisjak, D.F. and Starrett-Keller, C.M. (2014) Field anesthesia machine ventilator oxygen consumption in models of high and low pulmonary compliance. *Mil Med,* 179, 1465–1468.

Szpisjak, D.F., Lamb, C.L. and Klions, K.D. (2005) Oxygen consumption with mechanical ventilation in a field anesthesia machine. *Anesth Analg,* 100, 1713–1717.

Szpisjak, D.F., Javernick, E.N., Kyle, R.R. and Austin, P.N. (2008) Oxygen consumption of a pneumatically controlled ventilator in a field anesthesia machine. *Anesth Analg,* 107, 1907–1911.

Szypula, K.A., Ip, J.K., Bogod, D. and Yentis, S.M. (2008) Detection of inner tube defects in co-axial circle and Bain breathing systems: a comparison of occlusion and Pethick tests. *Anaesthesia,* 63, 1092–1095.

Venticinque, S.G. and Andrews, J. (2015) Inhaled anesthetics: delivery systems. In: Miller, R.D., Cohen, N.H., Eriksson, L.I., Fleisher, L.A., Wiener-Kronish, J.P. and Young, W.L. (eds). *Miller's Anesthesia,* 8th ed. Philadelphia, PA: Saunders, pp. 752–820.

Yilmaz, S. and Calbayram, N.C. (2016) Exposure to anesthetic gases among operating room personnel and risk of genotoxicity: a systematic review of the human biomonitoring studies. *J Clin Anesth,* 35, 326–331.

28

Equipment Cleaning and Sterilization

Cristina de Miguel Garcia and Kristen G. Cooley

School of Veterinary Medicine, University of Wisconsin, Madison, Wisconsin, USA

28.1　Introduction

Nosocomial or hospital-acquired infections (HAI) can be defined either as those developing after 2 days of hospital stay, or within 2 weeks of a previous hospitalization. These infections can originate from bacteria belonging to the endogenous flora of the patient or can be acquired from the hospital environment (De Man *et al.* 2001). Amongst environmental sources in human hospitals, those identified as reservoirs include inadequately decontaminated laryngoscope handles (Simmons 2000), thermometers (Van den Berg *et al.* 2000), bronchoscopes and endoscopes (Schelenz and French 2000; Cowen 2001), stethoscopes (Nunez *et al.* 2000), computer keyboards (Bures *et al.* 2000) and hospital staff acting as carriers (Lacey *et al.* 2001; Wang *et al.* 2001).

In veterinary medicine, early reports identified HAI as the origin for urinary tract infections, catheter site infections, surgical site infections, pneumonia and bacterial diarrheas (Boerlin *et al.* 2001; Johnson 2002; Lobetti *et al.* 2002). In animals, pathogens most commonly associated with nosocomial infections include Enterococcus spp., *E. coli*, Klebsiella spp., Staphylococcus spp., Enterobacter spp. and Pseudomonas spp. (Bernal-Rosas *et al.* 2015; Kuan *et al.* 2016). Furthermore, *E. coli* and *Staphylococcus aureus* have developed into Multidrug Resistant (MDR) *E. coli*, and Methicillin Resistant *Staphylococcus aureus* (MRSA) (Sanchez *et al.* 2002; Weese *et al.* 2004).

A recent survey by Benedict *et al.* (2008) revealed that 82% of 38 American Veterinary Medical Association accredited veterinary teaching hospitals had reported the incidence of HAI in the previous 5 years. Half of them had also identified zoonotic infections in their members of staff during the previous 2 years. In addition, Ruple-Czerniak *et al.* (2013) published a small animal multicenter evaluation of a standardized syndromic surveillance system to estimate rates of HAI among

critically ill dogs and cats. They found that in dogs having surgery and receiving anti-ulcer medication and antimicrobials, those with an indwelling urinary catheter and those whose hospitalization lasted longer than 6 days were at increased risk of HAI. Similarly, in the feline population, patients undergoing surgical procedures, those with urinary catheters and those receiving antimicrobial therapy, were at higher risk of nosocomial infections. In one multicenter study on equine HAI, the incidence of HAI was 19.7%, with the most commonly reported etiologies being surgical site and intravenous catheter site inflammation (Ruple-Czerniak *et al.* 2014).

Proper decontamination of equipment is essential to reduce HAI; however, methods of disinfection and sterilization when improperly or repeatedly carried out have the ability to compromise the integrity of equipment over time. Therefore, manufacturer's specifications should be consulted and equipment safety and functionality tests should be implemented before each use.

Other crucial factors in preventing HAI are to improve preventative measures and hygiene of personnel. Handwashing, alcohol-based hand sanitizers (Picheansathian 2004) or the use of disposable protective gear (Chen *et al.* 2006) can drastically reduce the transmission of pathogens between patients. The World Health Organization (WHO) (http://www.who.int/csr/resources/publications/standardprecautions/en/) has published infection control standard precautions and recommendations in healthcare. Enforcement of aseptic techniques and the use of single-patient, single-use equipment or sterile reusable equipment should be enforced whenever possible.

28.1.1　Risk Assessment

In 1968, Spaulding designed a strategy for the disinfection or sterilization of medical equipment and surfaces according to their degree of risk involved in their use

Veterinary Anesthetic and Monitoring Equipment, First Edition. Edited by Kristen G. Cooley and Rebecca A. Johnson.

(Table 28.1). Based on this, decontamination guidelines have been published by the Food and Drug Administration (FDA), the Environmental Protection Agency (EPA), the Centers for Disease Control (CDC), and other institutions, in order to decrease or prevent the risk of infection transmission by the use of these devices (Sehulster and Chinn 2003; Rutala *et al.* 2008). Contaminated medical devices can be classified according to three infection risk categories:

1) *High risk (critical items)*: These items are exposed to patients' uncontaminated tissues or the vasculature. These items must be sterile.
2) *Intermediate risk (semi-critical items)*: These items are exposed to mucous membranes or non-intact skin, but do not generally cross the blood barrier. No microorganisms but a small numbers of bacterial spores are acceptable, since intact mucous membranes are resistant to spores but susceptible to other agents, such as bacteria, mycobacteria and viruses.
3) *Low risk (non-critical items)*: These items encounter intact skin only.

The choice of decontamination method depends on several factors, including the origin and type of contamination (risk category), time required for the processing, type of material and manufacturer's specifications of the device, availability of the different methods, and potential hazards derived from the processing itself.

28.2 The Decontamination Process

28.2.1 Cleaning

For certain items, thorough cleaning could be sufficient for equipment reuse. However, in most cases cleaning takes place prior to disinfection or sterilization as it removes gross soil and reduces the bioburden, or population, of infectious agents. As such, residual organic load can inactivate some chemical germicides or protect microorganisms against disinfection or sterilization.

Cleaning involves washing with water and a detergent or enzymatic cleaner and may be achieved manually, mechanically, or by the combination of both. If equipment is not cleaned prior to disinfection, the present bioburden or retained soil may inactivate chemical germicides or afford microorganisms with protection. Blood and secretions or excretions should not be allowed to dry on a device, as it can make sufficient cleaning very difficult (Dorsch and Dorsch 2008). Clean tap or distilled water should be used as opposed to saline, as the latter can corrode metal instruments and devices (Dorsch and Dorsch 2008). Water temperature should not exceed 45 °C (113 °F), as higher temperatures can cause proteins

to coagulate and form a layer of protection for the microorganisms (Juwarker 2013). After cleaning, rinsing is essential to remove soil and leftover detergent. Drying of equipment should be exhaustive, as a humid environment will encourage microorganisms to grow and, if going for further processing, it can also react with the sterilant, creating toxic compounds (Buben *et al.* 1999). Wet items placed into a liquid disinfectant will dilute the agent and render it less effective. Many agents recommend using test strips to check the concentration after each use (Figure 28.1). Before cleaning an item, refer to the manufacturer's specifications for that item to avoid equipment damage.

This decontamination process should be carried out in an area separated from traffic, patients, general personnel, sterile equipment storage and other facilities to avoid cross contamination. Additionally, the area should be divided into clean and dirty areas, with non-recirculating heating and ventilation systems that minimize spreading of contaminants. This area should also be cleaned and disinfected daily.

28.2.2 Disinfection Versus Sterilization

Decontamination by heat is always favored over chemical disinfection; however, chemical disinfection is convenient, rapid and cost-effective. Nonetheless, it can result in production of toxic compounds, and be flammable, corrosive or chemically incompatible with certain materials. Following disinfection, items should be rinsed with water, thoroughly dried, and stored in a way that avoids recontamination (Figure 28.2). Furthermore, disinfection is preferred to sterilization whenever possible, as the latter may damage anesthetic equipment made of rubber and plastic by repeated processing. However, sterilization is always required for critical equipment exposed to mucous membranes, broken skin or used in invasive procedures.

28.2.3 Disinfection

Disinfection is a process that eliminates most disease-producing microorganisms, except bacterial spores. There are three levels of disinfection: low, intermediate and high:

1) Low-level disinfection kills most bacteria (except for mycobacteria and spores), some viruses and fungi. These products are EPA-registered hospital disinfectants without mycobactericidal action (chlorine-based products, phenols, ammonium quaternary compounds, 70–90% alcohol).
2) Intermediate-level disinfection destroys bacteria (not spores), mycobacteria, most viruses and fungi. These

Table 28.1 Spaulding classification of patient care items and environmental surfaces with examples of disinfections/sterilization method.

Device classification	Process	Microorganism inactivation	Method	Example
Critical or high-risk items that enter sterile tissues/vasculature	Sterilization	All microorganisms and spores	Steam autoclave Dry heat Ethylene oxide Gas plasma Chemical (GA >0.2%, HP 7.5%, paracetic acid 0.2%)	Instruments Catheters Cannulas
Semi-critical or intermediate-risk items that contact mucous membranes and non-intact skin	High-level disinfection	All microorganisms and spores (except high spore numbers)	Pasteurization Chemical (GA >0.2%, Orthophthalaladehyde 0.55%, HP 7.5%, AHP 0.5%)	Breathing systems AMBU bags Reservoir bags Tracheal tubes Endoscopes Bronchoscopes
Non-critical or low-risk items contacting intact skin	Intermediate-level disinfection	Bacteria (including mycobacteria), most viruses and fungi, no spores	Chemical	Pressure cuffs ECG leads Straps
	Low-level disinfection	Bacterial and some viruses, no mycobacteria or spores	Chemical	Surfaces Carts Cylinders Machines

GA = glutaraldehyde, HP = hydrogen peroxide, AHP = accelerated hydrogen peroxide (Rutala and Weber 2013).

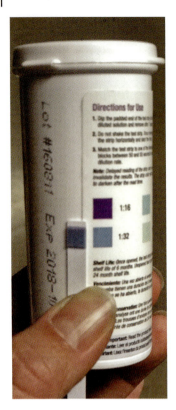

Figure 28.1 The use of a test strip to check the concentration of a disinfectant solution. This strip indicates a dilution of 1:32.

products are EPA-registered hospital disinfectants with mycobactericidal action (chlorine-based products and phenols).

3) High-level disinfection destroys all microorganisms, but not spores. Liquid immersion in chemical disinfectants is useful for thermo-sensitive equipment and entails soaking the equipment in a solution containing the disinfectant.

The normal cycle of high-level disinfection includes cleaning, rinsing, drying, disinfection, rinsing and drying. Most high-level disinfectants can also be used for sterilization purposes if enough exposure time is achieved.

28.2.3.1 Factors Affecting Disinfection

Many factors affect disinfection, including concentration, temperature, exposure time, evaporation and light exposure, bioburden, pH and the item itself.

Concentration of the Chemical Higher concentrations increase bactericidal activity. It is important to dry equipment before submerging it in the disinfectant/sterilization solution, as dilution will negatively affect the effectiveness of the process.

Temperature Higher temperatures will normally increase the performance of the agent, but can also

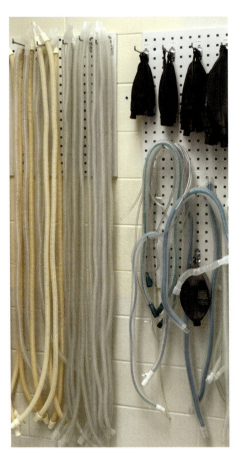

Figure 28.2 Correct storage of breathing hoses and reservoir bags to facilitate drying and avoid contamination.

increase losses, as they will decrease the concentration of the solution by evaporation.

Exposure Time Contact time for each agent needs to be met. As previously mentioned, some agents are high-level disinfectants or sterilants, depending on the exposure time.

Evaporation and Exposure to Light Concentration or efficacy of the chemical agents may be compromised if evaporation takes place or if the chemical is exposed to light.

Bioburden Organic material left on a device can inactivate disinfectant compounds, therefore thorough cleaning beforehand is recommended.

pH Biocidal activity can be affected by acidity or alkalosis of the solution.

Item Characteristics The composition of an item or device to be treated can affect disinfection.

Chemical disinfection/sterilization should be carried out in designated areas with adequate ventilation and personnel should wear appropriate protective gear. The solution should be stored in a tight container and careful manipulation is encouraged to avoid or minimize spillage.

28.2.3.2 Liquid Immersion Disinfection Agents

Glutaraldehyde (GA) Glutaraldehyde (GA) disinfectant is generally used as it has excellent biocidal activity, being effective against bacteria, fungi and viruses at room temperature. High-level disinfection is achieved with shorter exposure times (20–30 minutes), while sterilization requires between 3 and 10 hours. Despite evaporation and dilution during use, to ensure the disinfectant activity remains unchanged, concentrations of GA must remain between 1 and 1.5%. A disadvantage of this product is that it requires activation by alkalization to work and that it needs to be neutralized before disposal. Activated product has a use-life of 14–30 days (manufacturer-dependent). GA is highly toxic and exposure to fumes can cause headache, eye irritation and asthma-like symptoms (Baur *et al.* 2012). It is recommended that this product be used in a closed container in a well-ventilated area with an eyewash station within a 10-second walk. OSHA recommends exposure monitoring with a ceiling exposure limit of 0.05 ppm. Equipment disinfected with GA must be rinsed with copious amounts of water prior to re-use (Perry and Caveney 2012). Endotracheal tubes can be sterilized with either GA or ethylene oxide; however, the safety of the cuffs could be compromised with repeated processing (Yoon *et al.* 2007).

Ortho-phthalaldehyde (OPA) When using ortho-phthalaldehyde (OPA), high-level disinfection will be achieved after a 12-minute exposure at room temperature, although this time can be decreased if higher temperatures are used. It does not require activation, can generally be discarded through normal disposal, and does not emit any noxious fumes. It can be used to disinfect breathing system tubing and flexible fiber optic laryngoscopes; furthermore, the latter can also be effectively disinfected by the use of alcohol-based products (Chang *et al.* 2012). Metal laryngoscope blades and handles can be adequately sterilized, not only with aldehyde but also with aldehyde-free compounds (Telang *et al.* 2010). This product has a tendency to stain skin, mucous membranes, clothing and surfaces.

Quaternary Ammonium Compounds (Quats) Quaternary ammonium compounds (Quats) are low-level disinfectants at room temperature, as they have no sporicidal action; they are therefore useful for cleaning purposes. These compounds are also inactivated by organic material. Products like this are normally employed in sanitation of floors, furniture and walls; however, they can also be used for disinfecting medical equipment that contacts intact skin (e.g. blood pressure cuffs, ECG cables, oxygen masks, continuous positive airway pressure equipment).

Phenolic Compounds Considered to be low- to intermediate-level disinfectants, phenolic compounds do not destroy certain viruses and spores that are resistant to them. They are derived from carbolic acid and can be combined with detergents to create biocidal detergents. Generally, they are used for decontamination of surfaces and low-risk equipment.

Ethyl and Isopropyl Alcohols Ethyl and isopropyl alcohols are common solutions of low- to intermediate-level disinfectants used at 70–90% vol with a wet contact time of between 2–5 minutes. They are virucidal, fungicidal and gram-negative bactericidal, but with no sporicidal activity. An alcohol flush cycle is included in some disinfection processes, as it evaporates quickly, removing water contamination with it.

Chlorine Compounds The chlorine compounds group is inexpensive and quick acting. Amongst these we can find household bleach; however, due to their corrosive and irritant nature, they are not normally used to treat equipment, but as surface disinfectants.

Biguanides Chlorhexidine is the most common biguanide used in veterinary medicine. It is easily inactivated by the presence of organic material, so items must be cleaned prior to being placed in the recommended 0.5% solution for 10 minutes (Figure 28.3). After soaking, items must be rinsed with copious amounts of tap water. Biguanides are toxic to fish and should not be released into the environment (Perry and Caveney 2012). Although low-concentration chlorhexidine is frequently used as part of oral hygiene practices in veterinary medicine (Laverty *et al.* 2015), chlorhexidine at higher than clinically-useful concentrations (>0.5% vs. 0.15% or less) may cause oral ulcers, pharyngitis and tracheitis from endotracheal tubes disinfected with chorhexidine that are not thoroughly rinsed (https://veterinarypracticenews.com/the-pros-and-cons-of-scrubbing-with-betadine-chlorhexidine).

Hydrogen Peroxide (HP) Hydrogen peroxide (HP) solution is effective against all microorganisms and spores, and is therefore used in the plasma sterilization cycle. However, it cannot be used in equipment containing rubber and plastic and it may corrode some metals. It can otherwise be used as a low-level disinfectant at lower concentrations. Paracetic acid is sometimes added to HP solutions, since it is not deactivated by peroxidase and

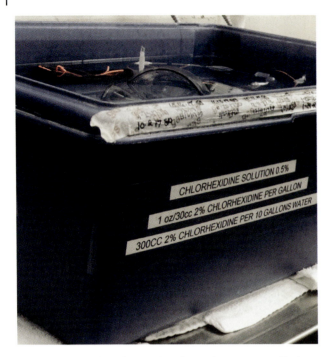

Figure 28.3 Chlorhexidine soaking bin with appropriate dilution instructions on the front.

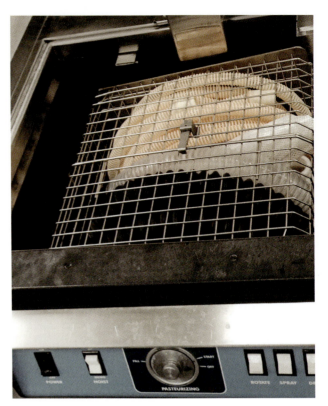

Figure 28.4 Pasteurizer loaded with anesthetic breathing hoses.

catalase will break down HP. Paracetic acid is also degraded to environmentally safe residues.

Accelerated Hydrogen Peroxide This formulation of accelerated hydrogen peroxide, also know as AHP (Virox Animal Health, Oakville, ON Canada), is a hydrogen peroxide mixture (it also contains surfactants, chelators and wetting agents), which is a non-irritating sporicidal, bactericidal and viricidal surface cleaner and low-level disinfectant. It is fume-free and safe to use around animals. A more concentrated product from the same company is capable of high-level disinfection and safe to use on most semi-critical items (Prevention HLD 2017).

Juwarkar (2013) has published other comparative properties of the different products. Furthermore, examples of FDA-cleared sterilants and high-level disinfectants can be found on the FDA website (www.fda.gov).

28.2.3.3 Thermal Washer Disinfector or Pasteurization

In thermal washers, equipment is frequently exposed to water below 100 °C (normally 70 °C for 30 min), although temperature may vary in an inversely proportional manner to the exposure time. Some pasteurizers also wash equipment. A protein dissolving soap can be added to the pasteurizer to help break down proteins and clean equipment. Breathing system tubes, endotracheal tubes, facemasks, laryngeal masks, stylets and laryngoscope blades are some of the equipment that can undergo this type of high disinfection process (Figure 28.4).

28.2.4 Sterilization

There are three different methods of sterilization: high temperature, low temperature and cold sterilization (liquid immersion). High temperature sterilization includes steam autoclaving of equipment or the use of dry heat sterilization. Low temperature methods include ethylene oxide and hydrogen peroxide gas plasma. Liquid immersion sterilization can be achieved with most disinfectant agents if enough temperature and time are allowed (see disinfectant agents above for more information).

28.2.4.1 High Temperature Sterilization

Steam sterilization (or autoclaving) uses saturated steam under pressure, as this technique transfers heat to materials much more rapidly than dry heat. Moreover, increasing the temperature dramatically decreases the time needed for sterilization (e.g. time required for sterilization at 115 °C is 30 min, but increasing the temperature to 134 °C will decrease the processing time to 3 min). Equipment undergoing autoclaving needs to be cleaned and packaged in material that can be easily penetrated by steam and must be dry before being removed from the sterilizer. Anesthetic equipment that can be sterilized by this method includes v-gels, laryngeal mask airways (LMA) and thermo-resistant components of respiratory equipment (Figure 28.5).

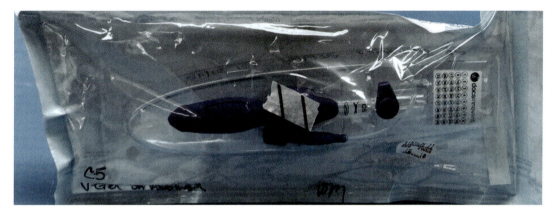

Figure 28.5 After thorough cleaning, the v-gel® can withstand the high temperatures of the steam autoclave (up to 121 °C) and can be reprocessed numerous times.

The advantages of this system is its effectiveness in destruction of microorganisms and spores, speed, ease of use, absence of toxic byproducts and that items are prepackaged so they can be used later in time. One of the major disadvantages is that it cannot be used for heat-sensitive items, as they could be damaged (Figure 28.6).

Steam sterilization monitoring is recommended and can be achieved by the use of indicators. Mechanical indicators denote time, temperature and pressure of the load being sterilized. Chemical indicators, like the autoclave tape, change color, indicating proper exposure to steam. Biological indicators, such as strips or ampules, can be placed in areas of the load that are more difficult to sterilize (Figure 28.7).

Dry heat sterilization is used for equipment that could be damaged or is incompatible with moisture; however, processing times take longer and require higher temperatures (160 °C for 120 min or 190 °C for 30 min). It is also the ideal technique for sterilization of oil-based or semi-liquid compounds such as glycerin, waxes, etc.

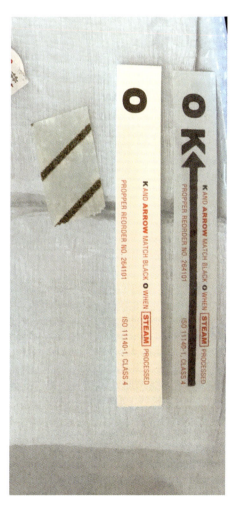

Figure 28.7 Examples of indicator strips that are used in the steam autoclave to indicate that the appropriate temperature was reached and that the items were sterilized. The right strip has been activated and the left strip has not. Autoclave tape is also used as a secondary indicator. In this image, the autoclave tape has been activated, as shown by the black lines on the small strip of tape. Indicators should be placed on the outside and within the item to ensure thorough sterilization.

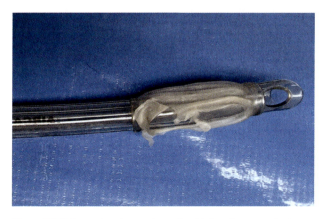

Figure 28.6 Example of an endotracheal tube after autoclaving Although this tube is intact, the cuff is significantly melted.

28.2.4.2 Low Temperature Sterilization

Ethylene oxide (EO) is a colorless and poisonous epoxy compound, soluble in water and easily liquefied at ordinary temperatures and pressures. It is available in pressurized tanks, ampules or cartridges, at a concentration no higher than 3%. EO is highly flammable and the vapors form explosive mixtures when mixed with air, in all proportions from 3–80 %vol. The explosion hazard is eliminated when the vapors are mixed with more than 7.15 times their volume of carbon dioxide (Jones and Kennedy 1930).

Cotton and Roark first described the biological activity of EO in 1928 and several reviews of its characteristics and properties have subsequently been published (Phillips and Kaye 1949; Mendes *et al.* 2007). Equipment undergoing EO sterilization needs to be disassembled, cleaned, dried and packaged in material permeable to gas and water vapor. Exposure time ranges from 1.5–6 hours, depending on temperature, which varies between 38 and 60 °C and a relative humidity of between 40 and 80%. Aeration is also required after processing, as EO can penetrate some materials (i.e. plastics and rubber) and can be retained in varying amounts.

The advantages of EO sterilization are that is very reliable and can be used in thermo-sensitive materials such as IV cannulas; however, processing time is long and costly and equipment inadequately processed can expose patients to residual EO or its byproducts, which are irritant and/or toxic, depending on exposure levels (Buben *et al.* 1999). In addition, there is risk of worker exposure to gases and explosions; therefore, strict adherence to operating instructions and recommendations is encouraged. The occupational safety and health administration regulations (OSHA) have established a limit exposure of 1 ppm for an 8-hour time weighted exposure or 5 ppm in short-term exposures. As with high temperature sterilization, the use of physical, chemical and biological indicators are recommended to ensure sterilization was optimal.

Gas plasma sterilization is carried out by applying energy to hydrogen peroxide to create a cloud of reactive ions that interact with the molecules essential for the metabolism and reproduction of living cells. Opposite to EO sterilization, there is lack of worker exposure and environmental contamination, as its products are water and oxygen. The temperature during the whole cycle does not increase over 50 °C, so it can be used for most heat-labile equipment, except for equipment with narrow lumens and materials containing cellulose, as such components absorb sterilant vapors, thus decreasing its concentration. Biological indicators are also recommended when using this method of sterilization.

28.3 Recommendations for Cleaning and Disinfecting Specific Items

28.3.1 Cleaning

All items used should first be cleaned with a mild detergent to remove all organic material (blood, mucus, etc.) and to decrease the bioburden in preparation for disinfection. After being thoroughly washed inside and out, items should be rinsed and dried prior to submerging into a disinfection solution. Placing wet items into the disinfectant may lead to dilution of the agent and render it ineffective. As previously mentioned, the use of test strips is recommended to test efficacy of the agent. Do not use solution past expiration dates, even if the test strips are indicating an effective concentration.

28.3.2 Semi-Critical Items

Semi-critical items (i.e. those that touch mucous membranes or non-intact skin) can be disinfected by accelerated hydrogen peroxide, based on ease of use (8 min contact time at 20 °C, no fumes or noxious odor, drain disposal, can be reused for up to 21 days, no activation or dilution required), microbial effectiveness (bacteria, viruses, spores, mycobacteria and fungi), and material compatibility (steel, plastics and elastomers) (Prevention HLD 2017).

28.3.2.1 Airway Equipment

Airway equipment (endotracheal tubes, tracheostomy tubes, supraglottic airways, V-gels, etc.) are often intended for one-time use only, therefore cleaning recommendations are not available from the manufacturer (Figure 28.8). Sterilization of these items is recommended; however, many are made out of polyvinyl chloride or silicone and cannot withstand the heat of an autoclave. All items must first be cleaned prior to disinfection/sterilization, and items should not be allowed to sit for any length of time before cleaning. Organic material that is dried onto an item is more difficult to effectively clean. When cleaning these items, gently inflate the cuff (if present) to smooth out any wrinkles that could harbor bacteria. Gently and thoroughly clean the inside and outside of the items with a mild detergent and warm water. The use of an endotracheal tube cleaning brush is recommended (Figure 28.9). After removing all organic material, rinse well and allow to dry. Once dry, place the airway into the high-level disinfectant (HLD) solution and allow to soak, fully submerged, for the necessary duration to achieve disinfection or sterilization. Rinse well with clean water or alcohol and allow to dry before storing.

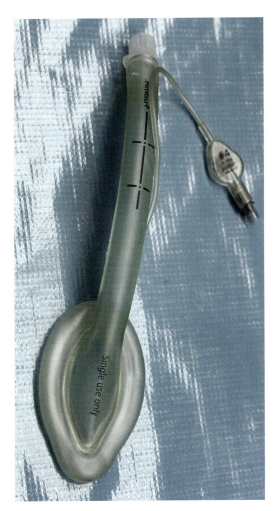

Figure 28.8 Example of an item (laryngeal mask airway) indicating that it is to be used one time only. It is best practice to discard these items. If reused, they must be properly cleaned and disinfected. As single use items, the integrity of the cuff, cuff inflation pilot and connections may be questionable after reprocessing. These items must be checked prior to reuse.

28.3.2.2 Adapters, Connectors, Mouth Gags, Specula, Bougies, Stylets, Facemasks

When cleaning adapters (e.g. end-tidal CO_2), connectors (elbows, swivels), mouth gags, specula, Bougies, stylets and facemasks (Figure 28.10), remove all organic debris by washing with a mild detergent and warm water after each use. Small brushes should be used to help remove organic material from small spaces. Once clean and dry, either steam sterilize (metal components such as the mouth gag, stylets or specula) or soak in HLD for the recommended amount of time to achieve either disinfection or sterilization. Rinse well with water or alcohol and allow to dry before storing. Some disinfectants may not be compatible with the rubber diaphragm common in facemasks, and some agents may discolor or make clear plastics cloudy – check the material compatibility of agent used.

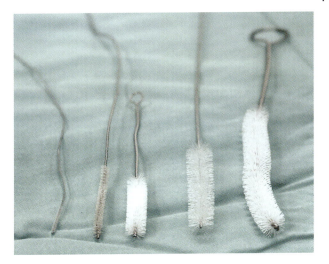

Figure 28.9 A variety of endotracheal tube brushes are available to facilitate the cleaning of the different-sized tubes. These brushes can also be used to clean the cracks and crevices of other types of equipment requiring decontamination.

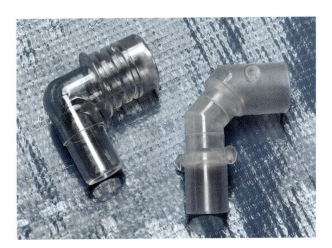

Figure 28.10 Many adapters and tube positioners contact mucous membranes and should be treated as semi-critical items. They require thorough cleaning and high-level disinfection.

28.3.2.3 Temperature

Semi-critical items, including probes, esophageal stethoscopes, transesophageal ECG, spray applicators, laryngoscope blade, pulse-oximeter probes, etc. pose a challenge for a variety of reasons, mostly attributed to the fact that they may not be able to withstand submersion into a liquid. Since these are reusable items, the manufacturer should provide advice on how best to clean and disinfect these pieces. Probe covers are an option but may affect the function of the item. After each use, the item should be cleaned with a mild detergent and care should be taken to remove organic material from creases and crevices (around the laryngoscope blade light source, tip of the spay applicator etc.; Figures 28.11 and 28.12).

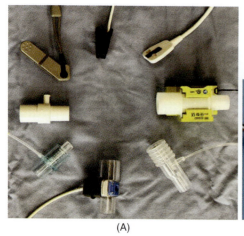

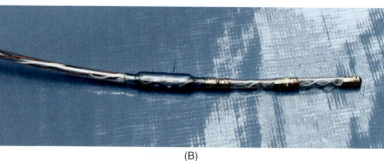

(A)   (B)

Figure 28.11 (A) Temperature probes, pulse-oximeter probes, mainstream capnometer adaptors, and esophageal monitors are considered semi-critical items because they contact mucous membranes. They can be a challenge to clean and disinfect because they may not be submersible. (B) Additionally, esophageal ECG leads also fall into this category.

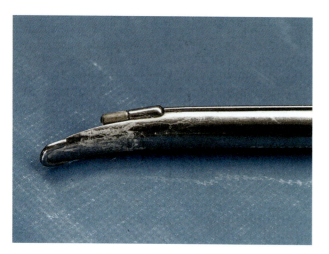

Figure 28.12 A laryngoscope blade contaminated with dried saliva.

Once dry, the items may then be gently wiped down with a suitable HLD wipe or 70% alcohol. Wipe down not only the portion that contacts the patient but also the length of the cord, tubing or handle. Please refer to the manufacturer's guidelines to avoid damaging the product during cleaning.

28.3.2.4   Breathing Hoses (Circle and Non-Rebreathing), Reservoir Bags, Y-pieces, Resuscitation Bags (AMBU)

These items do not typically contact mucous membranes or non-intact skin; however, they are often listed as semi-critical items. Hoses and bags are difficult to clean and challenging to dry. The only portion of these items that is exposed to mucous membranes (Y-piece

and patient end of hoses, resuscitation valve) should routinely be cleaned and disinfected using a HLD. If an item becomes contaminated with body fluids or blood, the item must be thoroughly cleaned and disinfected using a high-level disinfectant. Pasteurization is also an option, as is the regular use of bacterial-viral filters on the inspiratory limb of the breathing circuit, to protect patients from what might be contaminating the machine.

28.3.3   Non-Critical Items

Non-critical items are those items that encounter intact skin only. Non-critical items require low-level disinfection (LLD), such as 70% isopropyl alcohol or AHP.

28.3.3.1   Piezoelectric Crystals (Doppler Probes), ECG Clips and Leads, Blood Pressure Cuffs, Stethoscope Bells and Tubing

These items should be cleaned and disinfected after each use. If visibly soiled, clean non-critical items with mild detergent and warm water. After the removal of organic material, wipe the item down using the manufacturer's approved LLD (Figure 28.13).

28.3.3.2   Anesthesia Machine Parts

Anesthesia machine parts include unidirectional valves, dome caps, flutter discs, APL/pop-off valve, carbon dioxide absorber canister and ventilator bellows. The anesthesia machine should be disassembled and cleaned regularly based on use. Unidirectional valves, dome caps and flutter discs can be cleaned with a mild detergent and warm water rinsed and then wiped or soaked in an LLD and then rinsed and allowed

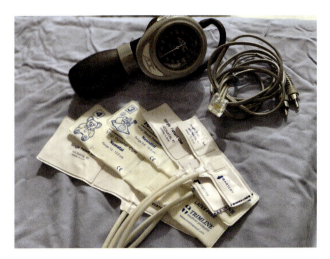

Figure 28.13 Piezoelectric crystals, blood pressure cuffs and sphygmomanometers contact intact skin only; therefore, low level disinfection is required.

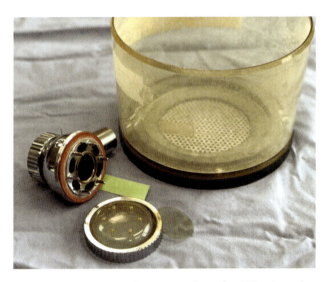

Figure 28.14 Machine and monitor surfaces should be cleaned and disinfected regularly using a low-level disinfectant. The machine can also be taken apart and cleaned at regular intervals and after a known contaminated case.

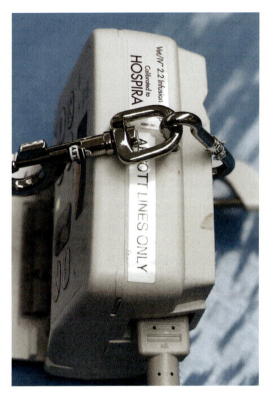

Figure 28.15 This fluid pump shows an area of contamination and illustrates the importance of wiping down all equipment after each anesthetic case.

28.3.3.3 Anesthesia Machine Surfaces

Personnel are often the source of contamination of anesthesia machine surfaces, such as monitors and knobs, ventilator housing, gas cylinder and drops, waste gas scavenging systems, pens, clipboards, chairs, etc. Appropriate hand hygiene can be challenging due to the nature and intensity of anesthesia care. As such, these areas should be cleaned of gross organic debris and then wiped down with a low-level disinfectant at the end of the day or when visibly soiled (Figure 28.15).

28.3.4 Hand Hygiene

The anesthetist's hands are easily contaminated during IV catheter placement and intubation, as well as during the anesthetic case. Hands should be washed with mild soap and warm water when visibly soiled, when contact with body fluids occurs, after known contamination or after using the restroom. It is acceptable to use an alcohol-based hand sanitizer when hands are not visibly soiled after patient contact and frequently throughout the day. Use an appropriate amount, so that all hand surfaces are wet and rub hands together until dry (CDC 2002).

to dry prior to reassembly (Figure 28.14). The APL/pop-off valve can be wiped with an LLD at the end of the day. The carbon dioxide absorber canister should be washed and wiped with an LLD whenever the exhausted granules are changed. Ventilator bellows should be cleaned periodically; consult the manufacturer's guidelines prior to doing so. When anesthetizing patients with known communicable bacterial or fungal infections, a bacterial-viral filter can be placed on the expiratory valve to protect the machine from contamination.

References

Benedict, K.M., Morley, P.S. and VanMetre, D.C. (2008) Characteristics of biosecurity and infection control programs at veterinary teaching hospitals. *J Am Vet Med Assoc*, 233, 767–773.

Bernal-Rosas, Y., Osorio-Muñoz, K. and Torres-García, O. (2015) *Pseudomonas aeruginosa*: an emerging nosocomial trouble in veterinary practice [*Pseudomonas aeruginosa*: un problema nosocomial emergente en veterinaria], *Revista MVZ Córdoba*, 20, 4937–4494.

Boerlin, P., Eugster, S., Gaschen, F., Straub, R. and Schawalder, P. (2001) Transmission of opportunistic pathogens in a veterinary teaching hospital. *Vet Microbiol*, 82, 347–359.

Buben, I., Melichercıkova, V., Novotna, N. and Svitakova, R. (1999) Problems associated with sterilization using ethylene oxide: residues in treated materials. *Cent Eur J Public Health*, 4, 197–202.

Bures, S., Fishbain, J.T., Uyehara, C.F., Parker, J.M. and Berg, B.W. (2000) Computer keyboards and faucet handles as reservoirs of nosocomial pathogens in the intensive care unit. *Am J Infect Control*, 28, 465–471.

Baur, X., Bakehe, P. and Vellguth, H.J. (2012) Bronchial asthma and COPD due to irritants in the workplace – an evidence-based approach. *Occup Med Toxicol*, 26, 7–19.

CDC (2002) Guideline for hand hygiene in health-care settings. *MMWR Morb Mortal Wkly Rep*, 51, 1–44.

Chen, T.H., Wong, K.L., Shieh, J.P., Chuang, Y.C., Yang, Y.C. and So, E.C. (2006) Use of condoms as blade covers during laryngoscopy, a method to reduce possible cross infection among patients. *J Infect*, 52, 118–123.

Chang, D., Florea, A., Rowe, M. and Seiberling, K.A. (2012) Disinfection of flexible fiberoptic laryngoscopes after *in vitro* contamination with *Staphylococcus aureus* and *Candida albicans*. *Arch Otolaryngol Head Neck Surg*, 138, 119–121.

Cotton, R.T. and Roark, R.C. (1928). Ethylene oxide as a fumigant. *Indust Eng Chem*, 20, 805.

Cowen, A.E. (2001) The clinical risks of infection associated with endoscopy. *Can J Gastroenterol*, 15, 321–331.

De Man, P., van der Veeke, E., Leemreijze, M., van Leeuwen, W., Vos, G. *et al.* (2001) Enterobacter species in a pediatric hospital: horizontal transfer or selection in individual patients? *J Infect Dis*, 184, 211–214.

Dorsch, J.A. and Dorsch, S.E. (2008) Cleaning and sterilization. In: *Understanding Anesthesia Equipment*, 5th ed. Philadelphia, PA: Lippincott, Williams & Wilkins, pp. 985–993.

Johnson, J.A. (2002) Nosocomial infections. *Vet Clin North Am Small Anim Pract*, 32, 1101–1126.

Jones, G.W. and Kennedy, R.E. (1930.) Extinction of ethylene oxide flames with carbon dioxide. *Indust Eng Chem*, 22, 146–147.

Juwarkar, C.S. (2013) Cleaning and sterilization of anaesthetic equipment. *Indian J Anaesth*, 57, 541–550.

Kuan, N., Chang, C., Lee, C. and Yeh, K. (2016) Extended-spectrum beta-lactamase-producing *Escherichia coli* and *Klebsiella pneumoniae* isolates from the urine of dogs and cats suspected of urinary tract infection in a veterinary teaching hospital. *Taiwan Vet J*, 42, 143–148.

Lacey, S., Flaxman, D., Scales, J. and Wilson, A. (2001) The usefulness of masks in preventing transient carriage of epidemic methicillin-resistant *Staphylococcus aureus* by healthcare workers. *J Hosp Infect*, 48, 308–311.

Laverty, G., Gilmore, B.F., Jones, D.S., Coyle, L., Folan, M. and Breathnach, R. (2015) Antimicrobial efficacy of an innovative emulsion of medium chain triglycerides against canine and feline periodontopathogens. *J Small Anim Pract*. 56, 253–263.

Lobetti, R.G., Joubert, K.E., Picard, J., Carstens, J. and Pretorius, E. (2002) Bacterial colonization of intravascular catheters in young dogs suspected to have parvoviral enteritis. *J Am Vet Med Assoc*, 220, 1321–1324.

Mendes, G.C.C., Brandao, T.R.S. and Silva, C.L.M. (2007) Ethylene oxide sterilization of medical devices: a review. *Am J Infect Control*, 35, 574–581.

Nunez, S., Moreno, A., Green, K. and Villar, J. (2000) The stethoscope in the emergency department: a vector of infection? *Epidemiol Infect*, 124, 233–237.

Perry, K. and Caveney, L. (2012) Chemical disinfectants. In: Caveney, J., Jones, B. and Ellis, K. (eds.) *Veterinary Infection Prevention and Control*. Ames, IA: Wiley-Blackwell, pp. 129–134.

Phillips, C.R. and Kaye, S. (1949) The sterilizing action of gaseous ethylene oxide: a review. *Am J Hyg*, 50, 270–279.

Picheansathian, W.A. (2004) A systematic review on the effectiveness of alcohol-based solutions for hand hygiene. *Int J Nurs Pract*, 10, 3–9.

Prevention, H.L.D. [package insert] (2017) *Virox Technologies*. Oakville, Ontario, Canada.

Ruple-Czeniak, A.A., Aceto, H.W., Bender, M.R., Paradis, M.R., Shaw, S.P. *et al.* (2013) Using syndromic surveillance to estimate baseline rates for healthcare-associated infections in critical care units of small animal referral hospitals. *J Vet Intern Med*, 27, 1392–1399.

Ruple-Czeniak, A.A., Aceto, H.W., Bender, M.R., Paradis, M.R., Shaw, S.P. *et al.* (2014) Syndromic surveillance for evaluating the occurrence of healthcare-associated infections in equine hospitals. *Equine Vet J*, 46, 435–440.

Rutala, W.A., Weber, D.J. and The Healthcare Infection Control Practices Advisory Committee (HICPAC) (2008) Guideline for disinfection and sterilization in healthcare facilities: recommendations of the CDC. *MMWR Morb Mortal Wkly Rep*, 1–158.

Sanchez, S., McCrakin-Stevenson, M.A., Hudson, C.R., Maier, M. *et al.* (2002) Characterization of multidrug resistant *Escherichia coli* isolates associated with nosocomial infections in dogs. *J Clin Microbiol*, 40, 2586–2595.

Sehulster, L. and Chinn, R.Y.W. (2003) Guidelines for environmental infection control in health-care facilities. Recommendations of CDC and Healthcare Infection Control Practices Advisory Committee (HICPAC). *MMWR Recomm Rep*, 52, 1–44.

Schelenz, S. and French, G. (2000) An outbreak of multidrug-resistant *Pseudomonas aeruginosa* infection associated with contamination of bronchoscopes and an endoscope washer disinfector. *J Hosp Infect*, 46, 23–30.

Simmons, S.A. (2000) Laryngoscope handles: a potential for infection. *J Am Assoc Nurse Anesth*, 68, 233–236.

Telang, R., Patil, V., Ranganathan, P. and Kelkar, R. (2010) Decontamination of laryngoscope blades: is our practice adequate? *J Postgrad Med*, 56, 257–261.

Van den Berg, R.W., Claahsen, H.L., Niessen, M., Muytjens, H.L., Liem, K. and Voss, A. (2000) *Enterobacter cloacae* outbreak in the NICU related to disinfected thermometers. *J Hosp Infect*, 45, 29–34.

Wang, J.T., Chang, S.C., Ko, W.J., Chang, Y.Y., Chen, M.L. *et al.* (2001) A hospital-acquired outbreak of methicillin-resistant *Staphylococcus aureus* infection initiated by a surgeon carrier. *J Hosp Infect*, 47, 104–109.

Weese, J.S.T., DaCosta, T., Button, L., Goth, K., Ethier, M. and Boehnke, K. (2004) Isolation of methicillin resistant *Staphylococcus aureus* from the environment in a veterinary teaching hospital. *J Vet Int Med*, 18, 468–470.

Yoon, S.Z., Jeon, Y.S., Kim, Y.C., Lim, Y.J., Ha, J.W. *et al.* (2007) The safety of reused endotracheal tubes sterilized according to Centers for Disease Control and Prevention guidelines. *J Clin Anesth*, 19, 360–364.

29

Unique Species Considerations: Dogs and Cats

Turi Aarnes

College of Veterinary Medicine, The Ohio State University, Columbus, Ohio, USA

29.1 Introduction

Dogs and cats are the most common species veterinary professionals anesthetize. As such, most standard equipment and monitors are discussed in the appropriate chapters elsewhere in this text. However, a few specific ideas associated with dogs and cats are addressed below.

29.2 Intubation

Maintenance of anesthesia using inhalant anesthetics is often best accomplished utilizing an endotracheal (ET) tube to ensure inhalant anesthetic delivery to the lungs. Additionally, endotracheal intubation can protect the airway from regurgitated gastric contents and subsequent aspiration.

It is advisable to choose the ET tube that best fits the trachea. An ET tube that is too small can increase resistance to breathing (McDonell and Kerr 2007), result in leakage of inhalant, and necessitate over-inflation of the cuff. Tracheal trauma due to cuff over-inflation has been well-documented (people, cats, dogs) and can result in tracheal tear, tracheal stenosis and tracheal necrosis (Alderson 2006). Alternatively, selection of an ET tube that is too large can result in laryngeal trauma during intubation.

Choosing an appropriately sized ET tube can be challenging. Experience is often utilized to determine ET tube size; however, for a novice anesthetist there are charts to aid in this determination (Table 29.1). Digital palpation of the outer diameter of the trachea has also been routinely utilized. However, digital palpation alone, and in combination with measurement of nasal septal width, has been associated with under-estimation of ET tube size (Lish *et al.* 2008).

Breed also has an effect on ET tube size selection. Phenotypic parameters associated with tracheal size have been investigated in different breeds of dogs. For example, the vertical length of the fourth digital pad in combination with body mass has been utilized to determine a formula for ET tube size in Dalmatians (Avki *et al.* 2006). Brachycephalic dogs have hypoplastic tracheas (Suter *et al.* 1972) and as such, their ET tubes tend to be smaller than in dogs of comparable weight. Dachshunds have a larger tracheal size and larger ET tube sizes should be chosen in this breed when likened to dogs of comparable weight (Crow *et al.* 2009).

Endotracheal intubation should be confirmed by visualizing the passing of the tube between the arytenoid cartilages. If this is not possible, the endotracheal tube should be connected to a capnometer to ensure that an appropriate waveform and end-tidal CO_2 is being detected. While detection of CO_2 is not a complete guarantee of endotracheal intubation, it is quick and technically easy to perform. A radiograph can also be obtained to visualize the ET tube in the trachea if certainty cannot be obtained.

After endotracheal intubation, the breathing circuit should be attached to the ET tube and the ET tube secured in place. The APL valve should be closed, the rebreathing bag squeezed to elicit an airway pressure of $20\ cmH_2O$, and the cuff inflated only if a leak is detected (i.e. gas heard passing around the ET tube, inhalant smelled, etc.). Ideally, a pressure manometer should be utilized to determine a cuff pressure of between 19 and 25 mmHg (Hartsfield 1996; Briganti *et al.* 2012). Remember to open the APL valve following this test.

Mechanical dead space associated with the ET tube should be minimized, especially in small patients, as excessive dead space can increase the work of breathing (Hartsfield 2007). For single-use tubes, this can be accomplished by cutting the end of the endotracheal tube at the incisors and replacing the adaptor on the tube. Alternatively, tubes can be cut to different sizes and reused, though this can make tube selection slightly

Veterinary Anesthetic and Monitoring Equipment, First Edition. Edited by Kristen G. Cooley and Rebecca A. Johnson.
© 2018 John Wiley & Sons, Inc. Published 2018 by John Wiley & Sons, Inc.

Table 29.1 Endotracheal tube size chart.

Body Weight of Patient	Endotracheal Tube mm I.D.
CATS	
1 kg	3.0
2 kg	3.5
3–4 kg	4.0
4–5 kg	4.5
DOGS	
2 kg	5.0
3 kg	5.5
4–5.5 kg	6.0
5.5–7 kg	6.5
7–9 kg	7.0–7.5
9–12 kg	8.0
13 kg	8.5
14–18 kg	9.0–10.0
16–20 kg	11.0
30 kg	12.0
40 kg	14.0
40+ kg	16.0

more difficult. as tube selection would have to take into account length as well as diameter.

Endotracheal intubation is associated with increased anesthetic risk in cats (Brodbelt *et al.* 2007). This is likely due to several factors, including laryngospasm and iatrogenic tracheal trauma. Cats are predisposed to laryngospasm and laryngeal trauma (Hall and Taylor 1994; Mitchell *et al.* 2000). The V-gel® system (Jorgensen Labs, Loveland, CO) is marketed for use in cats and allows for administration of inhalant and a protected airway, while also not requiring endotracheal intubation (see Chapter 14).

29.3 Breathing System

Although rebreathing circuits are routinely used in small animals, non-rebreathing systems are typically recommended for patients less than 3 kg, due to increased resistance to breathing and possible dead space in rebreathing systems. Non-rebreathing systems can be utilized in large patients, but there is an increased cost associated with their use due to higher fresh gas flows (oxygen and inhalant waste are increased) and contribution to waste anesthetic gas environmental pollution. Additionally, these high fresh gas flows may significantly reduce patient body temperature (Kelly *et al.* 2012).

29.4 Monitoring

The American College of Veterinary Anesthesia and Analgesia recommends monitoring of circulation, oxygenation, ventilation, temperature, neuromuscular blockade and recovery (ACVAA 2009). Monitoring techniques have also been discussed in detail elsewhere in this book.

29.4.1 Electrocardiogram (ECG)

An electrocardiogram (ECG) should be utilized to monitor heart rhythm in the peri-anesthetic period using at least a three-lead system. An ECG will also determine heart rate values based on amplitude of a waveform deviated from baseline. However, since only electrical activity is recorded, in many situations the ECG will be inaccurate in its assessment of heart rate and should not be utilized as a sole monitoring tool, as cardiac function is not assessed using this method. For further details, see Chapter 20.

29.4.2 Arterial Blood Pressure

Blood pressure measurement is used as an indirect indicator of cardiac output. Blood pressure monitors are discussed in detail in Chapter 19. In small animal patients, evaluations of non-invasive blood pressure monitors have determined that most are inaccurate in their determination of arterial blood pressure. However, trends in blood pressure measurements may be of value. The American College of Veterinary Internal Medicine has determined standards for minimum performance of blood pressure monitors, although it is important to distinguish that these standards apply to awake patients (Brown *et al.* 2007).

29.4.2.1 Non-Invasive Blood Pressure Monitoring

Oscillometric blood pressure monitors rely on oscillations of the artery after the occlusion of blood flow is relieved. In small patients, the arterial oscillations are typically small due to arterial size and the oscillations must travel the length of the tubing to the monitor. As a result, many oscillometric blood pressure monitors underestimate arterial blood pressure in small patients, such as cats (Caulkett 1998). Oscillometric blood pressure monitors may more accurately represent the mean arterial blood pressure in comparison with systolic and diastolic pressures (Aarnes *et al.* 2012).

A Doppler flow detector and sphygmomanometer can be utilized to determine systolic pressure non-invasively, but has also been demonstrated to underestimate systolic pressure (Caulkett *et al.* 1998). Recognition of the limitations of non-invasive blood pressure monitoring is important in determining the importance of accurate blood pressure monitoring as related to time and expense for placement of an arterial catheter to measure blood pressure invasively.

29.4.2.2 Invasive Blood Pressure Monitoring

Blood pressure can be monitored invasively using a catheter placed in a peripheral artery, a fluid-filled line, and a transducer attached to the monitor. Invasive blood pressure monitoring utilizing a peripheral artery is the gold standard for monitoring arterial blood pressure in clinical patients. However, there are limitations as placement of a catheter in a peripheral artery is a technical skill that must be mastered through repetition. In addition, arterial catheter location has been demonstrated to affect the measurement of blood pressure (Acierno *et al.* 2015).

29.4.3 Pulse Oximetry

A pulse oximeter is a non-invasive monitor that estimates oxygen saturation of hemoglobin in real time. Pulse oximetry is discussed in detail in Chapter 18. Briefly, red and infrared light passes through tissue and is transmitted to a photocell. The two different types of light are absorbed differently by oxyhemoglobin and reduced hemoglobin. The flow of red cells with each beat of the heart is detected as the red cells flow through vessels and the pulse oximeter utilizes this information to also display a heart rate.

The pulse oximeter utilizes absorption of light as an indicator of oxygen saturation of hemoglobin. As such, pigmented tissue can be a source of error for pulse oximeters. Pulse oximeters do not function well in times of poor perfusion, in low oxygen states and can be affected by patients with severe anemia. In small veterinary patients, the pulse oximeter clip can apply pressure to tissues that results in compression and decreased blood flow. However, pulse oximetry and pulse monitoring has been associated with decreasing risk of anesthetic-related death in cats and is always recommended in small animals (Brodbelt *et al.* 2007).

29.4.4 Body Temperature

Animals lose body heat through four mechanisms: evaporation, conduction, convection and radiation (see Chapter 22). Anesthetic drugs contribute to loss of body heat through suppression of internal heat retention mechanisms, alteration of the body's temperature "set point" and effects of vasculature (vasodilation, vasoconstriction) among others. Hypothermia is a common problem in veterinary anesthesia, and while transient, can increase the risk of general anesthesia via impaired coagulation, development of arrhythmias and decreased wound healing (Aarnes 2013).

Monitoring of body temperature is important in anesthetized small animal patients, due to their increased body surface area compared with large animal patients. Rectal temperature monitoring has been considered the standard in awake clinical patients, and esophageal temperature monitoring is commonly performed in anesthetized patients.

Axillary temperature monitoring has been investigated in awake animals, due to animal temperament or because of anal/rectal surgery in which rectal temperature monitoring may disrupt the surgical site. Unfortunately, axillary temperatures do not reliably correlate to rectal temperature in dogs and cats, and even when correlated, the large gradient between techniques results in lack of recommendation of the axillary temperature technique as a substitute for rectal temperature monitoring (Lamb and McBrearty 2013; Goic *et al.* 2014; Mathis and Campbell 2015).

29.3 Recovery

Patient monitoring is always recommended well into the recovery period. It should include specific monitoring of respiration, oxygenation and ventilation, as well as body temperature, circulation and level of pain (Bednarski *et al.* 2011). The goal of this monitoring is to ensure anesthetic recovery proceeds safely for the anesthetist and patient, and to ensure appropriate analgesia is employed. As many anesthetic drugs impair circulation and respiration, it is imperative that these parameters are assessed prior to and after administration of any sedation or analgesics. The post-operative period was determined to be the period of greatest risk for cats and dogs since, when peri-operative death occurred, 61% of cats and 47% of dogs died post-operatively (Brodbelt *et al.* 2008a).

29.6 Anesthetic Risk

Risk associated with anesthetic-related death is of concern for veterinarians. Recent studies have demonstrated that the overall risk of anesthetic- and sedation-related death was 0.17% in dogs and 0.24% in cats (Brodbelt *et al.* 2008a). These numbers are higher than the associated risks in people (~0.02–0.005%). Factors associated with anesthetic risk in small animal veterinary patients are sickness (increasing ASA status), decreased body weight, emergency procedures, age, and anesthetic duration, especially in dogs (Brodbelt *et al.* 2008b). Low body weight, endotracheal intubation and intravenous fluid administration were associated with an increased risk of death in cats (Brodbelt *et al.* 2007). Recognition of the factors associated with increasing anesthetic risk may help to decrease such risk in the future.

References

Aarnes, T.K. (2013) Temperature regulation during anesthesia: anesthetic-associated hypothermia and hyperthermia. In: Muir, W.W. III, Hubbell, J.A.E., Bednarski, R.M. and Lerche, P. (eds). *Handbook of Veterinary Anesthesia,* 5th ed. St Louis, MO: Elsevier Mosby, pp. 330–347.

Aarnes, T.K., Hubbell, J.A., Lerche, P. and Bednarski, R.M. (2012) Comparison of invasive and oscillometric blood pressure measurement techniques in anesthetized camelids. *Can Vet J,* 53, 881–885.

Acierno, M.J., Domingues, M.E., Ramos, S.J., Shelby, A.M. and da Cunha, A.F. (2015) Comparison of directly measured arterial blood pressure at various anatomic locations in anesthetized dogs. *Am J Vet Res,* 76, 266–271.

ACVAA (2009) Recommendations for monitoring anesthetized veterinary patients. Available from: http://www.acvaa.org [accessed October 2016].

Alderson, B., Senior, J.M. and Dugdale, A.H. (2006) Tracheal necrosis following tracheal intubation in a dog. *J Small Anim Pract,* 47, 754–756.

Avki, S., Yigitarslan, K. and Ozgel, O. (2006) Comparison of airway size with some phenotypic parameters in Dalmatian puppies: a practical method to estimate endotracheal tube size. *Vet Anaesth Analg,* 33, 24–27.

Bednarski, R., Grimm, K., Harvey, R., Lukasik, V.M., Penn, W.S. *et al.* (2011) AAHA anesthesia guidelines for dogs and cats. *J Am Anim Hosp Assoc,* 47, 377–385.

Briganti, A., Portela, D.A., Barsotti, G., Romano, M. and Breghi, G. (2012) Evaluation of the endotracheal tube cuff pressure resulting from four different methods of inflation in dogs. *Vet Anaesth Analg,* 39, 488–494.

Brodbelt, D.C., Blissitt, K.J., Hammond, R.A., Neath, P.J., Young, L.E. *et al.* (2008a) The risk of death: the confidential enquiry into peri-operative small animal fatalities. *Vet Anaesth Analg,* 35; 365–373.

Brodbelt, D.C., Pfeiffer, D.U., Young, L.E. and Wood, J.L.N. (2007) Risk factors for anaesthetic-related death in cats: results from the confidential enquiry into perioperative small animal fatalities (CEPSAF). *Br J Anaesth,* 99, 617–623.

Brodbelt, D.C., Pfeiffer, D.U., Young, L.E. and Wood, J.L.N. (2008b) Results from the Confidential Enquiry into Perioperative Small Animal Fatalities regarding risk factors for anesthetic-related death in dogs. *J Am Vet Med Assoc,* 233, 1096–1104.

Brown, S., Atkins, C., Bagley, R., Carr, A., Cowgill, L. *et al.* (2007) Guidelines for the identification, evaluation, and management of systemic hypertension in dogs and cats. *J Vet Intern Med,* 21, 542–558.

Caulkett, N.A., Cantwell, S.L. and Houston, D.M. (1998) A comparison of indirect blood pressure monitoring techniques in the anesthetized cat. *Vet Surg,* 27, 370–377.

Crow, S.E., Walshaw, S.O. and Boyle, J.E. (2009) Intubation. In: *Manual of Clinical Procedures in Dogs, Cats, Rabbits, and Rodents,* 3rd ed. Ames, IA: Wiley-Blackwell, pp. 177–216.

Goic, J.B., Reineke, E.L. and Drobatz, K.J. (2014) Comparison of rectal and axillary temperatures in dogs and cats. *J Am Vet Med Assoc,* 244, 1170–1175.

Hall, L.W. and Taylor, P.M. (1994) *Anaesthesia of the Cat.* London: Bailliere Tindall.

Hartsfield, S.M. (1996) Airway management and ventilation. In: Tranquilli, W.J., Thurmon, J.C. and Grimm, K.A. (eds). *Lumb and Jones' Veterinary Anesthesia and Analgesia,* 3rd ed. Ames, IA: Blackwell Publishing, pp. 515–556.

Hartsfield, S.M. (2007) Airway management and ventilation. In: Tranquilli, W.J., Thurmon, J.C. and Grimm, K.A. (eds). *Lumb and Jones' Veterinary Anesthesia and Analgesia,* 4th ed. Ames, IA: Blackwell Publishing, pp. 495–532.

Kelly, C.K., Hodgson, D.S. and McMurphy, R.M. (2012) Effect of anesthetic breathing circuit type on thermal loss in cats during inhalation anesthesia for ovariohysterectomy. *J Am Vet Med Assoc,* 240, 1296–1299.

Lamb, V. and McBrearty, A.R. (2013) Comparison of rectal, tympanic membrane, and axillary temperature measurement methods in dogs. *Vet Rec,* 173, 524–528.

Lish, J., Ko, J.C.H. and Payton, M.E. (2008) Evaluation of two method of endotracheal tube selection in dogs. *J Am Anim Hosp Assoc,* 44, 236–242.

Mathis, J.C. and Campbell, V.L. (2015) Comparison of axillary and rectal temperatures for healthy beagles in a temperature- and humidity-controlled environment. *Am J Vet Res,* 76, 632–636.

McDonell, W.N. and Kerr, C.L. (2007) Respiratory system. In: Tranquilli, W.J., Thurmon, J.C. and Grimm, K.A. (eds). *Lumb and Jones' Veterinary Anesthesia and Analgesia,* 4th ed. Ames, IA: Blackwell Publishing, pp. 117–152.

Mitchell, S.L., McCarthy, R., Rudloff, E. and Pernell, R.T. (2000) Tracheal rupture associated with intubation in cats: 20 cases (1996–1998). *J Am Anim Hosp Assoc,* 216, 1592–1595.

Suter, P.F., Colgrove, D.J. and Ewing, G.O. (1972) Congenital hypoplasia of the canine trachea. *J Am Anim Hosp Assoc,* 8, 120–127.

30

Unique Species Considerations: Ruminants and Swine

Denise Radkey[1]*, Lindsey Snyder*[2]*, and Rebecca A. Johnson*[2]

[1] *MedVet Medical and Cancer Center for Pets, Worthington, Ohio, USA*
[2] *School of Veterinary Medicine, University of Wisconsin, Madison, Wisconsin, USA*

Part I: Ruminants

30.1 Introduction

Ruminant anesthesia presents unique challenges, primarily due to their specialized alimentary tract, size variety and the potential difficulty in securing an airway with their individual head conformations. It is crucial for the anesthetist to have all necessary supplies and a good working knowledge of each species' individual requirements to provide the best medical care and the safest environment for not only the patient, but the personnel as well.

30.2 Handling and Restraint

Small ruminants (sheep and goats) and camelids are typically quite tractable and require limited restraint prior to administering premedications. A halter and lead rope are sufficient to transport the majority of animals to the induction area. Small ruminants and camelids frequently have uneventful inductions and, depending on their size, do not require more than light manual restraint before becoming sternally recumbent.

Larger ruminants, such as adult cows and bulls and camelids, require a bit more forethought, and depending on the particular animal's disposition, the approach to handling and restraint may be quite different. Mature dairy cows are generally well adjusted to humans and handling, and often can be led into the induction room with minimal encouragement. In contrast, adult breeding bulls may be "pushy" or even aggressive, and may require premedication prior to transport to the induction area. Beef cattle, especially cows with nursing calves, present a unique challenge. These animals are often less tractable and are handled infrequently, thus sedation

prior to entering the induction area is common. Many unhandled animals may even need sedation from a distance, with either a pole syringe or a dart gun, before transport to the induction area. Ideally, these patients would be secured in a head catch to contain them in a desired area (Figure 30.1).

Once an adult ruminant enters the induction area, they are positioned close to a padded wall; when anesthesia is induced, the patient can be pushed against the wall by several knowledgeable individuals or with a squeeze gate (Figure 30.2). If the patient is not positioned against a padded wall, they can be difficult to control once they progress to unconsciousness and the potential for patient and personnel injury becomes much greater. The same is done for procedures requiring the patient to be on a tilt table (i.e. distal limb, hoof, udder surgery, etc. (Figure 30.3); proper sedation is imperative to prevent patient and personnel injury while the animal is secured to the table.

Once sedated, safe to approach, and positioned in a controlled area (squeeze gate or tilt table), an intravenous (IV) catheter should be placed immediately for anesthetic induction and subsequent endotracheal intubation. Depending on the facility and the anticipated medical or surgical procedure, ruminants can be maintained on injectable anesthetics until they are transported to the surgical suite or procedure room for transitioning onto inhalant anesthetics.

Following anesthetic induction, intubation should be performed in sternal recumbency which, especially in very large ruminants, is easiest to achieve when they are squeezed against a wall or if they remain sternal against the table upon recumbency. It is important to keep them sternal until an airway is secured, as the transition to lateral recumbency greatly increases the chance of ruminal regurgitation.

Veterinary Anesthetic and Monitoring Equipment, First Edition. Edited by Kristen G. Cooley and Rebecca A. Johnson.
© 2018 John Wiley & Sons, Inc. Published 2018 by John Wiley & Sons, Inc.

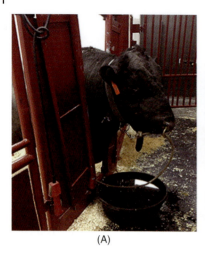

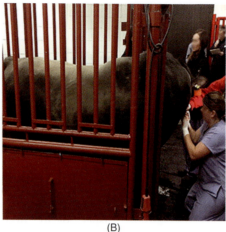

(A)   (B)

Figure 30.1 (A) Head catch secured to a squeeze chute used to safely handle bulls or other fractious ruminants. (B) IV catheter placement in a large fractious bull in a head catch and chute.

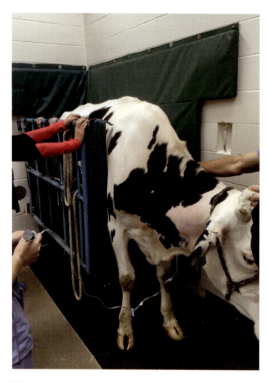

Figure 30.2 A squeeze gate used during large ruminant induction. Ample padding covers the wall and gate to prevent injury from any hard or sharp surfaces. The gate should be used to prevent the patient from rolling into lateral recumbency before intubation.

30.3 IV Catheterization

An indwelling IV catheter is a crucial aspect of every anesthetic event, especially those involving injection of irritating drugs, such as guaifenesin or thiopental (Figure 30.1). The jugular vein is most accessible in ruminants of all sizes, due to its large diameter and relative ease of catheter maintenance. Adult cattle, especially bulls, can have skin as much as 1 cm thick, therefore it is best to

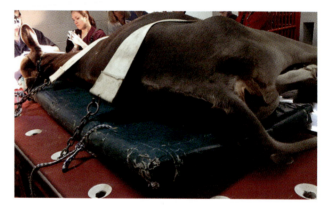

Figure 30.3 Adult Brown Swiss cow heavily sedated on a tilt table for an ophthalmic procedure. Note the large padding and restraint straps.

make an incision with a scalpel blade through an intradermal/subcutaneous bleb of local anesthetic solution such as 2% lidocaine.

Catheters come in a variety of options, but some of the most commonly used catheters in large ruminants are 14 gauge, 13 cm, over-the-needle or 14-gauge, 20 cm, over-the-wire. The same types of catheters in smaller diameters and lengths can be used in small ruminants. Over-the-wire catheters are placed by first advancing a short catheter into the vein, removing the stylet, and feeding the guide wire through the catheter lumen. The wire is removed and a dilator is advanced over the wire to dilate the skin and vascular entrance to an appropriate diameter. Once the dilator is removed, the catheter is placed over the wire and advanced into the vessel. At this point, the wire is removed and the catheter is capped and sutured into place.

Over-the-needle catheters (Mila International, Inc., Florence, KY) (Figure 30.4) are simpler to place, as they involve less components and procedural steps than do over-the-wire catheters. This type of catheter is placed by advancing the stylet with catheter through the skin

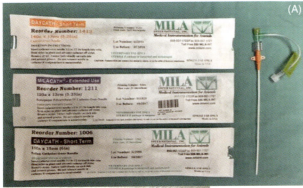

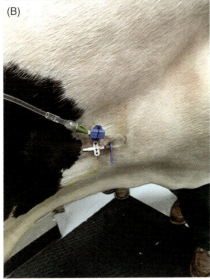

intersection of a line extending from the base of the ear and a line extending from the lower jaw provides the best entrance point for catheterization (Cerba *et al.* 2014) (Figure 30.5). The vein is distended by applying pressure under the ventral projection of the sixth cervical vertebra. Their skin can be very thick and a small incision should be made with a scalpel through a local anesthetic bleb before catheter placement. Catheters are placed as described above; however, the presence of vascular valves can prevent complete advancement of the catheter within the vessel lumen (Cerba *et al.* 2014). If valves are encountered, catheter advancement can be facilitated by holding off and distending the vessel at the distal aspect or by flushing the catheter as it is advanced forward.

30.4 Induction Equipment

Tracheal intubation is indicated in all ruminant species undergoing general anesthesia and even after sedation if heavy enough to cause loss of the protective laryngeal and pharyngeal reflexes. Tracheal intubation is especially

Figure 30.4 (A) Left: Over the needle catheters in a variety of shapes and sizes (10–14 gauge pictured). Right: 14-gauge MILA catheter attached to a t-port. The hub of the catheter comes with "wings" that can be sutured to the skin. (B) Large-bore over the wire IV catheter placed in the right jugular of a large (650 kg) dairy cow. Head is to the right.

incision and into the vessel. Once the vessel is penetrated by the stylet, the stylet and catheter are advanced slightly until the catheter is assuredly within the vessel lumen. Once the catheter is within the lumen, it is advanced forward off the stylet, a t-port or other cap is firmly attached, and sutures are placed to secure both the catheter and the t-port or cap to the skin.

Venous catheter placement is best performed using the jugular vein in adult llamas and alpacas as well; however, the anatomical differences in these species are unique. Appropriate restraint and stabilization of the head and neck greatly facilitates catheter placement. The right jugular vein should be evaluated first, as the esophagus may interfere with placement in the left jugular vein. The jugular vein is separated from the common carotid artery and vagosympathetic trunk by a cervical branch of the omohyoid muscle; the jugular is most superficial and easiest to palpate in this area. The

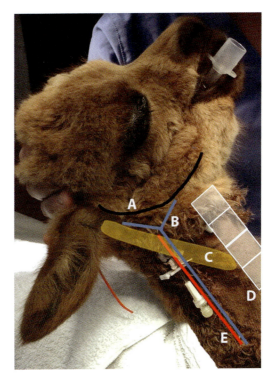

Figure 30.5 Camelid anatomic landmarks for intravenous catheter placement. The omohyoid muscle separates the jugular vein from the carotid artery just distal to the ramus of the mandible. More distal on the neck, the carotid artery and the jugular vein become intimately associated, which prevents safe catheterization beyond this point. (A) Ramus of the mandible, (B) jugular vein, (C) omohyoid muscle, (D) trachea, (E) carotid artery.

important in ruminants, due to their unique gastrointestinal anatomy, which increases risk of regurgitation and subsequent aspiration of rumen contents (Riebold 2007; Abrahamsen 2009). In general, intubation does not require sophisticated equipment. However, key anatomical differences may complicate intubation if the proper equipment is not available. The anesthetist must be familiar with and prepared to use a multitude of techniques to obtain a patent airway efficiently. For example, in sheep and goats, the larynx is easily visualized with a laryngoscope and the trachea directly intubated through the oral cavity. In contrast, large cattle and camelids may require manual intubation with use of a mouth gag. As previously mentioned, ruminants are most commonly intubated in sternal recumbency to maximize glottis position and possibly visualization, but also to reduce passive reflux of rumenal contents into the oropharynx and subsequent aspiration.

30.4.1   Mouth Speculums/Gags

Metal mouth gags, such as the Weingart Mouth Speculum (GerVetUSA, Albertson, NY) and the Günter Mouth Gag (KRUUSE, Langeskov, Denmark), are commercially available and are designed to sit on the lower incisors and rostral dental pad (Figure 30.6). The speculums work as a jack to open the mouth to its widest point allowed by the temporomandibular joint and soft tissues of the mouth. With the speculums in place, the anesthe-

tist can better visualize or palpate the tracheal entrance. Tracheal intubation can then occur with a stylet or the anesthetist can pass their arm into the patient's oral cavity to digitally palpate the larynx and arytenoid cartilages and manually guide the tube into place (Figure 30.7).

Calves and small ruminants such as sheep and goats are often too small to implement use of a mouth speculum/gag. In these patients, gauze ties or small diameter ropes are used to facilitate opening of the mouth (Hall 2001; Figure 30.8). One tie should be placed caudal to the lower incisors using care to avoid entrapping the tongue and the other on the dental pad. The holder can then carefully open the jaw to its widest point. This allows the anesthetist to then place a laryngoscope into the oral cavity to visualize the airway or to manually intubate the trachea.

30.4.2   Laryngoscopes

In small ruminants, a laryngoscope can be used to depress the tongue and aid in airway visualization. Depending on patient size and their oral cavity depth, longer or shorter blades may be required. It is best to depress the tongue with the blade remaining parallel to the patient's mandible to avoid obstructing the view with the blade itself. Care is taken to avoid touching and traumatizing the epiglottis. In the majority of cases, the use of a laryngoscope provides adequate visualization of the airway from which intubation can proceed.

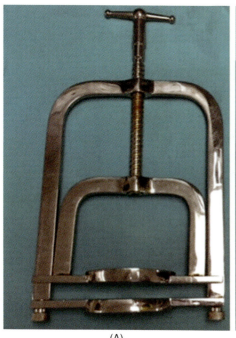 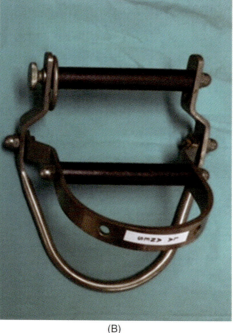

(A)   (B)

Figure 30.6 (A) Günter mouth gag. (B) Weingart mouth speculum.

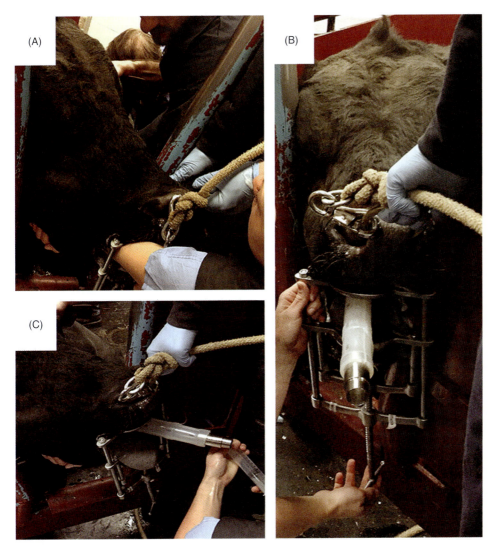

Figure 30.7 (A) Manual tracheal intubation using a Günter mouth gag. (B) Intubated bull showing removal of the speculum after successful intubation. (c) Air should be added to the endotracheal tube cuff immediately upon intubation in ruminants to prevent regurgitation and aspiration of ruminal contents.

Laryngoscopes consist of a handle and a blade, equipped with a replaceable light source and are used to facilitate endotracheal intubation in most species (see Chapter 13). There are many varieties of laryngoscopes and blades available on the market, most of which are designed for use in human patients. Most blades have a flange on the right side to aid in human intubation by a right-handed anesthetist (Figure 30.9B). However, in contrast to veterinary anesthesia, human intubation is performed with the patient on their back, while holding the laryngoscope handle and blade "upside-down". Thus, the flange is on the "wrong" side of the blade for veterinary anesthetists who are right-handed. Therefore, the flange, especially the more prominent one on the MacIntosh blade, can obscure visualization of the larynx and make intubation rather difficult. This is notably of concern when considering small ruminant intubation whose narrow oral cavity size can be an impediment. Blades designed for human use are shorter (205 mm) than desirable for use in ruminants. Miller laryngoscope blades come in a variety of sizes, 280–450 mm, and are helpful when intubating calves, camelids and other small ruminants (Figure 30.9A).

30.4.3 Stylets

In many small ruminants, it can be challenging to open their mouths more than 30–45 degrees. Their long, narrow oral cavity makes visualization of the larynx even more difficult. The use of a variety of stylets can be beneficial in facilitating intubation in these species (Figure 30.10). For example, a stylet made of two or three

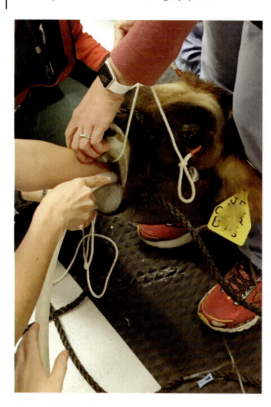

Figure 30.8 Calf intubation in sternal recumbency using ropes to hold the mouth open. One rope is placed on the dental pad and the other behind the incisors taking care not to entrap the tongue.

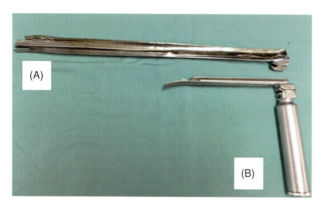

Figure 30.9 (A) An extended laryngoscope blade (450 mm) used in intubating large ruminants, which fits on a standard laryngoscope handle. (B) A standard large laryngoscope blade (205 mm) used when intubating smaller ruminants (calves, goats and sheep).

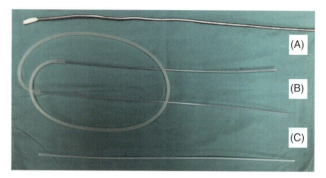

Figure 30.10 (A) Rigid stylet with the patient end covered with tape to prevent damage to the trachea in the event that it should extend beyond the endotracheal tube during intubation. Note that metal stylets are only intended to reside within the lumen of the endotracheal tube and can be bent to the appropriate conformation for each individual patient. (B) Double-ended stylet provides adequate length with additional flexibility in the center. (C) Soft polypropylene urinary catheters can be taped together in tandem to provide the desired length for each individual patient. Their ends are non-traumatic and therefore can be passed beyond the patient end of the endotracheal tube to aid intubation.

through the arytenoids and into the trachea with ease. It is imperative that stylets used in this manner are made from a soft, pliable material to avoid damage to the fragile laryngeal, pharyngeal and/or tracheal tissues. Once

polypropylene urinary catheters taped in tandem can be a valuable intubation tool (Figure 30.10C). The endotracheal tube is threaded over the stylet before attempting intubation to allow efficient passage of the endotracheal tube once the stylet is in place (Figure 30.11). The stylet should extend past the end of the endotracheal tube to a distance that allows the stylet to be advanced first

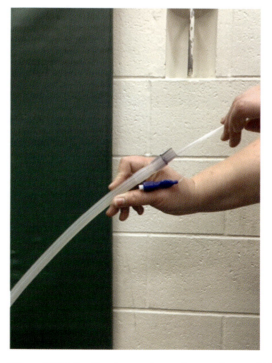

Figure 30.11 A soft polypropylene urinary catheter within the lumen of the endotracheal tube. It is important to maintain a length of stylet beyond the machine end of the endotracheal tube to prevent it from falling into the airway. It is helpful for a second person to hold the stylet while the endotracheal tube is threaded into the airway by the anesthetist.

the stylet is past the arytenoids and into the tracheal lumen, the endotracheal tube is advanced slowly over the top of the stylet while ensuring the proximal end of the stylet is anchored to avoid it slipping into the airway. Due to the narrow oral cavity in these patients, the laryngoscope may need to be removed prior to advancing the endotracheal tube over the stylet. Once the endotracheal tube is in place, the stylet is quickly removed to allow connection to the anesthetic circuit.

Stylets can also be made of metal; however, these stylets are intended for use entirely within the lumen of the endotracheal tube (Figure 30.10A). This type of stylet is used if the anesthetist desires a more rigid endotracheal tube that can be bent into a more useful conformation for that particular patient. Never should a metal stylet protrude beyond the distal end of the endotracheal tube and into the patient's airway, since significant damage to the larynx, pharynx or trachea may result. The proximal end of the stylet should extend beyond the machine end of the endotracheal tube and is secured to prevent it from slipping into the airway. Once the endotracheal tube is placed distal to the arytenoids, the tube is advanced into the trachea and the stylet is removed carefully.

In larger ruminants, where small diameter stylets are ineffective, an equine nasogastric tube can be used as a stylet. For example, the tube is passed as any other stylet would be, but it provides the additional length and relative rigidity required in larger patients. Once the endotracheal tube is advanced into the airway over the nasogastric tube, the nasogastric tube should be removed.

30.4.4 Laryngoscopy

Camelids and small ruminants can occasionally be difficult to intubate. In these situations, video endoscopy can be beneficial (Figure 30.12) as the endoscope itself can be

used as a stylet. The internal diameter of the endotracheal tube must be larger than the endoscope, allowing airflow to pass and the tube to be easily advanced off the end once in place. One person "drives" the endoscope while the person performing the intubation feeds the scope into the oral cavity. Once the tip of the endoscope is through the arytenoid cartilages, the endotracheal tube is passed over the scope and advanced into the trachea. Although somewhat technically challenging, in an emergency, this technique can prove invaluable.

30.4.5 Endotracheal Tubes

Many types of endotracheal tubes are available for ruminants and camelids. Most endotracheal tubes are manufactured for humans; however, there are veterinary-specific products available for patients requiring additional length and/or diameter (e.g. Surgivet, Smiths Medical, Dublin, OH; JorVet, Jorgenson Labs, Loveland, CO) (Figure 30.13). At a minimum, veterinary-specific tubes should have markings of internal and external/outer diameter (I.D., O.D.) and length. Additionally, some tubes marketed for veterinary use may have their sizes recorded using the French gauge scale, which may or may not always represent the internal diameter of the tube (Mosley 2015).

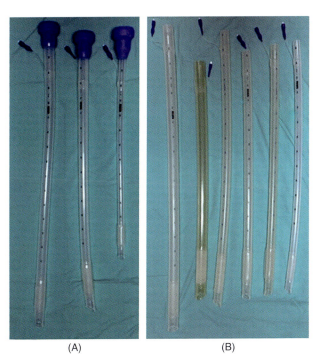

(A) (B)

Figure 30.13 (A) Funnel-shaped adapters can be ordered on all sizes of large animal endotracheal tubes. (B) Size 35 mm to 20 mm I.D. (left to right) endotracheal tubes for large animals. These tubes can be cut to size and fitted with a metal adapter to connect with the anesthesia circuit.

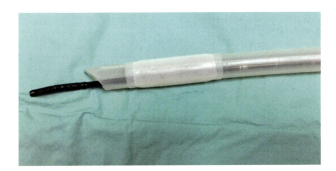

Figure 30.12 A video endoscope used as a stylet for patients who are difficult to intubate. The endoscope is fed through the lumen of the endotracheal tube and beyond the patient end into the oral cavity. The anesthetist guides the endoscope between the arytenoids and into the trachea, where the endotracheal tube can be advanced off and into place.

Generally, the largest tube that can fit the lumen of the patient's trachea without causing damage is desirable. The cuffed Murphy-type tube is the most common type used in ruminants (Mosley 2015). The machine end of the tube should not be advanced into the patient's airway past the incisors. The airway end of the tube should not be advanced beyond the thoracic inlet in any species, especially in ruminants and camelids due to the presence of a tracheal bronchus proximal to the bifurcation of the mainstem bronchi (Mosley 2015).

Endotracheal tube size can be approximated based on body weight (Table 30.1). For example, endotracheal tubes of 5–14 mm I.D. are used in small ruminants; tubes used in goats are generally 1 to 2 sizes smaller than those required for sheep of the same body weight (Gray and McDonnell 1986; Thurmon and Benson 1993; Valverde and Doherty 2008).

Small camelids have similar-sized airways compared to small ruminants. Orotracheal tube size varies from a 6-mm tube in a newborn cria to approximately 12–14-mm tubes for a large adult llama. It is advisable to have a range of tubes available if the anesthetist is unfamiliar with intubating these species (Cerba *et al.* 2014).

There are two types of tube cuff designs: high volume/low pressure and low volume/high pressure. Regardless of cuff type, tracheal ischemia and necrosis can result from excessive cuff pressures, even in ruminants. Tracheal wall pressures above 48 cmH$_2$O may impede capillary blood flow leading to ischemia of the tracheal mucosa, and pressures below 18 cmH$_2$O may increase the risk of aspiration (Stewart *et al.* 2003). Since ruminants have a large fermentation chamber full of fluid and incompletely digested fiber, and they produce a large amount of saliva, the pilot cuff is frequently inflated immediately after intubation to avoid aspiration of these fluids (Lin and Pugh 2002). Once the cuff is inflated and an adequate seal is present to maintain airway pressures of 20–30 cmH$_2$O, air can slowly be removed from the cuff until a leak is seen, at which point a small amount of air should be added back to recreate a complete seal. This method allows placement of only the minimum amount of pressure required to create a seal and helps to avoid tracheal injury.

The machine end of the endotracheal tube should contain a connector for attachment to the anesthetic circuit (Figure 30.14). Smaller endotracheal tubes (up to 16 mm) have a connector that is of uniform size (15 mm outer diameter [O.D.]) allowing connection to all standard anesthetic circuits. Tubes intended for use in large animals may have a silicone Funnel Fit adapter designed to fit over the large animal Y-piece (54 mm O.D.) (Figure 30.14B), or a removable metal connector (22 mm O.D.)

Table 30.1 Endotracheal tube size based on body weight.

Body Weight (kg)	Endotracheal Tube Size (mm)	
	Oral	**Nasal**
25–50	8–10	4–6
50–100	10–14	6–8
100–200	14–18	8–10
200–300	16–18	10–12
300–400	18–22	14–16
400–500	22–26	16–18
500–800	24–30	18–22
>800	30–35	20–22

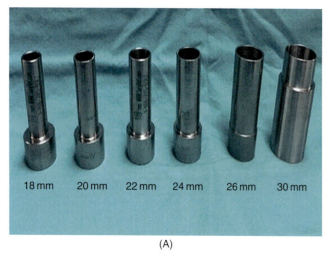

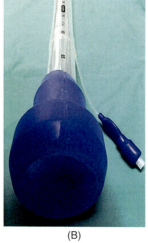

(A) (B)

Figure 30.14 (A) Metal endotracheal tube adapters for large animal tubes. Adapters are made to fit inside the Y-piece (22 mm O.D.). (B) Funnel-shaped adapters can be ordered for a variety of sizes of endotracheal tubes.

specifically made to fit the Bivona/Drager Tapered Adapters (Bivona adapter/funnel tube: Surgivet, Smiths Medical, Dublin, OH; Drager: DRE Veterinary, Louisville, KY) found on some large animal Y-pieces (Figure 30.14A).

30.4.6 Nasotracheal Intubation

Nasotracheal intubation is a useful technique for procedures in or around the oral cavity (e.g. jaw fractures, tooth extractions, laryngeal/pharyngeal surgeries, etc.), where a standard orotracheal tube may interfere with surgical access. This method is also used in sedated, conscious animals, who may require supplemental oxygen or are at high risk of aspiration. Induction and maintenance of anesthesia can also be performed via a nasotracheal tube in many species, including calves and llamas (Riebold *et al.* 1994; Quandt *et al.* 1996).

An ideal nasotracheal tube is one that has minimal curvature and is of a suitable length to extend intratracheally past the larynx (JorVet, Jorgenson Labs, Loveland, CO; Surgivet, Smiths Medical, Dublin, OH). Silicone or rubber nasotracheal tubes are preferred, due to their soft and flexible nature, an advantageous feature when attempting to navigate through delicate nasal passages (Figure 30.15). Ideally, a tube with thin walls is used to increase the internal diameter; however, a thin tube is at increased risk of compression or kinking (Quandt *et al.* 1996). Tube size is patient specific, although it generally will be smaller than that used for orotracheal intubation (Table 30.1).

Nasal intubation causes variable degrees of edema and swelling of the soft tissues, which when severe, can partially or completely obstruct airflow. Therefore, airflow should be assessed before intubation to ensure patency of flow bilaterally. If flow is not present through either nostril, nasal intubation should be avoided to prevent worsening of abnormal nasal airflow. This is especially important in species who are semi-obligate nasal breathers (i.e. camelids). Additionally, prior to intubation, the nares should be cleaned to prevent introduction of foreign material or debris into the trachea as the tube is advanced into the airway.

Nasal tubes should be passed ventral and medial through the nostril, ventral nasal meatus and larynx into the trachea. Lubrication of the tube is essential and the addition of 2% lidocaine to desensitize the highly innervated nasal tissues facilitates intubation, especially in non-sedated patients. The tube should be passed gently, knowing that some resistance is normally present; however, excessive force can cause damage and potentially hemorrhage.

Tube placement can be assessed by squeezing the air from a bulb syringe and attaching it to the end of the nasotracheal tube. If the bulb inflates, this suggests the tube is in the airway; however, if it fails to expand, the tube is likely located in the esophagus (Riebold 2007). Tube placement can also be established with a capnometer. Once appropriate placement is confirmed, the cuff should be checked for a leak in the standard fashion. Since a smaller diameter tube is required for passage through the nasal cavity, obtaining a seal at the cuff within the trachea could prove difficult. If a seal cannot be achieved, the patient should be re-intubated with either a larger nasotracheal tube if possible, or an orotracheal tube; the risk of aspiration in these species is far too great to proceed without a complete seal.

30.5 Tracheal Insufflation and Demand Valves

Tracheal insufflation should be provided whenever possible with enriched oxygen mixtures, since hypoxemia is common in large, recumbent ruminants. Since most heavily sedated and anesthetized ruminants are intubated, oxygen insufflation into the endotracheal tube is easily performed via a small-diameter hose connected to an oxygen flowmeter (Figure 30.16). The diameter of the insufflation tubing should be significantly smaller than the diameter of the endotracheal tube, so ventilatory resistance and the work of breathing does not considerably increase. If the patient is no longer intubated, for example in recovery, a stomach tube can be fed into the nares and into the nasopharynx to provide supplementation in compromised patients. Inspired flows can be delivered at a rate of 5 L/min in small ruminants and 15 L/min in large ruminants (Gabel *et al.* 1966).

In patients that exhibit apnea or hypoventilation in recovery, or have become too deeply sedated during a procedure, supplemental breaths can be administered with a demand valve through their endotracheal tube (Figure 30.17). These valves are designed to fit a standard endotracheal tube adapter (15 mm O.D.); however, adapters are made to attach the valve to the Funnel Fit Adapter (JD Medical, Phoenix, AZ) and 22 mm I.D. endotracheal tube adapters as well (Figure 30.18). They are designed to

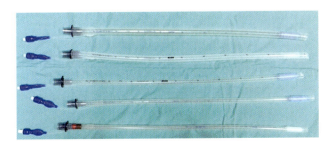

Figure 30.15 A variety of flexible, relatively thin-walled and long tracheal tubes sized 7–12 mm I.D. (top to bottom).

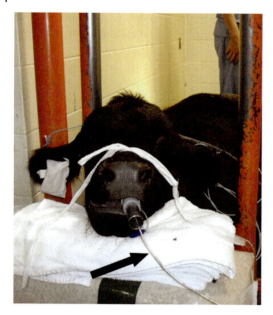

Figure 30.16 Bull with small diameter tubing (black arrow) providing oxygen insufflation during recovery from general anesthesia.

deliver oxygen from a supplied source when the patient begins to inspire, thus delivering a type of intermittent positive pressure ventilation. Demand valves, however, are designed for human use and can cause excessive resistance if left attached to the endotracheal tube in ruminants. Therefore, it is advisable to only use the valve manually to "sigh" the patient and then promptly remove it from the endotracheal tube adapter. These valves are manufactured as either high-flow or low-flow models. High-flow models deliver a maximum flow rate of approximately 160 L/min at 50 psi and low-flow models deliver 40 L/min (JD Medical, Phoenix, AZ; Smiths Medical, Dublin, OH) (Mosley 2015).

30.6 Padding and Positioning

Large patients may require a hoist to lift them into proper anesthetic positioning; many hoists can hold up to 2-ton loads, although this varies between manufacturers. If a hoist is required, hook and loop leg straps are placed distal to the fetlocks on all four limbs to distribute weight evenly. The patient is positioned as quickly as possible and as safely as possible to limit the time during which extreme force is placed on the distal limbs (Figure 30.19).

Improper positioning and padding of anesthetized horses are implicated as causes of significant post-anesthetic myopathies and neuropathies due to localized obstruction of blood flow (White 1982). It is reasonable to assume these may also occur in adult ruminants, although they are not as commonly encountered (Abrahamsen *et al.* 2009). Adult cattle should be placed on either a waterbed or a 10–15-cm thick foam pad. Pads 5 cm thick are sufficient for sheep, goats and camelids (Riebold 2007). When in dorsal recumbency, care should be taken to distribute weight evenly across the gluteal muscles to reduce points of increased pressure and all four legs should be in a flexed and relaxed position. When in lateral recumbency, a tire inner tube or padding with similar characteristics is placed under the down shoulder to provide further protection of the radial nerve. The down forelimb is pulled anteriorly to reduce the amount of weight placed on the humerus. Additionally, ample padding should be placed between the fore- and hind-limbs to maintain their position parallel to the table surface. Limb supports with copious padding are used in lieu of pads as they keep the limbs more stable and at the ideal angle to prevent injury to the brachial plexus, maintain venous drainage and minimize joint pain post-operatively. These techniques also help to

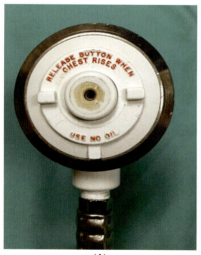

(A)

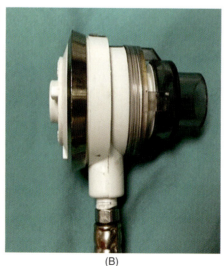

(B)

Figure 30.17 (A) The flush button on the front of the demand valve. (B) The oxygen inlet connection on the opposite side of the valve that fits into an adapter made for standard endotracheal tubes. It can also be used, although less effectively, on the cut end of an endotracheal tube to deliver a breath.

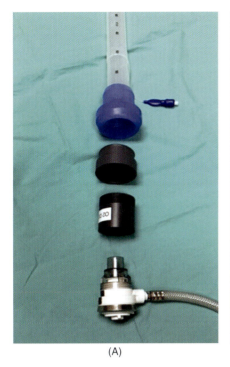
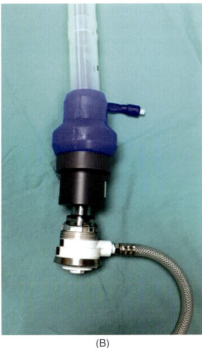

(A)   (B)

Figure 30.18 An adapter made specifically for attaching the demand valve to the funnel end of the endotracheal tube. This adapter allows efficient delivery of a breath. This adapter should be removed along with the demand valve between each breath.

minimize pressure on the radial, peroneal and femoral nerves on the dependent, as well as non-dependent limbs, and prevent nerve paralysis. Care should be taken to avoid extreme flexion or extension of the limbs in order to clear the operative sight. A "doughnut"-shaped pad or towel is placed beneath the down eye that should be generously lubricated. The eyelids should be closed to further prevent injury to the globe. This is especially important in camelids, whose eyes are rather prominent and prone to injury.

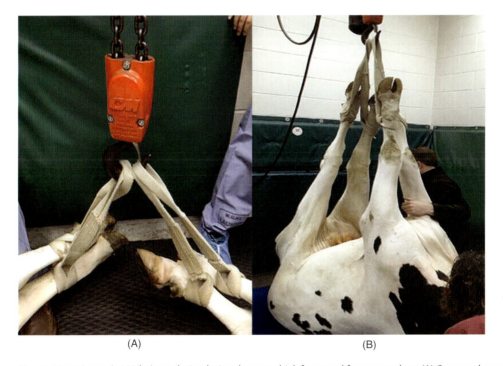

(A)   (B)

Figure 30.19 Large (~650 kg) cow being hoisted onto a thick foam pad for a procedure. (A) Correct placement of the leg straps. (B) Complete suspension of the cow in order to accomplish proper positioning. Animals of this size need to be promptly positioned to limit the time spent suspended by the straps.

Whether in dorsal or lateral recumbency, the patient's nose should be angled slightly downward to allow drainage of copious salivary secretions and any gastric contents, should regurgitation occur (Figure 30.20). Ideally, the drainage would flow off the end of the table to avoid wicking around the head and limit contamination of the eye. In smaller patients, use of a circulating warm-water blanket and/or convective warm air blowers can be implemented to avoid hypothermia.

30.7 Monitoring Equipment

Monitoring equipment used in any species should be specifically directed to the cardiovascular and respiratory systems at a minimum. Pulse rate, pulse pressure, mucous membrane color and capillary refill time should be monitored throughout anesthesia; however, these variables provide limited information about the patient's overall cardiovascular status. Thus, monitoring should include electrocardiography (ECG), invasive (preferably) or non-invasive blood pressure measurements, assessment of arterial hemoglobin O_2 saturation with pulse oximetry, inhalant and end-tidal CO_2 ($ETCO_2$), concentration assessment and analysis of arterial blood gases, thus allowing for an accurate assessment of anesthetic depth and cardiovascular, respiratory and central nervous system depression.

30.7.1 Electrocardiography (ECG)

An ECG should be placed with either standard limb leads (i.e. I, II, III) or a dipole (augmented) lead to detect arrhythmias and for improved views of morphology of the various complex components (i.e. p-wave, t-wave, etc.) (Mosley 2015). While an ECG provides partial information about electrical activity of the heart, it provides limited information regarding cardiac function.

30.7.2 Blood Pressure Measurement and Blood Gas Analysis

Arterial blood pressure measurement is elemental when a patient is under general anesthesia. The larger the patient, the more important it is to monitor blood pressure and treat hypotension. Decreased perfusion induced by anesthetic agents is catastrophic in horses, resulting in significant lameness and potential euthanasia (Grandy *et al.* 1987). Similar outcomes may also occur in large ruminants, although well-designed prospective or retrospective studies on anesthetic complications in ruminants are lacking. Oscillometric non-invasive blood pressure measurements can be performed if the properly-sized cuffs are available; however, studies have shown poor agreement between invasive (arterial catheter) and non-invasive (oscillometric) techniques in sheep, goats, cattle and camelids (Aarnes *et al.* 2012,

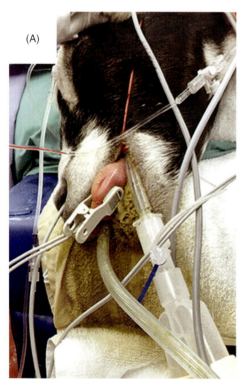
(A)

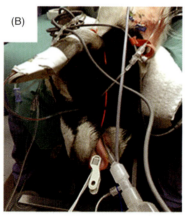
(B)

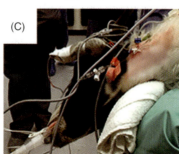
(C)

Figure 30.20 (A) Goat with a large amount of regurgitation and suction tubing. (B, C) The same goat in (A) repositioned to allow better and more complete drainage.

2013). Therefore, invasive monitoring via an arterial catheter and either a pressure transducer and amplifier or an aneroid manometer is recommended (Figure 30.21). A transducer system provides accurate measurement of systolic, diastolic and mean arterial blood pressure, whereas an aneroid manometer frequently only allows measurement of mean pressure.

Arterial catheterization is relatively simple in ruminants and camelids and is associated with limited complications (Riebold *et al.* 1980). As with any type of catheterization, the site should be sterilely prepared before placement. The caudal auricular artery, saphenous and common digital arteries are the most commonly catheterized vessels (Riebold 2007). Ruminants and camelids both tend to have very thick skin; therefore, puncturing the skin with an equal or larger gauge hypodermic needle prior to catheterization is recommended to avoid damaging the catheter during passage through the skin (Riebold *et al.* 1980). Once the catheter is in place, it should be flushed periodically with heparinized saline (2–4 units/mL) to prevent clot formation within the catheter. When the catheter is removed, direct compression of the insertion site should be maintained to prevent hematoma formation.

In addition to blood pressure monitoring, arterial catheters provide a source from which to obtain arterial blood gas samples. Blood gas analysis provides information from acid–base balance and metabolism to gas exchange and ventilation.

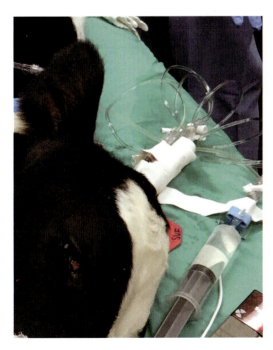

Figure 30.21 Calf with arterial catheter in auricular artery. The transducer is placed at the level of the left atrium and connected to a multiparameter monitor for measurement.

30.7.3 Gas Monitoring

30.7.3.1 End-Tidal CO_2 ($ETCO_2$)

At a minimum, respiratory monitoring should involve measurement of end-tidal CO_2 ($ETCO_2$) via capnography. Due to ruminants' impressive production of saliva as well as respiratory secretions, mainstream capnometry is not recommended. This type of capnometry is sensitive to condensation of secretions on the cuvette, which interferes with light transmission and hinders its ability to display accurate $ETCO_2$ values (Dorsch and Dorsch 2008). Not only will the $ETCO_2$ values be inaccurate under these conditions, but also the expensive optical sensor could be irreparably damaged.

A diverting or sidestream capnometer is recommended for use in ruminants; however, this configuration is not impervious to airway secretions. Sidestream capnometers work by continuously aspirating samples of end-tidal gas into the tubing attached to the adaptor at the machine end of the endotracheal tube. The sample is aspirated through the tubing into a special cuvette, where the sensor analyzes it and the results are reported on the digital monitor. While the monitor is aspirating air from the sampling site, it can also aspirate respiratory secretions, which are voluminous in ruminants. These airway secretions can obstruct the sampling line or the filter, which can cause inaccurate readings or prevent readings altogether. The sampling line, filter and water trap may all require changing during the anesthetic period, potentially numerous times. Attempts should be made to keep the sampling site in a position (upright), where gravity works against respiratory secretions, preventing them from draining directly into the tubing (Figure 30.22). Decreasing the amount of fluid entering the sampling line will conceivably decrease the frequency at which equipment must be replaced.

30.7.3.2 Anesthetic Agents

Anesthetic agent analyzers that use optical low-spectrum infrared measurement cannot distinguish between methane, halothane and isoflurane in the expired gas of herbivores (Moens *et al.* 1991; Mortier *et al.* 1998). Due to this inability, these types of gas analyzer will report falsely high concentrations of inhalants in the expired gas, potentially leading the anesthetist to believe their patient is receiving an inappropriately high level of inspired inhalant and prompting them to decrease the vaporizer setting and risking too light a plane of anesthesia. The presence of methane does not affect expired gas readings on analyzers using high-spectrum infrared measurement or piezoelectric measurement and these types of analyzers should be used when anesthetizing ruminants. However, if unavailable, low-spectrum analyzers can be used intermittently (every 15–30 min) by

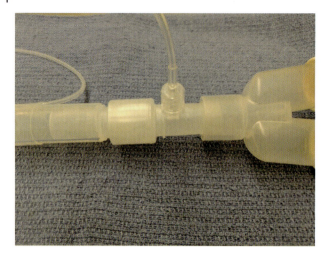

Figure 30.22 End-tidal CO_2 sampling port should be upright to prevent respiratory secretions from clogging the sampling line and preventing accurate measurement.

placing a container of activated charcoal in the sample path to absorb the expired anesthetic agent. The gases will pass through the charcoal that will not absorb the methane, but will absorb the anesthetic. Once the charcoal container is removed, the background methane concentration can be subtracted from the display value to determine the actual concentration of expired inhalant (Moens *et al.* 1991).

30.8   Commercial Anesthetic Machines

There are numerous commercial large animal machines and some that are no longer sold, but remain in use today (e.g. Dräger, DRE Veterinary, Lousiville KY; Vetland, Louisville, KY; Tafonius, Hallowell EMC, Pittsfield, MA; Mallard Medical, Redding, CA). The vast majority of these machines require electricity in order for the ventilator portion to function and require connection to oxygen and vacuum drops to deliver the anesthetic. While all machines can be outfitted with their own oxygen cylinders, their addition makes the machine bulky and difficult to transport.

30.9   Anesthetic Circuit

30.9.1   Breathing Hoses

Breathing circuit tubing is made out of corrugated plastic or rubber inspiratory and expiratory limbs. The internal diameter of the patient's endotracheal tube should be the smallest diameter within the breathing system; therefore, because the internal diameter of adult rebreathing hoses is 22 mm, patients with endotracheal tubes larger than 22 mm require a larger circuit. Large animal rebreathing hoses have an internal diameter of 50 mm and are normally required for all adult cattle and other large ruminants. Most large animal circuits incorporate the CO_2 sampling port into the Y-piece (Figure 30.23). When anesthetizing small ruminants, a small animal $ETCO_2$ adaptor should be used that has an internal diameter no smaller than the internal diameter of the endotracheal tube.

30.9.2   Reservoir Bag and Ventilator Bellows

The purpose of the reservoir or breathing bag is to provide a reservoir of gas available to deliver to the patient when assisted ventilation is desired or required. The breathing bag should have a volume that is approximately 5–10 times the patient's tidal volume (10–20 mL/kg) or the patient's minute ventilation. Too large a reservoir bag will contribute extra volume to the rebreathing anesthetic circuit and slow the rate of change in anesthetic concentration when the vaporizer output is changed. Reservoir bags come in a range of sizes from 0.5–30 L.

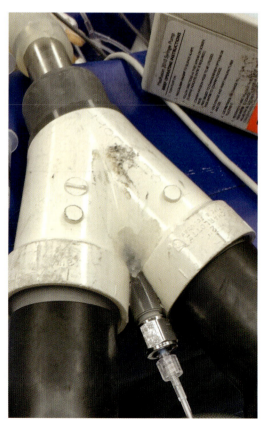

Figure 30.23 End tidal CO_2 sampling port mounted directly on the large animal Y-piece.

30.9.3 Ventilators

Adult cattle and small ruminants differ from their younger counterparts, since they have a fully developed rumen that is associated with a number of potential complications including bloating and aspiration. Thus, domestic ruminants tend to hypoventilate while anesthetized (Riebold 2007). Although a ventilator is not required to perform large animal general anesthesia, it is recommended when the procedure is estimated to be longer than 90 minutes (Riebold 2007). Any adult cow or bull in dorsal recumbency should be mechanically ventilated due to their sheer size, since it is difficult to maintain adequate arterial oxygen tension and safe arterial carbon dioxide tensions when spontaneously breathing. Additionally, these animals should be mechanically ventilated when anesthetized on an emergency basis, since proper fasting times have not been implemented and their rumen is full and very heavy.

Small ruminants (<100 kg) can be maintained on a small animal anesthesia machine and circuit with or without a ventilator. Small ruminants are much easier to ventilate with assisted breaths, by hand squeezing the reservoir bag if a mechanical ventilator is not available. A standard small animal anesthetic machine is also sufficient for most llamas and alpacas. A ventilator is not essential to maintain ventilation in most normal camelids, as they tend to maintain adequate ventilation if an appropriate level of anesthesia is maintained (Cerba *et al.* 2014).

Anesthesia machines vary with respect to which ventilatory parameters are manually controlled. For example, the Mallard Medical Model 2800 series anesthesia ventilator (Mallard Medical, Redding, CA) allows changes in the inspiratory flow, inspiratory time and respiratory rate. The tidal volume is controlled by adjusting the inspiratory flow until the desired tidal volume is achieved. The inspiratory:expiratory ratio is calculated based on the selected inspiratory time and respiratory rate (a short inspiratory time and a high respiratory rate would create a low ratio and vise-versa). This is in contrast to the Dräger Large Animal Anesthesia Ventilator (DRE Veterinary, Lousiville KY), which allows you to change the inspiratory:expiratory ratio directly, as well as the inspiratory flow (tidal volume) and respiratory rate.

Most large animal machines are classified as dual-circuit and time-cycled, pneumatically driven and electronically controlled with either an ascending or descending bellows configuration. The exception to this is the Hallowell Tafonius and Tafonius Junior machines (Hallowell EMC, Pittsfield, MA). These machines are piston-driven and computer controlled and can also be furnished with a patient monitoring module. This ventilator is capable of providing both controlled and assisted modes of ventilation. Tidal volume, respiratory rate, inspiratory time and maximal working pressure can be altered manually. The microprocessor will then automatically determine the inspiratory flow rate and expiratory time based on the above-mentioned settings.

30.9.4 Ventilator Bellows

Typical large animal ventilator bellows will deliver a tidal volume of up to 15–20 L, depending on the ventilator model. Ventilators can be configured with an ascending (standing) or descending (hanging) bellows. The terms ascending and descending refer to their motion during expiration; ascending bellows rise during expiration and a descending bellows fall.

The bellows are housed in clear plastic that allows observation of tidal volume delivery via a set scale on the side of the case. It is important to remember that the apparent tidal volume delivered when using the scale on the bellows housing is not necessarily an accurate representation of the actual tidal volume delivered. Many factors contribute to increase or decrease the actual tidal volume seen by the patient; however, the most relevant to large animal anesthesia are leaks in the circuit and decreased lung compliance causing a smaller tidal volume to be delivered.

The Tafonius large animal workstation ventilator (Hallowell EMC, Pittsfield, MA) is a veterinary-specific piston-driven ventilator. This machine has a cylinder, piston, linear actuator, two rolling diaphragms and positive/negative pressure relief valves. As the piston is actuated, it moves downward, decreasing the space below the lower diaphragm, which delivers a breath to the patient. During expiration, the piston moves upward in response to the measured airway pressure. No resistance is met to expiration normally; however, if this is desired, the settings can be changed to add a set amount of positive end expiratory pressure.

30.10 Anesthetic Recovery

To avoid ruminal tympany and regurgitation, all ruminants should be placed in sternal recumbency, with the endotracheal tube left in place and its cuff inflated, until swallowing and coughing reflexes are evident. If regurgitation had occurred during anesthesia, the oral cavity and pharynx should be lavaged and drained (Thurmon and Benson 1993; Riebold 2007) and the endotracheal tube removed with its cuff inflated in an attempt to remove any material that may have relocated to the trachea.

In patients with nasotracheal intubation, extubation should always be performed with the cuff deflated, so as not to damage the nasal passage upon tube removal. Ideally, the tube is removed with the patient in sternal recumbency with proper control over the head. Placing constant light pressure on the nasotracheal tube at the level of the nares in the ventromedial direction can help facilitate removal of the tube through the same route that it was placed (i.e. ventral nasal meatus). Removal of the tube in an abrupt or rough fashion can cause significant damage and hemorrhage. Always check for sufficient airflow through the nostrils following extubation, since laryngospasm and/or airway edema are commonly encountered; equipment and drugs for re-intubation should be easily accessible.

Because of the potential difficulty in securing an airway in smaller species such as llamas and alpacas, it is recommended to recover them in an area that is safe for the patient and anesthetist, but also close to supplies required for intubation in the case of an airway obstruction post-extubation. Once extubated, these patients are placed in a warm and well-padded stall without access to water until they are fully recovered.

Adult dairy cows with a typical calm demeanor are recovered either in a recovery stall or in their holding stall as long as both provide adequate padding. It is best to place these patients in sternal recumbency with their head on a pad that allows the nose to be tipped down to drain excess saliva and respiratory secretions (Figure 30.24). Deep bedding or a thick foam pad should

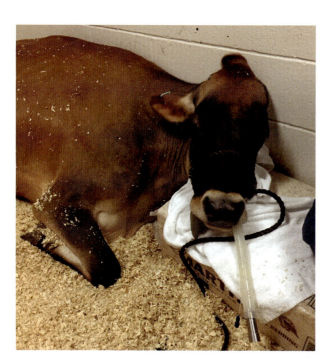

Figure 30.24 Adult Jersey cow recovering from general anesthesia in her stall. Ample bedding in provided to prevent compression injury and maintain sternal recumbency. Her head is supported on a shavings bale allowing drainage of saliva. The end of the endotracheal tube should be protected so the patient does not aspirate any shavings.

be placed under the animal while in the recovery stall. If placed on bedding, care should be taken so animals do not inhale bedding into the tracheal tube while still intubated. Cows typically have much calmer and smoother recoveries from anesthesia than do horses; therefore, it is not as prudent to remove the padding immediately once the cow stands.

Bulls and other less tractable patients are recovered in their holding stalls to avoid moving them once they are recovered, unless the facility provides a safe way to do this. These patients should be recovered in a similar manner as cows once in their stall.

30.11 Summary

In summary, although anesthetizing ruminants is associated with specific anatomical and physiological challenges, it can be safely performed with the correct equipment.

Part II: Swine

30.12 Introduction

Pigs present many unique challenges to the anesthetist. In general, pigs tend to be tenacious and require strict restraint in order to prevent injury to themselves or the personnel working with them. Additionally, there are several species–specific anatomical challenges faced by the anesthetist, including thick skin, relative lack of superficial veins for catheterization and drug administration, and the propensity for laryngeal spasm, which can be exacerbated by potentially difficult intubation associated with their unique laryngeal anatomy. A good working knowledge of this species' specific requirements will help the anesthetist to provide the best standard of care while keeping the patient and personnel safe.

30.13 Handling and Restraint

Typically, miniature, pot-bellied, and show pig breeds are accustomed to owner handling, but are very resistant to manual restraint. They may become nervous when approached in a cage or pen and will often bolt when catch attempts are made. It is advisable to approach these patients slowly to gain their trust before attempting to handle them. Once they are close enough to touch, pigs weighing approximately 10 kgs can be firmly grabbed around the abdomen/chest, lifted, and quickly tucked into both arms. It is important to be swift due to the potential for significant injury while evading capture.

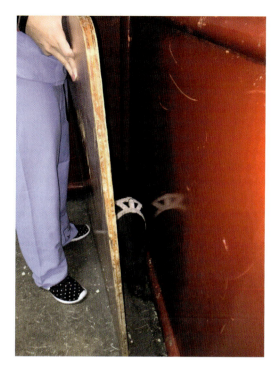

Figure 30.25 A wooden or hard plastic board can be used to secure the pig against a wall for premedication. The board should be taller and slightly longer than the patient to prevent the pig from escaping.

Normally they will be quite boisterous and vocal initially during this process, but quickly calm down once they feel they are no longer in danger. With larger pigs, a "pig board" can be used, which is a wooden, metal, or thick plastic board that is slightly taller than the patient and approximately the same length as the body (Figure 30.25). This board guides the patient into the corner and is used to squeeze them to the wall for premedication administration. Use of the board not only protects personnel from bites or being run over by the patient, but also prevents the patients from injuring themselves. Pigs have very sharp teeth; use of a towel or blanket over the pig's head can provide a barrier to prevent bites in smaller patients.

Regardless of the breed or size of patient, once premedicated, pigs should be watched closely, but left in a quiet room undisturbed to allow optimal sedation before being transported to the induction area.

30.14 Intravenous Catheter Placement

Intravenous injections and/or catheter placement can present a major challenge due to a lack of visible superficial veins in some breeds and pigs' general resentment of restraint.

30.14.1 Peripheral Catheters

Catheter placement in the auricular vein is easily achieved in some pigs (Figure 30.26); however, these patients are frequently sedated before catheterization. In smaller pig breeds, catheterization of the auricular vein is achieved with use of a 22–24 gauge over-the-needle intravenous catheter. In larger breeds with much larger ear veins, an 18–20 gauge catheter can be used. Following placement, the catheter should be taped, sutured or stapled to the ear to prevent dislodging. Cotton padding can be folded and used as a "stent" within the concave surface of the ear. Other sites for peripheral intravenous catheter placement include the cephalic and lateral saphenous veins, but these may be slightly more challenging to access.

30.14.2 Jugular Catheters

Catheterization of the external jugular vein in pigs is uniquely challenging due to their short necks and abundant jowls. Unlike other species, the jugular vein is not visible externally and is located blindly if an ultrasound is not used.

Using the blind method, the jugular vein is located in the jugular furrow, which is 0.5–1.5 cm cranial to the manubrium and 0.5–1.0 cm lateral to midline (Carroll *et al.* 1998). Catheter placement can be performed by using a Vacutainer tube (Becton Dickinson Vacutainer Systems, Franklin Lakes, NJ) attached to a needle, which automatically aspirates blood and through which a guide

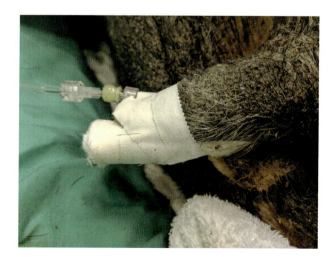

Figure 30.26 IV catheter placement is most easily achieved with a catheter in the auricular vein. Some patients will allow this without premedication; however, many will require sedation. Several pieces of gauze can be stacked and taped together to form a "stent" to which the catheter can be taped and secured. It should be positioned as deep into the ear as possible to avoid it slipping and pulling the catheter along with it.

wire is passed once the vein is punctured. Studies evaluating this technique found no signs of pain or discomfort, inflammation or infection associated with it in large and small pigs (Carroll and Hartsfield 1998; Matte 1999).

The ultrasound-guided method can also be used. Several studies have evaluated the usefulness and ease of jugular catheter placement with ultrasound guidance (Brederlau *et al.* 2008; Izer *et al.* 2017). The jugular vein is more easily compressed, thinner walled and more hypoechoic than the carotid artery and a 100% success rate was reported when veterinarians with only basic ultrasound knowledge performed the procedure (Izer *et al.* 2017).

30.14.3   Intraosseous Catheters

When intravenous catheterization attempts fail, intraosseus catheter placement is a viable option. Intraosseous catheters can be placed in long bones, similar to other species. Use of a commercially available placement kit is recommended, since the cortical surfaces of their bones can be very thick and require sharp instruments (Arrow® EZ-IO® Intraosseous Vascular Access System, Teleflex Medical, Research Triangle Park, NC; Figure 30.27).

30.15   Induction Equipment

Orotracheal intubation is recommended in all anesthetic procedures, due to the potential for loss of a patent airway and reduced protective laryngeal reflexes. Not only does proper placement of an endotracheal tube provide a secure and patient airway, it facilitates positive pressure ventilation, protects the lungs from fluid aspiration, and

prevents contamination of the procedure room with waste anesthetic gas.

30.15.1   Anatomy

Swine have a distinct set of anatomical features that can complicate orotracheal intubation. For example, their oral cavities do not open very wide and the epiglottis is often entrapped above an elongated soft palate. The base of the tongue is thick and can obstruct the view of the larynx, while the floor of the larynx has an acute curve within which the endotracheal tube can become lodged. In addition, there are blind soft tissue pouches where the endotracheal tube can be placed improperly. More specifically, the pharyngeal diverticulum is a long pouch (3–4 cm in adults, 1 cm in piglets), that lies above the epiglottis in the wall of the pharynx within which the endotracheal tube can be erroneously placed. The lateral ventricles also lie bilaterally within the wall of the proximal trachea. If the endotracheal tube is inadvertently passed into these structures and perforates the airway, the patient will develop pneumomediastinum and potentially pneumothorax.

30.15.2   General Intubation Techniques and Equipment

Intubation is performed with the patient in sternal recumbency, with their head and neck in a natural position (not hyperextended; Figure 30.28). The jaw can be held open with gauze ties or small ropes behind the canine teeth on the mandible and maxilla. It is helpful to have a tongue depressor or some other atraumatic tool to lift the soft palate off the epiglottis in

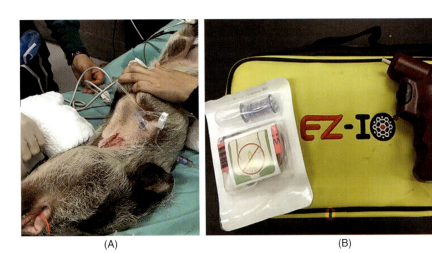

(A)   (B)

Figure 30.27 Intraosseous catheter placement in a humerus of a pot-bellied pig. A surgical approach to the jugular vein was attempted (incision on neck), but due to extreme hypovolemia, was unsuccessful. A commercially available kit (EZ-IO® System) was used for ease of placement.

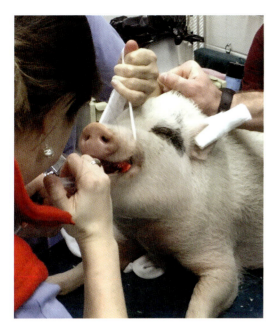

Figure 30.28 Pigs should be placed in sternal recumbency with their heads slightly elevated, taking care not to hyperextend the neck.

order to visualize the larynx. Swine can exhibit laryngeal spasm that can result in airway obstruction. Therefore, once the larynx is visualized, it is crucial to apply local anesthetic before attempting intubation. For example, lidocaine can be applied to the larynx topically using an atomizer (Mila International, Florence, KY; Figure 30.29) or a long red-rubber or polyurethane catheter.

Once the larynx is desensitized, intubation can be attempted. The tip of the endotracheal tube is passed between the arytenoid cartilages and once through, it will often hit the floor of the larynx due to the acute angle between it and the trachea. If the endotracheal tube cannot advance further, rotate it 180 degrees while applying gentle forward traction to avoid the blind

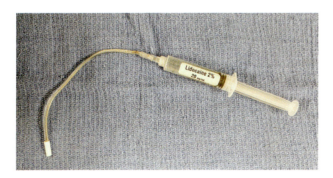

Figure 30.29 The larynx is very sensitive and prone to spasm; therefore, it should be desensitized with lidocaine prior to intubation. An atomizer sprays a fine mist and is very effective at covering a larger surface area than using a syringe tip or catheter.

pouches described above. Use of this method frequently allows for successful intubation.

30.15.3 Laryngoscopes

Use of a laryngoscope is crucial to successful orotracheal intubation in swine. The tip of the laryngoscope blade should be placed on top of the thick tongue at the base of the epiglottis. Firm downward force should be placed at this position to aid in visualization of the entire larynx. Depending on patient size, either a standard Miller (205 mm) or a modified Miller blade (up to 405 mm) can be used (see Chapter 13). Generally, in piglets and small pot-bellied pigs, the shorter of the two blades is useful; however, those larger than approximately 25 kg will likely require the additional length of the longer blade.

30.15.4 Stylets

In cases where direct visualization of the larynx is possible, but the positioning or angle for intubation is not ideal, use of a stylet can be advantageous. There are multiple types of stylets available, most of which can be homemade from common veterinary supplies. A single polypropylene urinary catheter or two in tandem provides a soft, pliable and atraumatic option that is fed into the trachea, followed by the endotracheal tube, which is threaded over the top. Stylets made of a harder, malleable material are also available, which allow the anesthetist to bend the endotracheal tube at an angle that better facilitates intubation. However, caution must be used to prevent these harder stylets from extending beyond the patient end of the endotracheal tube, as they can cause significant trauma to the fragile tracheal mucosa (see Figures 30.10 and 30.11).

30.15.5 Laryngoscopy

Video laryngoscopy should be readily available for all difficult swine intubations (see Figure 30.12). If a patient cannot be easily intubated, the endoscope can prove invaluable. The endoscope is used as a stylet; therefore, it is crucial that its diameter is not larger than the endotracheal tube's internal diameter. Before advancing the endoscope into the oral cavity, the endotracheal tube should be threaded onto it. If it is a tight fit, a small amount of sterile lube can be placed on the endoscope tip. This technique requires at least two people, one to "drive" the endoscope into the larynx and one to thread the endotracheal tube off and into the trachea. The tip of the endoscope should be advanced past the arytenoid cartilages before an attempt is made to pass the endotracheal tube into the trachea. Once the tube is placed, the endoscope is removed and the tube is secured.

30.15.6 Endotracheal Tubes

There are many types of endotracheal tubes available; some are manufactured for humans, but can be used in veterinary patients and some are veterinary-specific products (see Chapter 14). The various types of endotracheal tubes will have some combination of external markings indicating internal diameter (I.D.), outer diameter (O.D.) and length. Most endotracheal tubes are marked according to the O.D. and are of the cuffed, Murphy-type variety. The endotracheal tube should be selected based on the patient's lean body weight. It is important to keep in mind that many "pet" pigs are overweight, which can lead to selection of inappropriately large endotracheal tubes. Generally, piglets or mini-pigs weighing less than 5 kg will take a size 3–4 mm, weanlings 5–10 kg will take a size 4.5–6 mm, adult pot-bellied pigs will take a size 7–9 mm and market pigs can take up to a size 18 mm. Before intubation, the endotracheal tube should be measured such that the distal end does not extend past the thoracic inlet and that the machine end of the tube is not inserted distal to the incisors. It is especially important in swine that the endotracheal tube not be inserted distal to the thoracic inlet, due to the presence of a tracheal bronchus proximal to the bifurcation of the main-stem bronchi.

30.16 Monitoring Equipment

Standard monitoring equipment for continuous evaluation of the cardiovascular and respiratory systems is recommended during the entire anesthetic period for all species. Monitors should include electrocardiography (ECG), direct or indirect blood pressure measurement, end tidal concentration of CO_2, assessment of hemoglobin O_2 saturation (SpO_2) with pulse oximetry, and body temperature (Figure 30.30).

30.16.1 Electrocardiography (ECG)

ECG leads should be placed in a standard configuration (i.e. lead I, II, III). Swine have thick subcutaneous fat and delicate skin that may preclude use of alligator electrode clips due to bruising; however, there are many alternatives. Alligator clamps can be attached to the shaft of a small gauge needle inserted into the skin, manufactured small gauge needle electrodes are available, adhesive patches can be used, and esophageal ECG leads are available for use in swine.

30.16.2 Blood Pressure Measurement

Although some may consider blood pressure measurement an advanced monitoring technique, its use is crucial

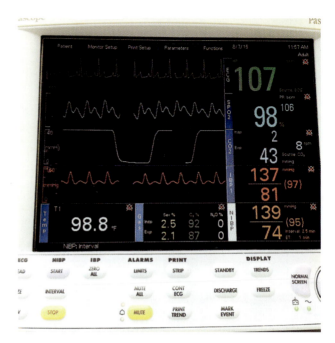

Figure 30.30 Example of a multi-parameter anesthetic monitor (Datascope Passport 2 Multiparameter Monitor, Soma technology, Inc., Bloomfield, CT) on a pot-bellied pig. The monitor incorporates simultaneous monitoring with an ECG, pulse oximeter, inspired and end-tidal inhalant, CO_2, O_2 and N_2O monitor, invasive and non-invasive blood pressure monitor, and body temperature. Each monitor has separate controls and sweep speeds, evident as the broken waveforms in the ECG, pulse oximeter, invasive blood pressure and capnometer, which is sweeping at a different speed than the other monitors. The pulse rate is 106 bpm, respiratory rate is 8 breaths/minute, end-tidal CO_2 is 43 mmHg and the mean blood pressure is 97 mmHg. Note the slight differences in blood pressure values between invasive and non-invasive monitors and in heart rate taken from the ECG (reads electrical complex frequency) and pulse oximetry (pulse rate).

during any general anesthetic event. Non-invasive methods include oscillometric and Doppler flow measurement. The cuff can be placed in multiple places; however, most commonly it is placed above the carpus or on the tail (Figure 30.31). The proper-sized cuff is approximately 40% the circumference of the body part. Doppler flow measurements have been shown to be within 2–2.5 mmHg of the direct arterial blood pressure measurement when the cuff is placed above the carpus and the Doppler flow probe on the radial artery (Chow 1999). Oscillometric methods have also shown good correlation with direct measurement when the cuff is placed on the tail (Hodgkin *et al.* 1982; Cimini and Zambraski 1985; Knaevelsrud and Framstad 1992).

Direct arterial blood pressure measurement requires catheterization of a peripheral artery, which can be more challenging and requires a higher skill level than is necessary in other species. As with any other catheter placement, the site of insertion and the surrounding area should be clipped and sterilely prepped before

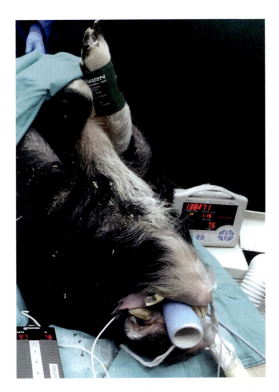

Figure 30.31 Non-invasive blood pressure monitoring requires placement of a cuff proximal to the carpus or the tail. Pictured is an anesthetized pig in dorsal recumbency with a size 6 cuff above the carpus and attached to an oscillometric monitor. Systolic, diastolic and mean arterial pressures are 138, 71 and 115 mmHg, respectively and the pulse rate is 75 bpm (Cardell Veterinary Monitor, Midmark Animal Health, Versailles, OH).

placement. The most superficial and easiest to visualize is the auricular artery; however, this is usually only an option in the larger pigs. The auricular artery courses down the middle of the ear, is very superficial, and can be cannulated with a 20–26 gauge catheter. The catheter can be secured with tape, staples or sutures and is connected directly to a pressure transducer and monitor. Other arteries available for cannulation are the medial saphenous, tail, femoral, radial and carotid arteries; however, these may require a surgical cut-down or ultrasound-guided placement and are associated with potential complications.

30.16.3   End-Tidal CO$_2$ (ETCO$_2$)

ETCO$_2$ provides vital information about ventilation and cardiac output and should be performed using capnography rather than a capnometer. Mainstream or sidestream monitors can be used; however, in larger swine, the internal diameter of mainstream monitors may be smaller than the internal diameter of the endotracheal tube and therefore, will increase breathing resistance. Normal physiologic ETCO$_2$ in swine is 35–45 mmHg

and any increase above these values indicates the need for intermittent or continuous positive pressure ventilation, especially in longer procedures. Acute and drastic increases in ETCO$_2$ could indicate the onset of malignant hyperthermia (Moon and Smith 1996), a pharmacogenetic disease seen in swine.

30.16.4   Body Temperature Monitoring

In many large animal species, monitoring temperature is not always performed. However, pigs may easily become either hypothermic or hyperthermic. For example, they tend to become hypothermic since they lack the insulating hair coat that most other species have. Additionally, some breeds of pigs have a higher percentage of offspring with a genetic mutation causing the syndrome of malignant hyperthermia, which is usually fatal if not detected early. For these two reasons, monitoring temperature in pigs is crucial. Core body temperature can be measured with rectal or esophageal thermistors attached to a digital monitor (Haskins 2015). A hot water blanket placed beneath the patient in combination with a forced warm air blanket is usually sufficient to prevent significant intra-operative hypothermia.

30.17   Anesthetic Circuit

30.17.1   Breathing Hoses and Reservoir Bags

The internal diameter of the patient's endotracheal tube should be the smallest diameter within the breathing system. In general, even adult market pigs will not require an endotracheal tube larger than 18–20 mm O.D. and therefore, a standard circle system could be used. Large animal rebreathing hoses have an internal diameter of 50 mm and therefore require a larger endotracheal tube adapter (22 mm O.D.) than is used on smaller breathing circuits (15 mm O.D.).

A breathing bag provides a reservoir of gas that is available to deliver the patient an assisted breath at any time. The size of the breathing bag should be 5–10 times the patient's tidal volume (10–20 mL/kg).

30.17.2   Ventilators

Swine tend to hypoventilate under general anesthesia, especially when in dorsal recumbency. Therefore, an appropriately-sized mechanical ventilator can be useful. In general, swine weighing less than 100 kg usually have tidal volumes between approximately 1.0 and 1.5 L and can be maintained on a small animal ventilator with a bellows volume up to 1500 mL. Those patients weighing more than 100 kg require a larger bellows, which can be found on various large animal anesthesia machines.

30.18   Anesthetic Recovery

During recovery, it is important to continue monitoring cardio-respiratory parameters. Ideally, all swine recoveries are near emergency equipment and all necessary tools to re-intubate in the event of an airway obstruction. It is prudent to have additional induction agent, a laryngoscope, stylets (± endoscope) and extra endotracheal tubes available. The endotracheal tube should be left in place until the patient is holding its head up and chewing/swallowing has returned. Smaller pigs can be recovered on the procedure table, but larger pigs should be placed on the ground with ample padding during recovery. Pigs may become very cold during procedures; therefore, it is wise to have external warming devices (Bair hugger, heat lamps, etc.) and blankets available.

Additionally, many domestic pigs have excessive body conditioning, which provides a large depot where many drugs will accumulate. Drug accumulation in combination with their propensity to become hypothermic can significantly prolong the recovery process.

30.19   Summary

Although pigs provide some unique challenges to the anesthetist, proper planning and preparation allow for safe and successful anesthetic events. Minimal specialized equipment is required; however, knowledge of the unique challenges they present, both with their anatomy and their disposition, is of the utmost importance.

References

Aarnes, T.K., Hubbell, J.A.E., Lerche, P. and Bednarski, R.M. (2012) Comparison of invasive and oscillometric blood pressure measurement techniques in anesthetized camelids. *Can Vet Journal*, 53, 881–885.

Aarnes, T.K., Hubbell, J.A.E., Lerche, P. and Bednarski, R.M. (2013) Comparison between invasive and non-invasive blood pressure measurement techniques in sheep, goats and cattle. *Vet Anesth Analg*, 41, 174–185.

Abrahamsen, E.J. (2009) Chemical restraint and injectable anesthesia of ruminants. *Vet Clin North Am Food Anim Pract*, 29, 209–227.

Brederlau, J., Muellenbach, R., Kredel, M., Schwemmer, U., Roewer, N. and Greim, C. (2008) Comparison of arterial and central venous cannulations using ultrasound guidance in pigs. *Vet Anaesth Analg*, 35, 161–165.

Carroll, G.L. and Hartsfield, S.M. (1996) General anesthetic techniques in ruminants. *Vet Clin North Am Food Anim Pract*, 12, 627–661.

Cerba, C., Anderson, D.E., Ahmed, T., Van Saun, R.J. and Willard-Johnson, L. (2014) Part 6: Anesthesia and analgesia. In: Cerba, C., Anderson, D.E., Ahmed, T., Van Saun, R.J. and Willard-Johnson, L. (eds). *Llama and Alpaca Care*, 1st ed. St Louis, MO: Elsevier, pp. 579–586.

Chow, P.K., Ng, T.H., Heng, D. and Mack, P.O. (1999) A simple method of blood pressure measurement in the pig using a neonatal cuff. *Ann Acad Med Singapore*, 28, 15–19.

Cimini, C.M. and Zambraski, E.J. (1985) Non-invasive blood pressure measurement in Yucatan miniature swine using tail sphygmomanometry. *Lab Anim Sci*, 35, 412–416.

Dorsch, J.A. and Dorsch, S.E. (2008) Gas monitoring. In: *Understanding Anesthesia Equipment*, 5th ed. Baltimore, MD: Lippincott Williams & Wilkins, pp. 679–753.

Gabel, A.A., Heath, R.B. and Ross, J.N. (1966) Hypoxia: its prevention in inhalation anesthesia in horses. In: *Proceedings of the 12th Annual Meeting of the American of the Association of Equine Practitioners*, Los Angeles, CA: pp. 179–196.

Grandy, J..L, Steffey, E.P., Hodgson, D.S. and Woliner, M.J. (1987) Arterial hypotension and the development of post-anesthetic myopathy in halothane-anesthetized horses. *Am J Vet Research*, 48, 192–197.

Gray, P.R. and McDonell, N.W. (1986) Anesthesia in goats and sheep. Part II: General anesthesia. *Compend Contin Educ Pract Vet*, 8(Suppl), S127–S135.

Hall, L.W. (2001) Anesthesia of sheep, goats and other herbivores. In: Hall, L.W., Clarke, K.W. and Trim, C.M. (eds). *Veterinary Anesthesia*, 10th ed. London: WB Saunders, pp. 341–366.

Haskins, S.C. (2015) Monitoring anesthetized patients. In: Grimm, K., Lamont, L., Tranquilli, W., Greene, S. and Robertson, S. (eds). *Lumb and Jones' Veterinary Anesthesia and Analgesia*, 5th ed. Hoboken, NJ: Wiley, pp. 86–109.

Hodgkin, B.C., Burkett, D.E. and Smith, E.B. (1982) Noninvasive measurement of systolic and diastolic blood pressure in swine. *Am J Physiol*, 242, 127–130.

Izer, J., Wilson, R., Hernon, K. and Ündar, A. (2017) Ultrasound-guided vessel catheterization in adult Yorkshire cross-bred pigs. *Vet Anaesth Analg*, 44, 133–137.

Knaevelsrud, T. and Framstad, T. (1992) Measurement of arterial blood pressure in the sow: a comparison between an invasive and an automatic oscillometric method. *Vet Anesth Analg*, 19, 10–12.

Lin, H.C. and Pugh, D.G. (2002) Anesthetic management. In: Pugh, D.P. (ed). *Sheep and Goat Medicine*, 2nd ed. Philadelphia, PA: WB Saunders, pp. 51–538.

Matte, J.J. (1999) A rapid and non-surgical procedure for jugular catheterization of pigs. *Lab Anim*, 33, 258–264.

Moens, Y., Gootjes, P. and Lagerweij, E. (1991) The influence of methane on the infrared measurement of halothane in the horse. *J Vet Anesth*, 18, 4–7.

Moon, P.F. and Smith, L.J. (1996) General anesthetic techniques in swine. *Vet Clin N Am Food Anim Prac*, 12, 663–693.

Mortier, E., Rolly, G. and Versichelen, L. (1998) Methane influences infrared technique anesthetic agent monitors. *J Clin Monit Comput*, 14, 85–88.

Mosley, C.A. (2015) Anesthesia equipment. In: Grimm, K., Lamont, L., Tranquilli, W., Greene, S. and Robertson, S. (eds). *Lumb and Jones' Veterinary Anesthesia and Analgesia, The Fifth Edition of Lumb and Jones.* Hoboken, NJ: Wiley, pp. 23–85.

Riebold, T.W., Brunson, D.B., Lott, R.A. and Evans, A.T. (1980) Percutaneous arterial catheterization in the horse. *Vet Med Small Anim Clin*, 75, 1736–1742.

Riebold, T.W., Engel, H.N., Grubb, T.L., Adams, J.G., Huber, M.J. and Schmotzer, W.B. (1994) Orotracheal and nasotracheal intubation in llamas. *J Am Vet Med Assoc*, 204, 779–783.

Riebold, T.W. (2007) Ruminants. In: Tranquilli, W. and Grimm, K. (eds). *Lumb and Jones' Veterinary Anesthesia and Analgesia*, 4th ed. Ames, IA: Blackwell, pp. 731–746.

Stewart, S.L., Secrest, J.A., Norwood, B.R. and Zachary, R. (2003) A comparison of endotracheal tube cuff pressures using estimation techniques and direct intracuff measurement. *AANA J*, 71, 443–447.

Thurmon, J.C. and Benson, G.J. (1993) Anesthesia in ruminants and swine. In: Howard, J.L. (ed.). *Current Veterinary Therapy*, 3rd ed. Philadelphia, PA: WB Saunders, pp. 385–422.

Quandt, J.E. and Robinson, E.P. (1996) Nasotracheal intubation in calves. *J Am Vet Med Assoc*, 209, 967–968.

Valverde, A. and Doherty, T.J. (2008) Anesthesia and analgesia in ruminants. In: Fish, R.E., Danneman, P.J., Brown, M.J. and Karas, A.Z. (eds). *Anesthesia and Analgesia in Laboratory Animals*, 2nd ed. London: Academic Press, pp. 385–411.

White, N.A. (1982) Postanesthetic recumbency, myopathy in horses. *Compend Contin Educ Pract Vet*, 4, 44–S52.

31

Unique Species Considerations: Equine

Carolyn Kerr

University of Guelph, Guelph, ON, Canada

31.1 Introduction

Providing safe and effective anesthesia to any species requires the purchase, assembly, set up and diligent maintenance of equipment. Unique equipment requirements exist for the equine patient due to the range in age of patients in which anesthesia may be required, the tremendous breadth of size within the species, the risks associated with anesthesia for both personnel and the patient, and the spectrum of facilities in which sedation and general anesthesia may occur.

Physiologic maturity and predisposition to specific complications varies substantially with age and size of the equine patient which, in turn, impacts the need for particular equipment. For example, neonatal foals presenting within the first few hours of life may require laboratory equipment to evaluate the adequacy of passive transfer and glucose status, while adult draft horses under anesthesia require extensive padding to avoid muscle ischemia. Select equipment and products available for human patients or companion animals can be used in the equine; however, equipment designed and manufactured specifically for the equine is required in most hospital facilities. A partial, yet not exhaustive list of current suppliers for equipment commonly used in the equine, whether specifically designed for the equine or other species, is provided for reference in Table 31.1.

In addition to the patient's demographics, the type of procedures performed and the intended location of a procedure will affect specific equipment requirements. For example, if a practice performs only standing sedation and short duration field anesthesia for elective surgery, equipment needs are relatively minimal compared to that required for a full service referral equine hospital that provides care for patients ranging from miniature horse foals to adult draft horses. Relative to other domestic species, the morbidity and mortality associated with general anesthesia in the equine is high.

Relatively aggressive hemodynamic monitoring, particularly during inhalant-based anesthesia in this species, is therefore standard practice. Various monitors routinely used in the equine are described below.

31.2 Sedation and Pre-Anesthetic Period Considerations

31.2.1 Pre-Operative Health Assessment

Equipment necessary to perform a thorough general physical examination are essential pieces of equipment. In addition to a stethoscope and thermometer, an electrocardiogram (ECG), ophthalmoscope, ophthalmic fluorescein stain, ultrasound, and radiographic equipment, as well as diagnostic lameness equipment, may be required prior to providing sedation or a general anesthetic to a patient when an abnormality is identified on general physical examination. For example, pre-operative ECGs, when deemed necessary, may be performed with a multi-parameter physiologic monitor that includes an ECG or a simple portable device designed for ECG monitoring only. Ideally, the monitor is equipped with a printout capacity to permit in-depth examination of the cardiac rhythm over time. Further details regarding desirable ECG monitor characteristics are discussed below.

31.2.2 Halter and Ropes

Irrespective of the facilities or location where general anesthesia or standing sedation occurs, an equine patient should be wearing an appropriately-sized, sturdy, well-constructed halter in good condition that has been well fitted. In some situations, it may be important to ensure there are no snaps on the halter to avoid it becoming connected to a fixture such as a ring at an inappropriate

Veterinary Anesthetic and Monitoring Equipment, First Edition. Edited by Kristen G. Cooley and Rebecca A. Johnson.
© 2018 John Wiley & Sons, Inc. Published 2018 by John Wiley & Sons, Inc.

Table 31.1 Partial list of equine equipment suppliers.

Equipment	Company and Contact Information	Equipment	Company and Contact Information
Weigh Scales			Radiometer 250 S. Kraemer Blvd Brea, CA 92821 USA www.radiometeramerica.com
	Rice Lake Weighing Systems 230 West Coleman St Rice Lake Wisconsin, WI 54868 USA https://www.ricelake.com/en-us/ support/contact-us		IRMA VET Blood gas analyzer LifeHealth, LLC 2656 Patton Road Roseville, MN 55113 USA www.lifehealthmed.com
Farrier Supplies			i-Stat Handheld Abbott 400 College Road East Princeton, NJ 08540 USA www.pointofcare.abbott.com
	Centaur Forge 117 N. Spring Street Burlington, WI 53105 USA www.centaurforge.com		epoc Blood Analysis System Epocal Inc 2060 Walkley Rd, Ottawa, ON K1G 3P5 www.alere-epoc.com
	Professional Farrier Supply 23 Coles Crescent Mono, Ontario L9W 5W2 Canada www.profarriersupply.com	Veterinary Glucometers	
Microhematocrit Centrifuge			AlphaTrak Zoetis 10 Sylvain Way Parsippany, NJ 07054 USA
	Vetlab Supply 18131 SW 98th Ct. Palmetto Bay, FL 33157 USA www.vetlab.com	Immunoglobulin G Assays (Point of Care)	
	Jorgensen Laboratories 1450 Van Buren Ave. Loveland, CO 80538 www.jorvet.com		SNAP Foal IgG Test Idexx One IDEXX Drive Westbrook, Maine 04092 USA www.idexx.com
Refractometers			Gamma Check E Plasvacc USA Inc, 1535 Templeton Road Templeton, CA 93465 USA www.plasvaccusa.com
	Jorgensen Laboratories 1450 Van Buren Ave. Loveland, CO 80538 www.jorvet.com	Vascular Access Catheters	
	Cole-Parmer 210-5101 Buchan St Montreal, QC H4P 2R9 Canada www.coleparmer.ca 625 Bunker Ct, Vernon Hills, IL 60061 USA www.coleparmer.com		BD Angiocath Becton Dickinson 9450 S State St, Sandy, Utah 84070 USA www.bd.com
Blood Gas Analyzers and Hemoximeters			Mila Long Term Catheters Mila International 7984 Tanner's Gate Lane Florence, Kentucky 41042 USA www.milainternational.com
	Nova Biomedical 200 Prospect Street Waltham, MA 02454-9141 USA www.novabio.us		

Equipment	Company and Contact Information	Equipment	Company and Contact Information
Oral Rinsing Syringe	Arrow Long Term Catheters 3015 Carrington Mill Boulevard Morrisville, NC 27560 USA www.telflex.com	Hobbles	ReCathCo, LLC 2853-106 Oxford Boulevard Allison Park, PA 15101 USA www.recathco.com
Urinary Catheters	Horse Dental Equipment ZI de Bellevue 14 rue Blaise Pascal 35220 Chateaubourg France McCarthy & Sons Service 87 Skyline Cres NE, Calgary, AB T2K 5X2 Canada www.mcandson.com	Foam Pads	Shank's Veterinary Products 505 E. Old Mill Street Milledgeville, IL 61051 USA http://www.shanksvet.com A & A Pad Co. 803 Wast Faye Drive Maryville, TN 37803 USA www.aapadco.com Dandy Products, Inc 3314 State Road 131 Goshen, OH 45122 USA www.dandyproducts.net
Tracheal Tubes	Smith Medical 5200 Upper Metro Place, Suite 200 Dublin, OH 43017 USA www.smiths-medical.com	Equine Slings	Shank's Veterinary Products 505 E. Old Mill Street Milledgeville, IL 61051 USA http://www.shanksvet.com CDA Products Potter Valley CA 95469 USA www.andersonsling.com
Equine Epidural Catheters	Benson Medical 151 Esna Park Drive, Markham, ON L3R 3B1 Canada www.bensonmedical.ca Kruuse Havretoften 4 DK-5550 Langeskov Denmark www.kruuse.com Patterson Veterinary 137 Barnum Road Devens, MA 1434 USA www.pattersonvet.com Smith Medical 5200 Upper Metro Place, Suite 200 Dublin, OH 43017 USA www.smiths-medical.com www.surgivet.com Med-Rx 2810 Coventry Road Oakville, Ontario L6H 6R1 Canada www.med-rx.ca		Hast Large Animal Rescue Equipment Hast, PSC 2787 Floyd Highway South Floyd, Virginia 24091-3055 USA www.rescue.hastpsc.com Liftex 48D Vincent Circle Ivyland, PA 18974 USA www.liftex.com Munks 503 SW Victoria Ct Gresham, OR 97080 USA www.wigginsinc.com

(Continued)

Table 31.1 (Continued)

Equipment	Company and Contact Information	Equipment	Company and Contact Information
Anesthetic Machines and Ventilators	Midmark Animal Health International 60 Vista Dr Versailles, OH 45380 USA http://www.midmarkanimalhealth.com/		Criticare Systems Inc N7W22025 Johnson Dr, Waukesha, WI 53186 USA www.criticareusa.com
	DRE Veterinary 1800 Williamson Court Louisville, KY 40223 USA www.dreveterinary.com		DRE Veterinary 1800 Williamson Court Louisville, KY 40223 USA www.dreveterinary.com
	Hallowell EMC 239 West Street Pittsfield, MA 1201 USA www.hallowell.com		GE Healthcare www3.gehealthcare.com
	Kruuse www.kruuse.com		Parks Medical Electronics, Inc 19460 SW Shaw Aloha, OR 97007 USA www.parksmed.com
	LAPD-1000 and LAV-3000 Ventilator JD Medical Dist. Co. Inc 1923 West Peoria Avenue Phoeniz, Arizona 85029 USA www.jdmedical.com		Patterson Veterinary 137 Barnum Road Devens, MA 1434 USA www.pattersonvet.com
	Mallard 2800C and 2800C-P Mallard Medical 20272 Skypark Drive Redding, CA 96002 USA www.mallardmedical.com		Smith Medical 5200 Upper Metro Place, Suite 200 Dublin, OH 43017 USA www.smiths-medical.com www.surgivet.com
	Smiths Medical 5200 Upper Metro Place, Suite 200 Dublin, OH 43017 USA www.smiths-medical.com www.surgivet.com	Recovery Hood	
Demand Valve	Equine Demand Valve JD Medical Dist. Co. Inc 1923 West Peoria Avenue Phoeniz, Arizona 85029 USA www.jdmedical.com		Shanks's Veterinary Equipment 505 E. Old Mill Street Milledgeville, IL 61051 USA http://www.shanksvet.com
Monitors	Benson Medical 151 Esna Park Drive, Markham, ON L3R 3B1 Canada www.bensonmedical.ca		

time. A thick cotton lead rope, with a solid snap, is recommended to connect to the halter. When additional ropes are required, cotton ropes of lengths suitable for the individual situation are also recommended. In some instances, it may be preferable to avoid snaps altogether and rely on knots to secure ropes.

31.2.3 Weigh Scales

Equine weight is ideally determined with calibrated scales. Desirable features include a weight range of 20–1500 kg, a ramp up to a solid and quiet platform with a non-slip surface, and quick performance. Construction should be such that it is waterproof and sand resistant. A variety of designs is available, ranging from stationary

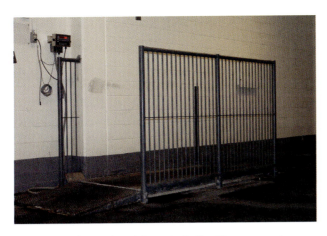

Figure 31.1 Electronic weight scales built with a ramp up to a platform, and nonslip surface in a hospital facility.

units that require electricity, to portable battery operated units (Figure 31.1).

31.2.4 Weigh Tapes

Equine weigh tapes have graduated markers with weight rather than distance. The most common require the user to measure the horse circumferentially at the girth. In adult horses, they provide a general estimate of the weight although they are considered inaccurate in ponies and foals.

31.2.5 Farrier Supplies

Ideally, horses are not shod at the time of general anesthesia to minimize risk of self-injury during recovery as well as to protect the surface of the recovery room. At some facilities, it is standard practice to remove shoes prior to general anesthesia. Purpose-made clinch cutters, a rasp, nail and shoe pullers, purchased from farrier supply sources, facilitate shoe removal.

31.2.6 Laboratory Equipment

Recommendations regarding peri-operative laboratory assessment of the equine patient, and therefore the need for laboratory equipment, varies. Short duration elective field anesthesia may require no on-site equipment, as pre-operative blood analysis, if deemed necessary, can be performed in advance using a remote diagnostic laboratory. Due to the relatively high incidence of hematological abnormalities in patients with underlying disease, the need for frequent re-assessment of critically ill patients, as well as the physiological alterations associated with non-elective or lengthy, elective anesthesia in the equine, on-site laboratory equipment is generally located within referral hospital facilities. While the equipment necessary

to perform a complete blood count and biochemistry profile may not be on-site, the ability to measure a patient's packed cell volume, total solids, blood gases, blood glucose and electrolytes is common.

31.2.6.1 Microhematocrit Centrifuge

A basic bench-top micro-hematocrit centrifuge with a capillary tube rotor is used to measure the packed cell volume from a small sample of blood. Desirable features of a micro-hematocrit centrifuge include a short-time interval to reach a speed of 12 000 RPM, a safety lid that locks when the rotor is moving, a built-in timer and a braking system. Although some centrifuges have a built-in scale on the rotor for reading the hematocrit, a separate hematocrit reader (in percent), that can be placed directly on a bench top, is recommended for ease of use.

31.2.6.2 Refractometer

A traditional, portable, handheld refractometer can be used to determine the total plasma protein from a serum or plasma sample. The refractive index of a solution is temperature dependent, therefore it is important to use a refractometer with automatic temperature compensation. Additional desirable features include the inclusion of a serum protein scale, which reads in g/dL or g/L, a focusing eyepiece with eyecup, and a means to calibrate.

31.2.6.3 Blood Gas Analyzers and Hemoximeters

Blood gas analyzers, either bench-top or point-of-care, with the capacity to measure blood gas tensions, pH, hemoglobin concentration, lactate, glucose and electrolytes including ionized calcium, are commonly used to assess equine patients peri-operatively. Most blood gas analyzers also calculate certain variables such as SaO_2. However, equations based on human blood are generally programmed into the instruments, which results in some inaccuracy.

Large hospitals are generally equipped with bench-top analyzers with a large range of analytes that regularly auto-calibrate. Point-of-care machines, such as blood gas analyzers with disposable single-use cartridges, are a portable and cost-effective alternative to a bench-top machine for monitoring some variables. Several different models are available and have been tested for use with equine blood (Grosenbaugh *et al.* 1998; Looney *et al.* 1998; Bardell *et al.* 2017). When considering the type of analyzer suitable for a given practice, consider the range of different analytes measured and calculated, the demonstrated accuracy and precision of results using the machine with equine blood, the storage temperature needs of the point-of-care machine cartridges, and the recommended working temperature of the analyzer, in addition to the per sample cost.

Hemoximeters, using photometric methods, measure hemoglobin in its various states, including oxygen carrying hemoglobin, non-oxygen carrying hemoglobin, carboxyhemoglobin, fetal hemoglobin and methemoglobin. These instruments are not routinely used clinically, although may prove valuable in cases with dyshemoglobinemias or when evaluating the accuracy of other devices designed to measure a patient's hemoglobin oxygen saturation, such as a pulse oximeter (Giguere *et al.* 2014). A portable co-oximeter has recently been introduced to the market and may prove useful in the future (Rainbow® Pulse Co-Oximetry; Masimo Corporation, Irvine, CA).

31.2.6.4 Glucometers

Critically ill neonatal foals have a high incidence of hypoglycemia (Hollis *et al.* 2008). Chemistry and blood gas analyzers are used to measure plasma or blood glucose; however, point-of-care glucometers can be used to verify repeated blood glucose levels at a low cost with small volumes of blood (Hackett and McCue 2010; Hug *et al.* 2013). Most glucometers on the market are designed for human use; however, units designed for veterinary species are also available. While some glucometers marketed for use with human blood have been shown to be inaccurate with equine blood, more recent models have shown better accuracy (Hug *et al.* 2013). Most models are supplied with test strips to run prior to use; however, when possible, the accuracy of an individual unit should be verified intermittently using a calibrated blood gas analyzer or standard chemistry analyzer. Continuous glucose monitoring systems have been evaluated in equine patients. While their set-up time and cost are current limitations, future product development may improve their value for clinical use in the equine (Wiedmeyer *et al.* 2003; Hug *et al.* 2013).

31.2.6.5 Immunoglobulin G (IgG) Assays

The ability to rapidly and accurately evaluation a foal's serum Immunoglobulin G (IgG) at 18–24 hours of age is also considered a necessity for equine practitioners. Unfortunately, serum total protein concentration is not an adequate estimate of IgG levels (Davis and Giguere 2005; Metzger *et al.* 2006). Commercial laboratories can measure serum IgG levels using various assays. However, due to the need for a timely diagnosis and treatment of failure of passive transfer, for facilities that perform non-elective surgeries, on-site ability to assess the IgG status in foals is recommended. Radial immunodiffusion is considered the gold standard method of measuring IgG levels in serum; however, the assay requires 24 hours to complete. This feature makes the latter assay less desirable for guiding initial treatment in a foal at risk of failure of passive transfer. Other more rapid assays available for

screening serum IgG levels use glutaraldehyde coagulation, latex agglutination, zinc turbidity, colorimetric immunoassays and enzyme-linked immunoassays. These assays are generally available in kits and can be performed stall-side. The recommended strategy for identifying failure of passive transfer is to choose a screening test with high sensitivity. Foals with failure of passive transfer as identified by the initial test can be retested with a second highly specific test to avoid unnecessary treatment. If only one test is used, a test with high sensitivity is recommended (Watson 2009).

31.2.7 Medical Supplies

A range of disposable supplies including needles and syringes, stored in an organized fashion that permits easy access is essential. In the field, this may be a simple portable case, while purpose-built anesthesia carts are available for in-hospital use (Figure 31.2). As sedative and anesthetic drugs are generally prepared in advance of a case, syringe labeling is essential as untimely and/or inappropriate administration of drugs can be dangerous to both horse and handlers. Syringe labels with drug names and concentrations can be purchased in a variety of colors to assist with easy identification of syringe contents. An inexpensive alternative are colored permanent

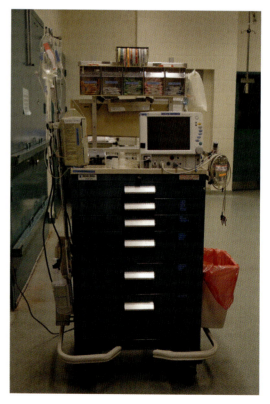

Figure 31.2 Mobile, purpose-built anesthesia cart showing supplies and equipment typically used in an equine hospital.

markers that can be used to write directly onto syringe barrels.

31.2.8 Vascular Access Catheters

Intravenous catheter placement for drug administration minimizes the risk of perivascular or intra-arterial injections. While sedative drugs are often not delivered via a catheter, constant rate infusions of sedatives to provide prolonged standing sedation are generally administered via an intravenous catheter. Placement of an intravenous catheter prior to general anesthesia is also routine, particularly in referral hospital settings (Wohlfender *et al.* 2015).

Vascular access catheters suitable for use in the equine vary in composition, design and size. Catheters made of polyurethane are most commonly used for long-term catheterization (up to 30 days), as they are relatively non-thrombogenic and resistant to kinking. A coating of silver zirconium phosphate, which inhibits bacterial growth, may be added to some polyurethane catheters. When the duration of catheterization is relatively short (<48 hours), catheters made of fluorinated ethylene propylene (FEP) polymers or polytetrafluoroethylene (Teflon) polymers are commonly used. The latter are generally more economical; however, they are relatively more thrombogenic and prone to kinking compared to the catheters made of polyurethane.

Catheter designs include over-the-needle, those supplied with a peel-away sheath, or with a guidewire for insertion. Over-the-needle FEP polymer or Teflon catheters are generally used for short-term venous or arterial access in the equine, as they are easy to place and are available in sizes from 10–24 gauge with varying lengths (Figure 31.3). Polyurethane over-the-needle catheters

are used for short- or long-term use. Catheters made of polyurethane, which are placed using an introducer sheath or guidewire, are generally supplied in a kit (Figure 31.4). The former contains a peel-away introducer, catheter and caps, while the latter contains an introducer needle, guidewire, vessel dilator, catheter and catheter caps. While over-the-needle catheters only have one lumen, other catheter designs may have more than one lumen, to permit the simultaneous administration of more than one drug or fluid without mixing.

The maximum flow rate through a catheter is inversely proportional to the length of the catheter, and the radius to the fourth power (r^4). As such, if the need for a rapid fluid rate is anticipated, the gauge of the catheter placed in a patient should be as large as possible. In adult horses, a 14-gauge, 5.25-inch catheter is commonly placed in the jugular vein for drug and fluid administration, while a 20-gauge, 2-inch catheter is placed in a branch of the facial artery for arterial blood sampling and pressure monitoring. In foals, a 16- or 18-gauge, 3.25-inch catheter is generally adequate for placement in the jugular vein and a 20- or 22-gauge, 1- or 2-inch catheter is placed in the facial or transverse facial artery.

Some catheters are supplied with wings on the proximal end to facilitate securing the catheter on the patient using suture material. If wings are not present, a circumferential suture can be placed around the catheter hub to secure it to the patient, or tape can be used to create wings on the catheter hub, which can be sutured to the patient. Fast drying adhesives are also effective at securing catheters while under anesthesia, although care should be taken to ensure no spillage onto the catheter itself or when working close to a patient's eyes.

Once placed in the patient, the proximal end of the catheter is capped with an injection cap or an extension set can be connected directly to the catheter to facilitate

Figure 31.3 Over-the-needle catheters made of FEP polymer in sizes ranging from 22-gauge to 14-gauge. The sizes displayed are typically used for short duration arterial and venous access in an equine patient.

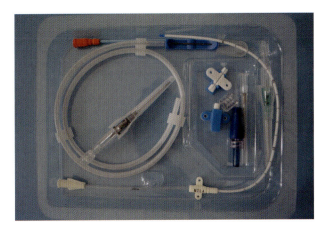

Figure 31.4 Catheter kit containing a polyurethane catheter placed with a guidewire. The kit includes an introducer needle, guidewire, vessel dilator, catheter and catheter caps.

drug or fluid administration. Caps and extension sets should be designed to screw onto the catheter to ensure they are securely fastened to minimize the risk of disconnection, which would allow air to enter, or blood to exit the catheter unimpeded. Some long-term polyurethane catheters come with integrated extension sets.

31.2.9 Oral Rinsing Syringes

Sturdy plastic syringes with a volume capacity of 250–400 mL, commonly referred to as dosing syringes, are useful tools to rinse an adult pony or horse's mouth prior to general anesthesia. The nozzle should have a blunt design and be constructed of a sturdy material such as brass to prevent breakage in the event of the patient biting down on the nozzle (Figure 31.5). Plastic, 60-mL syringes with a catheter tip are also suitable and less likely to inadvertently injure a foal when rinsing its mouth prior to anesthesia. Although intubation may not be planned for a short procedure, it is recommended that the oral cavity be rinsed as thoroughly as possible prior to anesthesia in the event that intubation is required.

31.2.10 Urinary Catheters

Urinary catheters are routinely placed in horses undergoing standing procedures that are anticipated to require a prolonged duration of sedation, particularly if infusions of alpha-2 adrenergic agonists are included in the sedative protocol. A 24 French (8.0-mm O.D.), 140–150-cm long catheter is generally suitable for adult male horses, while a similar-sized but shorter version is suitable for use in a mare. The proximal end of the urinary catheter is connected to tubing that is of adequate length, so that it can be directed into a pail or drain away from the horse or personnel. Advantages of performing urinary catheterization include maintaining optimal footing by preventing

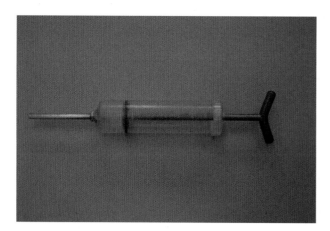

Figure 31.5 Oral rinsing syringe with a brass nozzle to reduce the chance of breakage when used.

urine collecting on the flooring underneath and surrounding the patient, prevention of posturing to urinate by the patient during standing surgery, and potentially decreased patient anxiety or discomfort associated with having a full bladder during sedation or recovery from anesthesia.

Male horses under general anesthesia placed in dorsal recumbency for a midline laparotomy generally have a urinary catheter placed to minimize risk of contamination of the incision and surgical field. In some hospitals, it may be customary for all horses to have a urinary catheter placed for prolonged general anesthesia.

31.2.11 Local Anesthetic Supplies

A range of spinal needles with varying gauges and lengths (20–22 gauge, 1.5-3 inch) are optimal to permit local anesthesia such as epidural injections or ophthalmic blocks. Epidural catheter kits with a 19-gauge catheter, 17-gauge, 3.5-inch Tuohy needle, a Tuohy Borst adapter, flat 0.22-micron filter and cap are suitable for use in the horse, to permit repeated epidural drug administration over a prolonged period of time (Martin *et al.* 2003; Figure 31.6A). The catheter should have graduated marks to assist with determination of length during insertion. The catheter can be secured to the patient using tape and protected by covering with a sterile adhesive bandage (Figure 31.6B).

31.2.12 Stocks

Equine stocks are often ideal locations for surgical, diagnostic or dental procedures. Many different designs of equine stocks exist and the style preference may vary according to the local horse population and the intended procedure. Desirable features include height adjustable front- and side-bars that can easily and quickly be removed in the event of an emergency, such as recumbency of the patient. Equally important to the stock design, is the footing and the location of the stock in a room. Ease of horse entry and exit from the stocks for both the safety of the horse and handler must be taken into consideration.

31.3 General Anesthesia

31.3.1 General Anesthesia Facilities

31.3.1.1 Induction Areas
Equine general anesthesia can be performed in many different styles of facilities. Irrespective of location, it is critical to have adequate space with non-slip footing and excellent lighting. Induction of anesthesia in the equine

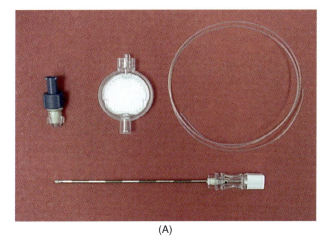

(A)

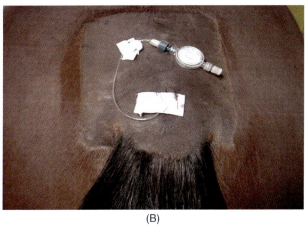

(B)

Figure 31.6 (A) Epidural kit contents containing a catheter, Tuohy needle, adapter and filter. The epidural catheter has graduated marks to assist with placement. (B) Epidural catheter placed in a horse and secured to the patient using butterfly tape sutured to the skin.

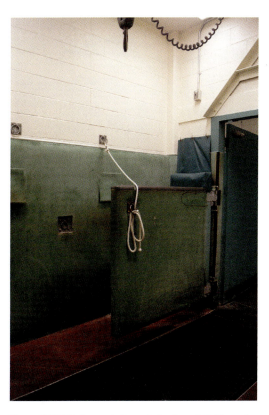

Figure 31.7 Swing gate in an induction stall. The gate measures 54 inches tall, 60 inches in length and is mounted 27 inches from the wall and 7 inches above the floor. Note the recessed ring on the wall and pad mounted at the end of the swing gate that can be removed to adjust to the size of the patient.

is most commonly performed using the free fall method or with a swing gate. The free fall method is common in the field setting or in hospital facilities when short-duration procedures will be performed in the location where the horse is induced and recovered. If performed indoors, non-slip flooring and padded walls free from hooks or shelves are ideal. In equine hospitals, anesthesia recovery rooms are frequently used for free fall inductions.

Anesthesia induction rooms with swing gates can provide additional control of the horse's location while it is achieving recumbency (Figure 31.7). Gates should have adequate clearance from the ground so that a limb cannot become trapped under the gate and should be of adequate length so that the horse's shoulder does not extend beyond the gate. A recessed wall mounted ring can provide a means to easily control the horse's head during induction. Running a rope through a ring on the handler side of the gate to a ring on the wall well above

the height of the gate can be used facilitate holding the gate against the patient during induction.

Equine tilt tables were historically popular in equine hospitals to facilitate anesthetic induction. While relatively uncommon at this time, tilt tables suitable for anesthesia induction and/or recovery of equine patients may remain in some equine hospitals and be used in special circumstances (Elmas *et al.* 2007; Figures 31.8A, B). Most tilt tables are designed to position the horse in lateral recumbency. The degree of padding on a tilt table may determine its suitability for prolonged use and in many cases, the horse must be transferred to a surgery table with padding if a prolonged surgery is scheduled.

Waterproof foam pads of various sizes and thicknesses are commonly placed under the patient if recumbency is anticipated to be greater than 15 minutes. Foam pad thickness recommended for a mature horse over 500 kg is generally 10–14 inches (25–36 cm). Air and water cushions are also available for equine use, although they are less popular for surgical patients due to greater patient instability. Horses placed in lateral recumbency for greater than 15 minutes should have their upper limb supported in a natural position parallel to the floor. Leg

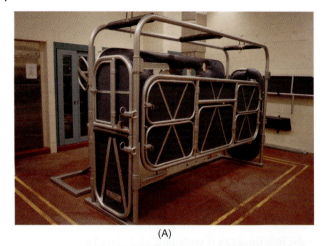

(A)

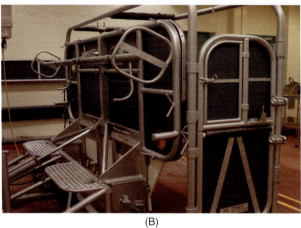

(B)

Figure 31.8 Two views (A, B) of a tilt table used during induction or recovery of a horse.

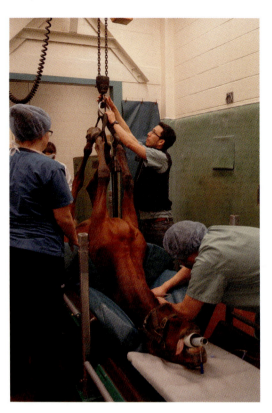

Figure 31.9 A horse being positioned on a surgery table using a hoist mounted on an overhead track system. Note the nylon hobbles used to attach the horse to the hoist.

supports are generally provided with equine surgical tables for this purpose.

Hoists are useful to lift and move horses onto or off of a surgery table. An electric chain hoist with a 2-ton capacity is suitable for lifting and positioning an anesthetized horse onto a surgery table. Ideally, the system is fast and is mounted on a track system to permit situating the hoist directly over the horse when it is in use (Figure 31.9). Hobbles are required to easily connect and disconnect the horse's limbs to the overhead hoist system. Nylon hobbles offer the advantage of being relatively easy to cut in the event of an emergency, such as a hoist failure.

Although pre-oxygenation of equine patients is not routine, access to oxygen delivered through a flowmeter capable of delivering up to 15 liters per minute may be advantageous for some patients (van Oostrom *et al.* 2017). If the oxygen source is via a bulk tank directed through a wall outlet, the latter should either be located outside of the induction room or at a height sufficient to prevent breakage by a patient or equipment.

31.3.1.2 Surgical Suite

While most anesthetic equipment used in the surgical suite are portable, the oxygen source, gas scavenging system and method of supporting intravenous fluid therapy are generally features of the room. Surgical suites should be equipped with an easy–to-access, yet safely stored, source of oxygen. Hospital bulk oxygen sources are commonly piped to wall or overhead connections. If oxygen tanks are used, they should be securely stored against a wall. A waste gas scavenging system should also be easily accessible within the surgical suite when inhalant anesthesia is used. While floor fluid stands can be used to deliver fluids, retractable overhead hooks can be used to minimize use of floor space.

31.3.1.3 Recovery Rooms and Systems

Horses may be recovered unassisted or using one of many different assisted recovery systems. The optimal size of the recovery room for use with unassisted recovery is unknown, although it is generally felt that too large a room may permit an ataxic horse to achieve an excessive speed during a failed attempt at standing, possibly predisposing to serious injury. A 12–14 square foot room with large angle or rounded corners is generally suitable for all but overly large draft horses. The flooring of a recovery room should most importantly have good grip and not be slippery even when wet. The degree of padding on the floor is highly variable; however, the walls of the stall should be padded.

In an unassisted recovery system, the use of a rapidly inflating and deflating air pillow in recovery was shown to result in a longer period of recumbency and a better quality of standing compared to a foam mat padded floor in one hospital setting (Ray-Miller *et al.* 2006). At least two doors suitable for human use only, should be situated strategically in the room to permit safe entry and exit of personnel and the means to view the horse in the recovery room from outside the stall is required. A hoist on a monorail system is a feature in many recovery rooms. The latter may be used to take a horse off a surgery table and permit the use of a sling to assist recovery.

For assisted recoveries, outcomes with a pool-raft recovery system, a hydropool system, a tilt table and a use of a sling have all been described, in addition to the rapidly deflating pad described above (Sullivan *et al.* 2002; Tidwell *et al.* 2002; Taylor *et al.* 2005; Elmas *et al.* 2007; Clark-Price 2013). While all of these systems offer advantages for high-risk patients, one of the more routinely used assisted recovery techniques involves simply using a head and tail rope. In most cases, the ropes are connected to a wall-mounted pulley system (Figure 31.10) and then directed outside of the recovery room through

holes, either high in the door or the wall above the doors, to permit personnel to assist remotely. Sling recoveries (e.g. Liftex large animal sling, Anderson sling, etc.) and tilt tables control the horse from recumbency until standing or weight bearing. These systems require trained personnel and a tolerant horse.

Hydropools are usually 12 ft long, 4 ft wide and 8.5 ft deep, with a hydraulic floor and heated (100°F) water (Figure 31.11). The floor is raised until the submerged horse is able to stand, then is further raised until it is at the level of the surrounding floor after which the horse walks out. Alternatively, a sling can be used to lift the horse from the pool. The pool-raft system requires the horse to be sling lifted into a raft with cut outs for the limbs in a pool (22 ft wide and 11 ft deep) as the head is placed on a smaller, floatable pad (Figure 31.12). As horses recover, they are lifted out of the pool by the sling to a recovery area. Major disadvantages of water-based systems are the cost of specialized equipment, trained personnel and pulmonary complications (i.e. pulmonary edema) (Richter *et al.* 2001; Sullivan *et al.* 2002; Clark-Price 2013).

In the hospital setting, an oxygen flowmeter with a 15-L/min capacity is generally attached to a wall outlet outside the recovery room (Figure 31.13). An oxygen line is routed into the stall through the ceiling or through a hole in the wall. Oxygen is delivered via a small flexible tubing placed inside the horse's airway in the early phases of recovery (Figure 31.14).

31.3.2 Mouth Specula and Gags

Inserting a mouth gag between the incisors or a wedge between the molars facilitates orotracheal intubation in

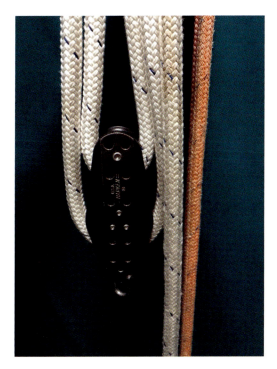

Figure 31.10 A strong pulley system used to rope-recover horses (photograph courtesy of Dr David Brunson, University of Wisconsin-Madison, WI).

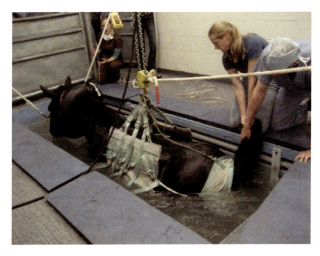

Figure 31.11 Example of a horse immersed in a hydropool during recovery. Note the padding surrounding the pool and the use of an inflatable device to keep the horses head elevated until the horse recovers (photo courtesy of Dr T. Grubb; with permission).

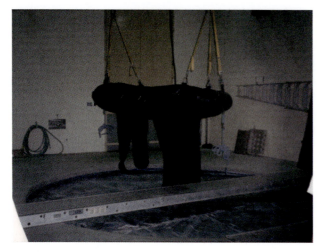

Figure 31.12 Example of a pool raft system where the horse is positioned onto the raft during, and is hoisted out, following recovery (photograph courtesy of Dr David Brunson, University of Wisconsin-Madison, WI).

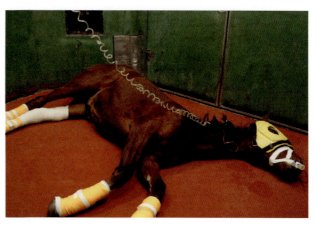

Figure 31.14 An oxygen insufflation line from an overhead supply placed into the orotracheal tube to supply enriched inspired oxygen levels during recovery. Note the padded helmet used to reduce trauma.

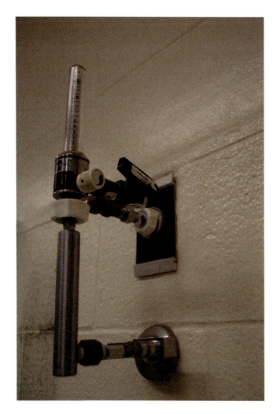

Figure 31.13 15 L/min oxygen flowmeter attached to a central gas supply of oxygen outside of a recovery stall.

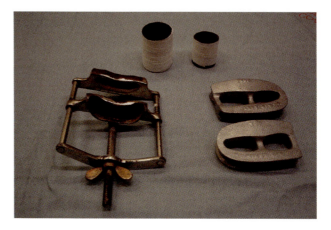

Figure 31.15 Sections of polyvinyl chloride piping, purpose-made metal mouth gags, and commercial wedges used to facilitate orotracheal intubation in the horse.

tubing and minimize slippage. A 5-cm diameter, 7-cm long PVC pipe placed between the upper and lower incisors will permit a standard 26–30 mm inner diameter tube to be inserted through its lumen. Stocking a range of sizes from 2–5 cm in diameter will permit the use of an optimally sized gag in a range of horses, ponies and foals.

31.3.3 Endotracheal Tubes

Tubes designed to be placed in the trachea of an equine patient may vary in numerous characteristics, including the materials of which they are manufactured, size, length, radio-opacity, presence of a cuff, cuff design, proximal end connection and distal tip design. Unlike supplies used in small animal patients that are frequently made for human use, the endotracheal tubes used for the equine are manufactured specifically for large animals, due to both their size and length requirements.

the equine. While metal gags and wedges are available, a section of polyvinyl chloride (PVC) pipe is a simple inexpensive alternative (Figure 31.15). The latter is easy to clean and unlikely to damage a patient's teeth during placement. Disposable tape can be used to cover the outside of the tube to improve grip on the surface of the

The most common tubes used for orotracheal or nasotracheal intubation in the equine are made of medical grade radiopaque silicone. They are primarily identified by their internal diameter (mm I.D.); however, the outer diameter (mm O.D.) and length (cm) are also identified on the side of the tube. All three measurements are included in the product specifications and should be considered when purchasing. Additional markings on the side of the tube include the manufacturer and graduated distance (in cm) from the tip of the patient end of the tube. For a given internal diameter, the outer diameter and length of a silicone tube may vary among suppliers. The wall thickness of silicone tubes is generally less than tubes made of red rubber, which permits maximization of internal tube size placement and therefore minimization of resistance to breathing. While the relatively flexible walls of silicone tubes are advantageous, tubes made of silicone are prone to kinking and can be damaged, particularly during anesthetic recovery.

Silicone tubes suitable for tracheal intubation range in sizes from 6–30 mm I.D. Neonatal pony foals may require tubes as small as 6–8 mm I.D. to permit nasotracheal intubation or 8–10 mm I.D. for orotracheal intubation. The length of these tubes is generally 50–55 cm, while similarly-sized tubes used in small animal patients are 32–36 cm. Adult large breed horses typically permit a 26–30 mm I.D. tube to be placed through the oral cavity into the trachea or a 22–24 mm I.D. tube to be placed nasotracheally. The length of these latter tubes is generally 90–100 cm.

Uncuffed silicone tubes may be purchased at a lower cost for use in equine recovery or in situations where a sealed airway is unnecessary. When used during inhalant anesthesia, or in a patient in which the need for positive pressure ventilation is anticipated, endotracheal tubes should have an inflatable cuff. Endotracheal tube cuffs are generally considered to be either high volume, low pressure or low volume, high pressure design with the latter being more common in the equine tubes available. When the latter style of cuff is deflated, the cuff has a low residual volume, thereby minimizing resistance during placement in a patient.

The inflation tube connecting the cuff to a proximally located pilot balloon is embedded into the wall of the endotracheal tubes for the majority of the distance between the cuff and pilot tube in most silicone tubes. This design feature minimizes the potential for breakage of the inflation line. Cuffs are generally filled with air, although specialty tubes that are designed to be filled with saline exist. The pilot balloon most commonly has a self-sealing valve system through which air can be injected using a standard syringe. When purchasing a tube, ensure that the cuff, line that connects the cuff to the pilot balloon, and pilot balloon are repairable or replaceable should they become damaged. Endotracheal tube cuff inflation should be performed with the least amount of air required, to prevent gas passing on the outside of the tube at peak airway pressures encountered during positive pressure ventilation.

The latter technique has been shown to prevent leakage of liquid material of similar density to water past the cuff into the distal trachea (Touzot-Jourde *et al.* 2005). However, excessive cuff inflation can result in high tracheal transmucosal pressures, which can produce ischemia of the tracheal muscosa (Touzot-Jourde *et al.* 2005). Tracheal perforation attributed to cuff over-inflation has also been reported in clinical cases (Saulez *et al.* 2009). Unfortunately, intracuff pressure is not an accurate measure of tracheal transmucosal pressure with low-volume high-pressure cuffs, as the pressure in the cuff has no relationship with the pressure exerted on a patient's trachea. If the cuff has been inflated with the least amount of air required to create a seal, monitoring intracuff pressure with a manometer (described below) may assist with identification of a loss of cuff pressure over time, assist with cuff re-inflation to an appropriate pressure, and minimize the risk of inadvertent cuff over-inflation.

Cole endotracheal tubes are uncuffed tubes with a stepped and tapered patient end. They are designed to create a seal at the larynx; however, they are more likely to result in a leak, are challenging to place and may result in a greater risk of laryngeal damage and as such, they are not in routine use in the equine.

The proximal ends of silicone tubes larger than 18 mm I.D. are commonly supplied with a funnel adapter that is designed to fit over the Y-piece on a large animal breathing circuit. The funnel can be removed and the end of the tube fitted with a 22 mm O.D. adapter suitable for insertion into the Y-piece of a large animal breathing circuit as well (Figure 31.16). Alternatively, tubes may be purchased without the funnel adapter, which can facilitate sampling of gases. Silicone tubes of 12 mm I.D. or less fit a 15 mm O.D. adapter that will insert into a standard small animal breathing circuit. In addition, the distal end of most silicone tubes has a beveled tapered end with a Murphy eye to reduce the risk of obstruction of the tube with secretions.

Historically, red rubber tubes were the preferred tubes designed for orotracheal intubation in the horse. These tubes have a curved design with a convex and concave side and are manufactured in a range of sizes with either a 15 or 22 mm O.D. adapter for the proximal end. As with the silicone tubes, they can be supplied with a cuff, and the distal tip of the tube generally has a Murphy eye. Unlike the silicone tubes, red rubber tubes, particularly in the larger sizes, are rigid due to their thick wall. While less popular than silicone tubes

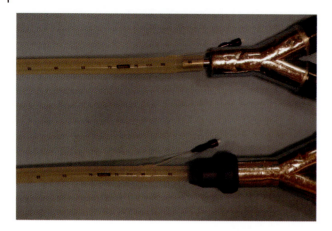

Figure 31.16 Silicone endotracheal tubes connected to a large animal breathing circuit with a funnel or metal adapters.

due to their rigidity and reduced lumen sizes relative to O.D., red rubber tubes are robust and not as prone to tears or kinking. Rubber tubes are generally not radiopaque.

Orotracheal intubation in the equine is generally performed blindly without a stylet or other means of assisting intubation. However, a flexible endoscope, if available, can be used to facilitate intubation in a patient in which pre-existing pathology in the oropharynx, larynx or trachea exists.

Routine cleaning of endotracheal tubes with cold disinfectant followed by thorough rinsing is recommended. Individual manufacturers and suppliers of endotracheal tubes generally indicate appropriate sterilization techniques such as autoclaving or low-temperature hydrogen peroxide gas plasma technology (STERRAD® Sterility Guide, Advanced Sterilization Products Division of Ethicon, Inc., Irvine, CA).

31.3.4 Endotracheal Tube Adapters

Endotracheal tube adapters permit connection of an endotracheal tube with a breathing circuit. The breathing circuit end of an adapter designed to connect to a small animal breathing circuit has a 15 mm O.D., while an adapter designed for a Y-piece on a large animal breathing circuit has a 22 mm O.D. at one end. The alternative end of an adapter fits into the proximal end of an endotracheal tube and, as such, a variety of sizes must exist to fit tubes of different sizes. It is important to use correctly fitting adapters to prevent leaks and inadvertent disconnections of the endotracheal tube to the breathing circuit. Misuse of medical tape to fit an adapter to an endotracheal tube has been reported to result in partial expiratory obstruction and rapid increase in airway pressures in a horse (Gregson and Clutton 2012).

31.3.5 Lubricant

Lubricating the outside of the endotracheal tube facilitates its advancement through the oral cavity or nasal passage of the horse. Water-soluble lubricating jelly is effective at reducing friction during use and is easily washed off the surface of tubes after use. It can be purchased in either small individual use packages or multi-use tubes and while not generally used in a sterile format, it is reported to be bacteriostatic.

A 2% lidocaine topical anesthetic in a viscous gel format is commercially available. It can be applied manually in a patient's ventral nasal meatus to minimize the sensation to and lubricate a nasotracheal tube as it is being placed.

31.3.6 Cuff Manometer

Simple pressure manometers can be used to measure the pressure within an endotracheal tube cuff following tube placement in a patient (see Chapter 14). In most commercially available units, the manometer can measure pressures in the range of 0–120 cmH$_2$O. As mentioned above, the measured intracuff pressure does not correlate with the pressure exerted by the cuff on the tracheal mucosa when using an endotracheal tube with a low-volume high-pressure cuff. However, the manometer can be used to trend changes in cuff pressure and assist in cuff re-inflation.

31.3.7 Tracheostomy Tubes

Tracheostomy tubes are available in a variety of materials, including metal and silicone, with the latter being available in a greater range of sizes (Figure 31.17). Tubes placed via a tracheostomy are generally smaller than

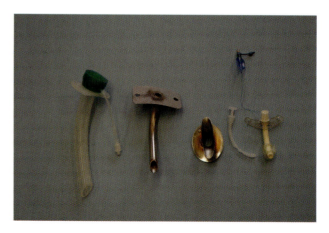

Figure 31.17 A variety of tracheostomy tubes including a cuffed silicone tube, metal Jackson trachea tube, metal self-retaining tube and cuffed plastic tube with a stylet.

those placed orotracheally due to the challenges of tube placement through the tracheal rings and musculature surrounding the trachea. Some tubes are provided with an insert to assist placement. For delivery of inhalant anesthesia, a cuffed silicone tracheostomy tube should be used with a suitable proximal end design that permits connection to the breathing circuit.

31.3.8 Eye Lubricant

Sterile eye ointment or eye drops are used on patients during general anesthesia to prevent corneal injury. Ointments may impair vision, which may be a concern if applied close to the anesthetic recovery period. Eye drops are therefore commonly used in patients under short-term general anesthesia or close to the recovery period.

31.3.9 Anesthetic Machines and Ventilators

Commercially available anesthetic machines are not routinely manufactured to deliver inhalant anesthesia in all patients ranging in size from 20–1200 kg; therefore, equine facilities must have anesthetic machines suitable for both small and large animals. Due to the range of equine patient sizes, large and small animal anesthetic machines with rebreathing circuits are common in equine facilities that provide inhalant-based anesthesia. When selecting a large or small animal machine for use in an equine patient, factors to consider include the weight of the patient, suitability of the ventilator support associated with each machine, and the size of the patient's endotracheal tube. Small animal anesthetic machines with rebreathing circuits are frequently suitable for miniature horses and foals of less than 125 kg, while large animal machines are optimally suited to patients above 125 kg. While equine patients that can accommodate up to a 12 mm I.D. endotracheal tube are generally connected to a small animal breathing circuit, patients with a 14 mm I.D. or 16 mm I.D. endotracheal tube can generally be connected to either a small or large animal breathing circuit, by using endotracheal tube adapters for either circuit. Patients with endotracheal tubes sized 18 mm I.D. or larger are generally connected to a large animal breathing circuit.

Two basic types of large animal machine design exist:

1) To-and-Fro system (Figure 31.18); and
2) Circle rebreathing system (see Chapter 4).

Machines with a To-and-Fro design are less common but are more portable; however, there is a greater risk that the patient will inhale dust from the carbon dioxide absorber and they are primarily suited to situations in which the horse is in lateral recumbency. Large animal

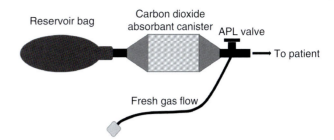

Figure 31.18 Schematic of a To-and-Fro anesthetic system for use in horses. Note that the carbon dioxide absorbant canister is in direct line with the patient's airway, increasing the chance of dust inhalation.

machines with circle rebreathing circuits are less portable, but are more suitable for use in a hospital setting, as they are easier to use with a horse in dorsal recumbency. Most modern equine anesthetic machines are designed with a circle rebreathing circuit and a built-in ventilator. Ventilators are commonly classified as either volume targeted or pressure cycled, based on the major control variable set by the operator (see Chapter 6). The Mallard (Model 2800, Mallard Medical, Redding, CA), Surgivet (Model LDS 3000, Smiths Medical, Dublin, OH) and Dräger (not currently manufactured) large animal ventilators are examples of volume-targeted ventilators designed for use in a controlled ventilation mode (Figures 31.19A–C). The ascending bellows design feature on the Mallard (Figure 31.19A) and Surgivet machines is a desirable feature, as it leads to improved identification of a leak in the circuit while in use, as well as facilitating drainage and drying of the inside of the bellows between uses. The JD Medical LAV-3000 and LAV-2000 (JD Medical Distributing Company, Inc., Phoenix, AZ) are pressure-cycled ventilators that use a modified mark-7 Bird ventilator with a descending bellows. These ventilators can be used in an assist, control or assist-control mode of ventilation. Tafonius (Hallowell EMC, Pittsfield, MA) is a computerized large animal machine with an integrated volume or pressure cycled ventilator. Rather than a bellows, a linear actuator moves a piston to generate a tidal volume that is delivered to the patient (Figure 31.19C).

Ideally, large animal anesthetic machines have a vaporizer with a large inhalant reservoir to minimize the need for refilling during prolonged anesthesia delivery.

Small animal anesthetic machines in routine use are designed with a circle rebreathing system. Most small animal anesthesia ventilators have bellows up to 1400–3000 mL. These ventilators generally connect to small animal anesthetic machines with a 22-mm diameter hose, while large animal ventilators generally connect to the anesthetic machine through a 5-cm hose. Some manufacturers provide machines with both small and large

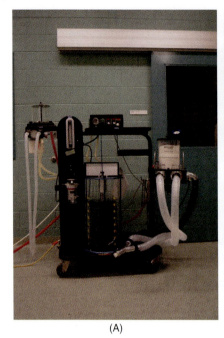
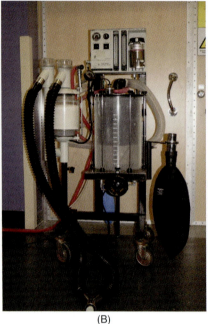
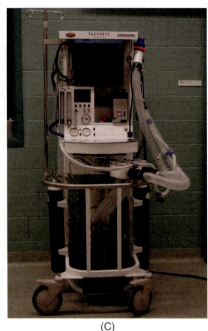

(A)   (B)   (C)

Figure 31.19 (A) Mallard anesthetic machine with both large and small animal breathing circuits in place and ascending ventilator bellows. (B) Drager anesthetic machine with descending ventilator bellows. (C) Tafonius anesthetic machine with piston-driven ventilation system.

animal breathing circuits and ventilators, which facilitates set up when dealing with patients of intermediate size (Figure 31.19A).

31.3.10 Demand Valves

A demand valve, connected to a compressed oxygen source, can be used to deliver oxygen to a patient via an endotracheal, nasotracheal or tracheostomy tube (Figure 31.20). An oxygen tank with a regulator or regulated bulk oxygen is required in addition to an appropriate range of adapters to permit a sealed connection with the proximal end of a tracheal tube.

In the equine, the demand valve is most commonly used to deliver intermittent positive pressure ventilation by manually triggering a valve to deliver a high flow of oxygen to the patient. The volume of oxygen delivered to the patient will depend on the flow of oxygen through the valve and the time that the operator maintains the valve open. As the valve creates excessive resistance to exhalation, it is generally disconnected from the patient's airway at the end of inspiration (Watney *et al.* 1985). In some models, the oxygen supply pressure may influence the maximum flow rate of oxygen delivered by demand valves. For equine use, it is recommended that the demand valve be capable of delivering a flow rate of 200–250 L/min (3.3–4.2 L/sec), allowing a relatively short inspiratory time in a mature horse (Riebold *et al.* 1980). Many demand valves currently available for purchase

deliver a maximum flow rate of 160 L/min. The latter flow rate is likely adequate if the valve is used to support ventilation for a short duration and the intent is not to achieve normocapnia in a patient.

31.3.11 Gas Supply

Most large hospitals rely on a large liquid oxygen tank or a bank of compressed gas tanks, while smaller hospitals may have several large gas cylinders. From the various regulated sources, oxygen can be delivered to the patient via an anesthesia machine, demand valve or flexible tubing attached to a flowmeter. Having a portable or mobile source of oxygen with a regulator and a delivery method such as a demand value is useful for managing emergencies throughout a hospital (Figure 31.20). In the field, portable E-cylinders with a regulator can be used to deliver oxygen via a demand value or flexible tubing attached to a flowmeter with a 15 L/min capacity (Figure 31.21). The use of a portable oxygen concentrator in the field setting has been described, although it is not commonly in use at this time (Coutu *et al.* 2015).

31.3.12 Anesthetic Monitors

31.3.12.1 Monitors

In the field setting, a stethoscope may be the sole hemodynamic monitor used, while referral equine hospitals are generally equipped with multiple types of anesthetic

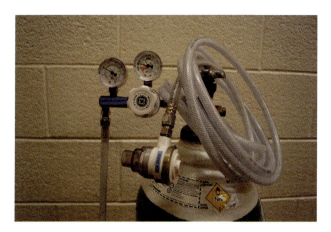

Figure 31.20 An oxygen demand valve with associated oxygen cylinder and regulator.

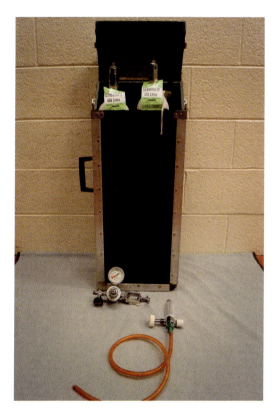

Figure 31.21 A portable oxygen tank system with a regulator and flowmeter.

monitors (Wohlfender *et al.* 2015). Monitors can be obtained from both veterinary and human equipment supply sources. As they can represent a substantial investment, investigation into warranties and service agreements prior to purchase is worthwhile. The mandatory safety and testing requirements for monitors approved for human use are highly regulated, while requirements for equipment used in veterinary medicine do not exist in many jurisdictions.

In some instances, more than one monitor may be used to collect the desired information from a patient, although multi-parameter monitors capable of measuring and displaying several variables, including an ECG, heart rate, systolic, diastolic and mean arterial pressure, SpO$_2$, inspired and expired oxygen and carbon dioxide as well as inhalant concentrations, are available and in common use. Multi-parameter monitors that include the ability to measure cardiac output using thermodilution, as well as perform spirometry, may also be located in tertiary referral settings.

Electrocardiogram (ECG) A monitor with a three-lead ECG is ideal for monitoring cardiac rhythm and rate (if used in conjunction with other monitors) during anesthesia in the equine. Desirable characteristics of an ECG for the equine include a lower heart rate recording range of 20–25 beats per minute, a long cable, printing capability and adjustable alarm settings. Monitors for human use often have relatively high lower heart rate recording values and default audible alarms may be set at unsuitable levels. The ECG leads are generally attached to an equine patient in a base-apex configuration with alligator clips, although adhesive pads can be used on short-haired or clipped horses.

Direct Arterial Pressure Monitoring Arterial blood pressure has been clearly shown to influence the incidence of complications and anesthetic outcome in equine patients maintained under anesthesia with inhalant agents (Grandy *et al.* 1987; Young and Taylor 1993). Combined with the high frequency of cardiovascular complications leading to anesthetic mortality, the current monitoring guidelines by the American College of Veterinary Anesthesia and Analgesia (Martinez *et al.* 2017) strongly recommend arterial blood pressure monitoring in horses when inhalation anesthesia is used (Johnston *et al.* 2002). In a recent international survey regarding equine anesthesia practices, monitoring of arterial blood pressure directly was routinely used by the majority of respondents, while over 20% of respondents also reported using indirect measurement of arterial blood pressure (Wohlfender *et al.* 2015).

With an arterial catheter in place, a simple manometer can be set up to read a patient's arterial blood pressure; however, hospitals that perform inhalant-based anesthesia are generally equipped with a monitor capable of measuring a patient's blood pressure directly using a disposable pressure transducer connected to an arterial catheter. This is accomplished using narrow bore (2.8 mm O.D. × 1.7 mm I.D.), noncompliant (high durometer), polyvinyl chloride tubing (Figure 31.22). The ease of performing direct arterial pressure monitoring, combined with its accuracy and continuity of the real-time

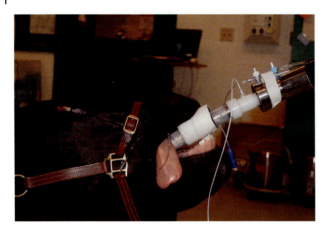

Figure 31.22 An arterial catheter placed in the facial artery and connected to a transducer through noncompliant polyvinyl chloride tubing for the purpose of monitoring direct arterial blood pressure. Note also the sidestream gas monitoring tubing, which takes the sample back to a monitor for further analysis.

information, make this method of monitoring a patient's blood pressure popular. Monitors generally display the waveform as well as provide a numerical display of the systolic, diastolic and mean pressure values. Calibration of the direct blood pressure monitors generally is performed by the manufacturer, although accuracy of the monitor and transducer can be verified in house using a mercury manometer.

Oscillometric and Doppler Blood Pressure Monitoring Non-invasive blood pressure monitoring using an oscillometric or Doppler ultrasonic monitor has been investigated in the adult horse and foal. The Doppler ultrasonic monitor has been used to non-invasively measure blood pressure by placing an occlusive cuff attached to a sphygmomanometer above the Doppler transducer on a horse's tail. In the adult horse, the accuracy of the method is dependent on the width of the cuff relative to the tail, with a 0.2–0.4 ratio of cuff width to tail circumference recommended. In the standing and laterally recumbent horse, the accuracy is clinically acceptable; however, in dorsally recumbent horses, the technique is unreliable (Bailey *et al.* 1994).

Non-invasive blood pressure monitors that utilize the oscillometric method have also been evaluated in anesthetized horses and foals in lateral recumbency. In both situations, the monitor was judged to be an acceptable method of measuring mean arterial blood pressure when using an appropriate cuff size on the tail (cuff width to tail circumference of 0.25) (Nout *et al.* 2002; Tearney *et al.* 2016). While the oscillometric method maintained acceptable accuracy over a range of hemodynamic conditions in one study in foals, studies evaluating the impact of position on the monitors accuracy have not been performed to date (Giguere *et al.* 2005).

Pulse Oximetry Pulse oximeters, with either transmission or reflectance probes, non-invasively measure hemoglobin oxygen saturation using the differential absorption of red and infrared light. They are available as a stand-alone monitor or the technology can be incorporated into a multi-parameter monitor. The reported accuracy of individual units and probes vary in horses and foals (Watney *et al.* 1993; Chaffin *et al.* 1996; Martinez *et al.* 1999; Koenig *et al.* 2003; Matthews *et al.* 2003; Giguere *et al.* 2014). Probes have been assessed on the lip, tongue, mandibular mucosa, ear, ventral aspect of the tail, and vulva. Unfortunately, in some studies performed in foals, the oxygen partial pressure was used to calculate oxygen saturation using a formula determined in adult horses versus measurement of hemoglobin saturation with a hemoximeter and therefore results may be flawed. In general, in the anesthetized equine, certain probes placed on the tongue or lip can provide a reliable assessment of oxygen saturation; however, the accuracy of the monitor may decrease with duration of anesthesia and the presence of underlying disease (Koenig *et al.* 2003; Matthews *et al.* 1994). As such, pulse oximeters are generally recommended as adjunctive anesthesia monitoring devices to be used with blood gas analyzers.

Capnography A capnograph can be used to sample airway gases and measure carbon dioxide using infrared absorption technology and display the results as a waveform as well as inspired and end-tidal values. They are available as either stand-alone units or more commonly, they are incorporated into multi-parameter anesthesia monitors. Mainstream (non-diverting) capnographs have a sensor that is placed between a patient's endotracheal tube and breathing circuit. Due to the sensor design, they are suitable only for patients connected to small animal breathing circuits. Sidestream (diverting) analyzers are used more frequently in equine hospitals, as the sampling line can be connected to adaptors located in either a small animal or a large animal breathing circuit (Figure 31.22). In general, capnographs can provide information regarding the placement of endotracheal tubes, airway and breathing circuit integrity, as well as providing an estimation of arterial carbon dioxide partial pressure. In the equine, end-tidal carbon dioxide levels tend to be 10–15 mmHg lower than arterial carbon dioxide levels. The patient position, duration of anesthesia, method of ventilatory support and hemodynamic status all influence the accuracy of end-tidal carbon dioxide measurements as a measure of arterial carbon dioxide values (Geiser and Rohrnach 1992; Neto *et al.* 2000; Koenig *et al.* 2003).

Volatile Anesthetic Gas Concentrations In addition to carbon dioxide, volatile anesthetics sampled from airway gases can be measured using infrared analysis. The accuracy of measured airway inhalant anesthetic concentration in the horse is dependent on infrared wavelength used during measurement. Specifically, methane in exhaled equine gas interferes with monitors that measure inhalant concentrations using a wavelength close to 3 μm, whereas those that use a wavelength within a range of 10–13 μm are not affected by methane (Dujardin *et al.* 2005).

Inspired and Expired Oxygen Many monitors that sample airway gas for carbon dioxide and inhalant gas measurements also measure oxygen. Rather than infrared analysis, oxygen is measured using a paramagnetic analyzer.

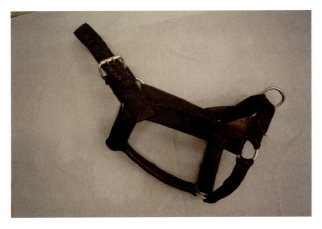

Figure 31.23 An equine recovery halter with D-ring positioned on the dorsal nasal area used for assisted recovery.

31.3.13 Fluid and Drug Delivery Devices

In a hospital setting, infusion pumps that regulate the flow of fluid through an intravenous fluid line or a syringe pump that connects to patient via a fluid line are both useful for administration of fluids and drugs during standing sedation or general anesthesia. Many different models of both infusion and syringe pumps with demonstrated accuracy are available. When selecting an infusion pump, consider the pump's ability to integrate with different fluid administration sets, range of flow rates that the pump can deliver, as well as alarm settings. Programmable wireless syringe pumps with a wide range of delivery volumes that can adapt to different syringe sizes are also useful additions to the anesthesia workstation.

31.4 Recovery Period

The type of equipment used during anesthesia recovery will vary according to the system used as discussed above. Padded helmets (Figure 31.14) are routinely placed on horses recovering unassisted, while nylon halters with a D ring on the noseband are used to connect a horse's head to ropes with an assisted recovery system (Figure 31.23).

In the event that a horse is unable to stand in the postanesthetic period, use of a purpose-built equine sling connected to an overhead hoist may permit a thorough assessment of the patient and improve outcome (Figure 31.24). Commercial slings are available in several different designs with varying complexity.

In addition to circulating water blankets, forced air warmers can facilitate rewarming of foals in the recovery period.

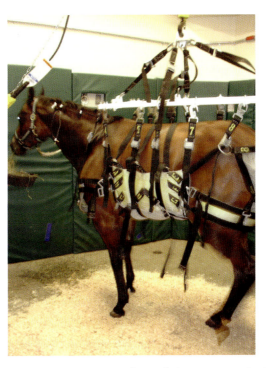

Figure 31.24 A horse standing with the assistance of a sling.

31.5 Medical Records

Requirements regarding the local standard of practice related to the medical record may vary across jurisdiction. A record of the pre-operative physical examination findings, client consent for the intended procedure, including sedation and/or anesthesia, drugs administered and the patient's physiological and behavioral response to sedation and/or general anesthesia, as well as the recovery from the latter, is generally a minimal requirement.

References

Bailey, J.E., Dunlop, C.I., Chapman, P.L., Demme, W.C., Allen, S.L. *et al.* (1994) Indirect Doppler ultrasonic measurement of arterial blood pressure results in a large measurement error in dorsally recumbent anaesthetised horses. *Equine Vet J*, 26, 70–73.

Bardell, D., West, E. and Senior, J.M. (2017) Evaluation of a new handheld point-of-care blood gas analyser using 100 equine blood samples. *Vet Anaesth and Analg, Epub ahead of print, doi*.10.1111.

Chaffin, M.K., Matthews, N.S., Cohen, N.D. and Carter, G.K. (1996) Evaluation of pulse oximetry in anaesthetized foals using multiple combinations of transducer type and transducer attachment site. *Equine Vet J*, 28, 437–445.

Clark-Price, S.C. (2013) Recovery of horses from anesthesia. *Vet Clin Equine*, 29, 223–242.

Coutu, P., Caulkett, N., Pang, D. and Boysen, S. (2015) Efficacy of a portable oxygen concentrator with pulsed delivery for treatment of hypoxemia during equine field anesthesia. *Vet Anaesth Analg*, 42, 518–526.

Davis, R. and Giguère, S. (2005) Evaluation of five commercially available assays and measurement of serum total protein concentration via refractometry for the diagnosis of failure of passive transfer of immunity in foals. *J Am Vet Med Assoc*, 227, 1640–1645.

Dujardin, C.L.L., Gootjes, P. and Moens, Y. (2005) Isoflurane measurement error using short wavelength infrared techniques in horses: influence of fresh gas flow and pre-anesthetic food deprivation. *Vet Anaesth Analg*, 32, 101–106.

Elmas, C.R., Cruz, A.M. and Kerr, C.L. (2007) Tilt table recovery of horses after orthopedic surgery: fifty-four cases (1994–2005). *Vet Surg*, 36, 252–258.

Geiser, D.R. and Rohrback, B.W. (1992) Use of end-tidal CO_2 tensions to predict arterial CO_2 values in isoflurane-anesthetized equine neonates. *Am J Vet Res*, 53, 1617–1621.

Giguere, S., Knowles, H.A., Valverde, A., Bucki, E. and Young, L. (2005) Accuracy of indirect measurement of blood pressure in neonatal foals. *J Vet Intern Med*, 19, 571–576.

Giguere, S., Sanchez, L.C and Shih, A. (2014) Accuracy of calculated arterial saturation in oxygen in neonatal foals and effects of monitor, sensor, site of sensor placement, and degree of hypoxemia on the accuracy of pulse oximetry. *J Vet Emerg and Crit Care*, 24, 529–535.

Grandy, J.L., Steffey, E.P., Hodgson, D.S. and Woliner, M.J. (1987) Arterial hypotension and the development of post-anesthetic myopathy in halothane-anesthetized horses. *Am J Vet Res* 48, 192–197.

Gregson, R. and Clutton, R.E. (2012) Near-fatal misuse of medical tape around an endotracheal tube connector during inhalation anesthesia in a horse. *Can Vet J*, 53, 978–982.

Grosenbaugh, D.A., Gadawski, J.E. and Muir, W.W. (1998) Evaluation of a portable clinical analyser in a veterinary hospital setting. *J Am Vet Med Assoc*, 213, 691–694.

Hackett, E.S. and McCue, P.M. (2010) Evaluation of a veterinary glucometer for use in horses. *J Vet Intern Med*, 24, 617–621.

Hollis, A.R., Furr, M.O., Magdesian, K.G., Axon, J.E., Ludlow, V. *et al.* (2008) Blood glucose concentrations in critically ill neonatal foals. *J Vet Intern Med*, 22, 1223–1227.

Hug, S.A., Riond, B. and Schwarzwald, C.C. (2013) Evaluation of a continuous glucose monitoring system compared with an in-house standard laboratory assay and handheld point-of-care glucometer in critically ill neonatal foals. *J Vet Emerg Crit Care*, 23, 408–415.

Johnston, G.M., Eastment, J.K., Wood, J.L.N. and Taylor, P.M. (2002) The confidential enquiry into perioperative equine fatalities (CEPEF): mortality results of Phases 1 and 2. *Vet Anesth Analg*, 29, 159–170.

Koenig, J., McDonell, W. and Valverde, A. (2003) Accuracy of pulse oximetry and capnography in healthy and compromised horses during spontaneous and controlled ventilation. *Can J Vet Res*, 67, 169–174.

Looney, A.L., Ludders, J., Erb, H.N., Glled, R. and Moon, P. (1998) Use of a handheld device for analysis of blood electrolyte concentrations and blood gas partial pressures in dogs and horses. *J Am Vet Med Assoc*, 213, 526–530.

Martin, C.A., Kerr, C.L., Pearce, S.G., Lansdowne, J.L. and Bouré, L.P. (2003) Outcome of epidural catheterization for delivery of analgesics in horses: 43 cases (1998–2003). *J Am Vet Med Assoc*, 222, 1394–1398.

Martinez, E.A., Carroll, G.L. and Hartsfield, S.M. (1999) Evaluation of the Nonin 8600V veterinary pulse oximeter in anesthetized horses. *J Vet Emerg and Crit Care*, 9, 13–18.

Martinez, E.A., Wagner, A.E., Driessen, B. and Trim, C. (2017) *Guidelines for Anesthesia in Horses*. Available from: http://acvaa.org/docs/Equine [accessed April 2017].

Matthews, N.S., Hartsfield, S.M., Sanders, E.A., Light, G.S. and Slater, M.S. (1994) Evaluation of pulse oximetry in horses surgically treated for colic. *Equine Vet J*, 26, 114–116.

Matthews, N.S., Hartke, S. and Allen, J.C. (2003) An evaluation of pulse oximeters in dogs, cats and horses. *Vet Anaesth Analg*, 30, 3–14.

Metzger, N., Hinchcliff, K.W., Hardy, J., Schwarzwald, C.C. and Wittum, T. (2006) Usefulness of a commercial equine IgG test and serum protein concentration as indicators of failure of transfer of passive immunity in hospitalized foals. *J Vet Intern Med*, 20, 382–387.

Neto, F.J., Luna, S.P.L., Massone, F., Thomassian, A., Vargas, J.L. *et al.* (2000) The effect of changing the mode of ventilation on the arterial to end tidal CO_2 difference and physiological dead space in laterally and dorsally recumbent horses during halothane anesthesia. *Vet Surg*, 29, 200–205.

Nout, Y.S., Corley, K.T.T., Donaldson, L.L. and Furr, M.O. (2002) Indirect oscillometric and direct blood pressure measurements in anesthetized and conscious neonatal foals. *J Vet Emerg Crit Care*, 12, 75–80.

Ray-Miller, W.M., Hodgson, D.S., McMurphy, R.M. and Chapman, P.L. (2006) Comparison of recoveries from anesthesia of horses placed on a rapidly inflating-deflating air pillow or the floor of a padded stall. *J Am Vet Med Assoc*, 229, 711–716.

Richter, M.C., Bayly, W.M., Keegan, R.D., Schneider, R.K., Weil, A.B. and Ragle, C.A. (2001) Cardiopulmonary function in horses during anesthetic recovery in a hydropool. *Am J Vet Res*, 62, 1903–1910.

Riebold, T.W., Evans, A.T. and Robinson, N.E. (1980) Evaluation of the demand valve for resuscitation of horses. *J Am Vet Med Assoc*, 176, 623–626.

Saulez, M.N., Dzikiti, B. and Voigt, A. (2009) Traumatic perforation of the trachea in two horses caused by orotracheal intubation. *Vet Rec*, 164, 719–722.

Sullivan, E.K., Klein, L.V., Richardson, D.W., Ross, M.W., Orsini, J.A. and Nunamaker, D.M. (2002) Use of a pool-raft system for recovery of horses from general anesthesia: 393 horses (1984–2000). *J Am Vet Med Assoc*, 221, 1014–1018.

Taylor, E.L., Galuppo, L.D., Steffey, E.P., Scarlett, C.C. and Madigan, J.E. (2005) Use of the Anderson Sling suspension system for recovery of horses from general anesthesia. *Vet Surg*, 34, 559–564.

Tearney, C.C., Guedes, A.G.P. and Brosnan, R.J. (2016) Equivalence between invasive and oscillometric blood pressures at different anatomic locations in healthy normotensive anaesthetized horses. *Equine Vet J*, 48, 357–361.

Tidwell, S.A., Schneider, R.K., Ragle, C.A., Weil, A.B. and Richter, M.C. (2002) Use of a hydro-pool system to recover horses after general anesthesia: 60 cases. *Vet Surg*, 31, 455–461.

Touzot-Jourde, G., Stedman, N.L. and Trim, C.M. (2005) The effects of two endotracheal tube cuff inflation pressures on liquid aspiration and tracheal wall damage in horses. *Vet Anaesth Analg*, 32, 23–29.

Van Oostrom, H., Schaap, M.W.H. and Van Loon, J.P.A.M. (2017) Oxygen supplementation before induction of general anesthesia in horses. *Equine Vet J*, 49, 130–132.

Watney, G.C., Watkins, S.B. and Hall, L.W. (1985) Effects of a demand valve on pulmonary ventilation in spontaneously breathing, anaesthetized horses. *Vet Rec*, 117, 358–362.

Watney, G.C.G., Norman, W.M. and Schumacher, J.P. (1993) Accuracy of a reflectance pulse oximeter in anesthetized horses. *Am J Vet Res*, 54, 497–501.

Watson, J.L. (2009) Assays for evaluation of failure of passive immunity. In: Robinson, N.E. and Sprayberry, K.A. (eds). *Current Therapy in Equine Medicine*, 6th ed. St Louis, MO: Saunders Elsevier, pp. 860–861.

Wiedmeyer, C.E., Johnson, P.J., Cohn, L.A. and Meadows, R.L. (2003) Evaluation of a continuous glucose monitoring system for use in dogs, cats, and horses. *J Am Vet Med Assoc*, 223, 987–992.

Wohlfender, F.D., Doherr, M.G., Driessen, B., Hartnack, S., Johnston, G.M. and Bettschart-Wolfensberger, R. (2015) International online survey to assess current practice in equine anaesthesia. *Equine Vet J*, 47, 65–71.

Young, S.S. and Taylor, P.M. (1993) Factors influencing the outcome of equine anaesthesia: a review of 1,314 cases. *Equine Vet J*, 25, 147–151.

32

Unique Species Considerations: Avian
Carrie Schroeder

School of Veterinary Medicine, University of Wisconsin, Madison, Wisconsin, USA

32.1 Introduction

Anesthesia of avian species can be a daunting task for the uninitiated; the published sedation and anesthetic-related mortality rates for birds range from approximately 1.75–16% (Brodbelt *et al.* 2008). A number of anatomical and physiological differences between mammalian and avian species exist and a thorough understanding of these differences is key in successfully providing anesthesia. A complete discussion of avian physiology is found in a number of textbooks dedicated solely to avian anesthesia, medicine and surgery. However, there are number of considerations related to anesthetic equipment that should be addressed as well. While some equipment has been developed solely for use in avian species, most of the equipment necessary to successfully anesthetize a bird is frequently the same as that used for mammals or can be easily adapted from equipment found in most veterinary practices.

32.1.1 Anatomy and Physiology

Briefly, the most striking difference in avian anatomy and physiology as related to anesthesia is the respiratory system. It is a system designed for marked efficiency in the face of high demand, such as during flight. The system consists of components designed for one of two jobs: ventilation or gas exchange. The ventilatory system is comprised of the larynx, trachea, primary and secondary bronchi, and air sacs, while the lungs, consisting of parabronchi and air capillaries, participate in gas exchange. In order to discuss the equipment necessary for anesthetizing a bird, it is important to highlight some of the most notable differences in the respiratory system.

32.1.2 Larynx, Trachea and Syrinx

The larynx of birds is considerably more rostral as compared to mammals, generally located at the base of the tongue. While there are species differences in appearance and ease of visualization, the glottis is usually easily located for endotracheal intubation, due to its rostal location and lack of an epiglottis (Figures 32.1A and B). It is important to note that the opening of the glottis is often larger than the diameter of the more distal trachea; excessively large endotracheal tubes may advance past the glottis but can induce damage to the tracheal mucosa (Heard 2016).

The avian trachea is generally much wider and longer than that of mammals. When compared to mammals, these differences result in comparable resistance, but significantly greater anatomical dead space (~4.5 times; McLelland 1989). Birds compensate for this increase in anatomical dead space with a relatively low respiratory frequency relative to body size. Different species of birds vary widely in the conformation of the trachea. For example, certain species such as cranes have evolved a long and convoluted trachea designed for loud vocalizations (Figure 32.2; Gaunt *et al.* 1987). Penguins variably have a septum within the trachea, while emu have a slit in the cervical trachea that connects to an expandable sac (McLelland 1989). With roughly 10 000 different species of birds, it is important to be aware of unique adaptations, such as variable tracheal morphology that may affect an anesthetic plan. However, one common factor among avian tracheae is the presence of complete tracheal rings. This is in contrast to mammalian tracheae, in which the trachealis muscle allows for gentle expansion of the trachea.

Avian species possess a unique anatomical variation at the tracheal bifurcation known as the syrinx. While vocalization in mammals originates in the larynx, the

Veterinary Anesthetic and Monitoring Equipment, First Edition. Edited by Kristen G. Cooley and Rebecca A. Johnson.
© 2018 John Wiley & Sons, Inc. Published 2018 by John Wiley & Sons, Inc.

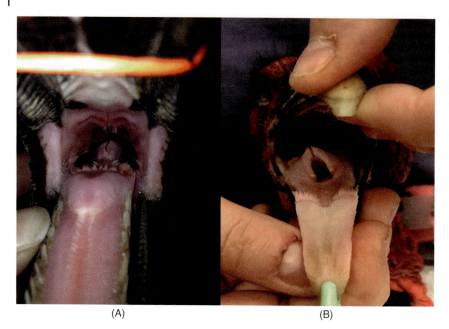

Figure 32.1 Closed glottis of a goose (*Anser domesticus*) (A); open glottis of a turkey (*Meleagris gallopavo*) (B). Note the ease of visualization and lack of an epiglottis. The tongue may be exteriorized using either fingertips or an atraumatic clamp (B).

(A)   (B)

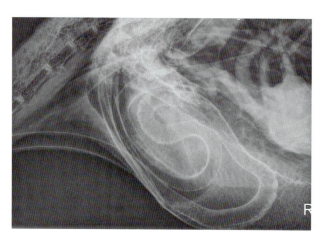

Figure 32.2 Convoluted anatomy of a crane trachea (whooping crane, *Grus americana*) as demonstrated on a radiograph. Multiple avian species have evolved a variety of tracheal conformations to allow for distinctive vocalizations (used with permission from Dr Rebecca Johnson, University of Wisconsin-Madison, WI).

syrinx is the source of vocalization in avian species. This is of clinical significance to the anesthetist as, unlike mammals that cannot vocalize while intubated, vocalization can occur in an anesthetized bird despite intubation.

32.1.3 Air Sacs and Lungs

Most avian species have nine air sacs distributed throughout the body and act as bellows for the conduction of inspired and expired gases (Figure 32.3A). Air sacs are minimally vascularized and do not participate significantly in gas exchange (Magnussen *et al.* 1976). Components of the avian skeleton variably connect with the air sacs, forming pneumatic bones, one of the evolutions for flight. This is clinically significant in that fractures of these bones will result in air escaping into subcutaneous tissue or, in the case of an open fracture, the environment. Surgical repair of a fractured pneumatic bone may require either judicious scavenging of waste anesthetic gasses or a purely intravenous anesthetic technique.

The lungs constitute the gas exchange system and are markedly different from mammalian lungs. They are relatively small and fixed in place; respiratory excursions observed in birds are a result of expansion of the air sacs, rather than the lungs. The tertiary bronchi, or parabronchi, contain perforations known as atria that lead to air capillaries (Duncker 1972). These air capillaries interlace with blood capillaries, a system analogous to the mammalian alveoli. In contrast to the alveoli of the mammalian lung, the gas composition along the length of the parabronchi is constantly changing. Therefore, the surrounding capillary blood contacts with variable partial pressures of oxygen and carbon dioxide. The result is a variable difference between the arterial and end-parabronchial partial pressure of oxygen and carbon dioxide (Scheid and Piper 1970). This effect is more notable during positive-pressure ventilation (Touzot-Jourde *et al.* 2005). Consequently, end-tidal carbon dioxide, as measured by capnometry, may not accurately estimate the arterial partial pressure of carbon dioxide ($PaCO_2$). Studies have found inconsistent results in the accuracy of capnometry in birds, largely depending on the ventilatory state (Edling *et al.* 2001; Touzot-Jourde *et al.* 2005; Desmarchelier *et al.* 2007; Pare *et al.* 2013).

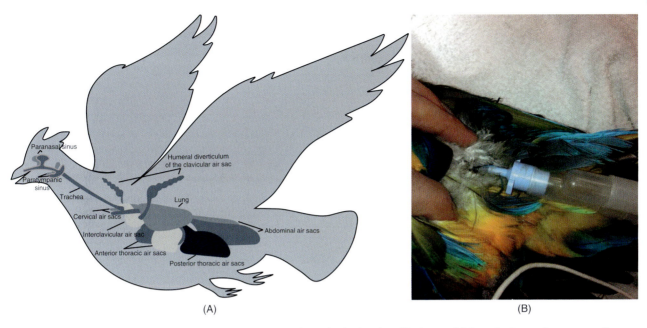

(A)   (B)

Figure 32.3 Distribution of air sacs in the bird (A). Sterilized endotracheal tube placed in the caudal thoracic air sac of a parrot to allow ventilation despite a tracheal obstruction (B). Image courtesy of Kristen Cooley, University of Wisconsin-Madison, WI.

32.1.4   The Respiratory Cycle

The complete avian respiratory cycle requires two separate cycles for complete passage of air through the respiratory system. Both inspiration and expiration are active processes, as birds lack a diaphragm and rely upon expansion and contraction of coelomic cavity volume for inspiration and expiration. Upon the first inspiration, inspired gases inflate the caudal air sacs; upon expiration, this volume in the caudal air sacs traverses across the lungs where gas exchange occurs. In the second inspiration, gases from the lungs move to the cranial air sacs and, upon expiration, these gases are exhaled through the mouth or nares via the trachea. Because of this respiratory pattern, clinicians can ventilate birds via a caudal air sac, which is of great advantage in the event of tracheal obstruction. The caudal thoracic or abdominal air sacs are cannulated via placement of a blunted endotracheal tube or commercially available air sac cannula (Figure 32.3B). Oxygen or anesthetic gases are delivered into the air sac and, due to the unique respiratory cycle, gases will flow over the lungs and be exhaled via the trachea. When administering anesthetic gases via this technique, it is important to scavenge waste gases escaping the trachea with either an endotracheal tube or tightly fitting mask.

32.2   Anesthetic Considerations

32.2.1   Anesthetic Masks

Following premedication, anesthetic induction of birds is commonly accomplished via mask induction rather than intravenous induction. The marked efficiency of the respiratory system coupled with a low functional residual capacity allow for rapid anesthetic induction with inhalational agents. The wide variation in beak and bill morphology can make mask selection and availability difficult. Smaller birds are induced by placing their entire head within a medium- to large-sized small animal mask. Birds with long beaks and bills may require modification of soda bottles (Figure 32.4). While it is unlikely that a bird will perfectly fit into the mask or mask diaphragm, it may be necessary to pack gauze or small towels into the orifice of the mask to prevent leakage of anesthetic gasses. A custom-made diaphragm is made with the palm of a latex glove stretched across the mask, with a small hole cut to size for the bird (Figure 32.5).

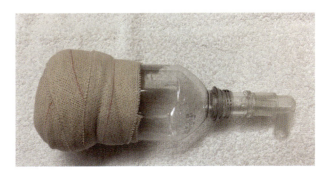

Figure 32.4 Modification of a 20-oz soda bottle for use as an anesthetic mask. Different sized adapters may need to be used in series as needed to provide the proper sized connection to an anesthetic circuit.

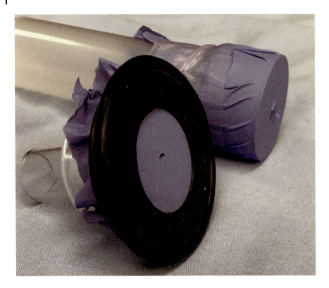

Figure 32.5 Modification of a commercially available facemask with a latex glove. The glove can be cut as needed to allow for a better fit on a beak or bill.

32.2.2 Endotracheal Tubes and Laryngoscopes

When intubating birds, it is important to remember the unique features of the avian proximal airway. Before anesthetic induction, be prepared with multiple sizes of endotracheal tubes. Smaller species may require specialized adaptations, as commercially available endotracheal tubes smaller than 2 mm internal diameter are generally unavailable. Intravenous catheters can be easily used as endotracheal tubes. The stylet is removed and an adapter from a 3.0 mm endotracheal tube can be fitted into the hub (Figure 32.6). It is important to note

that modified endotracheal tubes of this size are extremely flexible and are, therefore, prone to kinking. Furthermore, as the diameter of the endotracheal tube decreases, the more likely mucoid discharge can occlude the lumen. The presence of increased expiratory effort and/or lack of air sac deflation are signs of a mucous plug. The bird should be extubated and re-intubated with a clean endotracheal tube.

While laryngoscopes are useful in species with longer beaks or bills, visualization of the glottis is generally accomplished using any light source. Once the glottis is located, the endotracheal tube is gently inserted. Lubrication of the tube should be minimal to prevent inadvertent tube plugging. The endotracheal tube is secured with an elastic tie or can be taped to the beak or bill. Patients with large, strong beaks should have a syringe case, plunger or bite block secured in the beak to avoid inadvertent occlusion or severing of the endotracheal tube should anesthetic depth become too light (Figure 32.7).

Due to the complete tracheal rings, the avian trachea is rather non-expansible and is, therefore, more prone to pressure-induced damage or necrosis. To avoid excessive pressure on the tracheal lumen, endotracheal tube cuffs should remain un-inflated or minimally inflated. The use of uncuffed endotracheal tubes or Cole tubes is generally preferred (Figure 32.8). Tracheal damage may not be evident for several days following

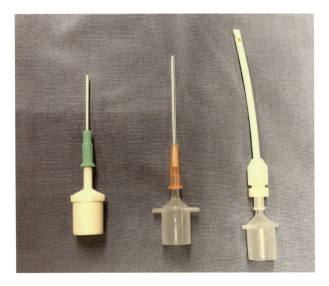

Figure 32.6 Adaptation of different sized intravenous catheters for use as endotracheal tubes. Adapters from a size 3.0-mm standard endotracheal tube may be used in the catheter hub to adapt the catheter to the anesthetic circuit.

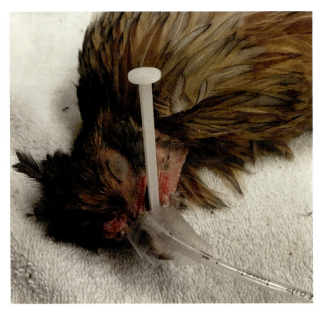

Figure 32.7 Syringe plunger used as a bite block in a rooster (*Gallus domesticus*) under isoflurane anesthesia. This is used to prevent biting down on the endotracheal tube upon emergence from anesthesia. Syringe cases and other materials may be used, provided they prevent occlusion of the endotracheal tube and do not hyperextend the beak in an open position.

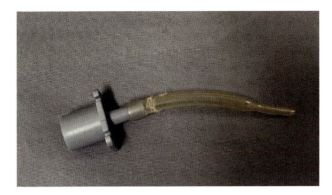

Figure 32.8 Cole endotracheal tube.

an anesthetic event. For example, clinical signs of post-anesthetic tracheal obstruction in birds of zoological collections were evident at 16 days post-anesthesia (Sykes *et al.* 2013); tracheal obstruction occurred in 1.8–3.25% of patients, despite being intubated with uncuffed endotracheal tubes, Cole tubes and intravenous catheters. This suggests that damage can also occur due to other factors such as irritation of the tracheal mucosa by dry anesthetic gases or chemical residue on the endotracheal tube, pressure from a stiff distal end of the endotracheal tube, or manipulation of the bird while being intubated.

Laryngeal mask airways (LMA) are a potential alternative to endotracheal intubation. While anecdotal reports of LMA use in birds are available, controlled studies in birds are not widely published (Zurawka *et al.* 2007). Due to the ease of endotracheal intubation and the relatively low incidence of complications, laryngeal mask airways are likely not the first choice

for airway devices in birds. However, it is extremely important to use great care in choosing the correctly sized endotracheal tube for the patient and manipulating the head and neck of an intubated patient with caution.

32.3 Venous Access

When feasible, intravenous catheterization for the administration of emergency drugs and fluid therapy should be attempted in all but the briefest of anesthetic events and smallest of avian patients. Catheterization technique is similar to mammals and commonly utilized venous access points are the right jugular vein, brachial and basillic veins of the wing, and the medial metatarsal vein of the legs (Figures 32.9A, B). Considerations unique to birds include an awareness of the considerably thinner and more delicate skin of the wing and neck; use caution with taping or stapling catheters in these locations. Use of Transpore tape (Transpore; 3M, Maplewood, MN) is generally preferred over thicker adhesive tape. Once an intravenous catheter is placed and secured, a balanced electrolyte solution is administered at a rate of 5–10 ml/kg/hr. In small birds, where intravenous catheterization may be challenging, or if intravenous catheterization is not feasible, intraosseous catheters may be placed in a non-pneumatized bone. Generally, the ulna or proximal tibiotarsus is the best choices. A spinal needle is the best choice as the stylet prevents plugging of the needle with fat or cortical bone. However, standard needles may be used if spinal needles are unavailable or too large (Figure 32.10).

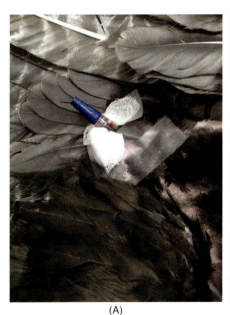
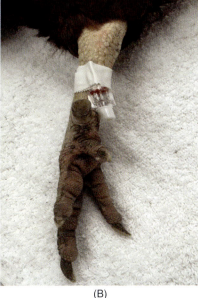

(A)   (B)

Figure 32.9 Intravenous catheters placed in the brachial (A) and medial metatarsal (B) veins. Note they are secured with clear tape to minimize trauma to the skin upon removal.

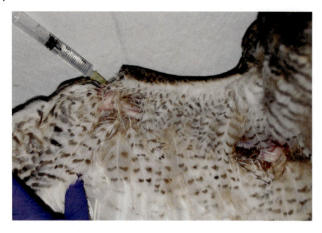

Figure 32.10 Intraosseous catheter placed in the distal ulna of a great-horned owl (*Bubo virginianus*) and attached to a syringe (photograph courtesy of Erin Lemley, CVT, CWR).

32.4 Anesthetic Monitors

When dealing with anesthetized birds, the simplest and most reliable monitors are the ears of the anesthetist via auscultation of a heartbeat and one's eyes to verify air sac excursions associated with breathing. However, adjunct monitors such as a Doppler flow probe, pulse oximeter, capnometer and electrocardiogram (ECG) will allow for a greater understanding of the cardiovascular and respiratory status of the animal.

32.4.1 Doppler Flow Probes

A Doppler flow probe placed over a peripheral artery, such as the ulnar artery of the wing or metatarsal artery of the medial tibiotarsus, allows audible evidence of blood flow and immediate detection of bradycardia, dysrhythmias and tachycardia. The probe is secured via Transpore tape or a clamp fashioned from two tongue depressors taped together at the end (Figure 32.11). If placed on a limb distal to a blood pressure cuff, blood pressure can be measured. However, comparisons of indirectly measured blood pressure using a Doppler probe as compared to directly measured blood pressure via arterial cannulation have demonstrated poor agreement between numbers in both awake and anesthetized birds (Acierno *et al.* 2008; Zehnder *et al.* 2009; Johnston *et al.* 2011). At best, indirect measurement of blood pressure in anesthetized birds approximates values between mean arterial pressure (MAP) and systolic arterial pressure (SAP) and can allow the anesthetist to monitor trends in blood pressure within a single patient.

32.4.2 Pulse Oximetry

A pulse oximeter is another valuable audible monitor that can signal the user to the presence or absence of

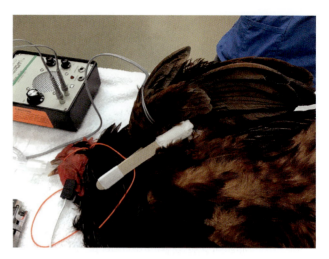

Figure 32.11 Doppler clamp fashioned from two tongue depressors. This simple tool can securely hold a Doppler crystal over an accessible artery.

blood flow, as well as changes in heart rate. Standard probes designed for human and small animal patients are utilized. Clamp-style probes, or transmittance probes, are placed across a wing, on a comb or wattle, or on the toes (Figures 32.12A, B). The tongue of larger species may be used, but great care is advised to avoid pressure-induced damage and this site is best avoided. Flat reflectance probes can be placed in the cloaca, upon the palate, or in the proximal esophagus of larger birds. However, it is important to note that the derived algorithm for SpO_2 is based upon the absorption of light of mammalian hemoglobin, not avian hemoglobin. When tested and compared to actual arterial saturation of oxygen (SaO_2) in pigeons and parrots, the pulse oximeter did not give an accurate value (Schmitt *et al.* 1998). The heart rate did however correlate well. This suggests that, like the Doppler flow probe, pulse oximetry may be more valuable in detecting the heart rate and pulsatile flow. It should be noted however that the Doppler flow probe is more reliable and less prone to artifacts, such that may occur from motion, ambient light or skin pigmentation. Detailed pulse oximetry is discussed in Chapter 18.

32.4.3 Capnometry

Capnometry is extremely valuable, since even with a perceived adequate respiratory rate, tidal volume is depressed in birds under anesthesia, resulting in significant hypoventilation (Ludders *et al.* 1990. 1995; Seaman *et al.* 1994). This is due to a direct depressant effect of the CNS by inhalational anesthetics, as well as the effect of muscle relaxation on respiratory musculature. Unlike mammals, both expiration and inspiration in birds are active processes and muscle relaxation from anesthetics can have significant consequences. However, as discussed above,

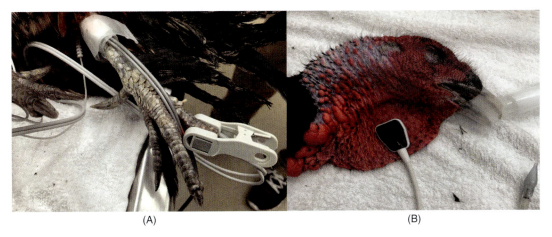

(A)   (B)

Figure 32.12 Different styles of pulse oximeter probes. Transmittance probe placed over the digit of a rooster (*Gallus domesticus*) (A); reflectance probe placed over the wattle of a turkey (*Meleagris gallopavo*) (B).

the respiratory system of birds is such that expired carbon dioxide levels are not always equivalent to arterial carbon dioxide partial pressures. It is also important to note that sidestream capnometers rely on aspiration of samples of expired gas that may exceed the tidal volume of small birds. The evaluated sample, therefore, may be an underestimation of the actual end-tidal carbon dioxide due to dilution with fresh gas flow. In general, however, the overall trend in end-tidal carbon dioxide levels over time is of value. For instance, an end-tidal carbon dioxide reading of 15–20 mmHg in a small- to medium-sized parrot is not uncommon and lower-than-expected end-tidal measurements are frequently seen in most species (Figure 32.13).

As anesthesia progresses and the reading increases to 30 mmHg, it may indicate hypoventilation due to excessive anesthetic depth. On the other hand, a decrease to 8 mmHg may indicate hyperventilation, but could also indicate other physiological perturbations such as hypothermia or a decrease in cardiac output. Sudden readings in the single digits or lack of end-tidal carbon dioxide should signal immediate evaluation and action. This may

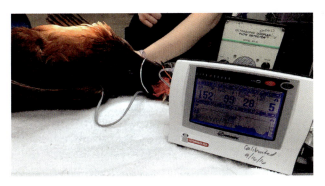

Figure 32.13 Falsely-low reading of end-tidal carbon dioxide in a rooster under isoflurane anesthesia (*Gallus domesticus*), due mainly to dilution by fresh gas flow. Temporarily decreasing the oxygen flow revealed an end-tidal carbon dioxide of 45 mmHg.

indicate apnea, dislodgement of the anesthetic circuit, extubation or cardiac arrest. For a more thorough discussion on the interpretation of capnography, please refer to Chapter 16.

32.4.4 Electrocardiography (ECG)

Electrocardiographs (ECGs) may be of use in evaluating the electrical activity of the heart (see Chapter 20). It is important to note that an ECG detects only electrical activity, not mechanical activity, of the heart. The avian myocardium has complete penetration of Purkinje fibers; the mean electrical axis is cranially oriented and the waveform is primarily negative in its orientation (Bailey and Pablo 1998). Three-lead placement is similar to that in mammals; the white and black forelimb leads can be placed on the carpus of the wing and the red lead can be placed over the tarsometatarsal region. Atraumatic clamps may be used, as ECG patches often do not work on feathered areas (Figure 32.14). Alternatively, 25-gauge needles can be placed in the subcutaneous tissue with the clamps attached to the needles. Interpretation of ECG tracings may be difficult due to the high heart rates of birds. It is common for the heart rate to exceed 250–300 beats per minute, especially in a light anesthetic plane or if analgesia is inadequate. If allowed by the monitor, slowing the paper speed to 50 or even 100 mm/sec may allow better evaluation.

32.5 Anesthetic Circuits

As in mammals, the choice of anesthetic circuit is largely dictated by patient size. In general, many birds anesthetized in clinical practice are rather small, easily less than 2 kg. Theoretically, the major advantage of a non-rebreathing system such as any Mapleson system or,

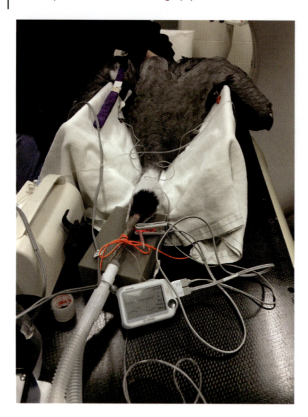

Figure 32.14 Atraumatic ECG clamps placed on a hooded crane (*Grus monacha*).

more specifically, a Bain coaxial system, is decreased resistance to spontaneous ventilation. This may be especially important in very small patients that may have a difficult time overcoming the resistance imparted by the one-way valves, carbon dioxide absorber and large size of the rebreathing system. Another advantage to non-rebreathing systems is the rapid adjustment of anesthetic depth, especially important in avian patients that may require a rapid transition from relatively high concentrations of inhalational anesthetics for induction to more moderate concentrations during the maintenance phase of anesthesia. A major disadvantage to the use of non-rebreathing systems is the relatively high gas flows that are required to avoid rebreathing, roughly 1.5–3 times the minute volume (Dorsch and Dorsch 2008). While this is wasteful in larger species, this "high flow" rarely exceeds 2 L/min in most bird species. Larger species, such as cranes and ratites, are easily maintained on a circle system in order to conserve oxygen flow.

32.6 Maintenance of Body Temperature

One of the anesthetic goals is to maintain the patient as close to homeostasis as possible. This can be difficult in

species that have a normal body temperature exceeding 104°F (40°C), as hypothermia sets in quickly. On the other hand, in birds with heavy plumage, body temperature may be well maintained or may even increase during anesthesia. Avian species vary in their normal body temperature and, once again, it is important to research species' reference values prior to undertaking anesthesia. Regardless of the normal body temperature, it is common for birds (especially companion, pet or small birds) to rapidly become hypothermic at the onset of anesthesia. A study evaluating thermal support in ringed turtle-doves found that birds without thermal support lost roughly 1°C within 10 minutes and 3°C within 25 minutes (Phalen *et al.* 1996). Much like in mammals, this can be attributed to multiple sources, including radiant loss of warmth to the environment, conductive heat loss to cooler surfaces, and evaporative loss to cold and dry anesthetic gasses. Peri-anesthetic hypothermia can lead to delayed drug metabolism and anesthetic recovery, impaired wound healing, coagulopathy and cardiac dysrhythmias (Fielder 2001). Post-anesthetic shivering can increase oxygen and glucose consumption, leading to hypoxemia and hypoglycemia.

It is extremely important to not only monitor cloacal temperature, but to provide thermal support. The extremely careful use of an external heat lamp on anesthetized birds helped to prevent anesthetic-associated heat loss, while the use of a warm-water blanket was found to be ineffective (Phalen *et al.* 1996). In addition, forced-air warming systems are effective in maintaining core body temperature in small patients such as birds. However, as with any warming device, it is important to avoid inducing hyperthermia. The large surface area-to-volume ratio of small birds, in addition to their small size, makes it easy to inadvertently induce hyperthermia. As previously stated, close monitoring of cloacal temperature is critical. Use great caution in providing external heat support by objects warmed in the microwave, as thermal burns are easily induced by this method of warming.

32.7 Anesthetic Recovery

As with all species, it is important to continue to monitor the patient closely upon conclusion of anesthesia. Oxygen should be supplemented until the patient is ready to be extubated. In most healthy birds, recovery from inhalational anesthetics is rapid. This, once again, is due to the efficiency of the respiratory system. Prolonged recovery should be investigated and may be due to hypothermia, hypoglycemia or adjunct anesthetic agents. Heart rate and rhythm should be monitored by auscultation or a Doppler flow probe until recovery is complete. Intravenous catheters are maintained until the patient is recovered and stable, so that emergency drugs and/or fluid support can be given, as needed. Upon discontinuation of inhalational anesthetic, the patient should be wrapped loosely in a towel and held so that the wings are gently restrained once the patient begins to move. Patients with strong jaws, such as large parrots and raptors, require close monitoring to avoid occluding or severing the endotracheal tube during recovery. Upon extubation, the patient can be placed in an incubator or warm recovery cage free of water to fully recover.

References

Acierno, M.J., da Cunha, A., Smith, J., Tully, T.N., Guzman, D.S. *et al.* (2008) Agreement between direct and indirect blood pressure measurements obtained from anesthetized Hispaniolan Amazon parrots. *J Am Vet Med Assoc,* 233, 1587–1590.

Bailey, J.E. and Pablo, L.S. (1998) Anesthetic monitoring and monitoring equipment: application in small exotic pet practice. *Semin Avian Exot Pet Med,* 7, 53–60.

Brodbelt, D.C., Blissitt, K.J., Hammond, R.A., Neath, P.J., Young, L.E. *et al.* (2008) The risk of death: the confidential enquiry into peri-operative small animal fatalities. *Vet Anaesth Analg,* 35, 365–373.

Desmarchelier, M., Rondenay, Y., Fitzgerald, G. and Lair, S. (2007) Monitoring of the ventilatory status of anesthetized birds of prey by using end-tidal carbon dioxide measured with a microstream capnometer. *J Zoo Wildl Med,* 38, 1–6.

Dorsch, J.A. and Dorsch, S.E. (2008) Mapleson breathing systems. In: Dorsch, J.A. and Dorsch, S.E. (eds). *Understanding Anesthesia Equipment,* 5th ed. Philadelphia, PA: Lippincott Williams & Wilkins, pp. 209–222.

Duncker, H.R. (1972) Structure of avian lungs. *Resp Physiol,* 14, 44–63.

Edling, T.M., Degernes, L.A., Flammer, K. and Horne, W.A. (2001) Capnographic monitoring of anesthetized African grey parrots receiving intermittent positive pressure ventilation. *J Am Vet Med Assoc,* 219, 1714–1718.

Fielder, M.A. (2001) Thermoregulation: anesthetic and peri-operative concerns. *AANA J,* 69, 485–491.

Gaunt, A.S., Gaunt, S.L., Prange, H.D. and Wasser, J.S. (1987) The effects of tracheal coiling on the vocalizations of cranes (Aves; Gruidae). *J Comp Physiol A,* 161, 43–58.

Heard, D. (2016) Anesthesia. In: Speer, B.L. (ed.). *Current Therapy in Avian Medicine and Surgery,* 1st ed. St Louis, MO: Elsevier, pp. 601–615.

Johnston, M.S., Davidowski, L.A., Rao, S. and Hill, A.E. (2011) Precision of repeated, Doppler-derived indirect blood pressure measurements in conscious psittacine birds. *J Avian Med Surg,* 25, 83–90.

Ludders, J.W., Mitchell, G.S. and Rode, J. (1990) Minimal anesthetic concentration and cardiopulmonary dose response of isoflurane in ducks. *Vet Surg,* 19, 304–307.

Ludders, J.W., Seaman, G.C. and Erb, H.N. (1995) Inhalant anesthetics and inspired oxygen: implications for anesthesia in birds. *J Am Anim Hosp Assoc,* 31, 38–41.

McLelland, J. (1989) Larynx and trachea. In: King, A.S. and McLelland, J. (eds). *Form and Function in Birds,* vol 4. London, UK: Academic Press, pp. 69–103.

Magnussen, H., Willmer, H. and Scheid, P. (1976) Gas exchange in air sacs: contribution to respiratory gas exchange in ducks. *Resp Physiol,* 26, 129–146.

Pare, M., Ludders, J.W. and Erb, H.N. (2013) Association of partial pressure of carbon dioxide in expired gas and arterial blood at three different ventilation states in apneic chickens (*Gallus domesticus*) during air sac insufflation anesthesia. *Vet Anaesth Analg,* 40, 245–256.

Phalen, D.N., Mitchell, M.E. and Cavazos-Martinez, M.L. (1996) Evaluation of three heat sources for their ability to maintain core body temperature in the anesthetized avian patient. *J Avian Med Surg,* 10, 174–178.

Scheid, P. and Piper, J. (1970) Analysis of gas exchange in the avian lung: theory and experiments in the domestic fowl. *Resp Physiol,* 9, 246–262.

Schmitt, P.M., Gobel, T. and Trautvetter, E. (1998) Evaluation of pulse oximetry as a monitoring method in avian anesthesia. *J Avian Med Surg,* 12, 91–99.

Seaman, G.C., Ludders, J.W., Erb, H.N. and Gleed, R.D. (1994) Effects of low and high fractions of inspired oxygen on ventilation in ducks anesthetized with isoflurane. *Am J Vet Res,* 55, 395–398.

Sykes, J.M., Neiffer, D., Terrell, S., Powell, D.M. and Newton, A. (2013) Review of 23 cases of post-intubation tracheal obstructions in birds. *J Zoo Wildl Med,* 44, 700–713.

Touzot-Jourde, G., Hernandez-Divers, S.J. and Trim, C.M. (2005) Cardiopulmonary effects of controlled versus spontaneous ventilation in pigeons anesthetized for coelioscopy. *J Am Vet Med Assoc,* 227, 1424–1428.

Zehnder, A.M., Hawkins, M.G., Pascoe, P.J. and Kass, P.H. (2009) Evaluation of indirect blood pressure monitoring in awake and anesthetized red-tailed hawks (*Buteo jamaicensis*): effects of cuff size, cuff placement, and monitoring equipment. *Vet Anaesth Analg,* 36, 464–479.

Zurawka, H.S., Berliner, A., Hofling, M.L. and James, S.B. (2007) Evaluation of three different anesthetic delivery systems in Indian peafowl (*Pavo cristatus*). *Proc. AAZV, AAWV, AZA/NAG Joint Conf,* 48, 166–167.

33

Unique Species Considerations: Rabbits
Katrina Lafferty

Wisconsin National Primate Research Center, University of Wisconsin, Madison, Wisconsin, USA

33.1   Introduction

Even with a comprehensive knowledge base in terms of anesthetic equipment and monitoring techniques, a veterinary professional may feel uneasy when handed a rabbit to anesthetize. Each year the number of pet rabbits increases and more of those rabbits are presenting for procedures requiring anesthesia. Ovario-hysterectomies, castrations, mass removals, diagnostic imaging, and even cancer treatment therapies are becoming increasingly commonplace.

33.2   Intubation

It is common for anesthesia personnel to "always intubate" whenever possible. Indeed, endotracheal intubation may increase the safety of an anesthetic procedure. As with any species, intubation facilitates a secure and patent airway, aids in appropriate delivery of inhalant anesthetic gases to the patient, reduces waste gas exposure to personnel and facilitates removal. In addition, it provides a means for positive pressure ventilation and may protect airways from fluid or foreign material. Intratracheal intubation also provides an alternative route for emergency drug administration and allows accurate use of capnometry monitoring.

However, with rabbits, intubation can be more difficult than in more traditional species. Rabbits have small oral openings with limited mandibular range of motion, fleshy and firmly attached tongues, narrow tracheas, a commonly-displaced glottis and large incisors (Worthley *et al.* 2000).

Although personnel can effectively and efficiently intubate most rabbits, caution is warranted since repeated attempts may cause laryngeal trauma and stimulate a vagal response in many rabbits, resulting in profound bradycardia (Lennox 2008). Additionally, rabbits are obligate nasal breathers and trauma to nasal tissues (with nasal intubation) causing nasal edema may lead to respiratory distress upon extubation (Lennox 2008). In a situation where intubation is unsuccessful, the patient may alternatively be maintained on a mask with extra-vigilant monitoring (Lennox 2008).

Most rabbits will require an endotracheal tube ranging from 2.0–3.5 mm outer diameter. Intubation is often blind and a smaller-than-expected endotracheal tube size is needed to achieve placement (Lichtenberger and Ko 2007). It is possible to intubate rabbits using orotracheal or nasotracheal intubation techniques. Although nasotracheal intubation is a viable intubation technique (Stephens Devalle 2009), it usually requires very small tubes and may be associated with nasal bacterial colonization and chronic inflammatory changes (Westergren *et al.* 1999). Regardless of intubation technique used, patient pre-oxygenation is recommended if possible (Figure 33.1). In addition, lidocaine (<2–5 mg/kg recommended) may be instilled on the glottis or down the center of the tracheal tube (when partially placed) to reduce laryngospasm. Adequate lubrication of the endotracheal tube will facilitate less traumatic passage. However, take care with over-zealous lubrication, as too much can plug the lumen of a small endotracheal tube or cause smearing of a camera scope if used. Equipment and methods are described for four common intubation techniques in rabbits, as well as for the laryngeal airway masks described below.

33.2.1   Direct Visualization Technique

For the direct visualization technique, the rabbit is placed in sternal recumbency with the head and neck fully extended. The mouth can be held open with gauze ties or IV tubing. The tongue is gently pulled forward and

Veterinary Anesthetic and Monitoring Equipment, First Edition. Edited by Kristen G. Cooley and Rebecca A. Johnson.
© 2018 John Wiley & Sons, Inc. Published 2018 by John Wiley & Sons, Inc.

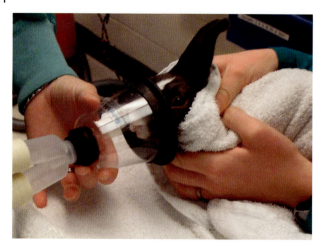

Figure 33.1 Pre-oxygenation with a tight fitting mask before intubation.

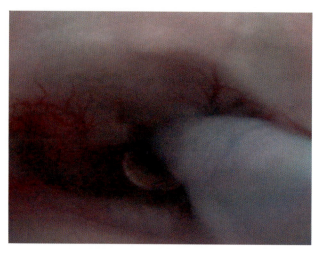

Figure 33.2 Endoscopic view of the trachea and arytenoids.

possibly to the side using a gauze square or cotton-tipped applicator. A laryngoscope with a pediatric blade or an otoscope with an adapted cone is used to depress the tongue and visualize the larynx and glottis. An issue with this technique it related to the size of oral cavity. For example, once the endotracheal tube is placed alongside the laryngoscope, it may be difficult to continue clear visualization of the tracheal opening. An introduction stylet, such as a Foley catheter or red rubber feeding tube, can be used as a guide for the endotracheal tube; the stylet is much smaller and should not block the field of view. The stylet is placed and the endotracheal tube is slid over top. Once the endotracheal tube is placed, the introduction stylet is removed (Macrae and Guerreiro 1989). This technique can be very difficult in small (<1 kg) patients. An important consideration when using this technique is to confirm beforehand that the endotracheal tube will easily slide over the stylet.

33.2.2 Indirect Visualization Technique

For the indirect visualization technique, a small, rigid or straight fiber-optic scope is required. Patients are placed in dorsal recumbency. As with the direct visualization technique, the mouth is held open and the tongue may be gently pulled to the side. The scope should be dampened with saline if possible to provide a less traumatic passage into the oral cavity. Once the glottis is visualized, an appropriately-sized endotracheal tube (with or without stylet) is passed next to the fiber-optic scope (Worthley *et al.* 2000). Endotracheal tube placement using this technique should be less traumatic, as ultimately there is good visualization of oropharyngeal anatomy (Figure 33.2). However, this technique does require endoscopic equipment correctly sized for small patients and competency with such equipment.

33.2.3 Blind Orotracheal Technique

For the "blind" orotracheal technique, the rabbit is placed in sternal recumbency with the head and neck hyperextended. For this type of intubation, more than any other, positioning is key to a successful, atraumatic intubation. With the head and neck in hyperextension, the trachea is straighter from the mouth to the thoracic inlet. For this method, it is not necessary to use ties to open the mouth (but still can be used if preferred), but the tongue should be pulled forward or off to the side to reduce the amount of tissue in the caudal oral cavity. The endotracheal tube is introduced between the incisors and gently advanced until condensation or "fogging" appears within the lumen of the endotracheal tube (Figure 33.3). The fogging appears with exhalation and the subsequent clearing of the tube indications inhalation. The endotracheal tube is advanced into the trachea with the clearing, or inhalation. Gentle rotation of the tube can be implemented to "nudge" the epiglottis aside and allow smoother passage. Placement of the endotracheal tube can be confirmed by auscultation of breath sounds and continued fogging in the endotracheal tube. However, the gold standard to confirm placement using the blind intubation technique is by using an end-tidal carbon dioxide monitor (Kruger *et al.* 1994). Some sources recommend "freezing" the endotracheal tubes beforehand to create a more rigid tube. However, chilled tubes may not show condensation, which can confuse the intubation attempt and warm quickly. In any case, this technique requires the least equipment and is quite successful.

33.2.4 Blind Nasotracheal Technique

Positioning for nasotracheal intubation is identical to that of "blind" orotracheal intubation. The endotracheal tube size will be smaller, typically size 2.0–2.5 mm outer

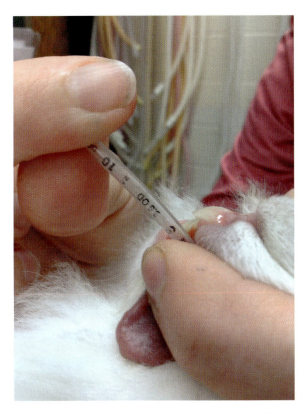

Figure 33.3 Fogging in the endotracheal tube on exhalation.

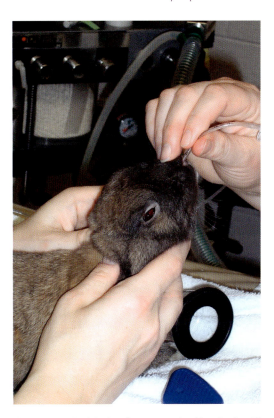

Figure 33.4 Positioning for nasotracheal intubation. The neck should be extended and tube passed ventro-medially through the nose and into the trachea.

diameter. Once positioned, the endotracheal tube is passed in a ventro-medial direction through the nasal canal (Figure 33.4). Some resistance is to be expected with this technique; however, there should never be a feeling of "crunchiness". If present, the tube is not passing through to the trachea, but rather has deviated into the nasal turbinates. As rabbits are obligate nasal breathers, only one side of the nose should be attempted for nasotracheal intubation. If both sides are used and suffer trauma or nasal edema, patients may have varying degrees of respiratory distress or respiratory obstruction (Devalle 2009). Adequate lubrication is essential for this technique; 2% lidocaine gel (Par Pharmaceuticals, Endo Company, Malvern, PA) may be used for this purpose.

33.2.5 Laryngeal Mask Airway (LMA) Technique

Laryngeal mask airway devices have been commonly used in human medicine for many years. Recently there has been an interest in manufacturing such a device that would be appropriately sized and have applications in veterinary medicine (V-gel®, Docsinnovent, London, England) (Figure 33.5). The laryngeal mask airway (LMA) consists of an airway tube similar to an endotracheal tube ending in a mask, which seat over the tracheal opening, allowing inhalant anesthetics to be delivered to the

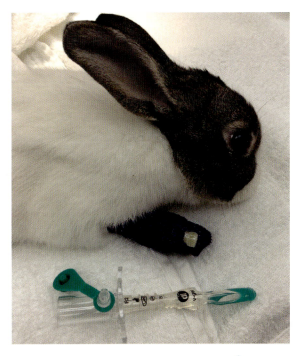

Figure 33.5 Correct laryngeal mask airway (V-gel®) size for a 1.5-kg rabbit.

patient. Early research suggests it can be a viable alternative to endotracheal intubations. In cats, the V-gel® can be placed at a lighter plane of anesthesia and may require a lower dose of induction agent in feline patients (Prasse *et al.* 2015). In rabbits, intubation with the V-gel® may affect hemodynamic responses less than endotracheal intubation (Toman *et al.* 2015). LMA devices are also used in pediatric non-human primates, as they may allow for a less traumatic intubation (Johnson *et al.* 2010).

Placement of the LMA is similar to traditional endotracheal tubes. The patient is placed in sternal recumbency with the head and neck extended. The mask portion is lubricated with water-soluble lubricant that may or may not contain lidocaine (Figure 33.6). The tongue is gently pulled to the side and the tip of the LMA inserted behind the incisors (Figure 33.7). The device is advanced through the oral cavity until some resistance is met. It may be necessary to rotate the tube slightly to move past the teeth and correctly seat the mask itself. An end-tidal carbon dioxide monitor should be used to confirm correct placement. A normal capnograph wave should be observed to ensure proper placement with no airway obstruction. Some advantages and disadvantages of using this technique include the following (Kazakos *et al.* 2007):

- Advantages of the V-gel® include ease of placement, which may be a consideration for less experienced personnel, less irritation of the laryngeal tissues, and less likelihood for tracheal trauma, as no tube contacts the tracheal mucosa. It is usually well tolerated and can be left in place well into recovery and facilitates accurate monitoring of end-tidal CO_2 levels.

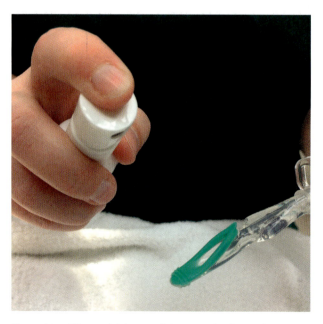

Figure 33.6 Water soluble spray lubrication for the mask portion of the V-gel® to facilitate placement.

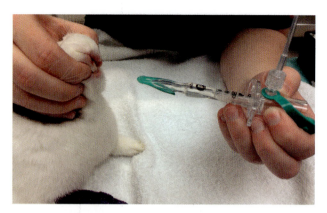

Figure 33.7 Rabbit positioning for placing a V-gel®. The neck should be extended and tongue moved laterally.

- Disadvantages of the V-gel® include the possibility of lingual cyanosis if the tongue is not carefully positioned. In addition, it may become dislodged with patient movement, causing inadequate control of airway or airway obstruction. If not seated properly, there is a less competent seal compared to an endotracheal tube, potentially resulting in more waste gas exposure and displacement or potential aspiration of foreign material. Mechanical ventilation is possible with this device, but may cause some gastric distension.

33.3 Breathing Circuits

Breathing circuits are discussed extensively elsewhere (Chapters 10 and 11). Many rabbits weigh under 5 kg and may be anesthetized using a non-rebreathing circuit. For example, Magill, Bain and Ayre's T-piece circuits can be used. Non-rebreathing systems are lighter and have less resistance to breathing due to lack of carbon-dioxide absorbent canisters and unidirectional valves. However, the lack of carbon-dioxide removal within the system must be compensated for by substantially higher oxygen flow rates; oxygen flow should be maintained at 1.5–3 times the patient's minute ventilation or approximately 150–200 mL/kg/min to remove carbon dioxide from the system (Johnson 2009).

Non-rebreathing circuits may be short and somewhat heavy and may subsequently pull on the endotracheal tube and delicate tracheal tissues of the patient. A device called a "mask stabilizer" can be used to hold down the breathing hose (Figure 33.8). The piece is weighted, may be magnetic and will prevent slippage of the tubing.

33.4 Monitors

All veterinary patients should be intensely monitored under anesthesia, regardless of species. Appropriate

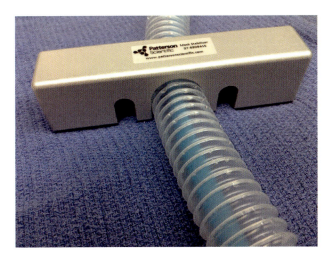

Figure 33.8 Mask stabilizer for securing lightweight breathing hoses.

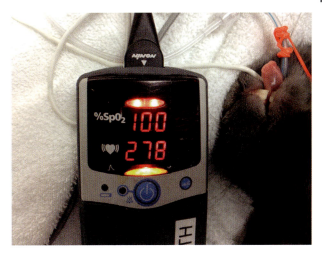

Figure 33.9 Correct pulse oximeter placement in a rabbit using a flat reflectance probe in the oral cavity. Note pulse rate of 278 bpm and a hemoglobin saturation with oxygen of 100%.

monitoring is a necessary and fundamental part of a safe anesthetic event, in order to detect and correct physiologic disturbances in a timely manner. Monitoring instrumentation in rabbits is similar to that required by small canine or feline patients (Heard 2014). Detailed breakdown and discussion of monitoring equipment is discussed elsewhere (Chapters 16–23). However, unique considerations for rabbits are detailed below.

33.4.1 Pulse Oximetry

A pulse-oximeter is a simple, rapid and non-invasive way to obtain pulse rate and track arterial oxygen saturation of hemoglobin in real time. The function and value of pulse oximetry is similar in rabbits as to most other species. However, pulse oximeters may be unable to obtain accurate parameters with heart rates over 300 beats per minute and in pigmented tissues. In addition, in conscious rabbits, pulse oximetry hemoglobin saturation values (SpO_2) were not significantly correlated to arterial hemoglobin saturation values (SaO_2) and tended to overestimate oxygen saturation by approximately 8% (Eatwell *et al.* 2013).

Another challenge is related to the anatomy of the rabbit and probe placement location. The rabbit tongue is small and firmly attached. Caution should be used in clamp or clip-style probes, as these can restrict blood flow to the lingual tissues. Other locations with sufficient pulsatile blood flow can be used, such as the toes, pinna, scrotum and vulva (Eatwell *et al.* 2013). Flat reflectance style probes can be used in the mouth, esophagus, rectum and within the base of the ear canal (Figures 33.9 and 33.10).

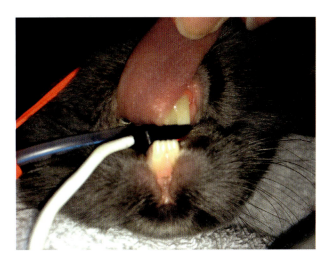

Figure 33.10 Close-up showing proper positioning of a reflectance pulse oximetry probe. The sensor can either be placed against the tongue or the oral mucosa.

33.4.2 Capnometry

Capnometry should be part of the monitoring plan for any species, rabbits being no exception. A capnometer acts as an early alert for changes in ventilation, circulation, endotracheal occlusion or incorrect tracheal tube or laryngeal mask placement. As with traditional species, a capnometer will give pertinent information regarding respiratory rate and hyper- or hypocapnia. Published ranges for normal end-tidal carbon dioxide ($ETCO_2$) and arterial CO_2 levels ($PaCO_2$) in rabbits are sparse, but normal $PaCO_2$ appears to be between approximately 25 and 40 mmHg (Eatwell *et al.* 2013). $ETCO_2$ values can approximate $PaCO_2$; however, $PaCO_2$ is approximately

5 mmHg higher than $ETCO_2$ in patients with normal pulmonary and cardiovascular function; this difference can be significantly increased in patients with respiratory disease (Nevarez 2005). In addition, recent evidence suggests that $EtCO_2$ is not as consistent as $PaCO_2$, and may be quite different for a given $PaCO_2$, even in conscious rabbits (Eatwell *et al.* 2013). In any case, $PaCO_2$ below 35 mmHg may constitute a degree of hyperventilation and above 45 mmHg may be considered hypoventilation (Schroeder and Smith 2011).

Two main types of capnometers exist (mainstream and sidestream) and are detailed in Chapter 16. Briefly, sidestream monitors consist of lighter pieces and are sometimes recommended above the bulky adaptors used in mainstream monitors for delicate species such as rabbits. Sidestream monitors can be attached to an endotracheal tube and used to aid and confirm intubation. However, some sidestream monitors draw a large sample volume (up to 150–200 mL/min) from the breathing system. In rabbits, this amount may constitute a large proportion of the normal breath. As a result, standard sidestream capnometers may provide slightly diluted, inaccurately low readings. There are commercially available micro-capnographs (Microcap™ Handheld Capnometer, Covidien, Boulder, CO) that sample volumes as small as 50 mL and will be more accurate for very small animals (Hawkins and Pascoe 2012).

Additional mechanical dead space associated with anesthetic monitors is a serious concern in small patients; the additional dead space added to the system by the capnometer should be considered. The capnometer airway adapters come in several sizes, including a pediatric version, which may be used on rabbits to minimize mechanical dead space (Figure 33.11; Smiths Medical ASD Inc., Dublin, OH).

Specifically made, low dead space CO_2 adapters are useful in cases where additional dead space is a concern (Figure 33.12, Welch Allyn, Skaneateles Falls, NY). The piece replaces the endotracheal tube adapter and has a

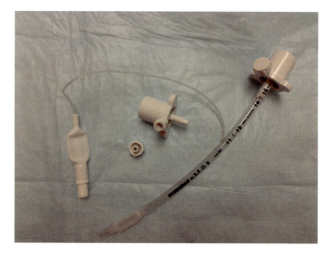

Figure 33.12 Adapter for use on the end of an endotracheal tube to minimize mechanical dead space on small patients.

side port where the sidestream monitor can be attached (Figure 33.13).

33.4.3 Non-Invasive Blood Pressure Monitoring

For rabbits, a Doppler ultrasonic flow detector is useful to detect a heartbeat. The probe can be placed over the radial artery, auricular artery or dorsal pedal artery to

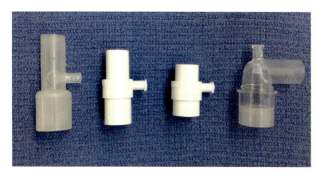

Figure 33.11 Several capnometer airway adapters illustrating the vast range of sizes.

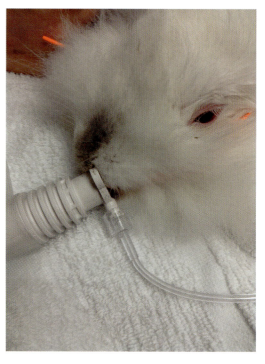

Figure 33.13 Orotracheally intubated rabbit with a minimal dead space adapter used to measure $ETCO_2$.

obtain heart rate, blood pressure (depending on the site – see below) and to listen for normal cardiac rhythm (Figures 33.14 and 33.15). In very small or hypovolemic/ hypotensive patients, it is possible to place the Doppler crystal directly over the carotid artery or the heart, but take care not to restrict ventilation when securing the crystal. The Doppler readings can also be used to verify the accuracy of the heart rate read by the pulse-oximeter. In some instances, respiratory sounds can also be heard on the Doppler, which is useful in small patients where it may not be possible to see chest excursions or rebreathing bag movement. While quite subjective, it is possible to detect (but not easily quantify) pressure changes when listening to the Doppler sound. For example, changes in the volume of the "whoosh" can indicate a change in blood pressure. When the ultrasonic flow probe is placed on a limb in combination with an appropriately-sized blood pressure cuff (~40% of the limb circumference), it is possible to obtain a systolic blood pressure measurement reading (Harvey *et al.* 2012). The systolic reading is generally within 8 mmHg of an auricular arterial reading and systolic blood pressure should be maintained above 90 mmHg while under general anesthesia (Harvey *et al.* 2012).

In some larger patients (those over 1–2 kg), oscillometric blood pressure monitors attached to blood pressure cuffs may also provide blood pressure readings (Figure 33.16). However, oscillometric monitors may not be able to read the high heart rates normally occurring in rabbit patients and may inaccurately read the blood pressures. In individual patients, accuracy of the non-invasive blood pressure measurements from a Doppler or other oscillometric monitor cannot be validated without use of an arterial catheter (which is not always practical), but can be useful in monitoring trends over the duration of the anesthetic episode (Bailey and Pablo 1998).

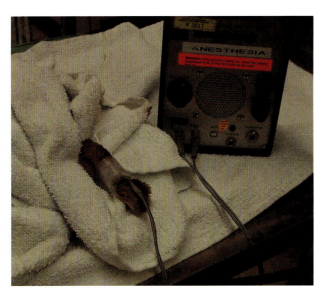

Figure 33.14 Doppler ultrasonic crystal placed on dorsal pedal artery to audibly detect pulse rate. When used with an appropriately sixed cuff, blood pressure can also be measured.

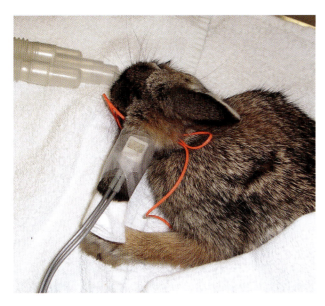

Figure 33.15 Doppler ultrasonic crystal placed on auricular artery to audibly detect pulse rate.

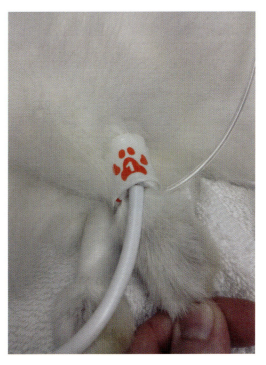

Figure 33.16 Size 1 blood pressure cuff on forelimb of a 1.5-kg rabbit. This can then be used with a Doppler probe or connected to an oscillometric device to obtain blood pressure.

33.4.4 Electrocardiography (ECG)

Electrocardiography (ECG) (see Chapter 20) has some, though limited, use in rabbit anesthesia monitoring. In rabbits, an ECG complex is made up of the same components (P, QRS, T) as a canine or feline complex. Unfortunately, there is limited information on normal/abnormal references. ECG placement will give additional heart rate confirmation and may show a respiratory wave. However, it is an electrical monitor and gives minimal information concerning heart function and the presence or absence of cardiac output.

Placement of the leads is the same as any other species; however, rabbits have friable skin. To minimize tissue damage caused by alligator clips, the teeth of the clips can be flattened. As an alternative, 25-gauge needles pierced through the skin with an alligator clip attached to the needle end can be used (Figure 33.17). In addition, some monitors have small, permanently affixed needles on the ECG cables, which is minimally traumatic to the skin (Vetcorder, Sentier, Brookfield, WI). There are also many types and brands of conductive adhesive ECG patches, which can be trimmed to an appropriate size and placed on the feet (Hawkins and Pascoe 2012).

33.5 Thermal Support

Due to their small size and increased surface area:volume ratio, rabbits are at an increased risk of hypothermia, which can occur quickly under general anesthesia. Hypothermia causes a decrease in drug metabolism that increases elimination and recovery times, affects clotting function and hemoglobin concentration, and increases morbidity and mortality (Staikou *et al.* 2011; see Chapter 22). Temperature should be confirmed at least every 15 minutes using a flexible rectal thermometer (with care due to fragile tissues) or an esophageal temperature probe.

Once cooled to a core temperature of 93 °F, many patients are no longer able shiver to warm themselves (Hanagata *et al.* 1995). Recovery is severely prolonged and the central nervous system function can be severely depressed. In rabbits, core temperatures below 90°F result in negative cardiac ionotropy, cardiac arrhythmias

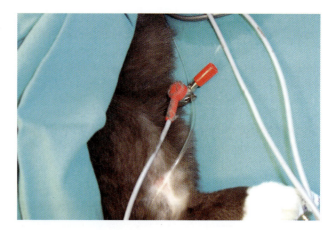

Figure 33.17 ECG placement in a rabbit using 25-gauge needles and alligator clips.

such as bradycardia, hypoxemia, thrombosis and death (Mattheussen *et al.* 1996). Many methods can be used to provide thermal support to rabbit patients including (Hawkins and Pascoe 2012):

- increasing temperature of preparation and surgical rooms;
- utilizing clear plastic drapes to provide an extra thermal barrier;
- minimizing surgical duration;
- minimizing patient preparation times;
- using warmed fluids for lavage;
- using circulating hot water blankets; and
- using forced air warming units.

Patients warm as quickly as they cool, especially if thick-furred, so monitoring for hyperthermia should occur as well. Vigilance in temperature monitoring is important for any patient under anesthesia, including rabbits (Heard 2014).

33.6 Summary

Most rabbit anesthetic and monitoring equipment can be found in the small animal hospital. However, rabbits do present some specific challenges concerning intubation and accurate monitoring. With experience, rabbit anesthetic techniques can be successful and straightforward.

References

Bailey, J.E. and Pablo, L.S. (1998) Anesthetic monitoring and monitoring equipment: application in a small exotic pet practice. *Semin Avian Exot Pet Med*, 7, 53–60.

Devalle, J. (2009) Successful management of rabbit anesthesia through the use of nasotracheal intubation. *J Am Assoc Lab Anim Sci*, 48, 166–170.

Eatwell, K., Mancinelli, E., Hedley, J., Benato, L., Shaw, D.J. *et al.* (2013) Use of arterial blood gas analysis as a superior method for evaluating respiratory function in pet rabbits (*Oryctolagus cuniculus*). *Vet Rec*, 173, 166.

Hanagata, K., Matsukawa, T., Sessler, D., Miyaji, T., Funayama, T. *et al.* (1995) Isoflurane and sevoflurane produce a dose-dependent reduction in the shivering threshold in rabbits. *Anesth Analg*, 81, 581–584.

Harvey, L., Knowles, T. and Murison, P. (2012) Comparison of direct and Doppler arterial blood pressure measurements in rabbits during isoflurane anaesthesia. *Vet Anaesth Analg*, 39, 174–184.

Hawkins, M.G. and Pascoe, P.J. (2012) Anesthesia, analgesia, and sedation of small mammals. In: Quesenberry, K.E. and Carpenter, J.W. (eds). *Ferrets, Rabbits, and Rodents: Clinical Medicine and Surgery*, 3rd ed. St Louis, MO: Elsevier Saunders, pp. 429–451.

Heard, D.J. (2014) Lagomorphs (rabbits, hares, and pikas). In: West, G., Heard, D. and Caulkett, N. (eds). *Zoo Animal and Wildlife Immobilization and Anesthesia*, 2nd ed. Ames, IA: Wiley Blackwell Publishing, pp. 879–891.

Johnson, C. (2009) Breathing systems and airway management. In: Welsh, L. (ed.). *Anaesthesia for Veterinary Nurses*, 2nd ed. Ames, IA: Wiley-Blackwell, pp. 90–120.

Johnson, J.A., Atkins, A.L. and Heard, D.J. (2010) Application of the laryngeal mask airway for anesthesia in three chimpanzees and one gibbon. *J Zoo Wildl Med*, 41, 535–537.

Kazakos, G.M., Anagnostou, T., Savvas, I., Raptopoulos, D., Psalla, D. and Kazakou, I.M. (2007) Use of the laryngeal mask airway in rabbits: placement and efficacy. *Lab Anim*, 36, 29–34.

Kruger, J., Zeller, W. and Schottmann, E. (1994) A simplified procedure for endotracheal intubation in rabbits. *Lab Anim*, 28, 176–177.

Lennox, A.M. (2008) Clinical technique: Small exotic companion mammal dentistry—Anesthetic considerations. *J Exot Pet Med*, 17, 102–106.

Lichtenberger, M. and Ko, J. (2007) Anesthesia and analgesia for small mammals and birds. *Vet Clin North Am Exot Anim Pract*, 10, 293–315.

Macrae, D.J. and Guerreiro, D. (1989) A simple laryngoscopic technique for the endotracheal intubation of rabbits. *Lab Anim*, 23, 59–61.

Mattheussen, M., Mubagwa, K., Van Akent, H., Wustent, R., Boutros, A. and Flameng, W. (1996) Interaction of heart rate and hypothermia on global myocardial contraction of the isolated rabbit heart. *Anesth Analg*, 82, 975–981.

Nevarez, J.G. (2005) Monitoring during avian and exotic pet anesthesia. *Semin Avian Exot Pet Med*, 14, 277–283.

Prasse, S.A., Schrack, J., Wenger, S. and Mosing, M. (2015) Clinical evaluation of the v-gel supraglottic airway device in comparison with a classical laryngeal mask and endotracheal intubation in cats during spontaneous and controlled mechanical ventilation. *Vet Anaesth Analg*, 43, 55–62.

Schroeder, C. and Smith, L. (2011) Respiratory rates and arterial blood gas tensions in healthy rabbits given buprenorphine, butorphanol, midazolam, or their combinations. *J Am Assoc Lab Anim Sci,* 50, 205–211.

Staikou, C., Paraskeva, A., Donta, I., Theodossopoulos, T., Anastassopoulou, I. and Kontos, M. (2011) The effects of mild hypothermia on coagulation tests and haemodynamic variables in anaesthetized rabbits. *West Indian Med J*, 60, 513–518.

Stephens Devalle, J.M. (2009) Successful management of rabbit anesthesia through the use of nasotracheal intubation. *J Am Assoc Lab Anim Sci*, 48, 166–170.

Toman, H., Erbas, M., Sahin, H., Kiraz, H.A., Uzun, M. and Ovali, M.A. (2015) Comparison of the effects of various airway devices on hemodynamic response and QTc interval in rabbits under general anesthesia. *J Clin Monit Comput*, 29, 727–732.

Westergren, V., Otori, N. and Stierna, P. (1999) Experimental nasal intubation: a study of changes in nasoantral mucosa and bacterial flora. *Laryngoscope*, 109, 1068–1073.

Worthley, S.G., Roque, M., Helft, G., Soundararajan, K., Siddiqui, M. and Reis, E.D. (2000) Rapid oral endotracheal intubation with a fibre-optic scope in rabbits: a simple and reliable technique. *Lab Anim*, 34, 199–201.

34

Unique Species Considerations: Rodents

Mario Arenillas Baquero[1] and Rebecca A. Johnson[2]

[1] *Veterinary Clinical Teaching Hospital, Complutense University of Madrid, Madrid, Spain*
[2] *School of Veterinary Medicine, University of Wisconsin, Madison, Wisconsin, USA*

34.1   Introduction

Rodents are diverse and include capybaras, muskrats, porcupines, chipmunks, woodchucks, prairie dogs, voles, hamsters, gerbils, squirrels, raccoons, rats, mice, beavers, guinea pigs, chinchillas, and many others. However, the most commonly anesthetized rodents are likely guinea pigs, chinchillas, rats and mice, as these species are both companion and laboratory animals. Although injectable anesthetic techniques have historically been used, especially in the laboratory setting, long-term injectable anesthesia is difficult to attain in certain situations, such as when the rodent is covered with drapes to maintain a sterile field or when the body position absolutely cannot change, such as during imaging studies. Furthermore, some injectable anesthetics are not rapidly reversible, may produce long recovery times, and so may increase the risk of anesthetic-associated complications. Compared to injectable anesthetics, inhalational anesthetics allow for rapid induction and recovery and a readily controllable anesthetic depth. Hence, inhalational anesthesia has become popular among researchers and veterinarians treating all rodent species in the last few decades (Richardson and Flecknell 2005) and familiarity with anesthetic and monitoring equipment is essential in these animals.

34.2   Anesthetic Machines

Anesthetic machines and breathing circuits provide oxygen and inhalants to the patient and remove waste gases. In most cases, 100% oxygen is used as a carrier gas for inhalants, but room air or mixtures of oxygen with air or nitrous oxide are also being used, especially in the research setting. Most machines are comprised of a flowmeter (or many flowmeters if multiple gases are spliced together) attached to a gas source, a vaporizer to control anesthetic vapor concentration, a breathing circuit which delivers anesthesia to the animal and some type of scavenging gas system. Fortunately, only a few types of breathing circuits are needed to accomplish a wide range of anesthetic tasks (Vogler 2008).

With larger rodent species (i.e. raccoons, skunks, etc.), circle or rebreathing systems can be used. However, many rodent species are quite small. Thus, rodent machines are comprised of very small circle/ rebreathing systems or, more frequently, lack all the components of a circle system, and are intended for use with non-rebreathing circuits designed similar to Mapleson D (Bain), E (Ayre T-piece) or F (Jackson-Rees) circuits, without a reservoir bag or APL valve. Additional features, such as multiple breathing circuits and provision for one or more induction chambers, are common (Volger 2008; Figure 34.1).

Many rodent anesthetic machines are commercially available that may connect to multiple breathing systems and conventional vaporizers (e.g. Table Top Research Animal Machine, V3000P (Parkland Scientific, Inc., Coral Springs, FL); DRE Compact Mini Rodent Anesthesia Machine (DRE Veterinary, Louisville, KY); Table-Top Single Animal Anesthesia Systems (Harvard Apparatus, Holliston, MA); VetFlo™ Traditional Anesthesia System (Kent Scientific Corporation, Torrington, CT); Hallowell Anesthesia WorkStation (Hallowell EMC, Pittsfield, MA)). In addition, one unique machine (SomnoSuite®, Kent Scientific Corporation, Torrington, CT) uses a digital, low-flow vaporizing system, with either room air or oxygen mixtures to provide controlled rodent anesthesia while producing less waste gas; this system easily integrates with ventilators and physiologic monitors (Damen *et al.* 2015; Figure 34.2). Although these commercially available rodent machines offer distinct advantages, it is also possible to create "in house" machines using separate

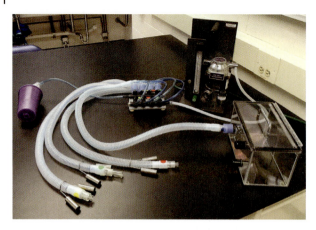

Figure 34.1 An anesthetic machine for research rodents with multiple breathing systems allowing simultaneous rodents to be anesthetized at once. Three non-rebreathing circuits are attached along with an anesthetic chamber and passive gas scavenger (purple). Rodent masks are seen at the end of the breathing systems and small, metal weights are used to keep the tubes in place.

flowmeters, vaporizers, tubing and scavenge systems, specifically designed for the user's needs (Figures 34.3A and B).

34.3 Anesthetic Induction Chambers

In rats, mice and other unique rodent species, anesthetic induction with volatile agents is often carried out

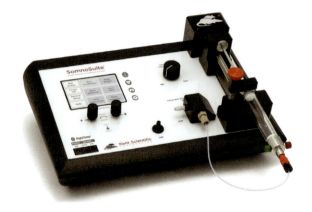

Figure 34.2 The Somnosuite® digitally controlled, low-flow rodent anesthesia system (photograph courtesy of Kent Scientific Corporation (Torrington, CT)).

in an anesthetic chamber (sometimes following premedication with a sedative and/or analgesic agent). Rapid unconsciousness is usually achieved using controlled levels of anesthetic vapor with low risk of injury to the operator (Gwynne and Wallace 1992; Flecknell *et al.* 1996; Wolforth and Dyson 2011). Chambers either can be purchased commercially or constructed "in house". They are usually made of acrylic, are suitable for the rodent's size and are transparent so the operator can observe the induction process (Flecknell 2009b). Induction chambers should contain a gas inlet and an outlet port for excess gas scavenging. The lid should fit tightly to prevent leaks and to reduce escape attempts;

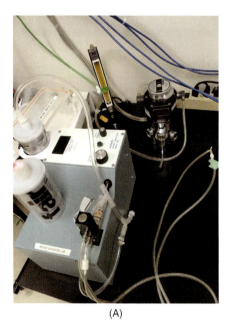 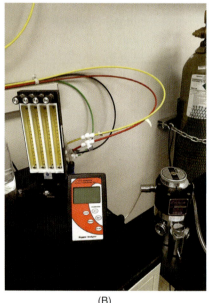

(A) (B)

Figure 34.3 Examples of anesthesia systems constructed "in house". (A) The flowmeter, vaporizer, ventilator, tubing and scavenge are all individual components of this system. (B) An anesthetic system with multiple flowmeters that splice inspired gas mixtures together with a separate vaporizer and an oxygen sensor.

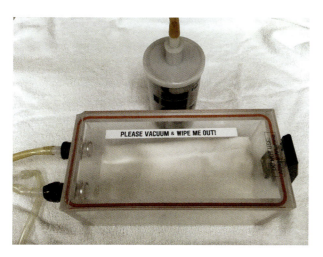

Figure 34.4 Example of a commercially available anesthetic chamber with an inlet for precise delivery of inhalant and an outlet to the scavenge system (f/air canister; Parkland Scientific Inc., Coral Springs, FL). Note the seal surrounding the top and the clamp to shut the lid tightly.

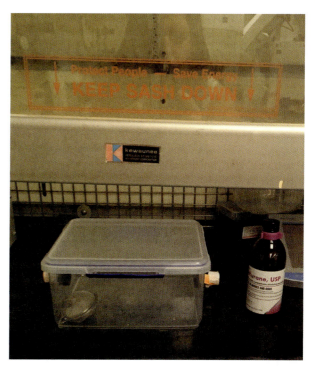

Figure 34.5 The use of an induction chamber in a fume hood to reduce personnel exposure to the inhalant once the lid is opened. Note the tea infuser containing anesthetic on a gauze used to avoid direct contact of the rodent with the inhalant while in the chamber.

many commercial designs are available and use a gasket and locking mechanism to ensure a tight seal (Volger 2008; Figure 34.4). One commercially available chamber has a "porthole" design to easily place the rodent into the chamber (DarvallVet/Advanced Anesthesia Specialists, Payson, AZ). However, some "in house" chambers are simply transparent, sealed boxes that are used in room air with the "hanging drop" technique (see below). Some chambers have a false bottom, usually a stainless metal grid, for easy clean up. Alternatively, paper towels or dry bedding can be used.

Use of an induction chamber is a simple and effective way to anesthetize rodents, as it avoids the requirement for a previously-placed intravenous catheter and manual restraint by simply placing the rodent inside and filling the container with a mixture of precisely measured isoflurane and oxygen delivered from a vaporizer. However, some anesthetists also practice the "hanging drop" technique, where a measured amount of inhalant is placed on a gauze that is put into the chamber filled with room air, while shielding the rodent from coming into direct contact with the inhalant by use of a mesh container or tea infuser (Figure 34.5). For example, 0.5 mL of inhalant placed into a 725-mL mouse induction chamber resulted in anesthetic induction at inspired concentrations of approximately 6.8% and 7.4% of isoflurane and sevoflurane, respectively. Induction time was approximately 36 seconds for isoflurane and approximately 46 seconds for sevoflurane (Risling *et al.* 2012). However, since inhalants are associated with dose-dependent respiratory depression, it is more desirable to use precisely delivered inhalant concentrations and enriched oxygen mixtures as the carrier gas instead of air and the "hanging drop" technique if feasible.

When the rodent becomes immobile and its breathing slows, the operator opens the chamber lid to retrieve the animal, at which time personnel may be exposed to large amounts of waste anesthetic gases. For this reason, chamber techniques are best performed in a fume hood (Figure 34.5) if available or chambers should be attached to a machine with a gas scavenger (Figure 34.1). Although evidence for adverse health effects associated with inhalants is not conclusive, working standards have been disseminated to alleviate occupational exposure to emitted halogenated anesthetics in light of effects engendered by the older agents (e.g. halothane, methoxyflurane). Recommended practices in operating rooms include the use of well-maintained anesthesia delivery systems equipped with gas-scavenging units, increased room ventilation, and regular air-quality monitoring (Smith and Bolon 2002). Scavenged anesthetizing chambers using a system with two boxes have been devised to remove the waste anesthetic gas in a controlled way, either actively routed out of the room or passively adsorbed using activated charcoal (Figure 34.3A). In addition, the development and testing of a portable system to reduce waste anesthetic gases that could be adapted to most portable and permanent anesthetic work stations has been reported (Wolforth and Dyson 2011). The system flushes anesthetic gas out of an induction chamber before operators open the chamber, without affecting the efficiency of the anesthetic system and may be beneficial to personnel with no access to a fume hood.

34.4 Masks

Commonly used rodent masks are usually designed with a cylindrical or funnel-shaped cone that fits over the animal's nose (and sometimes mouth, depending on species) to create a seal. A snug fit is usually achieved by including an anatomical shaping of the face of rodents or through an opening in a rubber diaphragm placed at the end of the mask where the nose may be introduced (Figures 34.1 and 34.6A, B). A quick technique to secure masks in rodent species with long incisors is to circumferentially attach a tracheal tube tie (Trinity Trach-Tube Ties, Fort Worth, TX) to the incisors and pull the ends through the connection between the mask and breathing tubes (Figure 34.7). Masks are meant to deliver oxygen or anesthetic mixtures to the animal and have become the standard method of general anesthesia for rodents in research and clinical cases, especially when endotracheal intubation is not possible or is not indicated (Figures 34.7 and 34.8).

When using a mask for maintaining anesthesia, mechanical dead space may be increased if it is too large. The mask design must shape the animal's nose to minimize mechanical dead space and reduce carbon dioxide rebreathing. However, this issue may be relatively less important in rodents than in larger species, since many anesthetic machines deliver an inspired flow rate signifi-

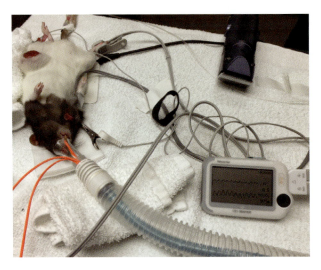

Figure 34.7 Use of a commercially designed rat mask to provide inhalational anesthetic. Note the use of tracheal tube ties around the incisors to secure the mask to the breathing tubes. Also note the use of a pulse oximeter and electrocardiogram (ECG).

cantly in excess of that actually required by small rodents. Thus, most systems that use a mask act as open systems and the dead space in the mask becomes relatively unimportant (Flecknell 2009a). Commercially available rodent masks have been developed to minimize rebreathing with streamlined gas flows and minimal dead space (DarvallVet/Advanced Anesthesia Specialists, Payson, AZ; Figure 34.9). Some masks set flat and have offset openings that can be turned, based on the height of the rodent's nose.

Keeping rodents on masks carries significant risks such as hypothermia and dehydration, and offers little

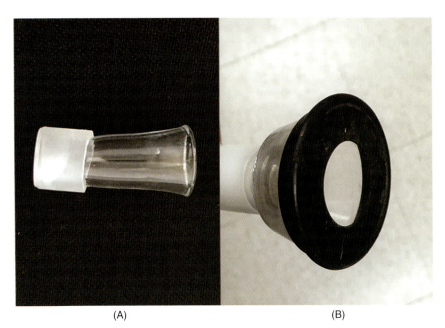

(A)   (B)

Figure 34.6 (A) Transparent rodent mask designed for a snug fit against a rat muzzle. Note that personnel would still have access to the head and eyes. (B) Slightly larger rodent mask with a diaphragm opening for the mouth and nose.

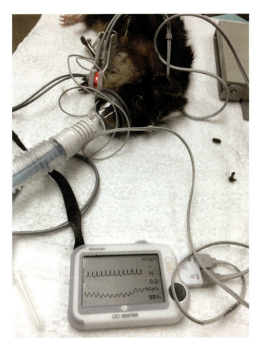

Figure 34.8 Use of a transparent mask snugly fitted over the nose of a guinea pig. Also note the use of a pulse oximeter and ECG.

help in case of airway collapse (Rivard *et al.* 2006). In addition, leaks around the mask are frequent; inclusion of a diaphragm modified mask adequately limited occupational exposure to waste isoflurane, but did not eliminate it, especially during prolonged studies in which multiple anesthesia procedures are performed (Smith and Bolon 2006). Other procedures used to reduce occupational exposure of laboratory animal personnel to waste inhalant emissions include improving the efficiency of gas-scavenging systems, increasing the air turnover rate in animal procedure rooms, and avoiding bench-top (no fume hood) use of induction chambers (Smith and Bolon 2002, 2006). Another way of reducing these drawbacks is endotracheal intubation (see Intubation below).

To help with waste gas scavenging, newer masks incorporate a coaxial design where the inner tube delivers

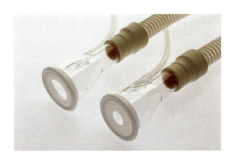

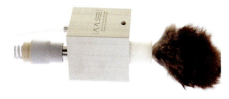

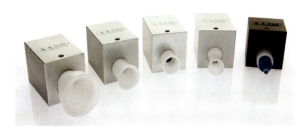

Figure 34.9 Examples of zero-dead space rodent masks to minimize rebreathing (ZDS Mask [top] and Qube [middle and bottom panels], DarvallVet/Advanced Anesthesia Specialists, Payson, AZ). The Qube has an offset opening that can be turned to adjust to the height of the animal's nose (image courtesy of DarvallVet/Advanced Anesthesia Specialists (Payson, AZ)).

fresh gas from the anesthesia machine and is closer to the nose, and the outer tube vents to the scavenge first and is connected to a suction source. This design is similar to some non-breathing hoses, which can be placed directly on the animal's nose (Vogler 2008) (Figure 34.10). Other designs consist of two separate tubes, one connected to the fresh gas outlet and another to the scavenge system. Low profile masks (Kent Scientific Corporation, Torrington, CT; Figures 34.6A and 34.7) provide limited opportunity for waste gas exposure and

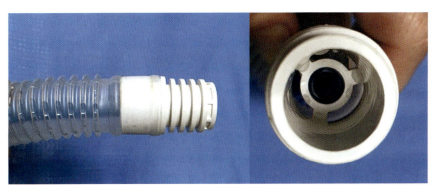

Figure 34.10 Example of a non-breathing tube that can be used as a coaxial mask. The inner tube supplies fresh gas flow and the waste gas exits via the outer tube.

allow anesthetic procedures with access to the eyes and head. In addition, anesthetists may create their own masks using available means, such as syringes, connectors or plastic bottles. These masks may fulfill the need of a specific experimental procedure (e.g. MRI) or surgical approach (e.g. craniotomy or dorsal laminectomy), since commercial products may hinder the procedure. Therefore, many masks with various shapes for different procedures that further reduce dead space, shorten operation time, allow removal of gases and improve survival, are being manufactured (Yuan *et al.* 2009).

Some procedures require minimal-to-no head movement of the animal. For these instances, stereotaxic stands available with anesthetic masks mounted on the incisor bar are used. They produce minimal personnel exposure to anesthetic gas and allow positioning of the rat for stereotaxic surgery (Stoelting Co., Wood Dale, IL; Figure 34.11). Various sizes and configurations are available from suppliers of stereotaxic equipment, including models with special restraint devices for use with neonates (Vogler 2008).

34.5 Endotracheal Intubation and Intubation Devices

34.5.1 Technique

Endotracheal intubation of larger rodents is similar to other domestic species and commercially available tracheal tubes and conventional techniques can be used. In smaller rodents, tracheal intubation is not always indicated, due to difficulty in the technique and anesthetic

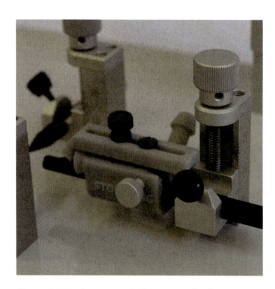

Figure 34.11 A stereotaxic frame attached to a mouse mask used for procedures where no movement can occur (photograph courtesy of Stoelting Co., Wood Dale, IL).

length. However, intubation is required for many procedures, such as repeated pulmonary function assessments, longitudinal imaging studies of the lung and abdomen, direct intratracheal aerosolization of various agents, and for procedures requiring assisted or mechanical ventilation, including prolonged surgical procedures (Rivera *et al.* 2005; Spoelstra *et al.* 2007). Rodent intubation can be difficult due to their physical size, small palate, oropharyngeal cavity, larynx and epiglottis, large incisors, vocal cords that move rapidly and a narrow trachea. Equipment to facilitate intubation has recently become commercially available at a reasonable cost. While the principles of intubation are similar to other larger animal species, the technical skills to intubate rats or mice are somewhat different. First attempts for non-experienced personnel are associated with an increase in complications such as esophageal intubation, mucus plugging, traumatic extubation, laryngo-epiglottic edema or laryngospasm (Rivard *et al.* 2006). However, with practice and the correct equipment, intubation can be atraumatic and readily achieved. Two critical steps that can determine the success and safety of rodent intubation are a clear visualization of oropharyngeal and laryngeal anatomy and passage of the endotracheal tube through the vocal cords (Su *et al.* 2016). Most of the methods originally devised for rats have subsequently been adapted to mice.

The rodent (most commonly a mouse or rat) is placed in dorsal recumbency on a flat or inclined platform to help maintain an easier position for intubation (e.g. Hallowell Rodent WorkStand, Hallowell EMC, Pittsfield, MA; Figure 34.12). The upper incisors are fixed using a rounded rubber or silk suture and the operator uses a cotton swab, laryngoscope blade, otoscope cone, or something similar to roll the tongue out of the mouth and to elevate the mandible. Following topical application of appropriate lidocaine doses on the larynx, intubation is performed using one of many techniques such as direct laryngoscopy or fiber optic laryngoscopy, with or without prior stylet placement (see below). An efficient way to produce targeted lidocaine delivery to the larynx is with a commercially available atomizer (LMA® MADamizer® Bottle Atomizer, Wolfe Tory Medical Manufacturers, Salt Lake City, UT; Figure 34.13).

34.5.2 Endotracheal Tubes

In larger rodents, size 2.0 and larger tracheal tubes can be used. In smaller animals, intravenous catheters are used as tracheal tubes attached to low dead space adapters for gas analysis (Figure 34.14). Soft catheters are preferred since they are more flexible, which minimizes tracheal trauma. However, tracheal tube kinking is common; one must be cautious when securing

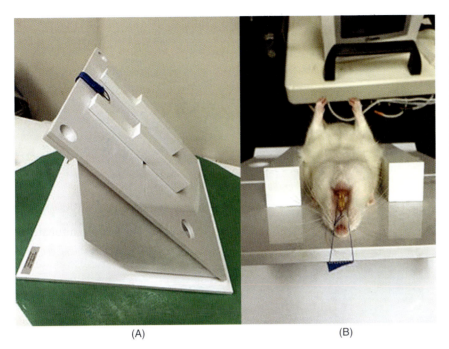

(A) (B)

Figure 34.12 (A) A tilted table to facilitate orotracheal intubation of small rodents. The teeth are attached to the circular suture and table tipped to help visualize the larynx (photograph courtesy of Hallowell EMC (Pittsfield, MA)). (B) Adult rat positioned on the table with the incisors secured using suture. Image is taken above the table looking toward the floor (photograph courtesy of Joel Weltman, DVM, DACVECC).

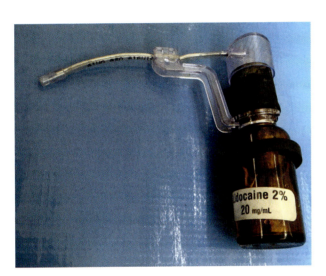

Figure 34.13 An atomizer that uniformly diffuses and directs the local anesthetic to the larynx.

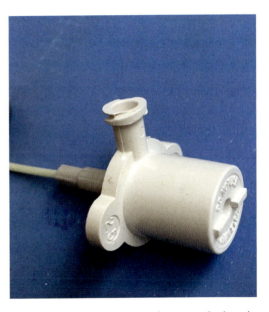

Figure 34.14 An intravenous catheter attached to a low dead space adapter for use as a tracheal tube and with a gas analyzer.

the tube to the rodent and positioning for the procedure. Several methods can be used to confirm intubation; for example, watching for fog in the tube or on a mirror placed near the tube opening, or by attaching a small bulb to the tracheal tube and observing synchronous thoracic motion as it is squeezed (Rivera *et al.* 2005; Figure 34.15). Other methods to confirm intubation are connection to a ventilator and observation of chest movements or attaching an extension tube to the endotracheal tube with a water column that will move accordingly to ventilation (Watanabe *et al.* 2009).

34.5.3 Fiber Optic and Endoscopic Intubation

Several methods to perform endotracheal intubation in rodents have been suggested and methods using direct light or lighted stylets are common. Historically, Vergari *et al.* (2003) used a small-bore, fiber optic arthroscope to intubate mice rapidly with minimal personnel training and no complications, even after re-intubation 4 and 8 weeks later. The major disadvantage of this method was the high equipment cost.

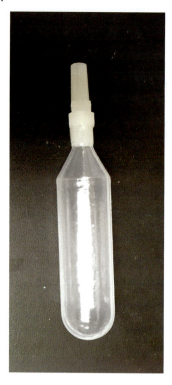

Figure 34.15 A small bulb that can be attached to the end of an intravenous catheter/tracheal tube. As it is squeezed, the thorax should expand to confirm tracheal intubation.

Newer, fiber optic methods use a cable transporting light from the illuminator to the fiber tip for visualization of the larynx and for use as a stylet (Rivera *et al.* 2005; BioLITE Intubation System, Braintree Scientific, Inc., Braintree, MA; Figures 34.16A and B). A modified MagLite flashlight (Mag Instruments, Inc., Los Angeles, CA) is used as the light source, with the lens and parabolic mirror removed and replaced with an aluminum disk to hold the fiber optic light. The delivery end of the fiber optic light fits into an intravenous catheter used as a tracheal tube. Similar to intubation in larger species, the tongue is retracted to one side and the larynx is visualized as the fiber optic light guide is advanced in the mouth. The fiber optic light is passed through the vocal cords and the catheter is glided over the guide. Another method to intubate rodents uses the endoscope system, "Tesala AE-C1" (AVS Company, Ltd., Tokyo, Japan; Konno *et al.* 2014a, b). The endoscope probe (AE-F07070) is used for capturing images and as a substitute stylet.

34.5.4 Direct Illumination and Laryngoscopy

Other methods using direct light in combination with laryngoscopes or mouth speculums are also common approaches to rodent endotracheal intubation (Costa *et al.* 1986; Linden *et al.* 2000; Spoelstra *et al.* 2007). These methods are similar to those in more traditional larger species. Some techniques use wire guides to introduce the endotracheal tube into the trachea with a standard or modified otoscope cone on a lighted and/or magnifying otoscope (Weksler *et al.* 1994; Kastl *et al.* 2004; Hamacher *et al.* 2008; Tomasello *et al.* 2016; Figures 34.17 and 34.18). Other techniques use specially designed fiber optic laryngoscopes for direct laryngeal visualization in small laboratory rodents (Alpert *et al.* 1982; Costa *et al.* 1986).

Surgical operating microscopes have also been used to magnify and light the oral cavity to facilitate the introduction of an endotracheal tube (Peña and Cabrera 1980). Other, useful methods to intubate rodents use trans-illumination of the ventral neck with a bright light source (Rivard et al. 2006; Figure 34.19) and thus, the cartilages from the larynx. Bright light directed from outside of the skin and focused on the pharyngeal region penetrates the skin, muscles and trachea and allows

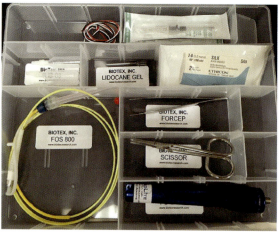

(A)

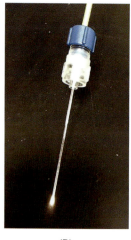

(B)

Figure 34.16 (A) A fiber optic intubation kit including all parts necessary for intubation. (B) Magnified image of the fiber optic tip that acts as a stylet for the tracheal tube. Note the lidocaine gel to aid with passage through the vocal cords. Be aware of the toxic lidocaine doses for each species.

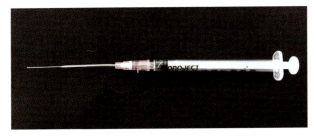

Figure 34.17 A syringe modified with a wire stylet inserted into the plunger. An intravenous catheter is placed over the wire and is easily advanced off the wire as the plunger is drawn back to remove the stylet.

(A)

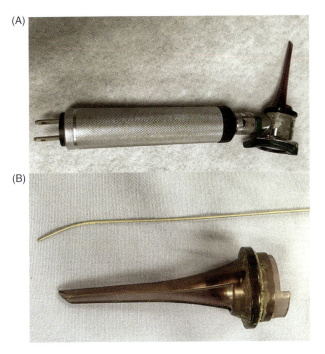

(B)

Figure 34.18 (A) A plug-in otoscope with a modified cone used for illumination and direct visualization of the rodent larynx. (B) Magnified view of a stylet and the modified cone. Note that part of the circular tube is removed to reduce obstruction of view.

direct visualization of the airway as the laryngeal cartilages open during inspiration and visual placement of the endotracheal tube through the oral cavity with an otoscope (Figure 34.20).

34.6 Ventilators

Conventional ventilators in larger rodents (see Chapter 6) can provide mechanical ventilation. However, due to their small respiratory volumes, specific rodent ventilators have been developed. Most current rodent ventilators are manually or microprocessor controlled, piston-driven, and can be set for various types of ventilation modes (e.g. MiniVet Ventilator/Small Animal

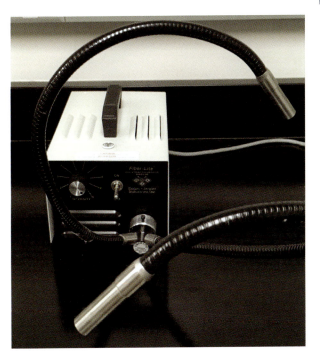

Figure 34.19 A fiber optic light source used to trans-illuminate the larynx and aid in airway visualization through the oral cavity.

Ventilator/MidiVent Ventilator (Harvard Apparatus, Holliston, MA); Numiovent BS (Numio Tecnologias, SL, Madrid, Spain); Merlin Small Animal Ventilator (Vetronic Services, Devon, UK)). Some are made for specific-sized rodents (e.g. MicroVent Ultralow Volume Ventilator for Prenatal Mice (Harvard Apparatus, Holliston, MA)), and some can be used in multiple rodent species (e.g. VentElite Small Animal Ventilator (Harvard Apparatus, Holliston, MA); Figure 34.21). Others can be used for normal ventilation strategies or be set to deliver high-frequency oscillations (e.g. MicroVent-1 (Hallowell EMC, Pittsfield, MA); Figure 34.22). In addition, one versatile machine that can be used for patients between 150 g and 7 kg, is equipped with a very small circle system and can be easily switched between its use as a respirator (with no inhalants) to an anesthetic ventilator to deliver inhalants (Anesthesia Workstation (Hallowell AMC, Pittsfield, MA); Figure 34.23). Although mechanical ventilation brings advantages and disadvantages (see Chapter 6), it can be useful in assessing extracellular fluid deficits in many species, including rodents (Lu *et al.* 2014).

34.7 Monitoring Equipment

When monitoring patients during an anesthetic procedure, the anesthetist should ensure a correct level of unconsciousness (i.e. depth of anesthesia), properly

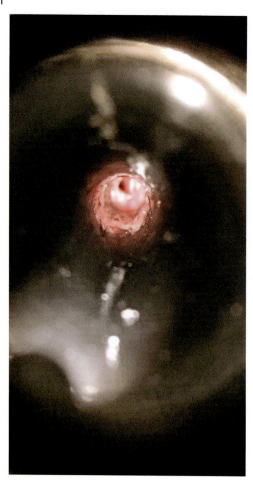

Figure 34.20 Visualization of a magnified rat larynx illuminated with a lighted otoscope. The rat is placed in sternal recumbency and the epiglottis can be seen at ~ 4:00-5:00 o'clock. The laryngeal cartilages appear on each side of the entrance to the trachea (small dark spot).

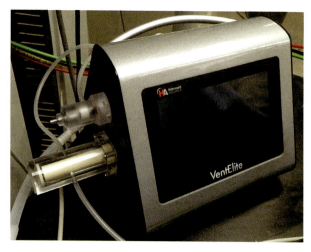

Figure 34.21 The VentElite Small Animal Ventilator (Harvard Apparatus, Holliston, MA) has a touch screen and can be used in patients from 10 g–1 kg (mice to guinea pigs).

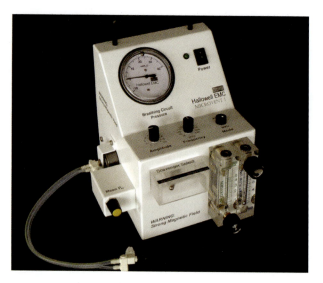

Figure 34.22 The Microvent 1 ventilator can be used for standard intermittent positive pressure ventilation or high frequency oscillation ventilation techniques in rodents (photograph courtesy of Hallowell EMC (Pittsfield, MA)).

interpret the complications that may arise, and be able to identify their cause to correct the problem. When small-sized animals are anesthetized, it is difficult to adapt and implement the anesthetic equipment used in larger species. However, some commercially available monitors do work well in many rodents (e.g. gas monitoring, see Chapter 16; pulse oximetry, see

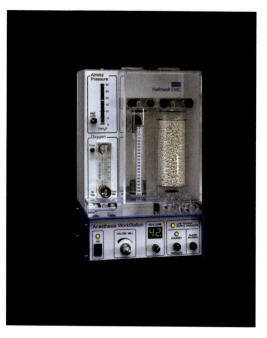

Figure 34.23 The Hallowell EMC Anesthesia Workstation can be used for patients from 150 g–7 kg and incorporates a very small circle breathing system (photograph courtesy of Hallowell EMC (Pittsfield, MA)).

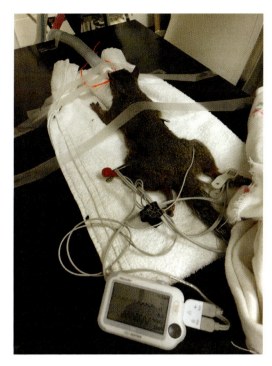

Figure 34.24 A Vetcorder (Sentier Connect, Brookfield, WI) used to monitor the electrocardiogram, pulse rate and hemoglobin saturation in a squirrel.

Chapter 18; blood pressure, see Chapter 19; electrocardiography, see Chapter 20) (Figures 34.7, 34.8 and 34.24). Others simply need simple adaptations, such as the use of low dead space adapters for capnography (Figure 34.14) or adjustable-tension pulse oximetry probes and very small needles (ZUMAYA™ ECG Electrode Kit (Sentier Connect, Brookfield, WI)) or

non-traumatic clips for electrocardiography leads (Figures 34.25A and B).

34.7.1 Specific Rodent Monitors

In the field of rodent research, it is not only important to monitor the patient's vital signs to ensure their welfare during the anesthetic procedure, but also for physiological stability to ensure valid experimental data and accurate interpretation (Smith and Danneman 2008). Thus, monitors specific for rodents have been developed with integrative devices to store the physiologic monitored data, aid in trend interpretation, add notable events during the procedures, extract relevant information and, ultimately, make a thorough study of all monitored variables. Ultimately, better research occurs when investigators tightly control anesthetic-induced changes in physiology. In fact, the most recent version of the *Guide for the Care and Use of Laboratory Animals* (2011) states that: "For anesthesia delivery, precision vaporizers and monitoring equipment (e.g. pulse oximeter for determining arterial blood oxygen saturation levels) increase the safety and choices of anesthetic agents for use in rodents and other small species". Although these monitors have been developed for use in research settings, clinical patients would benefit from their use as well. This chapter is not meant to be an exhaustive review of all commercially available rodent monitors. However, two validated examples are detailed below; many other excellent monitors may also be available to anesthetists and researchers.

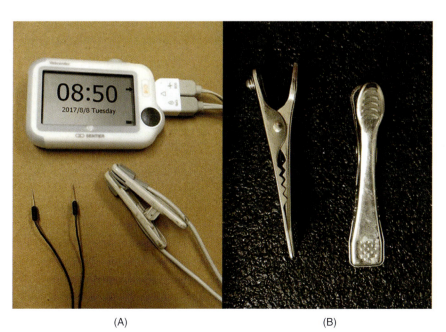

(A)   (B)

Figure 34.25 The Vetcorder (Sentier Connect, Brookfield, WI) uses an adjustable pulse oximetry probe and atraumatic clips as electrocardiograph (ECG) leads in rodents (A, B). Very small wires (ZUMAYA™ ECG Electrode Kit) can be used as ECG leads in very small species with delicate skin (A).

34.7.1.1 Multiparameter Monitors

Among multi-parameter monitors, the PhysioSuite® (Kent Scientific Corporation, Torrington, CT; Figure 34.26) is a rodent monitor that includes different modules with a real-time display, integrated digital controls, internal memory for data collection, and USB port for data output. Although an external computer is not required, there is an enabler for data streaming into LabChart (ADInstruments, Ltd, New South Wales, Australia), a data analysis software platform that allows recording of biological parameters, the analysis of trends, and application of advanced calculations while the experiment is being carried out. Modules include the MouseSTAT® for hemoglobin oxygen saturation (SpO_2), heart rate (up to 900 beats per minute), respiratory rate and perfusion index. It uses specially designed paw sensors for either mice or rats (also useful for rabbit ears and small rodent tongues) and MRI compatible sensors are available. The sidestream CapnoScan® module measures end-tidal CO_2 ($EtCO_2$) with a low sampling rate and compensates for changes in temperature, pressure and the presence of other medical (O_2, N_2O, helium) and anesthetic gases. The RightTemp® module maintains core body temperature using far-infrared light technology (FIR), which does not warm the air between the FIR source and the rodent. FIR waves resonate with organic matter and penetrate into the body, gently increasing the energy level of cellular water and warming the animal from the inside (see: www.kentscientific.com). In addition, a module developed to provide mechanical ventilation (RoVent®) is available.

34.7.1.2 Pulse Oximetry

The MouseOx® Plus (Starr Life Sciences Corp., Oakmont, PA; Figure 34.27) is a specifically designed small laboratory rodent pulse oximeter. It can be used in species with heart rates from 90–900 beats per minute

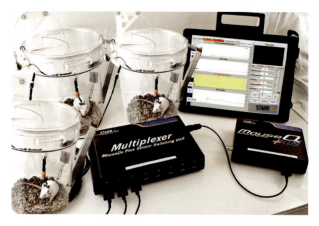

Figure 34.27 The MouseOx® Plus is specifically designed to be accurate in laboratory rodent species. Note the use of multiple rodents simultaneously (photograph courtesy of Starr Life Sciences Corporation (Oakmont, PA)).

(mice, rats, ferrets, guinea pigs, rabbits, voles, etc.) and measures SpO_2, pulse and respiration frequency and distensibility, temperature and motor activity. Some sensors are MRI compatible and some sensors form a collar around the animal, including neonates (Figures 34.27 and 34.28). Monitoring and data recording in multiple awake or anesthetized rodents is possible. The SpO_2 values are reportedly accurate at saturations of 100% to less than 20% (www.starrlifesciences.com), which may be advantageous because conventional pulse oximeters have been shown to be reasonably accurate in rodents at normal SpO_2 levels (80–99%), but become increasingly inaccurate as saturation falls (Flecknell 2009a). The MouseOx® Plus is also Bluetooth compatible and no wires are necessary; only the cable connecting the module with the platform used for the animal. There is also a stereotaxic adapter option including ear bars, a tooth bar and either a nose bar or an anesthesia mask.

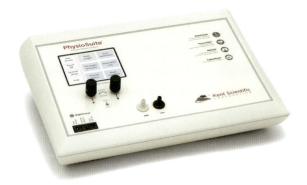

Figure 34.26 The PhysioSuite® is a rodent designed monitoring system in which specific modules can be added according to the anesthetists needs (photograph courtesy of Kent Scientific Corporation (Torrington, CT)).

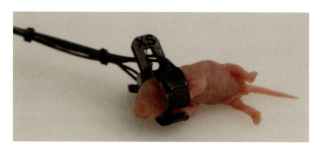

Figure 34.28 A pulse oximeter probe that acts as a collar on adult rodents, but can be used circumferentially around neonates. Care must be taken not to impede respiratory motion (photograph courtesy of Starr Life Sciences Corporation (Oakmont, PA)).

34.8   Warming Devices

In addition to conventional warming devices used on other species (see Chapter 22), many integrative rodent monitors are used that also include warming tools such as transparent plastic or metal warming surfaces (e.g. Heated Hard Pad (Braintree Scientific, Inc., Braintree, MA or Vetland Medical Sales and Services, LLC, Louisville, KY); Figure 34.29). In addition, other useful heating devices include large incubators that fit a complete rodent cage (ThermoCare (Paso Robles, CA); Figure 34.30). In any case, frequent body temperature monitoring is required. Many telemetry monitors also include core body temperature. However, if a rectal probe is used, care must be taken with the delicate rectal mucosa. Specific rectal probes are manufactured with small non-traumatic tips for rodent use (Rodent Rectal Probes (Braintree Scientific, Inc., Braintree, MA); Figure 34.31). In some cases, temperature monitoring devices that sense both at the Y piece and at the

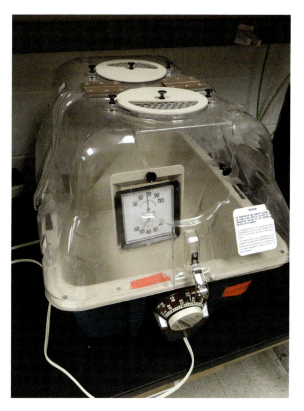

Figure 34.30   An incubator of sufficient size to house an entire rodent cage, so animals can continue normal activities while warming.

temperature probe can be used with a heated breathing circuit to warm the patient in a closed loop feedback system (SW Heated Breathing Circuit (DarvallVet/ Advanced Anesthesia Specialists, Payson, AZ); Figure 34.32). In addition, heated airway blocks that encompass low dead space masks or attach directly to standard

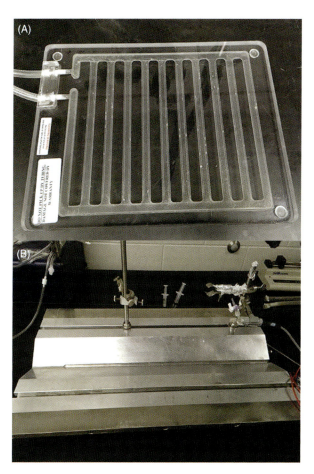

Figure 34.29   (A) Transparent warming pads or (B) heated metal tables used with circulating water to provide heat to experimental rodents.

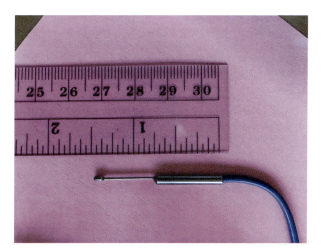

Figure 34.31   A very small tipped rectal probe for use in rats. The non-traumatic tip reduces rectal injury when placed.

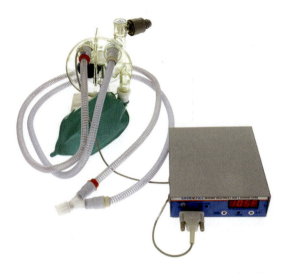

Figure 34.32 A heated breathing circuit as part of a closed-loop feedback system to prevent hypothermia in patients (image courtesy of DarvallVet/Advanced Anesthesia Specialists (Payson, AZ)).

endotracheal tubes can also be used (Qube, DarvallVet/ Advanced Anesthesia Specialists (Payson, AZ); Figures 34.9 and 34.33).

34.9 Summary

In summary, rodent anesthesia and monitoring are similar to those techniques used for other species. However, many products specifically made for rodents, especially research subjects, can offer distinct advantages in these species.

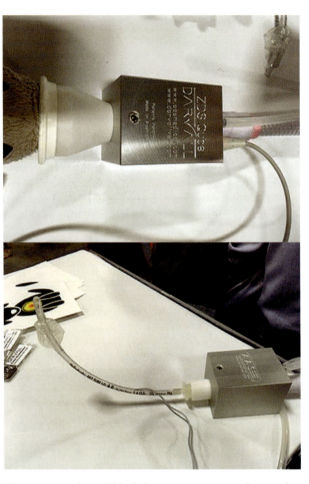

Figure 34.33 A heated block that encompasses a rodent mask (top) or attaches directly to endotracheal tubes (bottom) may help to reduce heat loss in patients (DarvallVet/Advanced Anesthesia Specialists, Payson, AZ).

References

Alpert, M., Goldstein, D. and Triner, L. (1982) Techniques of endotracheal intubation in rats. *Lab Anim Sci*, 32, 78–79.

Costa, D., Lehmann, J.R., Harold, W.M. and Drew, R.T. (1986) Transoral tracheal intubation of rodents using a fiberoptic laryngoscope. *Lab Anim Sci*, 36, 256–261.

Damen, F.W., Adelsperger, A.R., Wilson, K.E. and Goergen, C.J. (2015) Comparison of traditional and integrated digital anesthesia vaporizers. *J Am Assoc Lab Anim Sci*, 54, 756–762.

Flecknell, P.A. (2009a) Anaesthetic management. In: *Laboratory Animal Anaesthesia*, 5th ed. Burlington, MA: Academic Press, pp. 79–108.

Flecknell, P.A. (2009b) Preparing for anaesthesia. In: *Laboratory Animals Anaesthesia*, 5th ed. Burlington, MA: Academic Press, pp. 1–14.

Flecknell, P., Cruz, I.J., Liles, J.H. and Whelan, G. (1996) Induction of anaesthesia with halothane and isoflurane in the rabbit: a comparison of the use of a face-mask or an anaesthetic chamber. *Lab Anim*, 30, 67–74.

Guide for the Care and Use of Laboratory Animals (2011) Washington, DC: National Academic Press, p. 122.

Gwynne, B.J. and Wallace, J. (1992) A modified anaesthetic induction chamber for rats. *Lab Anim*, 26, 163–166.

Hamacher, J., Arras, M., Bootz, F., Weiss, M., Schramm, R. and Moehrlen, U. (2008) Microscopic wire guide-based orotracheal mouse intubation: description, evaluation and comparison with transillumination. *Lab Anim*, 42, 222–230.

Kastl, S., Kotschenreuther, U., Hille, B., Schmidt, J., Gepp, H. and Hohenberger, W. (2004) Simplification of rat intubation on inclined metal plate. *Adv Physiol Educ*, 28, 29–32.

Konno, K., Itano, N., Ogawa, T., Hatakeyama, M., Shioya, K. and Kasai, N. (2014a) New visible endotracheal intubation method using the endoscope system for mice inhalational anesthesia. *J Vet Med Sci*, 76, 863–868.

Konno, K., Shiotani, Y., Itano, N., Ogawa, T., Hatakeyama, M. et al. (2014b) Visible, safe and certain endotracheal intubation using endoscope system and inhalation anesthesia for rats. *J Vet Med Sci*, 76, 1375–1381.

Linden, R.D., Shields, C.B., Zhang, Y.P., Edmonds, H.L. and Hunt, M.A. (2000) A laryngoscope designed for intubation of the rat. *Contemp Top Lab Anim Sci*, 39, 40–42.

Lu, W., Dong, J., Xu, Z., Shen, H. and Zheng, J. (2014) The pleth variability index as an indicator of the central extracellular fluid volume in mechanically ventilated patients after anesthesia induction: comparison with initial distribution volume of glucose. *Med Sci Monit*, 20, 386–392.

Peña, H. and Cabrera, C. (1980) Improved endotracheal intubation technique in the rat. *Laboratory Anim Sci*, 30, 712–713.

Richardson, C. and Flecknell, P.A. (2005) Anaesthesia and post-operative analgesia following experimental surgery in laboratory rodents: are we making progress? *Altern Lab Anim*, 33, 119–127.

Risling, T.E., Caulkett, N.A. and Florence, D. (2012) Open-drop anesthesia for small laboratory animals. *Can Vet J*, 53, 299–302.

Rivard, A.L., Simura, K.J., Mohammed, S., Magembe, A.J., Pearson, H.M. et al. (2006) Rat intubation and ventilation for surgical research. *J Invest Surg*, 19, 267–274.

Rivera, B., Ince, C., Koeman, A., Emons, V.M., Brouwer, L.A. et al. (2005) A novel and simple method for endotracheal intubation of mice. *Lab Anim*, 41, 128–135.

Smith, J.C. and Bolon, B. (2002) Atmospheric waste isoflurane concentrations using conventional equipment and rat anesthesia protocols. *Contemp Top Lab Anim Sci*, 41, 10–17.

Smith, J.C. and Bolon, B. (2006) Isoflurane leakage from non-rebreathing rodent anaesthesia circuits: comparison of emissions from conventional and modified ports. *Lab Anim*, 40, 200–209.

Smith, J.C. and Danneman, P.J. (2008) Monitoring of anesthesia. In: Fish, R.E., Brown, M.J., Danneman, P.J. and Karas, A.Z. (eds). *Anesthesia and Analgesia in Laboratory Animals*, 2nd ed. London, UK: Academic Press, pp. 170–182.

Spoelstra, E.N., Ince, C. and Koeman, A. (2007) A novel and simple method for endotracheal intubation of mice. *Lab Anim*, 41, 128–135.

Su, C.S., Lai, H..C, Wang, C.Y., Lee, W.L., Wang, K.Y. et al. (2016) Efficacious and safe orotracheal intubation for laboratory mice using slim torqueable guidewire-based technique: comparisons between a modified and a conventional method. *BMC Anesthesiology*, 16, 1–7.

Tomasello, G., Damiani, F., Cassata, G., Palumbo, V.D., Sinagra, E. et al. (2016) Simple and fast orotracheal intubation procedure in rats. *Acta Biomed*, 87, 13–15.

Vergari, A., Polito, A., Musumeci, M., Palazzesi, S. and Marano, G. (2003) Video-assisted orotracheal intubation in mice. *Lab Anim*, 37, 204–206.

Vogler, G.A. (2008) Anesthesia delivery systems. In: Fish, R.E., Brown, M.J., Danneman, P.J., Karas, A.Z. (eds). *Anesthesia and Analgesia in Laboratory Animals*, 2nd ed. London, UK: Academic Press, pp. 127–169.

Watanabe, A., Hashimoto, Y., Ochiai, E., Sato, A. and Kamei, K. (2009) A simple method for confirming correct endotracheal intubation in mice. *Lab Anim*, 43, 399–401.

Weksler, B., Ng, B., Lenert, J. and Burt, M. (1994) A simplified method for endotracheal intubation in the rat. *Journal Appl Physiol*, 76, 1823–1825.

Wolforth, J. and Dyson, M.C. (2011) Flushing induction chambers used for rodent anesthesia to reduce waste anesthetic gas. *Lab Anim*, 40, 76–83.

Yuan, Y., Li, F., Wang, Y.M., Zhang, R.Q., Wei, L.P. and Wang, H.C. (2009) Respiratory face mask: a novel and cost-effective device for use during the application of myocardial ischemia in rats. *J Zhejiang Univ Sci B*, 10, 391–394.

35

Unique Species Considerations: Fish and Amphibians

Kurt Sladky

School of Veterinary Medicine, University of Wisconsin, Madison, Wisconsin, USA

35.1 Introduction

The application of safe and effective anesthetic techniques is essential for clinical veterinarians. Anesthetizing aquatic species, both with and without gills, presents a paradigm shift with respect to the methods and thought processes used when considering terrestrial animal anesthesia. Chemical restraint and anesthetic methods are commonly used in fish and amphibian patients, in order to facilitate animal transport, complete safe and thorough physical examinations, collect biologic samples, and perform other diagnostic and surgical procedures. The most efficient method for anesthetic delivery to most fish and amphibian species is by immersion bath, but other methods are also available. The objective of this chapter is to describe the anesthetic and monitoring equipment necessary for chemically immobilizing fish and amphibians in a clinical setting.

35.2 Fish and Amphibian Anesthesia: Induction and Maintenance

35.2.1 Bath Anesthetics

The most efficient method for anesthetic delivery to the majority of fish and amphibian species is by an immersion bath, which can be applied for short-term procedures using an induction container, or longer-term procedures using a recirculating water apparatus in fish (commonly referred to as a FADS; fish anesthetic delivery system (Figure 35.1), but also used for amphibians (Figure 35.2) (Lewbart and Harms 1999). Components of the FADS are readily available, economical and easy to assemble (Figure 35.3; Table 35.1). Most commonly, the main water-holding container is made from a commercial laboratory rodent cage made of durable plastic

(Table 35.1). The material can withstand abuse, including dropping on to hard surfaces, and can be cleaned in extremely hot water and almost any disinfectant (including commercial laboratory animal facility cleaning systems). An alternative is to use a standard, 10-gallon glass aquarium, but there is significantly less durability and thorough cleaning is difficult. Bath anesthetic methods require application of the anesthetic chemical in non-chlorinated water, such as MS-222 (tricaine methansulfonate), eugenol, isoeugenol or alfaxolone.

Anesthetic induction using a water-filled container (Figures 35.4 and 35.5) can provide short-term chemical immobilization, allowing for physical examination, common diagnostic procedures (e.g. gill, skin and fin biopsies), blood sample collection, and imaging. In fish and gilled amphibians, some minimally invasive procedures can be conducted directly in the induction container, partially submerged in water, allowing the animal to continue respiring. Gilled amphibians can remain submerged in the bath anesthetic solution during induction. It is important that non-gilled amphibians have their head above the anesthetic solution in order to prevent drowning.

For longer-term procedures and surgery, either the FADS, or a gas anesthetic in amphibians, are essential. Gas anesthetics can be used in some non-gilled amphibian species for maintenance. The FADS allows simultaneous anesthesia with flow of water over the gills in fish, allowing continuous oxygen exchange, in conjunction with the ability to keep the skin moist during prolonged procedures (Figure 35.6). The same bath anesthetic can be applied directly to the skin of non-gilled amphibians, in order to maintain an appropriate depth of anesthesia (Figure 35.7).

A number of different water-based chemicals have been evaluated as bath anesthetics in fish and amphibians. Tricaine methanesulfonate, or MS-222, is currently the only FDA-approved chemical for use as an anesthetic

Veterinary Anesthetic and Monitoring Equipment, First Edition. Edited by Kristen G. Cooley and Rebecca A. Johnson.
© 2018 John Wiley & Sons, Inc. Published 2018 by John Wiley & Sons, Inc.

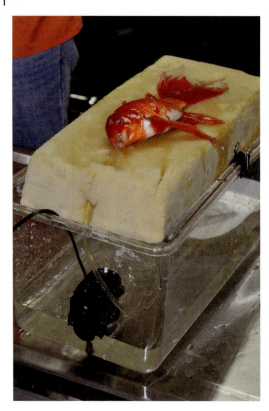

Figure 35.1 Fish Anesthesia Delivery System (FADS); anesthetized koi (*Cyprinus carpio*) in right lateral recumbency being maintained with MS-222 (100 mg/L).

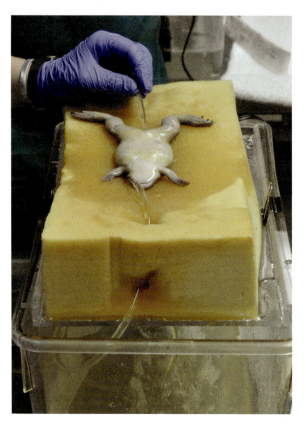

Figure 35.2 Fish Anesthesia Delivery System (FADS); anesthetized African clawed frog (*Xenopus laevis*) in dorsal recumbency being maintained with MS-222 (100 mg/L).

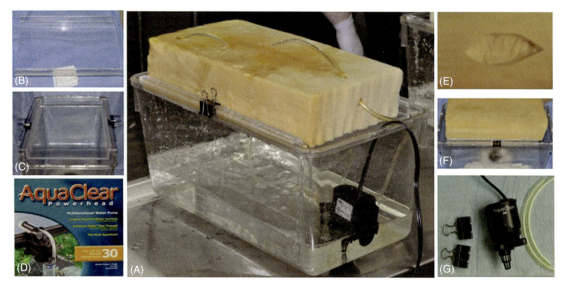

Figure 35.3 Components of a Fish Anesthesia Delivery System (FADS). (A) The complete FADS; (B and C) Plexiglas platform upon which the foam pad (E and F) is placed; (C) Allentown Microvent Rat Cage without top (Model: MBS10198MV, Allentown, NJ); (D) Hagen Aquaclear 310 powerhead; (E and F) Mattress foam cut to size with a wedge to conform to the fish; (G) Composite image of Hagen Aquaclear 310 powerhead, 2 large binder clips and 2 × 12–18″ of 1/4″ inner diameter aquarium plastic tubing (not shown, 6″ of 3/8″ inner diameter plastic tubing.

Table 35.1 Components of a fish anesthesia device for use in small- to medium-sized fish.

Plastic laboratory rodent cage without top (alternative is a 10-gallon glass aquarium)	Dimensions: 10 3/4"W × 19 1/4"D × 10 3/4"H. Allentown Microvent Rat Cage Model: MBS10198MV. Allentown, NJ 08501. Durable and easy to disinfect
Plexiglas platform	Available for custom order at most glass or plastic companies. Dimensions: 15 1/2"L × 8 3/4"W , with 2 "L"-shaped lips on each side (5/8" vertical glued to 5/8" horizontal). 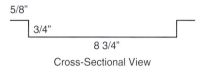 5/8" / 3/4" / 8 3/4" / Cross-Sectional View
310 Aquarium pump (Hagen Powerhead)	Available at most pet stores
Flexible aquarium plastic tubing	Available at most pet stores or hardware stores: 2 sets each of 12–18" of 1/4" inner diameter tubing; 6" of 3/8"
Rectangular mattress foam pad cut to fit the Plexiglas support top (a wedge can be cut in one side of the foam to accommodate a fish in dorsal recumbency)	Mattress companies frequently have residual foam mattress padding free of charge. Fabric or craft stores will sell foam
Binder clips	2 medium to large binder clips to bind the Plexiglas to the plastic rodent cage.
TOTAL COST	<$100.00

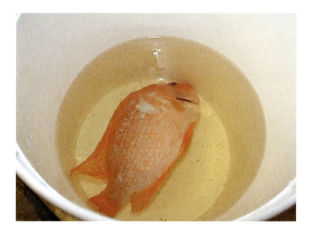

Figure 35.4 Koi (*Cyprinus carpio*) being anesthetically induced in MS-222 (200 mg/L) immersion bath in a clean, large plastic bucket.

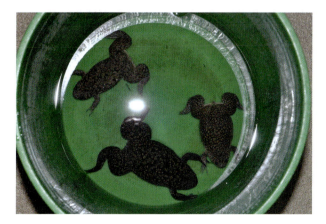

Figure 35.5 Three African clawed frogs (*Xenopus laevis*) being anesthetically induced in an MS-222 (500 mg/L) immersion bath in a clean, large plastic bucket.

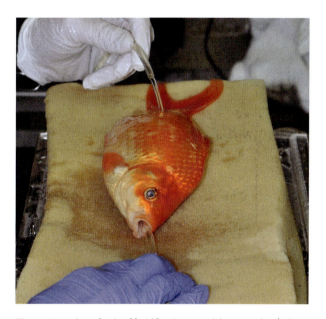

Figure 35.6 Anesthetized koi (*Cyprinus carpio*) on a recirculating anesthesia device (FADS). Notice that one plastic tube is inserted in the oral cavity to bathe the gills in anesthetic (MS-222) water, while the second plastic tube is used to keep the skin of the fish moist.

in fish, but requires a 21-day withdrawal period in food fish (Mylniczenko *et al.* 2014). MS-222 is a water-soluble, crystalline powder that can be used to produce a working stock solution of 10 mg/mL when mixed in clean, dechlorinated water and buffered appropriately. Since MS-222 is acidic, the stock solution should be buffered with sodium bicarbonate. A typical stock solution (10 mg/mL) recipe is as follows: 10 g of powdered tricaine methanesulfonate plus 5–10 g of sodium bicarbonate

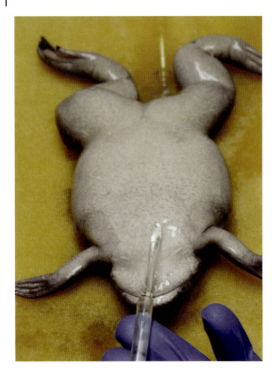

Figure 35.7 Anesthetized African clawed frog (*Xenopus laevis*) on a recirculating anesthesia device (FADS). Notice the two plastic tubes are used to continuously bathe the frog in anesthetic (MS-222) water.

usually anesthetize most species within a matter of 3 to 5 minutes (Mylniczenko *et al.* 2014). For sedation and induction of amphibians, the effective concentration varies dramatically, with tadpoles, gilled and other aquatic amphibians requiring approximately 500 mg/L and some terrestrial toads and salamanders requiring up to 5000 mg/L (Wright 2001).

A variety of methods can be used for anesthetic induction and recovery in fish and amphibians, and include the use of clean plastic buckets, plastic bags (e.g. Zip-Loc® bags), stainless steel dishes and buckets, plastic food containers and dishes, glass bowls, etc. (Figure 35.8). For manual restraint, the handler should wear powder-free gloves and use a net for capturing fish and aquatic amphibians (Figures 35.9 and 35.10). Once induced, the fish or amphibian patient can be maintained using the bath anesthetic or lunged amphibians can be intubated and maintained on a gas anesthetic machine (e.g. isoflurane or sevoflurane). Time to recovery from MS-222 bath anesthetic induction and maintenance is relatively rapid, with most fish regaining their righting reflex within 5 minutes, and appearing fully recovered within 10 minutes. Amphibians tend to recover more slowly than fish, depending on the duration of MS-222 exposure. Terrestrial amphibians should be placed on moist towels or in very shallow water during recovery, with the head propped up on moistened gauze pads during induction and recovery (Figure 35.11).

As mentioned above, MS-222 is considered to be the most widely-used bath anesthetic for fish and amphibians, but because of its cost and limited availability in some areas of the world, and because there is some evidence that it may cause retinal damage with prolonged use in fish, amphibians and humans (a single case) (Rapp and Basinger 1982; Bernstein *et al.* 1997), there has been con-

added to 1 L dechlorinated water (or aquarium water from which the fish is currently maintained). The stock solution should be stored in a glass bottle away from light at room temperature. When prepared and stored in this manner, the stock solution is good for approximately 30 days. For sedation and anesthetic induction of fish, final concentrations of between 100 and 200 mg/L will

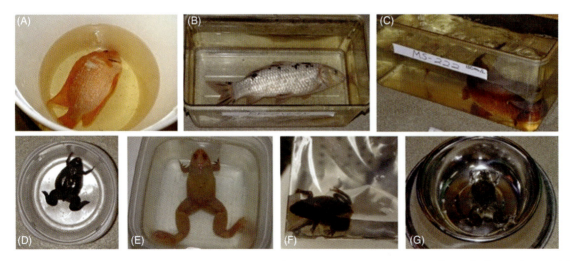

Figure 35.8 A composite image demonstrating a variety of readily available containers for inducing bath anesthesia in fish and amphibians. (A) Koi (*Cyprinus carpio*) in a standard plastic bucket; (B and C) Koi (*C. carpio*) in commercial rat cages; (D and E) Frogs (*Xenopus laevis*) in commercial plastic containers; (F) Frogs (*X. laevis*) in a plastic bag and in a stainless-steel dog dish (G).

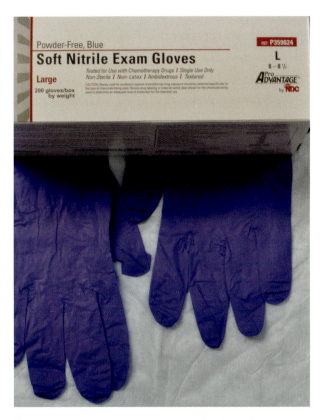

Figure 35.9 Example of powder-free, nitrile gloves for use in handling fish and amphibians.

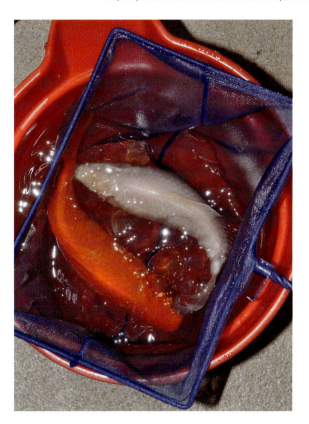

Figure 35.10 Two koi (*Cyprinus carpio*) being manually restrained from a plastic bucket using a net.

siderable interest in alternative bath anesthetics. Clove oil has recently become a widely-used alternative anesthetic agent to MS-222 in the commercial and "backyard" fish industries in the US and Japan (Sladky *et al.* 2001). It is also used in amphibians in clinical practice, as well as research. The active ingredient of clove oil is eugenol (4-allyl-2-methoxyphenol), a phenolic compound. It is an attractive anesthetic substance for use in fish and amphibians, because it is commercially available, inexpensive and is considered a GRAS (generally regarded as safe) substance by the USFDA (the USFDA does *not*, however, condone its use in food fish) (Sladky *et al.* 2001). Clove oil is available as an over-the-counter product (~84% eugenol) at most pharmacies, or as a 100% eugenol chemical grade from Sigma Chemical Company® (Sigma-Aldrich, St Louis, MO). Eugenol is an oil, which is not soluble in water and should be diluted with ethanol at a ratio of 1:10 (1 mL clove oil:9 mL ethanol) to yield a working stock solution of 85–100 mg/mL, depending on the source of the eugenol (over-the-counter clove oil is typically 84% eugenol, whereas the chemical product is 100% eugenol). Concentrations of 50–100 mg/L are effective for anesthetic induction in most fish species, but higher concentrations are necessary in amphibians (200–500 mg/L) (Baitchman and Stetter 2014). One should be cautious

when using eugenol, however, as the margin of safety is narrow, so death can occur more rapidly if the animal is not well monitored. In addition, recovery is significantly prolonged when compared with MS-222 anesthesia.

Similar in mechanism of action to eugenol, isoeugenol (Aqui-S®, Aqui-S New Zealand, Lower Hutt, NZ) is a

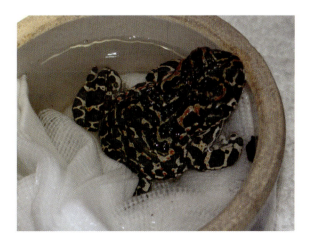

Figure 35.11 Moroccan midwife toad (*Alytes maurus*) in a dish containing MS-222. In amphibians with lungs, it is important to maintain the animal's head above the anesthetic immersion bath water in order to prevent aspiration.

pre-mixed bath anesthetic product approved for use in fish in many countries. Isoeugenol is widely being used globally as a fish anesthetic due to its approved use in many European, and South and Central American countries, as well as Australia and New Zealand, and is currently under consideration for approval by the US FDA (Investigative New Animal Drug). Aqui-S® is a 50% isoeugenol solution, while Aqui-S®20E is a 10% isoeugenol solution, and both can be added directly to non-chlorinated water for use in fish and amphibians. Aqui-S®20E is currently under review by the FDA for approval in fish. Isoeugenol was demonstrated to be an effective anesthetic in several fish species (Young 2009; Gladden *et al.* 2010). One significant caution about using eugenol products in fish and amphibians is that there are no systematically-derived data demonstrating analgesia, and therefore, performing invasive procedures while the animal is under eugenol-based anesthesia cannot be considered ethical. Therefore, an analgesic drug, preferably a mu-opioid receptor agonist (e.g. morphine) should be administered prior to performing fish surgery while using a eugenol-based product (Baker *et al.* 2013).

Alfaxalone was recently demonstrated to be an effective and safe anesthetic when administered as a bath in Oscar fish (Bugman *et al.* 2016) and koi (Minter *et al.* 2014), but was not considered safe or effective when administered intramuscularly in koi (Bailey *et al.* 2014). In amphibians, alfaxolone immersion appears to be most effective for sedation or induction in gilled species, but the effects are highly variable for induction in non-gilled amphibian species (Posner *et al.* 2013; Adami *et al.* 2016). Similarly, alfaxalone administered intramuscularly had variable results in those amphibian species tested (Posner *et al.* 2013). Propofol can be administered as a bath anesthetic or administered intravenously in fish. In koi, propofol immersion was effective for anesthesia, but 1 out of 9 koi died during the study, so it appears to have a narrow margin of safety (Oda *et al.* 2014). In amphibians, propofol as an immersion preparation does not appear to be effective or safe for sedation or anesthetic induction (Guénette *et al.* 2008).

35.2.2 Inhalational Anesthetics for Amphibians

For non-gilled amphibians, inhalational anesthetic agents can be used topically or administered as a gas absorbed transcutaneously, or delivered via the pulmonary system with endotracheal intubation achieved on larger, lunged species. Isoflurane and sevoflurane have been used topically to induce anesthesia with moderate to good success, depending on the technique employed. Isoflurane-saturated topical patches (0.03–0.06 mL/g) worked well in one study to induce anesthesia in African clawed frogs

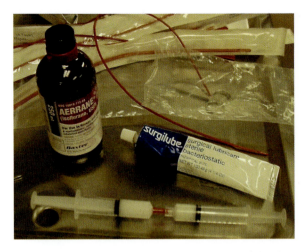

Figure 35.12 Isoflurane (or sevoflurane) can be mixed with water and sterile lubricating gel to produce an anesthetic gel for skin application in amphibians.

(Mitchell 2009). Transcutaneous isoflurane administration has been successfully applied to a variety of frog species by either dripping on isoflurane liquid to effect or by mixing isoflurane or sevoflurane with water and lubricating gel (Figures 35.12 and 35.13) (Mitchell 2009; Stone *et al.* 2013). However, there are a number of reports of skin sloughing in amphibians after application of isoflurane or sevoflurance liquid; therefore, this method should be used with caution. Isoflurane or seveoflurane in gas form can be effective and safe when applied using an anesthetic mask or chamber, preferably by putting the entire individual within an appropriately sized mask or chamber (Figure 35.14) (Mitchell 2009). However, with this method, the time to induction can be significantly prolonged, depending on the species being anesthetized. Once induced, amphibian species with lungs can be intubated with an appropriately sized, uncuffed endotracheal tube (Figure 35.15). The glottis is at the base of the tongue,

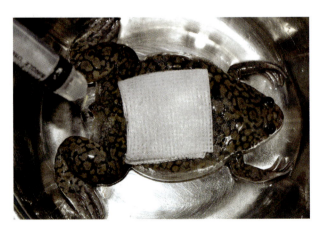

Figure 35.13 African clawed frog (*Xenopus laevis*) with isoflurane gel applied to the dorsum and covered with a small gauze pad.

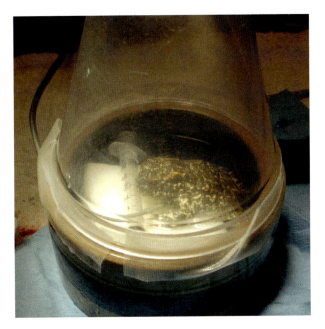

Figure 35.14 Moroccan midwife toad (*Alytes maurus*) being anesthetically induced with inhaled isoflurane using a standard large facemask.

much like reptiles, but the trachea is extremely short, so care must be taken so as not to advance the tube too far, causing intubation of a primary bronchus or doing damage to the trachea. Use of a Cole tube can be of benefit and provides a limited length of the tube entering the short trachea. Isoflurane has been administered to amphibians subcutaneously, intracoelomically and intramuscularly, but with generally unfavorable results.

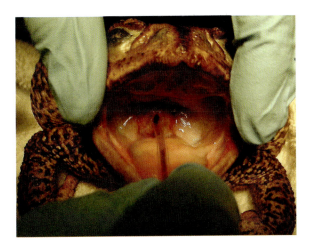

Figure 35.15 Endotracheal intubation of an unknown *Bufo* species. In amphibian species with lungs, endotracheal intubation, only using an uncuffed tube, is relatively simple, with the glottis located at the base of the tongue. Due to the short trachea prior to primary bronchi bifurcation, one should be cautious with depth of endotracheal tube placement. A Cole tube may be useful, as it limits the length of the tube passing beyond the glottis.

35.3 Anesthetic Monitoring

Monitoring anesthetized fish and amphibians is relatively straightforward and minimal equipment is required. The most significant problem with respect to the interpretation of anesthetic monitoring is that the hearts of fish and amphibians have intrinsic pacemakers, which may keep the heart beating beyond successful resuscitation of the animal.

35.3.1 Respiratory Rate Monitoring

Respiratory rate is measured in fish by monitoring opercular movements, which can be counted and indicated as opercular rate per minute (Figure 35.16). In amphibians, respiratory rate is measured by counting gular movements, or the inward and outward movements of the tissue in the intermandibular space (Figure 35.17). In larger amphibians with lungs, thoracic and coelomic movement may be observed during inspiration and expiration, in addition to gular movement. In gilled amphibians, the external gills grossly move regularly when respiring, and the movements can be counted.

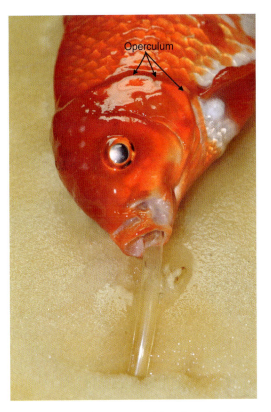

Figure 35.16 Koi (*Cyprinus carpio*) under recirculating bath anesthesia with MS-222 in right lateral recumbency. The left operculum is shown (black arrows), which can be monitored for respiratory rate in teleost fish species.

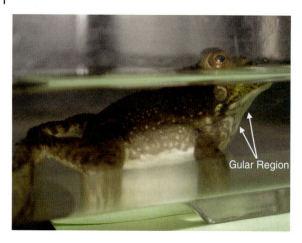

Figure 35.17 Conscious American bull frog (*Lithobates catesbeianus*) in a hospital transport aquarium. The gular region is shown (white arrows), which can be monitored for respiratory rate in many amphibian species.

35.3.2 Cardiac Function Monitoring

35.3.2.1 Stethoscope

Cardiac auscultation using a stethoscope is the most straightforward method for monitoring heart rate in amphibians, but is more difficult in fish due to the location of the heart and the noise of the water flowing over the gills when the fish is on a recirculating anesthesia machine. In smaller amphibians, the heart can be visualized grossly when the amphibian is in dorsal recumbency.

35.3.2.2 Doppler Flow Probe

An excellent alternative to the stethoscope for monitoring heart rate is to use a Doppler flow probe, which is an important piece of equipment to have when monitoring fish and amphibians under anesthesia. Proper placement of the Doppler flow probe allows audible monitoring of blood flow through the heart. Contact gel can be placed on the concave side of the probe, and the probe is placed over the region of the heart. In fish, the heart is relatively small and is located on the ventrum, approximately where the right and left opercula meet ventrally on the midline of the fish (Figure 35.18). Water flow from a recirculating anesthesia machine may be audible from the Doppler speaker, and in this case, a slight cranial adjustment of the probe will be required. In amphibians, the Doppler flow probe can be placed on the ventral midline at the level of the pectoral girdle, much like reptiles (Figure 35.19).

35.3.2.3 Ultrasound Probe

In those species of fish where it is not practical or possible to listen to the heart using a Doppler flow probe, a portable ultrasound probe can be used to locate the heart and monitor heart rate.

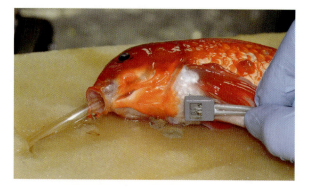

Figure 35.18 Koi (*Cyprinus carpio*) under recirculating bath anesthesia with MS-222 in right lateral recumbency. For evaluating heart rate in teleost fish species, the Doppler flow probe should be placed on the ventral midline, just caudal to the area in which the operculae meet. Coupling gel should be placed on the concave side of the probe prior to placement.

35.3.2.4 Electrocardiography (ECG)

Cardiac rhythm monitoring using an ECG may also be useful in both fish and amphibian patients (Baitchman and Stetter 2014; Mylniczenko *et al.* 2014). Standard mammalian leads can be used, but it may be necessary to attach the leads to the fins/skin using alligator clips clamped onto either hypodermic needles or stainless steel sutures passed through the fins/skin (Figures 35.20 and 35.21). In addition, atraumatic clips and leads directly attached to fine needles may be used (ZUMAYA™ ECG Electrode Kit, Sentier Connect, Brookfield, WI). In most amphibians, the cranial electrodes can be placed in the prescapular region and the caudal electrodes just cranial to the hind limbs. In limbless amphibians (e.g. caecilians), the electrodes should be placed as with snakes; two heart-lengths cranial and

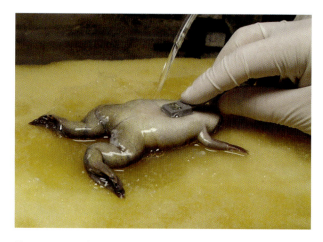

Figure 35.19 African clawed frog (*Xenopus laevis*) under recirculating bath anesthesia with MS-222 in dorsal recumbency. For evaluating heart rate in most amphibian species, the Doppler flow probe should be placed on the ventral midline, just caudal to the pectoral girdle. Coupling gel should be placed on the concave side of the probe prior to placement.

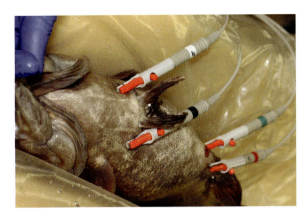

Figure 35.20 Smallmouth bass (*Micropterus dolomieu*) under recirculating bath anesthesia with MS-222 in dorsal recumbency. For evaluating heart rate and rhythm, a 4-lead, electrocardiogram (ECG) is attached near the pectoral and anal fins of the fish (photograph courtesy of the University of Wisconsin).

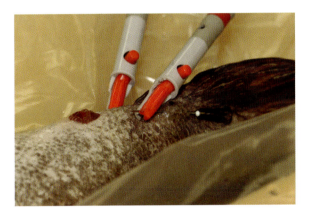

Figure 35.21 A close-up of the Smallmouth bass (*Micropterus dolomieu*) in Figure 35.20 demonstrating the use of hypodermic needles placed through the skin near the pectoral and anal fins; the ECG alligator clamps are attached to the hypodermic needles for best results (photograph courtesy of the University of Wisconsin).

caudal to the heart. In fish, three electrodes can be placed at the base of the pelvic fins and at the base of the anal fin. If attempting to use the newer, portable, hand-held, 2-lead ECGs, the leads can be placed on one pectoral fin and the anal or tail fin of fish, or the hind limb and fore limb of limbed amphibians (Figures 35.22 and 35.23).

35.3.3 Pulse Oximetry

Pulse oximetry is used to monitor both aspects of the respiratory system, but relies on pulsatile blood flow from the cardiovascular system. A pulse oximeter measures pulse rate and indirectly estimates arterial oxygen hemoglobin saturation. However, it is calibrated based on the oxygen-hemoglobin dissociation curve in humans. In mammals, pulse oximetry values are subject to error due to poor peripheral vascular perfusion, dark skin pigmentation and muscle movement, etc. In fish and amphibians, small cloacal probes may be the most practical, since finger and other clip probes are not particularly adaptable to fish anatomy, and the anatomy of some amphibian species. However, pulse oximeters may not be particularly useful in most fish and amphibian species, because it is extremely difficult to impossible to achieve an accurate reading and consistently interpret the true meaning of the measured value.

35.3.4 Blood Gas Analyses

Measuring blood gases in fish and amphibians using a portable clinical analyzer (e.g. iSTAT®, Abbott Laboratories, Abbott Park, IL) may provide some useful information regarding trends in venous (or mixed venous-arterial) PO_2 over time using multiple samples, but a single value at one time point is meaningless (Figure 35.24). While there is ongoing debate as to whether results from an iSTAT must

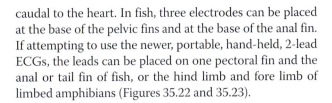

Figure 35.22 Koi (*Cyprinus carpio*) under recirculating bath anesthesia with MS-222 in dorsal recumbency. For evaluating heart rate and rhythm, a 2-lead, portable electrocardiogram (ECG) (Sentier Vetcorder®, Sentier, Brookfield, WI) is attached to the fins of the koi; one lead is attached to a pectoral fin and the second lead is attached to the tail fin.

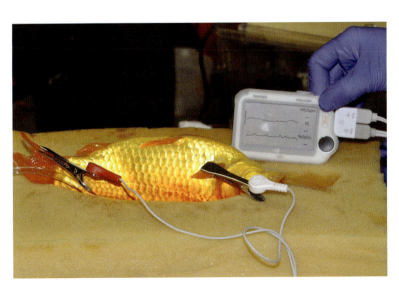

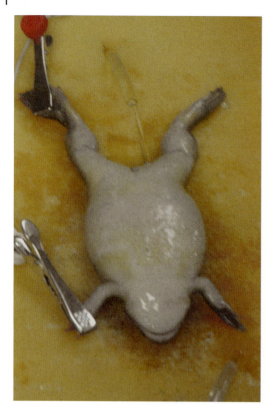

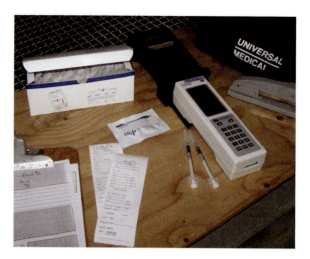

Figure 35.24 An iSTAT® handheld, portable point-of-care blood biochemical analyzer can be used for serial monitoring of mixed arterial-venous blood gases and biochemicals in fish and venous blood gases and biochemicals in amphibians during prolonged procedures. A single value is meaningless in fish and amphibians, but multiple samples over time can provide useful monitoring trends. In this image, a yellow perch (*Perca flavescens*) blood sample is being analyzed for blood gases, lactate and glucose using a CG4+ cartridge (photograph courtesy of Dr C. Hanley, DACZM).

Figure 35.23 African clawed frog (*Xenopus laevis*) under recirculating bath anesthesia with MS-222 in dorsal recumbency. For evaluating heart rate and rhythm, a 2-lead, portable electrocardiogram (ECG) (Sentier Vetcorder®, Sentier, Brookfield, WI) is attached to the limbs of the frog; one lead is attached to a fore limb and the second lead is attached to the hind limb.

be temperature corrected for the fish or amphibian species, in most research projects, iSTAT blood gas values are measured at 37°C and corrected for the body temperature of the fish or amphibian, or the water temperature (Sladky *et al.* 2001). In addition, other blood biochemical parameters, such as glucose and lactate, can be measured using the iSTAT, depending on the type of cartridge selected. There is evidence that significantly elevated blood lactate concentrations (e.g. >10 mmol/L) may be predictive of poor prognosis for survival with prolonged anesthetic or surgical procedures in some fish species (Hanley *et al.* 2010).

References

Adami, C., d'Ovidio, D. and Casoni, D. (2016) Alfaxalone versus alfaxalone-dexmedetomidine anaesthesia by immersion in oriental fire-bellied toads (*Bombina orientalis*). *Vet Anaesth Analg*, 43, 326–332.

Bailey, K.M., Minter, L.J., Lewbart, G.A., Harms, C.A., Griffith, E.H. and Posner, L.P. (2014) Alfaxalone as an intramuscular injectable anesthetic in koi carp (*Cyprinus carpio*). *J Zoo Wildl Med*, 45, 852–858.

Baitchman, E. and Stetter, M. (2014) Amphibians. In: West, G., Heard, D. and Culkett, N. (eds). *Zoo Animal and Wildlife Immobilization and Anesthesia*, 2nd ed. Ames, IA: Blackwell, pp. 303–312.

Baker, T., Baker, B., Johnson, S.M. and Sladky, K.K. (2013) Comparative analgesic efficacy of morphine and butorphanol in koi (*Cyprinus carpio*) undergoing gonadectomy. *J Am Vet Med Assoc*, 243, 882–890.

Bernstein, P.S., Digre, K.B. and Creel, D.J. (1997) Retinal toxicity associated with occupational exposure to the fish anesthetic MS-222. *Am J Ophthalmol*, 124, 843–844.

Bugman, A.M., Langer, P.T., Hadzima, E., Rivas, A.E. and Mitchell, M.A. (2016) Evaluation of the anesthetic efficacy of alfaxalone in oscar fish (*Astronotus ocellatus*). *Am J Vet Res*, 77, 239–244.

Gladden, J.N., Brainard, B.M., Shelton, J.L., Camus, A.C. and Divers, S.J. (2010.) Evaluation of isoeugenol for anesthesia in koi carp (*Cyprinus carpio*). *Am J Vet Res*, 71, 859–866.

Guénette, S.A., Beaudry, F. and Vachon, P. (2008) Anesthetic properties of propofol in African clawed frogs (*Xenopus laevis*). *J Am Assoc Lab Anim Sci*, 47, 35–38.

Hanley, C.S., Clyde, V., Wallace, R., Paul-Murphy, J., Patterson, T.A. *et al.* (2010) Effects of anesthesia and elective ovariectomy on serial blood gases and lactates in yellow perch (*Perca flavescens*), walleye pike (*Sander vitreus*), and koi (*Cyprinus carpio*): can lactate predict post-operative survival? *J Am Vet Med Assoc*, 236, 1104–1108.

Lewbart, G.A. and Harms, C.A. (1999) Building a fish anesthesia delivery system. *Exotic DVM*, 1.2, 25–29.

Minter, L.J., Bailey, K.M., Harms, C.A., Lewbart, G.A. and Posner, L.P. (2014) The efficacy of alfaxalone for immersion anesthesia in koi carp (*Cyprinus carpio*). *Vet Anaesth Analg*, 41, 398–405.

Mitchell, M.A. (2009) Anesthetic considerations for amphibians. *J Exotic Pet Med*, 18, 40–49.

Mylniczenko, N.D., Neiffer, D.A. and Clauss, T.M. (2014) Bony fish (lungfish, sturgeon and teleosts). In: West, G., Heard, D. and Culkett, N. (eds). *Zoo Animal and Wildlife Immobilization and Anesthesia*, 2nd ed. Ames, IA: Blackwell, pp. 209–260.

Oda, A., Bailey, K.M., Lewbart, G.A., Griffith, E.H. and Posner, L.P. (2014) Physiologic and biochemical assessments of koi (*Cyprinus carpio*) following immersion in propofol. *J Am Vet Med Assoc*, 245, 1286–1291.

Posner, L.P., Bailey, K.M., Richardson, E.Y., Motsinger-Reif, A.A. and Harms, C.A. (2013) faxalone anesthesia in bullfrogs (*Lithobates catesbeiana*) by injection or immersion. *J Zoo Wildl Med*, 44, 965–971.

Rapp, L,M. and Basinger, S.F. (1982) The effects of local anesthetics on retinal function. *Vision Res*, 22, 1097–1103.

Sladky, K.K., Swanson, C.R., Stoskopf, M.K., Loomis, M.R. and Lewbart, GA. (2001) omparative efficacy of MS-222 (tricaine methanesulfonate) and clove oil (eugenol) in red pacu (*Piaractus brachypomus*). *Am J Vet Res*, 62, 337–342.

Stone, S.M., Clark-Price, S.C., Boesch, J.M. and Mitchell, M.A. (2013) Evaluation of righting reflex in cane toads (*Bufo marinus*) after topical application of sevoflurane jelly. *Am J Vet Res*, 74, 823–827.

Wright, K. (2001) Restraint techniques and euthanasia. In: Wright, K. and Whitaker, B.R. (eds). *Amphibian Medicine and Captive Husbandry*. Malabar, FL: Krieger, pp. 111–122.

Young, M.J. (2009) The efficacy of the aquatic anaesthetic AQUI-S for anaesthesia of a small freshwater fish, *Melanotaenia australis*. *J Fish Biol*, 75, 1888–1894.

36

Unique Species Considerations: Reptiles

Christoph Mans

School of Veterinary Medicine, University of Wisconsin, Madison, Wisconsin, USA

36.1   Introduction

Reptiles are a highly diverse group of ectothermic animals. They provide unique challenges to the anesthetist due to their anatomy and physiology, which varies widely amongst different groups. Standard anesthetic equipment can often be used to induce and maintain anesthesia in reptiles, although using standard anesthetic monitoring equipment such as pulse oximetry or capnography is more controversial; these devices are not validated for most reptile species.

36.2   Anesthetic Induction

Anesthetic induction using inhalant anesthesia is frequently performed in snakes as well as small lizards (e.g. geckos), which are difficult to restrain. Snakes can be restrained and induced in a snake tube (Figure 36.1) covered with a facemask (Figures 36.2 and 36.3).

Different diameter snake tubes are commercially available (Figure 36.1) or can be made from clear plastic tubing. Snakes will advance through the snake tube, but are unable to turn around if an appropriate sized tube is chosen. The snake should be restrained at the caudal end (Figure 36.3) once it has moved far enough into the tube. Once anesthetic induction has been achieved, the snake may be removed from the tube, or may remain restrained within the tube if access to the oral cavity is necessary and can be achieved (Figure 36.4).

Alternatively, snakes and small lizards can be induced in standard induction chambers or larger face masks (Figure 36.5), which allow free movement of the reptile, in comparison to snake tubes.

Snakes are often transported in cloth bags, and may be placed directly in the induction chamber with prior removal from the bag. This technique is commonly used in venomous species, since direct contact and risk of injury is minimized. The limitation of placing the cloth bag into the induction chamber is the lack of visualization of the snake, and therefore only limited assessment on the anesthetic depth of the patient is possible until an adequate anesthetic depth is achieved. Once the righting reflex has been reduced, the snake should be removed from the cloth bag and continued anesthetic gas delivery performed by an endotracheal tube.

Small snakes and lizards can be induced using self-sealing plastic bags (i.e. plastic zippered bags; Figure 36.6). The animal is placed in an appropriately sized bag and the bag is filled with anesthetic gas delivered in 100% oxygen (Figure 36.6). The bag is then sealed and the patient visualized until anesthetic induction has occurred.

Mask induction is less frequently performed, in larger lizards (Figure 36.7A), for which injectable induction agents are deemed inappropriate. Delivery of anesthetic gases by mask may also be used to deepen anesthesia prior to endotracheal intubation, if the injectable induction agents did not reach the desired anesthetic depth (Figure 36.7B).

36.3   Airway Intubation

Endotracheal intubation is recommended for all reptiles that do not breathe spontaneously and have no protective airway reflexes. The mouth should be opened carefully in reptiles, due to the risk of iatrogenic trauma to the teeth and gingiva. Iatrogenic tooth fractures are a common complication, especially if force is applied. Snakes can regrow damaged teeth, while many lizard species with acrodont teeth (e.g. bearded dragons, chameleons) cannot. Kitchen spatulas (Figure 36.8A), plastic cards (e.g. credit cards) or tongue depressors (Figure 36.8B) can be used to open the mouth for

Veterinary Anesthetic and Monitoring Equipment, First Edition. Edited by Kristen G. Cooley and Rebecca A. Johnson.
© 2018 John Wiley & Sons, Inc. Published 2018 by John Wiley & Sons, Inc.

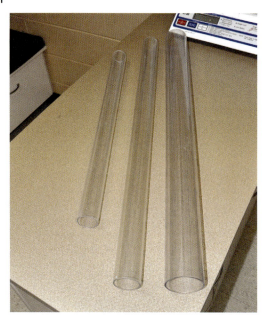

Figure 36.1 Clear plastic snake tubes of various sizes.

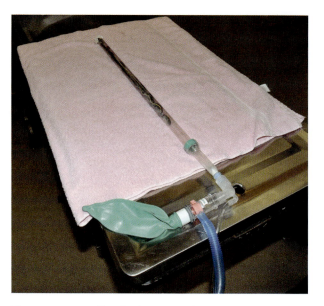

Figure 36.2 A small snake during anesthetic induction in a snake tube. Note that the adapter connecting the snake tube with the non-rebreathing circuit has been made from a syringe case and latex glove. The snake is small enough to fit into the snake tube, and the tube has been sealed caudally with masking tape.

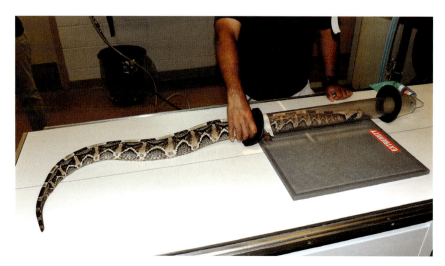

Figure 36.3 Venomous Gabon viper anesthetized in a snake tube for radiographs. Note how the snake is restrained caudally in order to avoid movement.

intubation. Alternatively, elastic or plastic straps or ties (Figure 36.8C) or gauze strips can be used, which carry lower risk of iatrogenic trauma.

Chelonians (i.e. turtles and tortoises) have closed tracheal rings (and short tracheas prior to bifurcation), whereas squamates (i.e. lizards and snakes) have incomplete tracheal rings (Schumacher and Mans 2014). Only uncuffed endotracheal tubes are recommended in chelonians, small lizards and snakes. If uncuffed tubes are not available, cuffed tubes can also be used; however, cuffs should not be inflated or if inflation is necessary, should be done with extreme caution to minimize tracheal pressure. In larger squamates, cuffed and inflated tubes can

be used with caution. Uncuffed tubes come in small sizes (Figure 36.9A) and Cole tubes (Figure 36.9B) may be used to avoid accidental intubation of a major bronchus in chelonians, since the trachea bifurcates early.

If an endotracheal tube of appropriate size is not available, then intravenous catheters (Figure 36.10) or red-rubber catheters with the tip cut off and smoothed can be used instead. Care should be taken not to kink any small diameter endotracheal tubes, since it will lead to occlusion of the tube. This risk is particularly high with intravenous catheters.

Securing the endotracheal tubes after intubation can be challenging in reptiles, particularly in, snakes. Tape is

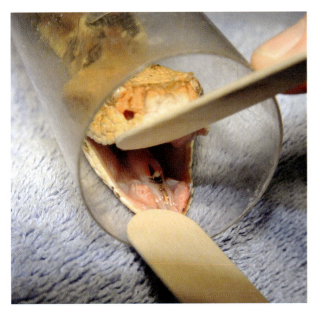

Figure 36.4 Safe access to the oral cavity for endotracheal intubation of an anesthetized venomous snake located in a snake tube.

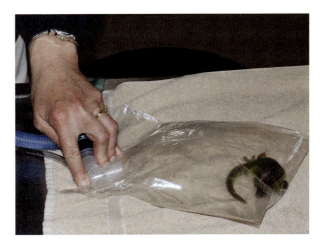

Figure 36.6 Madagascar day gecko in a Ziploc bag for anesthetic induction. The bag is filled with anesthetic gas delivered in oxygen and the bag is sealed.

(Figure 36.11C). Small lizards and snakes along with their endotracheal tube can be taped to a tongue depressor to avoid tube movement (Figure 36.12A).

36.4 Anesthetic Monitoring

36.4.1 Ultrasonic Doppler Devices

Ultrasonic Dopplers are the most reliable method to monitor heart rate in reptiles (Sladky and Mans 2012). Flat probes are more widely available and used in reptile anesthesia, since they can be secured onto the patient for continuous monitoring (Figures 36.12A and 36.13). Pencil probes (Figure 36.12B) can also be used, but are difficult to secure to the patient, and are therefore most commonly used for intermittent monitoring of the heart rate. The ultrasonic Doppler probe can be placed directly

usually the most effective method of securing endotracheal tubes (Figures 36.11A, B). The tape should first be applied around the endotracheal tube itself, before securing it to the head of the reptile patient to reduce the risk of the tube slipping. Use of two tongue depressors to "sandwich" the endotracheal tube also greatly enhances tube security (Figure 36.11B). The tongue depressors should be secured to the endotracheal tube itself first, and then to the patient. In lizards, elastic straps can also be used to secure the endotracheal tube. However, care should be taken not to obstruct small-diameter tubes by placing straps directly around the tube. Instead, tongue depressors or a small syringe should be taped to the tube and then the straps used to secure it to the patient

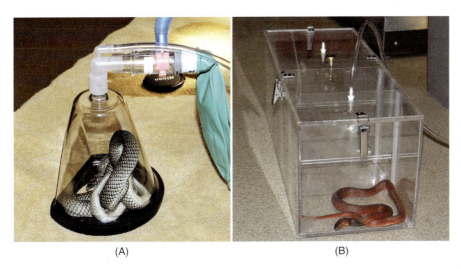

(A)   (B)

Figure 36.5 Anesthetic induction of a snake in a canine face mask (A) and in a commercially available induction chamber (B).

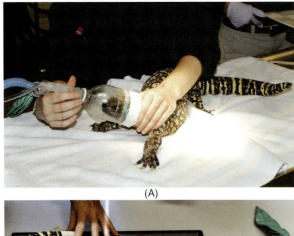

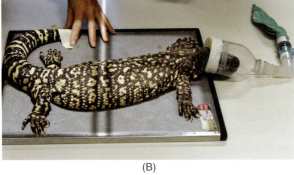

Figure 36.7 Mask induction (A) and anesthetic maintenance of a Mexican beaded lizard undergoing radiography (B).

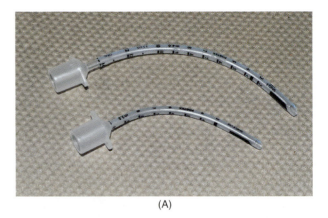

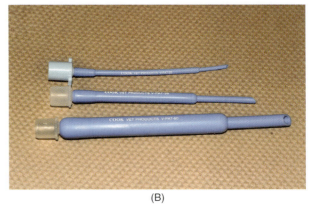

Figure 36.9 Uncuffed endotracheal tubes (A) and Cole tubes (B) suitable for intubation of a variety of reptiles.

over the heart in snakes and lizards, or the carotid arteries in lizards and chelonians. In lizards, the heart is located cranially between the forelimbs (except in monitor lizards and tegus), and the probe can either be positioned ventrally on the chest or in the axillary region. In chelonians, the placement of a Doppler probe for heart

rate measurement can be more challenging, since the heart cannot be directly accessed. Instead a flat or pencil probe can be placed over the carotid artery at the level of the thoracic inlet (Figure 36.14). Alternatively, the heart rate

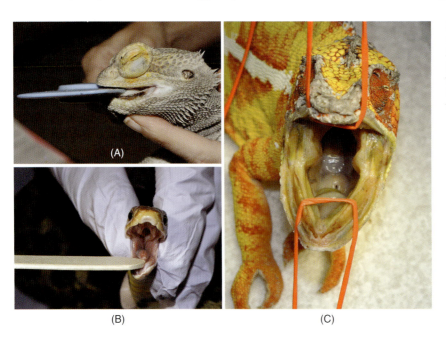

Figure 36.8 Opening the mouth of reptiles for endotracheal intubation. A spatula (A) will result in less iatrogenic injury of the gingiva and teeth, compared to a tongue depressor (B). Elastic strips can be used to hold the mouth open in order to perform endotracheal intubation (C).

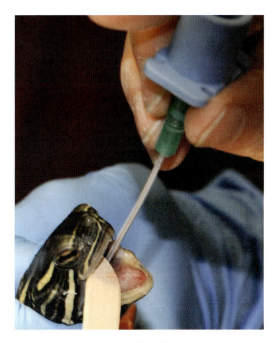

Figure 36.10 Endotracheal intubation in a freshwater turtle using an intravenous catheter.

can be monitored by echocardiography using appropriately sized probes and monitoring for myocardial contractions (Sladky and Mans 2012).

36.4.2 Indirect Blood Pressure Monitors

Indirect blood pressure monitoring in reptiles is poorly correlated with direct arterial blood pressure and therefore is minimally useful for monitoring of cardiovascular function (Chinnadurai *et al.* 2010). Direct blood pressure measurement by placement of arterial catheters is challenging in reptiles and therefore not routinely performed in clinical cases.

36.4.3 Electrocardiography (ECG)

ECG monitoring can be used in reptiles to monitor heart rate and rhythm (Figures 36.13 and 36.14). The reptilian ECG is similar to a mammalian ECG with a P, QRS and T wave, and in some species, an SV wave is present before the P wave. Low electrical amplitudes may make interpretation of a reptilian ECG challenging. ECGs are easily applied in all reptiles. For example, leads should be attached in snakes, two heart lengths cranial and caudal to the heart. In lizards and chelonians, leads may be placed in the cervical region instead of the front limbs (Kik and Mitchell 2005). In larger species, an esophageal ECG can be placed. Persistent baseline ECG and heart rate can also be detected in

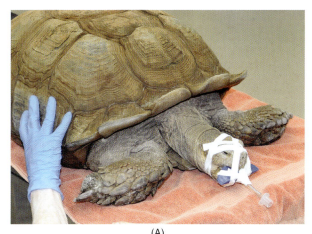

(A)

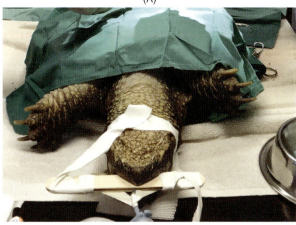

(B)

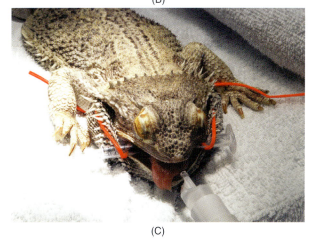

(C)

Figure 36.11 Securing endotracheal tubes in reptiles. Medical tape can be used to secure the tube to the head (A, B). The tube should be protected from biting using a commercially available bite block (A) or two tongue depressors (B). Elastic bands can also be used to secure tubes (C). Note the use of a 1-ml syringe as a bite block.

reptiles following CNS death; therefore, ECG as a monitor of cardiac activity for anesthetized reptiles is of limited value (Schumacher and Mans 2014).

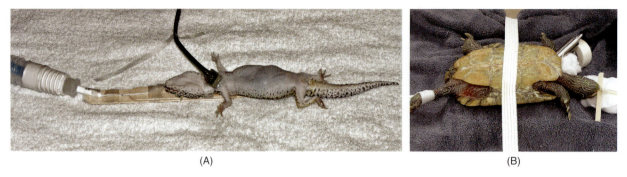

Figure 36.12 Use of an ultrasonic Doppler flat probe (A) and pencil probe (B).

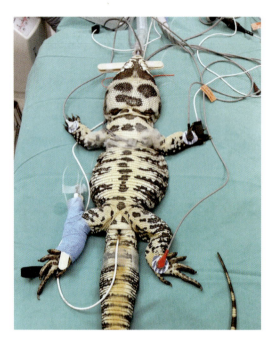

Figure 36.13 Anesthetized tegu lizard, with an intraosseous catheter (right tibia), ECG, cloacal pulse oximetry and Doppler flat probe used for anesthetic monitoring.

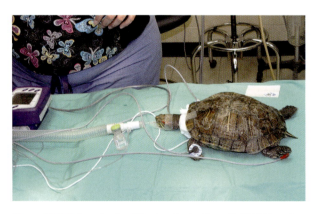

Figure 36.14 Anesthetized freshwater turtle, with ECG, Doppler flat probe and capnography used for anesthetic monitoring.

36.4.4 Pulse Oximetry

Pulse oximetry is routinely used in mammalian patients to calculate relative arterial oxygen hemoglobin saturation (SpO_2). Accuracy of pulse oximetry is influenced by poor tissue perfusion as well as pigmentation of the skin. In reptile anesthesia, use of pulse oximetry is associated with several concerns and potential erroneous readings (Schumacher and Mans 2014). For example, many pulse oximeters are calibrated based on the human oxygen hemoglobin dissociation curve and SpO_2 values are calculated, which affect pulse oximeter readings in reptiles. Additionally, high levels of methemoglobin have been reported in reptiles and will also interfere with accurate pulse oximeter readings, always shifting the reading to approximately 85% without the use of a co-oximeter. Further concerns are the pronounced differences in respiratory physiology and function among reptile species. Therefore, reference values derived from one taxa may be of limited accuracy in other taxa. However, if applied, reflectance pulse oximeter probes are most useful and can be placed into the esophagus at the level of the carotid artery, or in the evacuated cloaca (Figure 36.13) to provide continuous monitoring of arterial blood oxygen saturation and heart rate. Specific studies indicate that in anesthetized green iguanas, a comparison of arterial blood oxygen saturation as determined by pulse oximetry (SpO_2) versus arterial blood gas analysis (SaO_2) showed no significant differences between the two monitoring modalities over time (Hernandez-Divers *et al.* 2005). In addition, oxygen hemoglobin in conscious green iguanas calculated by pulse oximetry (86 ± 6%) was lower than the SaO_2 (92 ± 5%) indicated by arterial blood gas analysis; baseline SaO_2 values in conscious iguanas were reported to be more than 90% (Hernandez *et al.* 2011).

36.4.5 Blood Gas Analysis

Arterial blood gas analysis is rarely performed in clinical reptile anesthesia. Venous blood gases will give an assessment of metabolic status, and are affected by local tissue metabolism and low blood flow. However, in humans, venous blood gas analysis can predict arterial blood gas values for pH, PCO_2 and bicarbonate concentrations in some situations (Schumacher and Mans 2014). Baseline venous blood gas values in green iguanas are similar to those reported in humans and domestic animals (Hernandez *et al.* 2011). In reptiles, clinical interpretation of blood gas parameters is challenging, due to the lack of normal reference values in all taxa, as well as physiological features such as intra-cardiac or intra-pulmonary shunting, the ability to tolerate varying degrees of hypoxia, and the capability to convert to anaerobic metabolism (Schumacher and Mans 2014). In reptiles, many factors will influence normal arterial blood gas composition, including taxonomic differences (e.g. aquatic versus. terrestrial species), inspired concentration of oxygen and temperature.

At present, clinical application of interpretations based on mammalian blood gas values in reptiles is considered inaccurate, since reptiles have been shown to be more tolerant to changes in arterial partial pressures of oxygen and carbon dioxide. As mentioned above, intra-cardiac shunting and ventilation/perfusion mismatching (intra-pulmonary shunts) in reptiles may also result in inaccurate interpretation of arterial blood gases (Schumacher and Mans 2014). Circadian changes in arterial PO_2 and SaO_2 have been reported in green iguanas with values being significantly lower in the morning than in the afternoon. In most studies, blood gas values are determined at 37°C and corrected for the body temperature of the reptile (Hernandez *et al.* 2011).

36.4.6 Capnography

Capnography in reptiles is also associated with several limitations that may provide erroneous results (Figure 36.13). End-tidal CO_2 ($ETCO_2$) concentrations will provide an estimate of arterial CO_2 tensions; however, this technique has not been validated for reptiles (Schumacher and Mans 2014). Right to left intra-cardiac and intra-pulmonary shunts make this monitoring modality difficult to interpret. Another concern in small reptiles relates to the use of sidestream units with high sampling rates, which are likely to produce inaccurate results due to sample dilution with fresh gas (Schumacher and Mans 2014). Portable sidestream capnography units are available with low sampling rates adequate for even small patients, while pediatric mainstream units avoid the complication of sidestream dilution altogether. $ETCO_2$ appears to underestimate $PaCO_2$ in reptiles, but is a useful tool to monitor trends in arterial CO_2 tension (Schumacher and Mans 2014).

36.5   Summary

Reptile anesthesia is as diverse as the species being anesthetized. However, conventional equipment and monitors can work in these instances, especially with some slight modifications.

References

Chinnadurai, S.K., DeVoe, R., Koenig, A., Gadsen, N., Ardente, A. and Divers, S.J. (2010) Comparison of an implantable telemetry device and an oscillometric monitor for measurement of blood pressure in anaesthetized and unrestrained green iguanas (*Iguana iguana*). *Vet Anaesth Analg*, 37, 434–439.

Hernandez-Divers, S.M., Schumacher, J., Stahl, S. and Hernandez-Divers, S.J. (2005) Comparison of isoflurane and sevoflurane anesthesia after premedication with butorphanol in the green iguana (*Iguana iguana*). *J Zoo Wildl Med*, 36, 169–175.

Hernandez, S.M., Schumacher, J., Lewis, S.J., Odoi, A. and Divers, S.J. (2011) Selected cardiopulmonary values and baroreceptor reflex in conscious green iguanas (*Iguana iguana*). *Am J Vet Res*, 72, 1519–1526.

Kik, M.J.L. and Mitchell, M.A. (2005) Reptile cardiology: A review of anatomy and physiology, diagnostic approaches, and clinical disease. *Seminars in Avian and Exotic Pet Medicine*, 14, 52–60.

Schumacher, J. and Mans, C. (2014) Anesthesia. In: Mader, D. and Divers, S. (eds). *Current Therapy in Reptile Medicine and Surgery*. St Louis, Missouri: WB Saunders, pp. 134–153.

Sladky, K.K. and Mans, C. (2012) Clinical anesthesia in reptiles. *J Exot Pet Med*, 21, 158–167.

37

Unique Species Considerations: Non-Human Primates
Stephen Cital

Silicon Valley Veterinary Specialists, San Jose, California, USA

37.1 General Anatomy

Primates across the numerous different species have, in general, the same classic primate profile of a torso, arms with hands ending with longer digits, legs with feet ending in longer digits, a head, and for some species of primates, a tail. The leading variable when working with primates is the enormous size differences depending on species; for example, from the 30-g mouse lemur to the 340-kg male gorilla.

37.2 Taxonomy

The primate order consists of two major groups. Strepsirrhini (Prosimians) includes lemurs, pottos, bush babies and lorises, and Haplorrhini, which is broken down further into groupings such as the Tarsiiforms (tarsiers) and the Simiformes (anthropoids). The simian infra-order consists of further order and family breakdowns which, when simplified, consists of monkeys and apes. Monkeys represent over 200 species of Old World (Africa and Asian continents) and New World (American continents) specimens. Apes comprise of only six major species (not including humans), including siamangs, gibbons, chimpanzees, bonobos, gorilla and orangutans. Subspecies of apes do exist for these major specie groups, but are still commonly referred to by their major species name (Clutton-Brock 2002).

37.3 Immobilizing Equipment

Unlike many cats and dogs, primates can pose a challenge for initial pre-medication and induction as a wild species. Often with wild animals or those kept in large enclosures, practitioners will dart an animal for sedation or tranquilization with either a CO_2-powered gun or a blow dart. While this method is still readily used in the zoo or field setting, primates are one of the few species that can easily remove a dart and even toss it back at you due to their opposable thumbs and a higher level of problem-solving skills. It is always advisable to encourage positive reinforcement training for captive primates for injections whenever possible. This will help eliminate stress associated with darting, a more controlled and reliable means of medication administration and the training for the technique being a good bridge for the human–animal bond.

In the biomedical research setting, squeeze cages are often used (Figure 37.1). This allows a single person to pull the back of a specially designed cage forward and lock it in place, sandwiching the patient between the front of the cage and the back panel. Then the practitioner can easily and safely administer an intravenous or intramuscular injection of a sedative to the patient.

37.4 Anesthetic Machines

The typical small animal anesthetic machines are appropriate for a majority of primate species. It may be appropriate to use a large animal anesthetic machine for very large ape specimens, such as male gorillas or orangutans, based on their size and lung volumes. Non-rebreathing units will be necessary for very small or micro-species, similar to any other type of animal. Some micro-species or neonates may benefit from specialized anesthetic machines more commonly used in the biomedical research setting for mice and rats.

Protecting anesthetic machines from potential pathogens, such as tuberculosis, is something to consider when working with primates. Anesthesia circuit filters can be purchased and placed between the circuit hosing and anesthetic machine to eliminate or reduce pathogen infiltration into the machine where decontamination is more

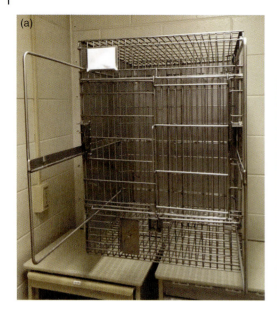
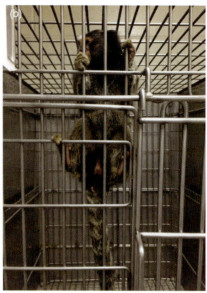

Figure 37.1 Example of a squeeze cage used for primates. (A) demonstrates the handles used to pull an animal forward to the front of the cage. (B) demonstrates a primate at the front of the cage, readily accessible to veterinary personnel.

challenging. The filters are also advantageous when working in biomedical or zoo settings, to prevent cross infection between primate species (see Chapter 28).

37.5 Monitors

Monitoring techniques used in non-human primates are similar to their use in other species. Specific considerations are discussed below.

37.5.1 Pulse Oximetry

Pulse oximetry is standard in most veterinary facilities, especially those performing anesthetic procedures. Pulse oximetry should be used for primate species as well, with common application sites echoing other species, such as the ear, tongue and lip (Figure 37.2). The benefit of working with primates and using this piece of monitoring equipment is primate anatomy. Most of the monitoring equipment used for veterinary patients was originally designed for use on humans. Utilizing application sites for the infrared sensor such as the fingers or toes, like in humans, is convenient and reliable. Other sites include the tail for monkey and prosimian species. For microspecies, the whole forearm or distal leg can be used, similar to applying the sensor to a finger.

The largest complication when using pulse oximetry in primates is pigmentation. Primate skin tones range from very fair to completely black. Many pulse oximeters have difficulty attaining reliable readings from heavily pigmented species. In this situation, the rectum or esopha-

gus is useful when reflective sensors are available (Ølberg and Sinclair 2014).

Certain brands of pulse oximeters (Masimo Corporation, Irvine, CA USA), are specially designed to accommodate heavily pigmented people and thus work

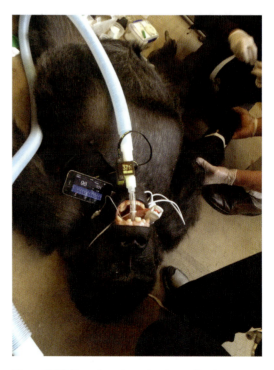

Figure 37.2 Use of a pulse oximeter and mainstream capnography in an anesthetized gorilla. The end-tidal CO_2 is measured at 37 mmHg with a pulse rate of 101 bpm and oxygen hemoglobin saturation of 98%.

better for heavily pigmented veterinary species as well (Shah and Modi 2012).

37.5.2 Electrocardiography (ECG)

Electrocardiography (ECG) is used in the same way in primates as in other small animal patients. Application of 3–6 lead electrodes are the same as in small animals, frequently placing leads in the axillary and proximal leg regions. Frequently, adhesive electrode pads are used on the palms and bottom of the feet, secured with tape whenever possible (Figure 37.3). This reduces electrical interference and mitigates using alligator clips that can cause minor soft tissue damage.

Esophageal ECG probes are also useful in primates, with size being the limiting factor for practical use. Depending on the species of primate, the monitor may need to be set to pediatric or small animal modes to accommodate high heart rates.

37.5.3 Blood Pressure Monitoring

Similar to other species, primates may have profound physiological responses to anesthetics and analgesics, such as opioids and gas anesthesia. Thus, it is imperative that reliable monitoring of blood pressure is used correctly in every anesthetized patient to follow physiological trends and intervene as necessary.

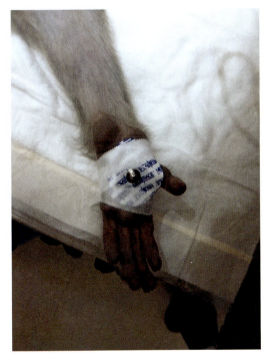

Figure 37.3 An example of an ECG patch taped to a primate limb; ECG clips are attached to the patch, reducing trauma to the skin.

37.5.3.1 Doppler Ultrasonographic Flow Monitoring

The use of Doppler ultrasonic monitoring for acquiring the systolic blood pressure in primates utilizes the same techniques used in small animals. The blood pressure cuff should be 30–40% the width of the appendage it will be secured around. The preferred site for placement of the blood pressure cuff is at the bicep or upper arm; the radial artery is then used when placing the Doppler crystal. The radial artery pulse can be found by application of ultrasound gel on the anterior aspect of the wrist. Starting at midline, move the Doppler crystal laterally until the pulse is audible.

If the thoracic limb is unavailable, a tail can also be used, if the patient has one. The cuff can be placed at the base of the tail, closest to the body. A small area of the ventral tail can be shaved and the Doppler crystal with ultrasound gel should be placed medially on the ventral aspect of the tail. If the patient does not have a tail, the pelvic limb can be used as an alternative. Placing the cuff on the quadriceps or thigh region is ideal. Larger or heavily muscled patients may cause the cuff to slip at this site. To place the Doppler crystal, utilize the tibial artery. The tibial artery initially starts medial at the posterior knee. As the artery continues down the leg, it branches and becomes more medial toward the ankle.

37.5.3.2 Oscillometric and High Definition Oscillometric (HDO) Automated Machines

Automated blood pressure machines are fairly reliable implements when attaining serial blood pressures during an anesthetic event in primates, due to similar cardiovascular anatomy and physiology to humans (Aiello and Wheeler 1995). Again, the blood pressure cuff should be 30–40% the width of the appendage it will be secured around. The upper arm, thigh and even the upper distal leg, just under the knee, are appropriate sites for cuff placement (Figure 37.4). The tail can also be utilized if the appropriate sized cuff is available. In large primates, such as apes, fingers can be used with small blood pressure cuffs; however, for accuracy reasons, this method should be a last option. When placing the blood pressure cuff, placing the transducer tubing over the artery provides the most reliable data. Commercial products are available, such as the oscillometric Cardell Veterinary Monitor, model 9402 (Midmark, Tampa, FL USA) and the HDO Vet BP Monitor (Memo Diagnostic, S and B MedVet, Babenhausen, Germany). High definition oscillometric monitors offer a real-time look at pulsatile waves and date collection of more minute BP changes.

37.5.4 Respiratory Monitoring

Similar to most species, primates often hypoventilate under general anesthesia. Apnea is a concern for any

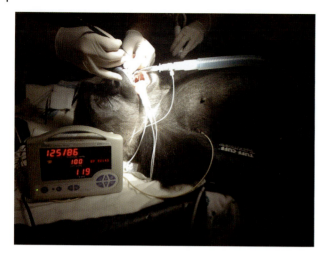

Figure 37.4 An oscillometric (Cardell) monitor with the appropriate sized cuff placed around the bicep of a female gorilla. Systolic, diastolic and mean blood pressure values are 125, 86 and 100 mmHg, respectively; the pulse rate is 199 bpm.

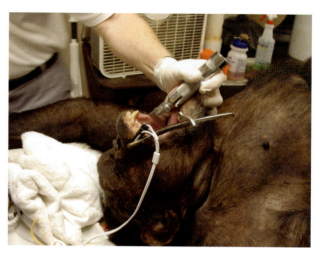

Figure 37.5 An anesthetized chimp showing correct placement of a laryngoscope prior to orotracheal intubation.

patient, but is common in primates due to their unique respiratory physiology (Patterson and Talbot 1969). All the typical methods used with small animal respiratory monitoring can be applied to the non-human primate patient. Minimizing mechanical dead space and proper tracheal intubation are key in successful maintenance of the respiratory tract of primates. For example, when intubating, it is pivotal for the person placing the endotracheal tube (ETT) to understand the specific species upper airway and bronchial anatomy. Primates have particularly short necks compared to other mammalian species and laryngoscopes are frequently used "upside-down", similar to the techniques used in humans, to successfully intubate primates (Figure 37.5). They also have a shorter distance from the arytenoids to the bronchial bifurcation, making it easy for one-sided intubation into either the right or left primary bronchi (Cerveny and Sleeman 2014; Ølberg and Sinclair 2014). In addition, primates have highly variable tracheal sizes, dependent on the species. A smaller primate, such as New World monkeys that have loud howling calls, may require a surprisingly larger ETT than one may anticipate, whereas larger apes may only require a size 6–8.5 mm ETT for larger-sized animals. However, commercially available ETTs are frequently used.

Capnometry or capnography techniques echo methods used in canine and feline species (see Chapter 16). Waveforms, such as the "shark fin" tracing, are not uncommon for patients with obstruction, a history of asthma or chronic obstructive pulmonary disease (COPD), which may be more prevalent in primates than in some other commonly dealt-with species. Thus, capnometry should always be performed whenever possible (Figure 37.2).

37.5.5 Post-Operative Monitoring

For animal and practitioner safety, some species, especially apes, will need to be recovered in a secure location. With the endotracheal tube cuff deflated, the observer may have to quickly pull the ETT and secure the animal in the enclosure with minimal to no monitoring attached to the patient (Figure 37.6).

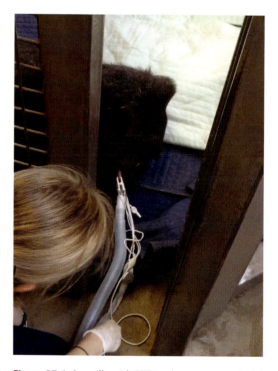

Figure 37.6 A gorilla with ETT in place, oxygen administration and minimal anesthetic monitoring (pulse oximetry) that can all be easily removed as the animal recovers behind the safety of a closing gate.

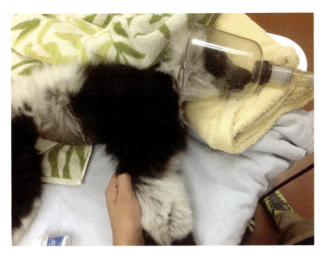

Figure 37.7 Use of a small animal mask to deliver flow-by oxygen in a lemur.

During recovery, it is recommended to provide oxygen supplementation by either mask, flow-by methods or a demand valve (Figure 37.7). Whenever possible, a portable pulse oximeter should be used to monitor the pulse rate and hemoglobin oxygen saturation of the recovering animal. Post-operative respiratory monitoring can be challenging, but is crucial when opioids are used during profound respiratory depression in primates. The Masimo Corporation (Irvine, CA USA) makes a device that allows the user to monitor respiratory rates via acoustic technology. A sticky pad with a sensor is placed on the neck near the trachea and the monitor senses the vibration of each breath and calculates the respiratory rate (Figures 37.8 and 37.9). The author has used this device in multiple primate species with good success. This is an ideal tool during recovery, especially since the patient does not have to be intubated. The device also has pulse oximetry incorporated, making it an ideal monitor for this type of situation.

37.6 Summary

In summary, non-human primates use similar equipment to human patients. However, they differ greatly from our domestic species. Knowledge of their physiology can aid in choosing correct equipment for each non-human primate patient.

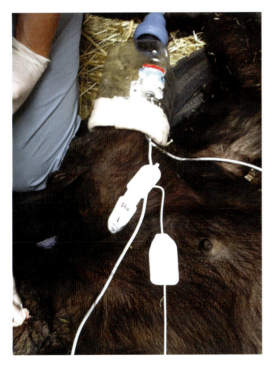

Figure 37.8 Use of an acoustic respiration sensor in a recovering chimpanzee. Note the sensors placed near the trachea and on the chest.

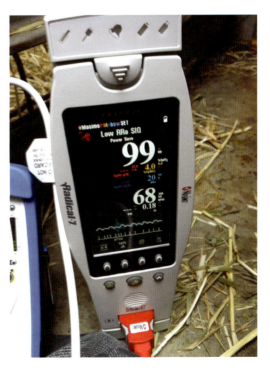

Figure 37.9 The digital display of the Masimo Radical-7 with the acoustic respiration and pulse oximetry modules. The respiratory rate is 20 breaths per minute, heart rate is 68 bpm and the hemoglobin oxygen saturation is 99%.

References

Aiello, L.C. and Wheeler, P. (1995) The expensive-tissue hypothesis: the brain and the digestive system in human and primate evolution. *Current Anthropology*, 36, 199–221.

Cerveny, S. and Sleeman, J. (2014) Great apes. In: West, G., Heard, D. and Caulkett, N. (eds). *Zoo Animal and Wildlife Immobilization and Anesthesia*, 2nd ed. Ames, IA: John Wiley & Sons, pp. 560–571.

Clutton-Brock, J. (2002) *Mammals; Smithsonian Handbook*. New York: DK Dehi, pp. 97–121.

Patterson, R. and Talbot, C.H. (1969) Respiratory responses in subhuman primates with immediate type hypersensitivity. *J Lab Clin Med*, 73, 924–933.

Ølberg, R.A. and Sinclair, M. (2014) Monkeys and gibbons. In: West, G., Heard, D. and Caulkett, N. (eds). *Zoo Animal and Wildlife Immobilization and Anesthesia*, 2nd ed. Ames, IA: John Wiley & Sons, pp. 549–559.

Shah, N. and Modi, D. (2012) Performance of Pronto-7 noninvasive hemoglobin pulse CO-oximeter in a dark skinned population. In: *Proceedings of the American Society of Anesthesiologists*. Washington, DC, A573.

Index

Veterinary Anesthetic and Monitoring Equipment, First Edition. Edited by Kristen G. Cooley and Rebecca A. Johnson.
© 2018 John Wiley & Sons, Inc. Published 2018 by John Wiley & Sons, Inc.